Handbook of
    Systemic Autoimmune Diseases

Volume 7

# The Kidney in Systemic Autoimmune Diseases

# Handbook of Systemic Autoimmune Diseases

**Series Editor: Ronald A. Asherson**

| | |
|---|---|
| Volume 1 | The Heart in Systemic Autoimmune Diseases<br>*Edited by: Andrea Doria and Paolo Pauletto* |
| Volume 2 | Pulmonary Involvement in Systemic Autoimmune Diseases<br>*Edited by: Athol U. Wells and Christopher P. Denton* |
| Volume 3 | Neurologic Involvement in Systemic Autoimmune Diseases<br>*Edited by: Doruk Erkan and Steven R. Levine* |
| Volume 4 | Reproductive and Hormonal Aspects of Systemic Autoimmune Diseases<br>*Edited by: Michael Lockshin and Ware Branch* |
| Volume 5 | The Skin in Systemic Autoimmune Diseases<br>*Edited by: Piercarlo Sarzi-Puttini, Andrea Doria, Giampiero Girolomoni and Annegret Kuhn* |
| Volume 6 | Pediatrics in Systemic Autoimmune Diseases<br>*Edited by: Rolando Cimaz and Thomas Lehman* |
| Volume 7 | The Kidney in Systemic Autoimmune Diseases<br>*Edited by: Justin C. Mason and Charles D. Pusey* |

# Handbook of Systemic Autoimmune Diseases

Volume 7

# The Kidney in Systemic Autoimmune Diseases

Edited by:

**Justin C. Mason**
*Rheumatology Unit Hammersmith Hospital*
*Imperial College London*
*London, United Kingdom*

**Charles D. Pusey**
*West London Renal and Transplant Centre Hammersmith Hospital*
*Imperial College London*
*London, United Kingdom*

Series Editor
**Ronald A. Asherson**

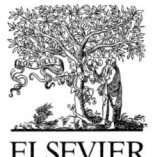
ELSEVIER

Amsterdam – Boston – Heidelberg – London – New York – Oxford
Paris – San Diego – San Francisco – Singapore – Sydney – Tokyo

Elsevier
Radarweg 29, PO Box 211, 1000 AE Amsterdam, The Netherlands
Linacre House, Jordan Hill, Oxford OX2 8DP, UK

First edition 2008

Copyright © 2008 Elsevier B.V. All rights reserved

No part of this publication may be reproduced, stored in a retrieval system
or transmitted in any form or by any means electronic, mechanical, photocopying,
recording or otherwise without the prior written permission of the publisher

Permissions may be sought directly from Elsevier's Science & Technology Rights
Department in Oxford, UK: phone (+44) (0) 1865 843830; fax (+44) (0) 1865 853333;
email: permissions@elsevier.com. Alternatively you can submit your request online by
visiting the Elsevier web site at http://www.elsevier.com/locate/permissions, and selecting
*Obtaining permission to use Elsevier material*

Notice
No responsibility is assumed by the publisher for any injury and/or damage to persons
or property as a matter of products liability, negligence or otherwise, or from any use
or operation of any methods, products, instructions or ideas contained in the material
herein. Because of rapid advances in the medical sciences, in particular, independent
verification of diagnoses and drug dosages should be made

**Library of Congress Cataloging-in-Publication Data**
A catalog record for this book is available from the Library of Congress

**British Library Cataloguing in Publication Data**
A catalogue record for this book is available from the British Library

ISBN: 978-0-444-52972-5
ISSN: 1571-5078

For information on all Elsevier publications
visit our website at books.elsevier.com

Printed and bound in The Netherlands

08 09 10 11 12    10 9 8 7 6 5 4 3 2 1

Working together to grow
libraries in developing countries

www.elsevier.com | www.bookaid.org | www.sabre.org

ELSEVIER    BOOK AID International    Sabre Foundation

# Preface

Systemic autoimmune disease encompasses a wide range of conditions demonstrating multi-organ involvement, in which renal disease is common and life threatening. This volume in the "Handbook of Systemic Autoimmune Disease" series brings together an international group of clinicians and clinical scientists to contribute to a state-of the-art review of underlying pathogenic mechanisms, methods of clinical assessment, classification and diagnosis of renal disease, combined with a detailed overview of treatment strategies. The section concerning pathogenic mechanisms will be of particular interest to both basic and clinician scientists. Patients with autoimmune disease are treated by a variety of clinicians and this book will, therefore, be of direct relevance to internal medicine physicians, nephrologists, rheumatologists, pediatricians, clinical immunologists, and general practitioners.

This volume is divided into four parts. In the Introduction, Ron Falk provides an authoritative overview of the contents of this volume and the current state of the field and speculates on what the future might hold. Part II contains a detailed review of pathogenesis including the role of autoimmune mechanisms in renal disease. Chapters on the role of complement activation, soluble factors such as cytokines, cellular mechanisms, and the renal cell response to immune injury are included. The final chapter in Part II addresses mechanisms underlying the renal toxicity of drugs used to treat autoimmune disease. Part III is focused on the disease mechanisms, clinical features, and treatment of the systemic vasculitides that may affect the kidney. Part IV adopts a similar approach for the renal disease associated with systemic lupus erythematosus, systemic sclerosis, and other important connective tissue diseases.

In summary, this volume will provide an essential reference source for all those involved in the care of patients with renal involvement in systemic autoimmune disease, and for those contributing to research into the underlying pathogenic mechanisms in these disorders.

Justin C. Mason and Charles D. Pusey

# Series Editor

## Prof. Ronald A. Asherson

Professor Ronald A. Asherson, MD, FACP, MD (Hon) (London), FCP (SA), FACR, is Professor of Immunology (Hon), at the School of Pathology, University of the Witwatersrand, as well as being Consultant Rheumatologist at the Rosebank Clinic in Johannesburg, South Africa. He is also a Visiting Professor at the Systemic Autoimmune Diseases Unit at the Hospital Clinic, Barcelona, Spain where he regularly visits and coordinates research projects.

Professor Asherson qualified in Medicine at the University of Cape Town in 1957 and, after completing his internship, became H/P to Professor Sir Christopher Booth at the Hammersmith Hospital, London, in 1960. In 1961 he accepted a Fellowship at the Columbia Presbyterian Hospital in New York, returning in 1962 to become Registrar and then Senior Registrar until 1964 at Groote Schuur Hospital in Cape Town. After 10 years as a Clinical Tutor in the Department of Medicine, he returned to the United States and was appointed as Assistant Clinical Professor of Medicine at the New York Hospital—Cornell Medical Centre under the late Professor Henry Heineman. From 1981 to 1986 he was associated with the Rheumatology Department at the Royal Postgraduate Medical School of London. It was at that time that he developed his interest in Connective Tissue Diseases and Antiphospholipid Antibodies.

In 1986 he moved to the Rayne Institute and St. Thomas' Hospital in London, where he was appointed Honorary Consultant Physician and Senior Research Fellow. In 1991 he took a sabbatical at St. Luke's Roosevelt Hospital Center in New York, working with Professor Robert Lahita. In 1992 he returned to South Africa for private practice in Johannesburg.

In 1998 he was elected as Fellow of the American College of Physicians (FACP) as well as a Founding Fellow of the American College of Rheumatology (FACR). From 1988 to 1991 he served on the Council of the Royal Society of Medicine in London. In 1992 he was co-winner of the European League Against Rheumatism (EULAR) Prize and in 1993 was the co-recipient of the International League Against Rheumatism (ILAR) Prize, both for his research on antiphospholipid antibodies. In 1994 he was elected a Fellow of the Royal College of Physicians (FRCP) of London. In 2002 he was awarded an Honorary Doctorate in Medicine from the University of Pleven in Bulgaria.

Professor Asherson has been an invited speaker at many universities and International conferences both in the USA and in Europe. He is the author of more than 300 papers on connective tissue diseases and has contributed to more than 30 textbooks of medicine, rheumatology, and surgery as well as having co-edited "*Problems in the Rheumatic Diseases*", the "*Phospholipid Binding Antibodies*", two editions of "*The Antiphospholipid Syndrome*" and "*Vascular Manifestations of the Systemic Autoimmune Diseases*". He is currently engaged in research on connective tissue diseases, particularly on the antiphospholipid syndrome together with colleagues in the USA, Spain, France, and Israel and is in clinical practice in South Africa. In 1999, he was the co-recipient of the Juan Vivancos Prize in Spain and in 2003 was the co-recipient of the Abbott Prize, awarded at the European League Against Rheumatism (EULAR) International Meeting, held in Lisbon, Portugal.

His original description of the "Catastrophic Antiphospholipid Syndrome" and the publishing of more than 40 papers on this new disease was rewarded by the attachment of the eponym "Asherson's Syndrome" to this condition at the November 2002 International Phospholipid Conference held in Sicily. He has established the first International Committee to study survivors of this syndrome.

He is currently editing a series of 12 volumes entitled "The Handbook of Systemic Autoimmune Disease" (Elsevier,) and in September of 2003 was Co-Chairman of the First Latin American Congress on Autoimmunity, held in the Galapagos Islands, Ecuador. He co-chaired and participated in a Session at the Milan Conference on "Heart, Rheumatism and Autoimmunity" held in February 2004.

He was awarded an Honorary Fellowship of the Slovakian Rheumatology Association in 2005.

# Volume Editors

### Justin C. Mason

Justin Mason is Reader in Vascular Rheumatology in the Faculty of Medicine at Imperial College London and Honorary Consultant in Rheumatology at the Hammersmith Hospital, London. He graduated in Medicine in 1986 from the University of London and trained in Rheumatology at the Kennedy Institute of Rheumatology, Charing Cross Hospital London and at the Royal Postgraduate Medical School, Hammersmith Hospital, London. Following award of a Medical Research Council Training Fellowship in 1992 and subsequently a PhD degree in 1996 from Imperial College London, he was awarded an Arthritis Research Campaign Senior Research Fellowship in 2000.

He is a member of the British Society for Rheumatology, American College of Rheumatology and a Fellow of the Royal College of Physicians in London and of the Association of Physicians of Great Britain and Ireland. He has a long-standing experience and interest in the management of systemic connective tissue diseases and large vessel vasculitis with a specific focus on systemic lupus erythematosus and Takayasu's arteritis.

Dr. Mason leads a basic science research group investigating molecular mechanisms involved in vascular injury and cytoprotection in systemic rheumatic diseases. In addition, he is actively involved in clinical research that aims to optimize clinical assessment and treatment of large vessel vasculitides and understand the relationship between chronic endothelial dysfunction and accelerated atherosclerosis. He is co-author of 50 original articles, 11 book chapters, and invited reviews.

He is an ad hoc reviewer for many journals including: *Rheumatology, Arthritis and Rheumatism, Blood, FASEB J., Annals of the Rheumatic Diseases, Arthritis Research and Therapy, Clinical and Experimental Rheumatology, Arteriosclerosis Thrombosis and Vascular Biology, Clinical and Experimental Immunology, Immunology, Molecular and Cell Biology, European Journal of Pharmacology, Journal of Vascular Research, Proteomics, American Journal of Physiology*, and the *Journal of Immunological Methods*.

### Charles D. Pusey

Charles Pusey is currently Professor of Medicine, Head of the Department of Renal Medicine, and Head of Postgraduate Medicine at Imperial College London. He is also Honorary Consultant Physician and Lead Clinician in the West London Renal and Transplant Centre, and Director of Research and Development at Hammersmith Hospitals NHS Trust. He qualified from Cambridge University and Guy's Hospital London and, after early appointments at Guy's, joined the Royal Air Force, where he gained experience in General Practice, General Medicine, and Renal Medicine. On leaving the RAF, he moved to Hammersmith Hospital as Senior Registrar in Renal and General Medicine to Professor Keith Peters. He started his clinical research on a MRC Training Fellowship and was subsequently awarded a Wellcome Trust Senior Fellowship. This led to his appointment as Senior Lecturer at the Royal Postgraduate Medical School, later merged with Imperial College London.

Professor Pusey remains active in clinical practice in all aspects of renal medicine, and leads a large multidisciplinary vasculitis service. He has pursued both clinical and laboratory-based research in parallel, and his work has focused on the causes and treatment of glomerulonephritis and systemic vasculitis. He has published over 300 articles on renal disease and contributed chapters to the standard textbooks on renal and general medicine. He is on the Editorial Board of several international journals, including the *Journal of the American Society of Nephrology* and *Nephrology Dialysis Transplantation*. He has a wide range of teaching commitments at undergraduate and postgraduate levels, and regularly supervises several PhD students. He has a particular interest in clinical academic training, and served as Academic Registrar at the Royal College of Physicians of London. He has been President of the Nephrology Section of the Royal Society of Medicine and Chairman of Kidney Research UK. He was elected to the Fellowship of the Academy of Medical Sciences in 2002.

# List of Contributors

**Gerald B. Appel**
Professor of Clinical Medicine, Columbia
University, College of Physicians and Surgeons,
Director of Clinical Nephrology, Columbia
University Medical Center, New York,
NY 10032, USA

**Ramzi Abou Ayache**
Service de Néphrologie, Hémodialyse et Transplantation Rénale, CHU de Poitiers, Université de Poitiers, 2 rue de la Milétrie, 86021 Poitiers, France

**Frank Bridoux**
Service de Néphrologie, Hémodialyse et Transplantation Rénale, CHU de Poitiers, Université de Poitiers, 2 rue de la Milétrie, 86021 Poitiers, France

**Menna R. Clatworthy**
Cambridge Institute for Medical Research and the Department of Medicine, University of Cambridge, School of Clinical Medicine, Addenbrooke's Hospital, Hills Road, Cambridge CB2 2XY, UK

**Michel Cogné**
Laboratoire d'Immunologie, CNRS UMR 6101, Faculté de Médecine, Université de Limoges, 2 rue du Dr. Marcland, 87025 Limoges, France

**H. Terence Cook**
Department of Histopathology, Faculty of Medicine, Imperial College, London
W12 ONN, UK

**David D'Cruz**
The Lupus Research Unit, The Rayne Institute, St. Thomas' Hospital, London SE1 7EH, UK

**Lars-Peter Erwig**
Department of Medicine and Therapeutics, Institute of Medical Sciences, University of Aberdeen, Aberdeen AB25 2ZD, Scotland, UK

**Ronald J. Falk**
University of North Carolina at Chapel Hill, Division of Nephrology and Hypertension, Department of Medicine, CB#7155,
349 MacNider Building, Chapel Hill,
NC 27599-7155, USA

**Carlos Garcia-Porrua**
Rheumatology Division, Hospital Xeral-Calde, c/Dr. Ochoa s/n, 27004, Lugo, Spain

**Julian D. Gillmore**
National Amyloidosis Centre, Centre for Amyloidosis and Acute Phase Proteins, Department of Medicine, University College London, Hampstead Campus, Rowland Hill Street, London NW3 2PF, UK

**Miguel A. Gonzalez-Gay**
Rheumatology Division, Hospital Xeral-Calde, c/Dr. Ochoa s/n, 27004, Lugo, Spain

**Timothy H.J. Goodship**
The Institute of Human Genetics and School of Clinical Medical Sciences, University of Newcastle upon Tyne, Central Parkway, Newcastle upon Tyne, NE1 3BZ, UK

**Jean Michel Goujon**
Service d'Anatomie Pathologique, CHU de Poitiers, Université de Poitiers, 2 rue de la Milétrie, 86021 Poitiers, France

**Olivier Harari**
UCB Celltech, Bath Road, Slough SL1 3WE, UK

**Philip N. Hawkins**
National Amyloidosis Centre, Centre for Amyloidosis and Acute Phase Proteins, Department of Medicine, University College London, Hampstead Campus, Rowland Hill Street, London NW3 2PF, UK

**Lorna Henderson**
Renal and Autoimmunity Group, Centre for
Inflammation, University of Edinburgh, Hugh
Robson Building, George Square, Edinburgh
EH8 9XD, Scotland, UK

**Peter Hewins**
University of North Carolina at Chapel Hill,
Division of Nephrology and Hypertension,
Department of Medicine, CB#7155,
349 MacNider Building, Chapel Hill,
NC 27599-7155, USA

**Gary S. Hoffman**
Center for Vasculitis Care and Research,
Department of Rheumatic and Immunologic
Diseases/Desk A50, The Cleveland Clinic
Foundation, 9500 Euclid Avenue, Cleveland, OH
44195, USA

**Stephen R. Holdsworth**
Centre for Inflammatory Diseases, Monash
University, Department of Medicine and Monash
Institute of Medical Research, Monash Medical
Centre, 246 Clayton Rd., Clayton, Vic. 3168,
Australia

**Anikphe E. Imoagene-Oyedeji**
Renal Electrolyte and Hypertension Division,
Department of Medicine, University of
Pennsylvania School of Medicine, Philadelphia,
PA 19104, USA

**Arnaud Jaccard**
Service d'Hématologie Clinique, CHU de Limoges,
Université de Limoges, Avenue Martin Luther King,
87025 Limoges, France

**David Jayne**
Renal Medicine, Renal Unit, Department of Medicine, Addenbrooke's Hospital, Cambridge CB2
2QQ, UK

**Cees G.M. Kallenberg**
Department of Rheumatology and Clinical
Immunology, University Medical Center
Groningen, University of Groningen, 9700 RB
Groningen, The Netherlands

**Menaka Karmegam**
Section of Nephrology, Department of
Renal Medicine, University of Chicago,
5841 S. Maryland Ave., MC5100 Chicago,
IL 60637, USA

**A. Richard Kitching**
Centre for Inflammatory Diseases, Monash
University, Department of Medicine and Monash
Institute of Medical Research, Monash Medical
Centre, 246 Clayton Rd., Clayton, Vic. 3168,
Australia

**Liz Lightstone**
West London Renal and Transplantation Centre,
Imperial College London, Hammersmith Hospital,
London W12 ONN, UK

**Michael P. Madaio**
Nephrology and Kidney Transplantation Section,
Temple University School of Medicine,
Philadelphia, PA 19140, USA

**Jose A. Miranda-Filloy**
Rheumatology Division, Hospital Xeral-Calde,
c/Dr. Ochoa s/n, 27004, Lugo, Spain

**Eamonn S. Molloy**
Center for Vasculitis Care and Research, Department of Rheumatic and Immunologic Diseases/
Desk A50, The Cleveland Clinic Foundation,
9500 Euclid Avenue Cleveland, OH 44195, USA

**Marianne Monahan**
Professor of Clinical Medicine, Columbia
University, College of Physicians and Surgeons,
Director of Clinical Nephrology, Columbia
University Medical Center, New York,
NY 10032, USA

**Haralampos M. Moutsopolous**
Department of Pathophysiology, School of Medicine,
National University of Athens, 115 27 Athens, Greece

**Heiko Mühl**
Pharmazentrum Frankfurt/ZAFES, Klinikum der
Johann Wolfgang, Goethe-Universität, Frankfurt
am Main D-60590, Germany

**Claes Nordborg**
Department of Pathology, Sahlgrenska University Hospital, SE-413 45 Göteborg, Sweden

**Elisabeth Nordborg**
Department of Rheumatology, Sahlgrenska University Hospital, SE-413 45 Göteborg, Sweden

**Mariana Noris**
Mario Negri Institute for Pharmacological Research, Clinical Research Centre for Rare Diseases, Aldo e Cele Dacco, Villa Camozzi, Bergamo, Italy

**Josef Pfeilschifter**
Pharmazentrum Frankfurt/ZAFES, Klinikum der Johann Wolfgang, Goethe-Universität, Frankfurt am Main D-60590, Germany

**Richard J. Quigg**
Section of Nephrology, Department of Renal Medicine, University of Chicago, 5841 S. Maryland Ave., MC5100, Chicago, IL 60637, USA

**Giuseppe Remuzzi**
Mario Negri Institute for Pharmacological Research, Clinical Research Centre for Rare Diseases, Aldo e Cele Dacco, Villa Camozzi, Bergamo, Italy

**Andrew J. Rees**
Department of Medicine and Therapeutics, Institute of Medical Sciences, University of Aberdeen, Aberdeen AB25 2ZD, Scotland, UK

**Alan D. Salama**
Renal Section, Division of Medicine, Imperial College London, Hammersmith Hospital, London W12 ONN, UK

**Michael Samarkos**
Department of Pathophysiology, School of Medicine, National University of Athens, 115 27 Athens, Greece

**Liliana Schaefer**
Pharmazentrum Frankfurt/ZAFES, Klinikum der Johann Wolfgang, Goethe-Universität, Frankfurt am Main D-60590, Germany

**Christophe Sirac**
Laboratoire d'Immunologie, CNRS UMR 6101 Faculté de Médecine, Université de Limoges, 2 rue du Dr. Marcland, 87025 Limoges, France

**Kenneth G.C. Smith**
Cambridge Institute for Medical Research and the Department of Medicine, University of Cambridge, School of Clinical Medicine, Addenbrooke's Hospital, Hills Road, Cambridge CB2 2XY, UK

**Virginia D. Steen**
Division of Rheumatology, Immunology and Allergy, Department of Medicine, Georgetown University, 3800 Reservoir Road, NW-LL, Gorman, Washington, DC 20007, USA

**Guy Touchard**
Service de Néphrologie, Hémodialyse et Transplantation Rénale, CHU de Poitiers, Université de Poitiers, 2 rue de la Milétrie, 86021 Poitiers, France and INSERM ERM 324, CHU de Poitiers, Université de Poitiers, 2 rue de la Milétrie, 86021 Poitiers, France

**Neil Turner**
Renal and Autoimmunity Group, Centre for Inflammation, University of Edinburgh, Hugh Robson Building, George Square, Edinburgh EH8 9XD, Scotland, UK

**Heather Wilson**
Department of Medicine and Therapeutics, Institute of Medical Sciences, University of Aberdeen, Aberdeen AB25 2ZD, Scotland, UK

# Contents

| | |
|---|---|
| Preface | v |
| Series Editor | vii |
| Volume Editors | ix |
| List of Contributors | xi |

## I Introduction

| | |
|---|---|
| Introduction<br>*Peter Hewins, Ronald J. Falk* | 3 |

## II Pathogenic Mechanisms

| | |
|---|---|
| Pathogenesis of Renal Diseases: Autoimmunity<br>*Anikphe E. Imoagene-Oyedeji, Michael P. Madaio* | 23 |
| Pathogenesis of Renal Disease: Complement<br>*Menaka Karmegam, Richard J. Quigg* | 43 |
| Pathogenesis of Renal Disease: Cytokines and Other Soluble Factors<br>*Stephen R. Holdsworth, A. Richard Kitching* | 63 |
| Pathogenesis of Renal Disease: Cellular Mechanisms<br>*Lars-Peter Erwig, Heather Wilson, Andrew J. Rees* | 81 |
| Pathogenesis of Renal Diseases: Renal Cell Response to Injury<br>*Josef Pfeilschifter, Heiko Mühl, Liliana Schaefer* | 93 |
| Renal Toxicities Associated with Immunomodulatory Drugs<br>*Alan D. Salama* | 107 |

## III The Vasculitides

| | |
|---|---|
| ANCA-Associated Systemic Vasculitides: Mechanisms<br>*Cees G.M. Kallenberg* | 123 |
| ANCA-Associated Vasculitis: Clinical Features and Treatment<br>*David Jayne* | 139 |
| Large and Medium Vessel Vasculitis: Mechanisms<br>*Elisabeth Nordborg, Claes Nordborg* | 159 |
| Large and Medium Vessel Vasculitis: Clinical Features and Treatment<br>*Eamonn S. Molloy, Gary S. Hoffman* | 175 |

Anti-GBM Disease: Mechanisms, Clinical Features, and Treatment   195
*Lorna Henderson, Neil Turner*

Renal Disease in Cryoglobulinemic Vasculitis   215
*Frank Bridoux, Christophe Sirac, Arnaud Jaccard, Ramzi Abou Ayache, Jean Michel Goujon, Michel Cogné, Guy Touchard*

Henoch-Schönlein Purpura   241
*Miguel A. Gonzalez-Gay, Carlos Garcia-Porrua, Jose A. Miranda-Filloy*

Hemolytic Uremic Syndrome/Thrombotic Thrombocytopenic Purpura   257
*Marina Noris, Giuseppe Remuzzi, Timothy H.J. Goodship*

## IV The Connective Tissue Diseases

Systemic Lupus Erythematosus: Mechanisms   285
*Menna R. Clatworthy, Kenneth G.C. Smith*

Systemic Lupus Erythematosus: Renal Involvement   311
*H. Terence Cook, Liz Lightstone*

Systemic Lupus Erythematosus: Treatment   323
*Marianne Monahan, Gerald B. Appel*

The Antiphospholipid Syndrome   333
*David D'Cruz*

Renal Involvement in Sjögren Syndrome   349
*Michael Samarkos, Haralampos M. Moutsopoulos*

The Kidney in Systemic Sclerosis   363
*Virginia D. Steen*

Amyloidosis   383
*Julian D. Gillmore, Philip N. Hawkins*

Inflammatory Arthritis, Behçet's Syndrome, and Sarcoidosis   397
*Olivier Harari*

Subject Index   407

# PART I:

# Introduction

# Introduction

Peter Hewins, Ronald J. Falk*

*Division of Nephrology and Hypertension, Department of Medicine, UNC Kidney Center, University of North Carolina at Chapel Hill, Chapel Hill, NC 27599-7155, USA*

The compilation of this volume coincides with two notable anniversaries in autoimmunity as it impacts upon the kidney. Anti-double stranded DNA antibodies were first characterized 50 years ago and it is 25 years since anti-neutrophil cytoplasm antibodies were discovered (Davies et al., 1982; Isenberg et al., 2007). Befittingly, the anniversaries coincide with a growing enthusiasm for the use of B-cell targeted therapies in proliferative lupus nephritis and systemic ANCA-vasculitis, the diseases with which these autoantibodies are respectively linked (Walsh and Jayne, 2007). The clinical utility of testing for autoantibodies is immediately apparent but even robust associations between specific immunoglobulins and particular autoimmune diseases or patterns of organ involvement do not guarantee a causal link. In order to determine pathogenic connections, we must turn to the wealth of human and experimental research in this field and so by way of an introduction to this comprehensive book, we highlight just some of the research most relevant to current understanding of how autoimmunity (exemplified by autoantibody-mediated disease) may arise and how we might potentially best salvage organ function and restore immunological normality.

The diversity of the autoantibody repertoire associated with SLE is well-recognized but anti-dsDNA antibodies, first eluted from the kidneys of patients some 40 years ago, are widely presumed to be pathogenically important (Koffler et al., 1967; Krishnan and Kaplan, 1967). Numerous human and animal studies support the hypothesis that lupus nephritis is an immune complex disease and signal the potential therapeutic benefit of suppressing autoantibody production which is clinically apparent (Austin et al., 1986; Shlomchik et al., 1994, 2001; Jacobi et al., 2003; Schwartz, 2006; Ahuja et al., 2007). In rodents, the existence of antibody secreting cells (ASC), principally plasma cells, that are refractory to deletion by conventional immunosuppressants has long been recognized and although the precise phenotype and location of pathogenic autoantibody secreting cells associated with human SLE is still uncertain, high rates of relapse following cyclophosphamide-based treatment suggest that autoreactive lymphocytes are not readily suppressed or deleted in this disease (Miller and Cole, 1967; Illei et al., 2002; Mok et al., 2004). Indeed, recurrence of anti-nuclear autoantibodies has been observed even after stem-cell transplantation which underscores the necessity of developing less toxic alternative methods to control autoantibody production (Traynor et al., 2000; Burt et al., 2006). During the 1970s, cyclophosphamide was adopted for necrotizing systemic vasculitis (diseases subsequently recognized as ANCA-associated) and rescued many patients from certain demise but its limitations once again became most apparent in patients who relapsed (Fauci et al., 1979; Cupps et al., 1982; Hoffman et al., 1992; Booth et al., 2004a; Hogan et al., 2005). Rather more recently, the pathogenicity of anti-myeloperoxidase antibodies in pauci-immune necrotizing vasculitis and

---

*Corresponding author.
Tel.: 919-966-2561; Fax: 919-966-4251
E-mail address: ronald_falk@med.unc.edu

glomerulonephritis has been confirmed by two separate animal models (Xiao et al., 2002; Little et al., 2005). These observations are not only paradigm to our knowledge of the mechanisms that direct "pauci-immune" injury of the vasculature but in addition, they have focused attention on the autoreactive B-cell as a credible therapeutic target. In the last 10 years, mycophenolate mofetil and rituximab (B-cell depleting, anti-CD20 antibody) have emerged as alternative treatments to control autoreactive lymphocytes in patients with life or organ-threatening forms of SLE or ANCA-vasculitis and, importantly, serious adverse-effects may be less frequent than with cylcophosphamide (Joy et al., 2005; Stassen et al., 2007; Walsh et al., 2007; Walsh and Jayne, 2007). Whilst major trials of MMF and rituximab treatment are still ongoing for both diseases, it does not seem overly naive to believe that these agents and related therapies in development offer the prospect of a significant shift in our approach to treatment. The role of autoantibody removal through plasmapheresis is also becoming more clearly established, particularly in ANCA-vasculitis with severe renal dysfunction (Jayne et al., 2007).

Do these developments herald an end to the need for investigation of the "effector arm" of the autoimmune response in systemic autoimmune diseases affecting the kidney? Clearly this is not the case since whilst the role of autoreactive B-cells has certainly been reaffirmed, many aspects of pathogenesis remain undetermined in both diseases. Pathogenic function(s) of autoreactive B-cells may still yet prove to be related to antigen presentation or other aspects of their interdependent relationship with autoreactive T lymphocytes rather than to autoantibody production per se (Chan et al., 1999a; Lipsky, 2001; Yan et al., 2006; Harvey et al., 2007). However, this issue remains contentious; B-cells that are unable to secrete immunoglobulin were previously proven to be sufficient for autoimmune injury in a murine model of SLE but more recently in a BAFF/BLys overexpressing mouse, lupus-like disease was convincingly demonstrated to be wholly T-cell-independent (Chan et al., 1999b; Groom et al., 2007). The important consequences of lymphocyte modulation in SLE and ANCA-vasculitis may be distinct, particularly as rituximab depletes B-cells from the peripheral blood and appears efficacious in both diseases, but the suppression of autoantibody titers is more uniform in ANCA-vasculitis disease (Walsh and Jayne, 2007). Additionally, the longer term outcomes associated with these newer treatments are uncertain and it is already apparent that an innate propensity to relapse often persists just as it did with cyclophosphamide (Smith et al., 2006). Interrupting the initiation of autoimmunity or promoting genuine and sustained tolerance surely therefore remain the ultimate goals of translational-autoimmune research.

If the composite of experimental data, clinical observation and encouraging therapeutic responses does persuade us of the central importance of autoantibodies in the pathogenesis of glomerular injury for SLE and/or ANCA-vasculitis, then it also signals a fundamental need to unravel the identity of the key autoreactive B-cells. Similar perturbations of B-cell populations appear to exist in the peripheral blood of patients with SLE and ANCA-vasculitis, in particular the presence of a subset of $CD19^{HI}CD27+$ memory B-cells that may be linked to autoantibody production (Culton et al., 2007). Furthermore, patients with SLE have an expanded CD27− memory B-cell population that may be involved in maintenance of autoantibody titers (Wei et al., 2007). Whilst autoantibody secreting cells are detectable in the peripheral blood, it is likely that the majority of such cells are sequestered in tissue (Clayton and Savage, 2003; Grammer et al., 2003; Radbruch et al., 2006). Long-lived plasma cells (probably able to survive for years or decades) predominantly reside in the bone marrow and smaller numbers are present in the spleen but inflamed tissues, notably both human and murine kidneys affected by lupus nephritis and the nasal mucosa of patients with Wegener's granulomatosis, also support at least short-lived B-cells, plasma cells, and antibody production (Sze et al., 2000; Cassese et al., 2001; Hutloff et al., 2004; Voswinkel et al., 2006). Intriguingly, following their differentiation in secondary lymphoid tissues, ASC may be programmed to home (via chemokine receptors and adhesion molecules) to the tissue in which B-cell activation originally occurred (Moser et al., 2006b).

Locating autoantibody secreting cells might therefore offer clues as to the site and identity of the inciting antigen exposure.

Relocation of plasmablasts to inflamed sites likely depends upon IFN$\gamma$ since this cytokine (generated by T lymphocytes (Th1 cells) and professional APCs) not only up-regulates CXCR3 expression on human B-cells and maturing plasma cells as well as murine plasmablasts, but also induces expression of the corresponding chemokine ligands (CXCL9, CXCL10, and CXCL11) in inflamed tissue (Muehlinghaus et al., 2005). Indeed, CXCL10 expression has been identified in renal biopsies from patients with glomerulonephritis (Romagnani et al., 2002). Furthermore, IFN$\gamma$ treatment of B-cells enhances their migration towards CXCL9 in vitro. In contrast, plasma cell precursor homing to the bone marrow likely involves CXCR4 expression (Hargreaves et al., 2001).

Homing capacity is, however, short-lived since plasmablasts rapidly down regulate chemokine receptors (Hauser et al., 2002). Transient migratory competence may in fact permit the maintenance of contemporaneous humoral immunity by promoting competitive displacement of older plasma cells which lack homing capacity (Moser et al., 2006a). In the context of autoimmunity, this might suggest that the persisting presence of autoantigen would facilitate expansion of an autoreactive repertoire and conversely, reducing availability of the autoantigen (or whatever exogenous antigen triggered the initiating immune response) might be therapeutically useful. Long-lived plasma cells that are not competitively displaced readily survive without antigenic challenge and antibody production can be initiated through indiscriminate polyclonal activation (Manz et al., 1998; Bernasconi et al., 2002).

By fortuitous paradox, rituximab treatment can suppress autoreactive B-cells and autoantibody production without interfering with "appropriate" humoral immunity. Thus serum IgG is maintained and immunocompetency towards exogenous antigens (at least those previously encountered) is preserved, presumably reflecting the longevity and CD20– phenotype of bone marrow plasma cells. As noted above, current data suggest that the correlation between administering rituximab, disease remission and autoantibody suppression is stronger for ANCA-vasculitis than SLE, although anti-dsDNA antibody reduction has also been reported (Cambridge et al., 2006a). Furthermore, it remains possible that pathogenically important autoantibodies with other specificities are modulated by rituximab treatment in SLE. Autoantibody titers may be suppressed by rituximab because they derive from short-lived ASC that are ordinarily replenished from CD20+ precursors. Recent studies of rheumatoid factor generation support the concept that short-lived plasmablasts are the predominant source of autoantibody production (William et al., 2005). Additionally, there are plasma cells that remain CD20+ and sensitive to rituximab; these have been definitively characterized in the tonsil and they may also exist in the spleen and other secondary lymphoid organs although their contribution, if any, to autoantibody production is unknown (Medina et al., 2002; Withers et al., 2007).

Whilst these data may suggest why autoantibody secreting cells can exhibit a heightened sensitivity to rituximab, there is also evidence that long-lived plasma cells contribute to autoantibody production which might explain variability in autoantibody suppression and the tendency to relapse. Thus long-lived (non-dividing, CD20–) plasma cells comprise around 40% of the antibody secreting cells in the spleens of NZB/W lupus-prone mice and contribute to autoantibody production (Hoyer et al., 2004). Furthermore CD20+ autoreactive B-cells may resist deletion by residency in specific compartments. In transgenic mice expressing human CD20, B-cells in splenic marginal zones and germinal centers are comparatively resistant to anti-CD20 antibody therapy (Gong et al., 2005). Treatment resistance appears not to be a function of diminished exposure to anti-CD20 antibody or an intrinsic property of specific B-cell lineages but rather it reflects expression of survival factors such as BAFF/BLyS and retention of B-cells in their locality which avoids their presentation to hepatic macrophages. Complement and Fcgamma receptor mediated killing of anti-CD20 antibody coated cells also appear important (Gong et al., 2005). BAFF/BLys acting in concert with IL-21, has recently been demonstrated to promote differentiation of IgG+ve marginal zone B-cells into plasma cells in human spleens and antibody production in an antigen dependent manner (Ettinger et al., 2007). Studies of the BAFF−/− NZM 2328 mouse also demonstrate the dependence of splenic ASC upon BAFF (Jacob et al., 2006). Moreover, this genotype results in reduced total IgG and circulating autoantibodies in young animals and sustained attenuation of renal injury at all ages (Jacob et al., 2006). Unexpectedly, older BAFF−/− NZM 2328 mice exhibited similar autoantibody titers to those seen in BAFF+/+ NZM 2328 mice despite the continued protection from severe glomerular injury, a reminder of the functional complexities of autoantibody-mediated disease.

All antibody secreting cells depend upon "survival niches" and a reduction in inflammatory cytokines (IL-5, IL-6, and TNFalpha) may help to reduce the availability of such niches (Moser et al., 2006a, b). Recent data have also indicated that T-cell depletion may compromise B-cell survival in secondary lymphoid tissues (Withers et al., 2007). Accordingly it seems prudent to remain cognizant of the combination of immunosuppressant agents that are administered with rituximab since their synergistic action could promote egress of autoantibody secreting cells as local inflammation is attenuated and novel combination therapies such dual anti-BLyS/anti-CD20 antibody treatment may prove to have increased potency (Stohl and Looney, 2006).

Even when autoreactive B-cells can be seemingly efficiently deleted, the potential for autoimmunity to recur may clearly persist. Naive B-cells appear to form the majority of B-cells that reconstitute the peripheral blood after rituximab in rheumatoid arthritis and relapses of rheumatoid arthritis are reported to be more frequent in patients whose peripheral blood B-cell population reconstitutes with a larger proportion of memory cells, which might reflect ineffective deletion of memory cells from solid organ pools (Leandro et al., 2006). Similarly in a small number of rituximab-treated SLE patients, sustained clinical remission has been reported to correlate with an extended suppression of circulating and tonsillar memory (CD27+) B-cells and an increase in transitional (immature) B-cells, although interestingly germinal centers were detected in tonsils and the magnitude of memory cell suppression was greater in peripheral blood than in tissue (Anolik et al., 2007). Beyond these studies, there is little indication of the origins of re-emerging autoantibody secreting cells where autoantibody production was initially suppressed following rituximab treatment; autoreactive cells might derive from a memory pool that escaped deletion or naive autoreactive B-cells exposed to antigen anew. It appears that the size and composition of the plasma cell population in the bone marrow is ordinarily regulated by plasma cell apoptosis induced via FcgammaRIIb ligation (Xiang et al., 2007). As yet it is unclear whether all ASC populations are similarly regulated but the finding may have particular relevance to autoimmune disease since plasmablasts from lupus-prone mouse strains were resistant to FcgammaRIIb-mediated deletion. This observation adds to several other proposed mechanisms by which a reduction in FcgammaRIIb expression on B-cells from mice and humans with SLE may contribute to disease pathogenesis (Fukuyama et al., 2005; Mackay et al., 2006). Accordingly, autoreactive B-cells and the autoantibody secreting cells to which they give rise seem poised to remain the focus of much attention in autoimmune research.

If cutting off the supply of autoreactive B-cells and autoantibodies offers an effective albeit potentially temporary mechanism to interrupt autoimmune injury, how best can we promote the effective resolution of damage already initiated? Recently, the fundamental importance of *active* resolution has come to the fore in inflammation research and these insights may yet prove to be relevant to autoimmune disease (Serhan et al., 2007). Moreover, since resolution is initiated by early pro-inflammatory signals ("the beginning programs the end"), it is possible that injudicious use or timing of anti-inflammatory therapy could actually aggravate tissue damage by interrupting the restoration of tissue homeostasis (Serhan and

Savill, 2005). The contrast between acute post streptococcal glomerulonephritis (APSGN) which typically heals spontaneously without scarring and the extensive glomerulosclerosis and tubular atrophy that can result from ANCA-vasculitis or lupus nephritis despite intense immunosuppression, is well-recognized (Savill, 2001). Differences in the nature and duration of the initiating stimulus likely contribute to the final outcome of glomerular injury but apoptosis and clearance of apoptotic cells are probably key events in effective resolution of inflammation and restoration of normal glomerular structure and function, irrespective of the original insult (Watson et al., 2006; Ferenbach et al., 2007). Infiltrating neutrophils do not emigrate from inflamed glomerulus but rather undergo apoptosis and must be taken up by macrophages which then exhibit an "anti-inflammatory" phenotype although the situation is clearly complex, since synchronous exposure to apoptotic neutrophils and LPS (TLR ligands) differentially modulates cytokine secretion by macrophages over 24 h compared to either stimulus alone (Savill et al., 2002; Lucas et al., 2003). This type of macrophage programming may ordinarily facilitate an appropriate, bimodal response with early pro-inflammatory and late pro-resolution (TGFbeta, IL-10) cytokine profiles which orchestrate an effective innate immune response. In autoimmune disease, an initial inflammatory response to exogenous stimuli could be appropriate but, by definition, subsequent responses are aberrant.

Proximal defects in the classical complement pathway, leading to aberrant clearance of apoptotic cells are well understood as potential initiators of autoimmune disease and in particular SLE, but these defects also directly amplify immune-complex mediated renal injury as demonstrated by the impact of C1q deficiency on accelerated nephrotoxic nephritis (Robson et al., 2001). Other defects of apoptotic cell clearance, such as CD14 deficiency, are not sufficient in themselves to incite autoimmunity but their influence upon independently initiated immune-mediated injury remains to be determined (Devitt et al., 2004). In ANCA-vasculitis, macrophages which have engulfed apoptotic neutrophils appear to be diverted away from a non-phlogistic phenotype and this may contribute to the failure of effective healing (Moosig et al., 2000; Harper et al., 2001). Additionally, the presence of ANCA accelerates neutrophil apoptosis without promoting concomitant externalization of phosphatidylserine which likely impairs neutrophil clearance and promotes secondary necrosis, amplifying tissue damage (Harper et al., 2000). In other circumstances, accelerated neutrophil apoptosis can actually defer progression from acute to chronic inflammation and reduce tissue scarring; *R*-Roscovitine, a cyclin-dependent kinase inhibitor, promotes caspase-dependent neutrophil apoptosis and attenuated tissue damage in several settings including a chronic model of bleomycin-induced lung injury (Rossi et al., 2006). Inhibition of ERK1/2 similarly promotes neutrophil apoptosis and inflammation resolution (Sawatzky et al., 2006).

Current anti-inflammatory strategies focus on suppression of pro-inflammatory mediators which belies a dearth of engineered pro-resolving approaches although some of the oldest "anti-inflammatory" drugs, notably aspirin and glucocorticoids, also turn out to enhance resolution (Serhan et al., 2007). Aspirin, through the acetylation of COX2, generates epimers of lipoxins, resolvins, and protectins, families of lipid mediators that are now appreciated as integral to the resolution process (Ariel and Serhan, 2007). Endogenous members of these same three eicosanoid families are rapidly generated during the interaction of macrophages and apoptotic neutrophils and enhance the macrophage's phagocytic capacity in addition to modulating further neutrophil influx (Schwab et al., 2007). Although it has not been studied in the kidney, generation of lipid mediators in other inflamed tissues depends upon transcellular biosynthesis which harnesses both infiltrating leukocytes and resident cells such as endothelial cells or interstitial fibroblasts. Thus one potential approach would be to identify or develop drugs that target stromal cells in order to promote resolution. The capacity of glucocorticoids to promote non-phlogistic clearance of apoptotic neutrophils has been recognized for some time and recent data indicate that this relates, at least in part, to annexin-1 which is released by not only dexamethasone treated macrophages but also neutrophils undergoing spontaneous apoptosis (Maderna et al., 2005; Scannell et al., 2007). Although annexin-1 is a peptide, it binds the lipoxin-A4 receptors on macrophages and enhances apoptotic cell uptake.

Currently, the specific relevance of these emerging concepts of active resolution to autoimmune renal disease is uncharted but it seems improbable that they will prove irrelevant particularly as exogenous protectins and resolvins are already known to attenuate renal ischemia-reperfusion injury (Duffield et al., 2006). It is already apparent that macrophages present in inflamed tissue are complex and pleiotropic; in addition to facilitating clearance of apoptotic cells they can direct various aspects of immune-mediated injury and promote scarring. These divergent roles are linked to phenotypic and temporal characteristics: macrophage subsets that broadly promote tissue destruction or repair/remodeling (classical and alternatively activated, respectively) can be identified to varying degrees by their cytokine profiles and by the chronology of tissue injury (Gordon and Taylor, 2005, Mantovani et al., 2007).

Specific to the kidney, glomerular injury is ameliorated by conditional ablation of macrophages during the progression of established nephrotoxic nephritis which implies that, overall, macrophages have a negative impact by enhancing crescent formation, myofibroblast proliferation, and matrix deposition (Duffield et al., 2005b). Similarly, deficiency of CCR2 (believed to be the major chemokine receptor for trafficking of inflammatory monocytes into tissue) reduces renal injury in the MRL/lpr model of lupus nephritis (de Lema et al., 2005). In contrast, macrophages manipulated ex vivo to exhibit an alternative phenotype have been reported to transiently attenuate renal injury in nephrotoxic nephritis and to mediate a sustained (4 week) amelioration of adriamycin induced nephropathy (Kluth et al., 2001; Wang et al., 2007). Meanwhile, macrophage ablation during the course of carbon-tetrachloride induced liver fibrosis elegantly demonstrates that timing is all important; deletion during the period of injury attenuates its severity whilst deletion after cessation of toxin injection prevents spontaneous resolution of fibrosis (Duffield et al., 2005a). Macrophage phenotype is clearly complex and very likely represents a continuous spectrum that changes according to the prevailing cytokine milieu in the microenvironment but, at present, something that is most clearly lacking is a systematic characterization of macrophages in autoimmune renal disease both in human tissue and in appropriate animal models where chronology may be more easily assessed. Given that animal models do not always provide informative surrogates for the complexities of human disease, it may be that an appreciation of the significance of these processes will also suggest a need for serial protocol biopsies in human disease, particularly if interventions that promote resolution become better understood and can be clinically utilized. As a corollary, the exploration of the role of macrophages in renal injury and recovery should remind us that single agents or monophasic therapies are unlikely to be the basis of successful treatment for autoimmune disease and that we should not discount "conventional" agents such as corticosteroids since they may have underappreciated effects. Clearly, optimized usage to minimize side-effects or development of alternatives that target the same effectors, remain important (Chapman et al., 2006).

If APSGN provides one example of a mechanism for the control of immune-mediated renal injury, then other diseases may also reveal useful processes. Anti-glomerular basement membrane (GBM) disease is devastating if unrecognized or when treatment is delayed, typically resulting in irreversible renal failure and the risk of pulmonary hemorrhage but, unlike ANCA-vasculitis and lupus nephritis, the risk of relapse following treatment for anti-GBM disease is generally very low. Recent evidence indicates that this is a consequence of the development of regulatory T-cell subsets (adaptive Tregs) (Salama et al., 2003). In contrast, regulatory T-cells may be dysfunctional in SLE and ANCA-vasculitis (Abdulahad et al., 2007; Valencia et al., 2007).

The origins of this dysfunction are unknown although interestingly in the SAMP1/YitFc mouse model of Crohn's disease, Treg function appears to be impaired by an expanded B-cell population which might have relevance to the efficacy of B-cell depleting therapies if the same phenomenon applies in other autoimmune diseases (Olson et al., 2004). It remains to be determined whether relevant subsets can be therapeutically promoted and what impact current treatment strategies may have upon this potential but it would not be surprising to discover that pan- immunosuppressive or ablative strategies do not engender their survival. Animal models indicate the feasibility of adoptive transfer of regulatory T-cells programmed ex vivo and importantly, this approach would not be dissimilar, for example, from existing protocols for the transfer of CMV specific CTLs in stem-cell transplant recipients (Scalapino et al., 2006). Moreover, it is now apparent that human regulatory T-cells can be efficiently expanded ex vivo using antigen-pulsed dendritic cells and that donor regulatory T-cells, transferred during liver transplantation, mediate a functional allosuppressive effect (Jiang et al., 2006; Demirkiran et al., 2007). A primary obstacle to the therapeutic use of Tregs in human autoimmunity is the lack of clearly identified pathogenic T-cell autoepitopes in diseases such ANCA-vasculitis. Intriguingly, a single histone-derived peptide that is recognized not only by Th cells capable of inducing B-cell autoreactivity and anti-DNA antibody production in lupus-prone SNF1 mice but also by T-cells from patients with SLE, can be used to tolerize SNF1 mice towards a range of lupus-autoantigens (Hahn et al., 2005). This process expands regulatory T-cells, reduces titers of various autoantibodies, and mitigates the severity of nephritis. Administration of low-dose peptide to mice with established glomerulonephrits halts disease progression and as such represents an alternative strategy to induce regulatory T-cells without the need for ex vivo expansion. More recently, this same peptide has also been shown to induce a Foxp3 expressing CD8+ T regulatory subset that suppresses autoantibody production (Singh et al., 2007). Interestingly, Foxp3 expression and TGFbeta production (which mediate immunomodulatory function) are interdependent in these CD8 Tregs. The efficacy of tolerogenic peptides has also been demonstrated in a rodent model of anti-GBM nephritis (Reynolds et al., 2005). A further experimental strategy for the expansion of Tregs may be the adoptive transfer of alternatively activated monocytes which was recently demonstrated to attenuate experimental autoimmune encephamyelitis (EAE) through expansion of Tregs and concomitant reduction of Th2 and Th17 cells (see below) (Weber et al., 2007).

Apart from their potential relevance to sustained remission, regulatory T-cells (natural Tregs) likely help to block the initiation of autoimmunity. Indeed, murine and human Foxp3 deficiency blocks Treg development and leads to lethal autoimmune disease and, similarly, in vivo ablation of Tregs triggers autoimmune disease in mice (Kim et al., 2007; Zheng and Rudensky, 2007). Further, a reduction in circulating Tregs has recently been observed in human CD40L deficiency, a condition associated with autoimmunity, and interestingly this was associated with an expanded autoreactive naive B-cell repertoire denoting impaired peripheral B-cell tolerance (Herve et al., 2007). However, unpicking the relevance of this type of observation to autoimmunity in the wider population is difficult: individuals who are genetically deficient and exhibit an extreme phenotype may or may not hold clues to the perturbation of immune regulation in other circumstances. This leads us to the third and perhaps least penetrable vista in autoimmune therapeutics, the capacity to intervene in those mechanisms which drive the inception of autoimmune disease. This concept is problematic since patients rarely present themselves for medical attention before the onset of overt autoimmune disease and furthermore, our understanding of what initiates disease continues to lag behind our knowledge of the effector mechanisms that direct injury. Nevertheless, illuminating these processes may ultimately offer the prospect of curative therapy in autoimmunity.

A little over 20 years ago, the Th1/Th2 paradigm was conceived and rapidly adopted as the presumed basis for perturbed immune regulation in many autoimmune diseases (Gutcher and Becher, 2007; Steinman, 2007). Specifically, Th1 responses were considered to promote various autoimmune processes, not least of all crescentic nephritis, and a considerable weight of evidence from animal models supports this contention although the polarity of the Th response in human diseases such as Wegener's granulomatosis is less clear (Balding et al., 2001; Voswinkel et al., 2005; Tipping and Holdsworth, 2006). More recently, seemingly incompatible data from disease models that were presumed to be Th1-mediated have prompted a re-evaluation and a new T-cell subset, the Th17 (IL-17 secreting) cells, has emerged as a more likely culprit in at least some organ-specific autoimmune diseases (Afzali et al., 2007; Furuzawa-Carballeda et al., 2007; Steinman, 2007). Notably, deficiency of key Th1 cytokines IFN$\gamma$ and TNFalpha, does not bestow a protective effect in autoimmune diseases such as EAE whereas mice are protected by interruption of Th17 cell development. The relevance of Th17 cells has also recently been demonstrated in the SKG mouse model of rheumatoid arthritis (Hirota et al., 2007). The role of Th1 cells in autoimmunity has not been wholly discredited since deficiency of the transcription factor T-bet, upon which Th1 differentiation and IFN$\gamma$ production are dependent, renders mice resistant to EAE but the picture is muddied by conflicting data on the influence of T-bet upon Th17 cells (Mathur et al., 2006; Gocke et al., 2007). T-bet deficiency does block autoantibody class switching and ameliorate glomerulonephritis in lupus-prone mice although in part this reflects T-bet function in B-cells (Peng et al. 2002). Another transcription factor ROR$\gamma$t, is clearly required for Th17 cell development and ROR$\gamma$t deficiency significantly impairs the development of EAE (Ivanov et al., 2006; Annunziato et al., 2007). It may transpire that Th1 and Th17 can cooperate to trigger autoimmune disease.

Differentiation of Th17 cells is intertwined with that of Tregs since the combination of TGF$\beta$ and IL-6 drives naïve murine T-cells towards the Th17 phenotype whereas TGF$\beta$ alone induces Foxp3 expression and Treg differentiation (Bettelli et al., 2006). In fact, murine Tregs can act as the source of TGF$\beta$ to drive differentiation of naïve cells into Th17 cells in the presence of IL-6 and, more intriguingly, Tregs can actually be transformed into Th17 cells by the autocrine action of TGF$\beta$ in the presence of IL-6 (Xu et al., 2007). Additionally, IL-6 independent differentiation of naïve murine T-cells to Th17 is possible (Kimura et al., 2007). Meanwhile IL-23 drives expansion of Th17 cells and IL-17 secretion from activated memory T-cells whereas IFN$\gamma$ and IL-4 down-regulate Th17 cell proliferation (Bettelli et al., 2006, 2007). It is becoming apparent that the signals which drive differentiation and proliferation of Th17 cells in humans differ to at least some extent from those delineated in mice but there are already descriptions of the involvement of Th17 cells in human Crohn's disease and autoimmune uveitis (Hoeve et al., 2006; Acosta-Rodriguez et al., 2007a, b; Amadi-Obi et al., 2007; Annunziato et al., 2007; Sato et al., 2007). At present there is very little information on what function if any Th17 cells might perform in autoimmune renal diseases, although Th17 cells have been identified infiltrating the kidneys of SNF1 mice with glomerulonephritis and patients with both active SLE and ANCA-vasculitis have elevated serum IL-6 levels (Booth et al., 2004a, b; Ripley et al., 2005; Kang et al., 2007). Whether the apparent deficits in Tregs associated with ANCA-vasculitis and SLE indicate a reciprocal expansion of the Th17 subset remains to be determined.

Other insights into the origins of autoimmunity are emerging through investigations of the mechanisms that maintain peripheral tolerance amongst B-cells (Ferry et al., 2006). Random Ig gene rearrangement and mutation generate antibody diversity but risk engendering autoreactivity (Townsend et al., 1999). Central and peripheral B-cell tolerance are believed to regulate the B-cell repertoire: central mechanisms most likely divert or remove B-cells with high-affinity for autoantigens through receptor editing and deletion (apoptosis) whilst lower affinity autoreactivity may be handled through induction of B-cell anergy (Cambier et al., 2007). However, anergy is not an irreversible state and there appear to be a number of potential aberrations in the maintenance of tolerance through which pathogenic autoimmunity can arise (Phan et al., 2003).

The frequency of autoreactivity amongst early immature B-cells (pre-B-cells) in the bone marrow of healthy individuals is remarkably high; 75% of cloned Ig genes were autoreactive in one study with 58% producing anti-nuclear staining of human epithelial (Hep2) cells (Wardemann et al., 2003). This type of autoreactivity frequently occurs in the context of polyreactivity towards a range of foreign and self nuclear antigens. Central tolerance eliminates many such cells but nonetheless a high proportion of immature B-cells emigrating from the bone marrow are still potentially autoreactive. In the main they recognize cytoplasmic Hep2 antigens which are not clearly linked to pathogenic autoimmunity but 7% are truly polyreactive, often with anti-ssDNA or dsDNA specificity. Further counter-selection occurs before entry into the mature naive pool where 4% remain polyreactive. Studies of B-cells cloned from the peripheral blood of small numbers of patients with SLE reveal that tolerance may be defective resulting in expanded numbers of autoreactive mature naïve B-cells (Yurasov et al., 2005, 2006). B-cells with antinuclear reactivity were not increased overall in the newly emigrant B-cell pools of SLE patients but neither were they depleted from the mature naïve cell pool to the same extent as in healthy donors. Furthermore, the expansion of polyreactive mature naïve B-cells was greatest in patients with active disease but did not fully reverse with clinical remission, suggesting that this might contribute to disease predisposition. In all likelihood, there will be heterogeneous breaches of tolerance including central abnormalities in some individuals, as well as peripheral defects of the type described.

Differentiation into autoantibody secreting cells is ordinarily very uncommon and there is additional counter-selection of mature naïve autoreactive B-cells preventing entry into the IgM memory pool in healthy individuals (Tsuiji et al., 2006). IgM memory cells likely represent the product of T-independent immune responses initiated through antigen exposure in splenic marginal zones. Human splenic marginal zone IgG memory cells were also recently described but, in the main, IgG memory cells originate from T-dependent immune responses in germinal centers and studies of one autoreactive B-cell population (bearing the 9G4 idiotype) ordinarily detectable in the mature naïve pool but only associated with a corresponding plasma cell population and circulating autoantibody titers in the context of SLE, indicate that germinal center exclusion is one mechanism that curtails B-cell autoreactivity (Cappione et al., 2005; Ettinger et al., 2007). Based upon analysis of tonsils and spleens, this process appears to be defective in patients with SLE in whom 9G4 cells accumulate within GCs and populate the isotype switched memory pool (in contrast GC exclusion operated as normal in patients with RA) (Cappione et al., 2005). Late-stage checkpoints also regulate other autoreactive B-cells; maturation of anti-ribonucleicprotein Smith B-cells is halted at the early pre-plasma cell stage in non-autoimmune mice but continues to terminal plasma cell differentiation (and autoantibody secretion) in MRL/lprlpr mice (Culton et al., 2006). Whilst these mechanisms may regulate particular B-cell populations, there seems to be overall enrichment for anti-nuclear (and poly-) reactivity in the human IgG memory B-cell pool of healthy donors despite an absence of circulating ANA (Tiller et al., 2007). Reversion of autoreactive B-cell clones to germ line Ig gene sequences, elegantly demonstrated that this autoreactivity mainly arose through somatic hypermutation (indicating an antigen driven process) (Meffre et al., 2001). Similarly, germ line reversion of patient-derived anti-dsDNA antibody hybridomas wholly abrogates autoreactivity, indicating that pathogenic autoimmunity is probably antigen-driven (possibly initiated through recognition of cardiolipin on apoptotic cells by the germ line Ig) (Wellmann et al., 2005). Thus B-cells entering GCs may be positively selected and driven towards dangerous autoreactivity, perhaps after BCR triggering by antigens presented on follicular dendritic cells. Alternatively, somatic hypermutation of autoreactive B-cells may be occurring outside of GCs at the T zone-red pulp border in the spleen (William et al., 2002).

Regardless of the precise location at which it occurs, antigen driven maturation implies that stochastic events shape the autoreactive repertoire which again highlights the relevance of determining the identity and origins of the inciting auto/foreign antigens. In a departure from conventional theories regarding the origins of autoautoimmunity, we have recently proposed that autoimmune disease is triggered by a foreign antigen related to an autoantigen through amino acid sequence "complementary." By definition, a protein translated from what would ordinarily be the antisense of the autoantigen mRNA is termed complementary but in practice complementarity to an autoantigen (and more specifically an autoepitope) as defined by sequence or perhaps structure could be a characteristic of either an endogenous or exogenous protein. The concept arose from identification of antibodies in the sera of PR3-ANCA positive patients which were reactive against a protein derived from the antisense RNA of the PR3 gene and, importantly, these antibodies also bound PR3-ANCA (denoting an idiotype, anti-idiotype relationship) (Pendergraft et al., 2004). Accordingly, the *Theory of Autoantigen Complementarity* proposes that autoimmunity begins with exposure to an antigen that is complementary to the autoantigen. The primary humoral immune response to this non-self antigen is followed by a secondary response directed against the idiotope of the primary immunoglobulin which is immunogenic by virtue of its non-germline-encoded antigen-binding site (Munthe and Bogen, 1999; Dembic et al., 2000; Munthe et al., 2004). This second anti-idiotypic antibody reacts with the idiotope of the primary antibody and as a consequence of biochemical properties conferred by complementarity, is also reactive against the autoantigen (Pascual et al., 1989). Accordingly, mice immunized with peptide complementary to human PR3 not only developed antibodies against the immunogen, but also anti-human PR3 antibodies (Pendergraft et al., 2004). Likewise, immunization of mice with a La/SSB– complementary peptide elicited antibodies against the immunogen and anti-idiotypic antibodies that reacted with the sense autoantigen (Papamattheou et al., 2004). Mechanistically, how this occurs is not well understood but there is great interest in understanding how *complementary* protein pairs affect biological systems and it is notable that anti-idiotypic antibodies are also being used to break tolerance against tumor antigens (de Cerio et al., 2007; Heal et al., 2002). If autoreactive B-cells can emerge as a consequence of initial exposure to complementary proteins as this theory suggests, then it is reasonable to suppose that their subsequent survival and expansion could be determined by the varied influences that we have described herein.

It is also interesting to note that the availability of autoantigens that promote maturation of autoreactive IgG memory and antibody secreting cells may be influenced by the coexistence of autoreactive IgM B-cells. Autoreactive IgM antibodies could actually facilitate clearance of autoantigen through the C1q pathway and hence reduce the likelihood of further B-cell maturation, a possibility that sounds another cautionary note over the wisdom of pan-B-cell depletion.

The mechanism(s) that prevent autoantibody production by autoreactive memory B-cells in healthy individuals probably include anergy: a state of hyporesponsiveness to BCR stimulation that is associated with a survival disadvantage and reduced half life (Ferry et al., 2006). In fact, anergy probably operates at a number of checkpoints during B-cell maturation and is considered to be a major regulator of peripheral tolerance (Cambier et al., 2007). Anergic B-cells were first characterized in transgenic mouse models where B-cell expression can be induced in the context of pre-specified antigen exposure and genetic background. The recent demonstration of anergic ("T3" or An1) transitional B-cells in the spleens of non-autoimmune B6 mice and the selective reduction in this population in lupus-prone NZB/W mice suggest that these observations have physiological and perhaps pathophysiological relevance, although the selective reduction of T3 B-cells was not evident in other lupus-prone strains which underscores how varied the key processes which maintain tolerance in a given scenario are likely to be (Merrell et al., 2006; Teague et al.,

2007). Further studies in transgenic strains emphasize a requirement for continuous exposure to antigen in maintaining an anergic phenotype amongst splenic B-cells (Rui et al., 2003). One implication of this is observation is that variation in the concentration or pattern of tissue-expression of certain autoantigens might have paradoxical effects. On the one hand, cellular injury, death, or activation may expose sequestered (intracellular) autoantigens and in so doing initiate the maturation of autoreactive B-cell and sustain autoantibody production by short-lived plasmablasts as eluded to earlier but, at the same time, resolution of cellular damage or removal of stimulation may promote maturation of transitional autoreactive cells that were held in developmental arrest (anergy) as a consequence of chronic antigen exposure.

Importantly, it appears that BAFF may orchestrate the selective survival disadvantage and maturation block imposed upon anergic B-cells in the periphery. Mice that overexpress BAFF exhibit expanded immature B-cell (T1) populations and develop autoimmunity (Mackay et al., 1999; Batten et al., 2000; Groom et al., 2007). Similarly, serum BAFF concentrations are elevated in patients with some autoimmune diseases including SLE (Stohl et al., 2003). In immunoglobulin transgenic mice (such as the hen egg lysozyme (HEL) model) where peripheral tolerance of intermediate affinity self-reactive B-cells is maintained through anergy, BAFF overexpression allows transitional B-cells to enter and mature in follicles and splenic marginal zones and seemingly reverses their anergic phenotype (Thien et al., 2004). Moreover, autoreactive B-cells in Ig transgenic mice demonstrate an increased BAFF dependency for survival and a competitive disadvantage in a mixed B-cell repertoire when the availability of BAFF is limited (leading to reduced survival) (Lesley et al., 2004). Modulation of BAFF levels (circulating and in tissue) can exaggerate or override this competitive disadvantage and skew the survival of autoreactive cells. These observations are of particular interest since they not only signal the potential utility of antagonizing BAFF (e.g., using Belimumab) but also imply that autoreactive B-cells re-emerging in a lymphopenic environment (after cyclophosphamide or rituximab treatment) may have a greater chance of survival. Moreover, rituximab therapy actually engenders increased serum BAFF levels (Cambridge et al., 2006b). High-affinity autoreactive B-cells appear not to depend on BAFF for survival and are ordinarily regulated through central tolerance.

Finally, the importance of co-stimulatory signals delivered through pattern recognition receptors and in particular Toll-like receptors (TLRs), for the initiation of pathogenic autoimmunity is now apparent (Christensen and Shlomchik, 2007; Ehlers and Ravetch, 2007). Most attention has focused on the roles of TLR7 and TLR9 which can be stimulated with ssRNA and CpG DNA (microbial or less potent endogenous CpG DNA), respectively. TLR7 and TLR9 signal through MyD88. More recently, it has become apparent that other members of the TLR family activated by specific bacterially derived ligands (including TLR2 and TLR4) contribute to immune-mediated glomerular injury through their expression on intrinsic and infiltrating cells (Brown et al., 2006, 2007). Furthermore, TLR-triggered autoimmune disease exhibits a functional redundancy since TLR3 activation incites anti-dsDNA autoimmunity and glomerulonephritis in MyD88−/− MRL/lpr mice (Sadanaga et al., 2007). TLR7 and TLR9, are located in the endosomal compartment and consequently can only be activated by endocytosed or phagocytosed ligands. Their relevance to autoimmunity was first recognized through studies of rheumatoid factor-specific B-cells where BCR ligation by immune complexes comprising IgG and chromatin allows internalization, processing, and delivery of a TLR9 ligand which results in B-cell proliferation. Importantly, B-cells responding to this co-stimulatory TLR-signal typically have BCRs of sufficiently low affinity to escape regulation by the usual mechanisms including tolerance. In humans, both class switched and unswitched memory B-cells constitutively express TLRs and generate ASC in vitro in response to isolated TLR9 ligand stimulation (enabling polyclonal activation) whereas naive B-cells express TLRs 9 and 10 only after BCR triggering and require dual activation through TLR9 and BCR to secrete antibody (Bernasconi et al., 2002, 2003). Anergic autoreactive cells (derived from the HEL transgenic model) are resistant to TLR9 signaling as a consequence of continuous antigen exposure (activating via ERK) and selective uncoupling of BCR-signaling from a calcineurin-dependent pathway (Rui et al., 2003). In patients with active SLE, expression of TLR9 by memory and plasma cells is increased and correlates with anti-dsDNA antibody positivity (Rui et al., 2003). Genetic manipulation of TLR9 expression in MRL/lprlpr mice also demonstrates the role of this receptor in anti-DNA antibody responses whereas anti-RNA antibody production is tied to TLR7 activation (Christensen et al., 2005; Lau et al., 2005; Berland et al., 2006; Ehlers et al., 2006; Pisitkun et al., 2006). However, TLR involvement in autoimmunity is complex: young MRL/lprlpr mice injected with CpG develop an accelerated and severe lupus-like disease at an age before they would ordinarily develop autoantibodies or organ damage but TLR9 deletion has also been reported to exacerbate autoimmune injury in MRL/lprlpr mice (Christensen et al. 2006; Pawar et al. 2006). In contrast, MRL/lprlpr TLR7−/− mice exhibit attenuated organ damage. The basis for these discrepancies is presently undetermined.

Lineage-specific deletion demonstrates that B-cell TLRs mediate nucleic acid stimulated antibody production but TLRs are widely expressed, including by dendritic cells (DC) which notably secrete type I interferons (the "lupus signature") following TLR7 or TLR9 ligation (Christensen and Shlomchik, 2007). Myeloid DCs activated by chromatin-IgG immune complexes that can bind FcgammaRIIa and then activate intracellular TLRs, also secrete BAFF. Consequently activation of DC-TLRs likely amplifies autoimmune responses. What may be of particular relevance is the potential of TLR-induced signaling to promote both T-cell dependent and independent antigen responses. In fact, it has been suggested that appreciation of the functions of TLRs challenges the conventional distinction of T-dependent from -independent immune responses (Lanzavecchia and Sallusto, 2007). This might be relevant to autoimmune diseases, such as ANCA-vasculitis where it has proved difficult to conclusively, identify autoantigen-specific T-cells despite evidence of class-switched B-cell autoreactivity, although target autoantigens in ANCA-vasculitis are not nuclear and their capacity to activate TLRs is unknown. Nonetheless it is intriguing to speculate whether the concept of an antigen that can deliver dual signals to an immune cell (either in isolation or as some form of complex) is restricted to the nuclear antigen repertoire. Recent evidence derived in the THP-1 cell line, suggests that PR3 does in fact prime for responsiveness to various TLR ligands although the mechanism requires clarification (Uehara et al. 2007).

In conclusion, both basic and translational research efforts are expanding our understanding not only of the usual mechanisms of humoral immune regulation but importantly how these may be subverted or disrupted so as to trigger and perpetuate autoimmune disease. Once pathogenic autoimmunity is initiated, there are a host of potential means to halt it and an increasing number are reaching the clinic but we are still some way away from "holistic" therapies that will restore homeostasis to both the injured tissues and the immune system. How durable contemporary concepts and hypotheses will prove to be remains uncertain, in all likelihood not all of them will meet the benchmark set by Clemens Freiherr von Pirquet 100 years ago when he unveiled his seminal work hypothesizing that antigen–antibody complexes ("toxic bodies") initiated a spectrum of organ damage in conditions such as the measles exanthema and serum sickness (Silverstein, 2000). There are indisputably significant deficiencies in the current knowledge base and it is plausible that rectifying these will require us to depart radically from current immunological dogma in order to understand what really initiates and sustains pathogenic autoimmunity in humans. The chapters of this book draw together many of today's leading investigators in the areas of autoimmune disease and the kidney to cover a remarkably wide-ranging body of research: the result is a fascinating overview of the subject matter which will assuredly stand the test of time.

## Key points

- ANCA-vasculitis and proliferative lupus nephritis are important causes of auto-antibody-mediated systemic autoimmune disease that targets the kidney.
- During the last 35 years, suppression of autoreactive B-cells has mainly relied on cyclophosphamide and high-dose steroids which are not only associated with significant side effects but frequently fail to induce sustained, relapse-free survival.
- Newer B-cell targeted therapies such as rituximab seemingly afford disease control with fewer side effects although their capacity to achieve sustained remission remains to be determined. Modulation of BAFF/BLyS may also be therapeutically useful.
- Concurrently, there is now a renewed interest in the origins, location, and longevity of autoantibody producing B-cells.
- B-cell autoreactivity is a frequent phenomenon in the normal human B-cell repertoire whereas autoantibody production is rare. Defective or dysregulated B-cell tolerance mechanisms probably predispose to autoimmunity but antigen-driven affinity maturation is also evident within IgG+ve autoreactive memory B-cells. The exact identity of inciting immunogens in most autoimmune responses remains elusive.
- Sustained remission of autoantibody-mediated disease may be achievable through promotion of appropriate regulatory T-cell subsets.
- The importance of active resolution of inflammation, involving lipid mediators and "alternatively activated" macrophages is becoming better understood and may well apply to autoimmune kidney diseases.

# References

Abdulahad, W.H., Stegeman, C.A., van der Geld, Y.M., et al. 2007. Functional defect of circulating regulatory CD4+ T cells in patients with Wegener's granulomatosis in remission. Arthritis Rheum. 56, 2080.

Acosta-Rodriguez, E.V., Napolitani, G., Lanzavecchia, A., et al. 2007a. Interleukins 1[beta] and 6 but not transforming growth factor-[beta] are essential for the differentiation of interleukin 17-producing human T helper cells. Nat. Immunol. 8, 942.

Acosta-Rodriguez, E.V., Rivino, L., Geginat, J., et al. 2007b. Surface phenotype and antigenic specificity of human interleukin 17-producing T helper memory cells. Nat. Immunol. 8, 639.

Afzali, B., Lombardi, G., Lechler, R.I., et al. 2007. The role of T helper 17 (Th17) and regulatory T cells (Treg) in human organ transplantation and autoimmune disease. Clin. Exp. Immunol. 148, 32.

Ahuja, A., Shupe, J., Dunn, R., et al. 2007. Depletion of B cells in murine lupus: efficacy and resistance. J. Immunol. 179, 3351.

Amadi-Obi, A., Yu, C.-R., Liu, X., et al. 2007. TH17 cells contribute to uveitis and scleritis and are expanded by IL-2 and inhibited by IL-27/STAT1. Nat. Med. 13, 711.

Annunziato, F., Cosmi, L., Santarlasci, V., et al. 2007. Phenotypic and functional features of human Th17 cells. J. Exp. Med. 204, 1849.

Anolik, J.H., Barnard, J., Owen, T., et al. 2007. Delayed memory B cell recovery in peripheral blood and lymphoid tissue in systemic lupus erythematosus after B cell depletion therapy. Arthritis Rheum. 56, 3044.

Ariel, A., Serhan, C.N. 2007. Resolvins and protectins in the termination program of acute inflammation. Trends Immunol. 28, 176.

Austin, H.A., III, Klippel, J.H., Balow, J.E., et al. 1986. Therapy of lupus nephritis. Controlled trial of prednisone and cytotoxic drugs. N. Engl. J. Med. 314, 614.

Balding, C.E.J., Howie, A.J., Drake-Lee, A.B., et al. 2001. Th2 dominance in nasal mucosa in patients with Wegener's granulomatosis. Clin. Exp. Immunol. 125, 332.

Batten, M., Groom, J., Cachero, T.G., et al. 2000. BAFF mediates survival of peripheral immature B lymphocytes. J. Exp. Med. 192, 1453.

Berland, R., Fernandez, L., Kari, E., et al. 2006. Toll-like receptor 7-dependent loss of B cell tolerance in pathogenic autoantibody knockin mice. Immunity 25, 429.

Bernasconi, N.L., Onai, N., Lanzavecchia, A. 2003. A role for Toll-like receptors in acquired immunity: up-regulation of TLR9 by BCR triggering in naive B cells and constitutive expression in memory B cells. Blood 101, 4500.

Bernasconi, N.L., Traggiai, E., Lanzavecchia, A. 2002. Maintenance of serological memory by polyclonal activation of human memory B cells. Science 298, 2199.

Bettelli, E., Carrier, Y., Gao, W., et al. 2006. Reciprocal developmental pathways for the generation of pathogenic effector TH17 and regulatory T cells. Nature 441, 235.

Bettelli, E., Oukka, M., Kuchroo, V.K. 2007. TH-17 cells in the circle of immunity and autoimmunity. Nat. Immunol. 8, 345.

Booth, A.D., Jayne, D.R.W., Kharbanda, R.K., et al. 2004a. Infliximab improves endothelial dysfunction in systemic vasculitis: a model of vascular inflammation. Circulation 109, 1718.

Booth, A.D., Pusey, C.D., Jayne, D.R. 2004b. Renal vasculitis—an update in 2004. Nephrol. Dial. Transplant. 19, 1964.

Brown, H.J., Lock, H.R., Sacks, S.H., et al. 2006. TLR2 stimulation of intrinsic renal cells in the induction of immune-mediated glomerulonephritis. J. Immunol. 177, 1925.

Brown, H.J., Lock, H.R., Wolfs, T.G.A.M., et al. 2007. Toll-like receptor 4 ligation on intrinsic renal cells contributes to the induction of antibody-mediated glomerulonephritis via CXCL1 and CXCL2. J. Am. Soc. Nephrol. 18, 1732.

Burt, R.K., Traynor, A., Statkute, L., et al. 2006. Nonmyeloablative hematopoietic stem cell transplantation for systemic lupus erythematosus. J. Am. Med. Assoc. 295, 527.

Cambier, J.C., Gauld, S.B., Merrell, K.T., et al. 2007. B-cell anergy: from transgenic models to naturally occurring anergic B cells? Nat. Rev. Immunol. 7, 633.

Cambridge, G., Leandro, M.J., Teodorescu, M., et al. 2006a. B cell depletion therapy in systemic lupus erythematosus: effect on autoantibody and antimicrobial antibody profiles. Arthritis Rheum. 54, 3612.

Cambridge, G., Stohl, W., Leandro, M., et al. 2006b. Circulating levels of B lymphocyte stimulator in patients with rheumatoid arthritis following rituximab treatment: relationships with B cell depletion, circulating antibodies, and clinical relapse. Arthritis Rheum. 54, 723.

Cappione, A., III, Anolik, J.H., Pugh-Bernard, A., et al. 2005. Germinal center exclusion of autoreactive B cells is defective in human systemic lupus erythematosus. J. Clin. Invest. 115, 3205.

Cassese, G., Lindenau, S., de Boer, B., et al. 2001. Inflamed kidneys of NZB/W mice are a major site for the homeostasis of plasma cells. Eur. J. Immunol. 31, 2726.

Chan, O.T., Madaio, M.P., Shlomchik, M.J. 1999a. The central and multiple roles of B cells in lupus pathogenesis. Immunol. Rev. 169, 107.

Chan, O.T.M., Hannum, L.G., Haberman, A.M., et al. 1999b. A novel mouse with B cells but lacking serum antibody reveals an antibody-independent role for B cells in murine lupus. J. Exp. Med. 189, 1639.

Chapman, K.E., Coutinho, A., Gray, M., et al. 2006. Local amplification of glucocorticoids by 11beta-hydroxysteroid dehydrogenase type 1 and its role in the inflammatory response. Ann. N. Y. Acad. Sci. 1088, 265.

Christensen, S.R., Kashgarian, M., Alexopoulou, L., et al. 2005. Toll-like receptor 9 controls anti-DNA autoantibody production in murine lupus. J. Exp. Med. 202, 321.

Christensen, S.R., Shlomchik, M.J. 2007. Regulation of lupus-related autoantibody production and clinical disease by Toll-like receptors. Semin. Immunol. 19, 11.

Christensen, S.R., Shupe, J., Nickerson, K., et al. 2006. Toll-like receptor 7 and TLR9 dictate autoantibody specificity and have opposing inflammatory and regulatory roles in a murine model of lupus. Immunity 25, 417.

Clayton, A.R., Savage, C.O. 2003. Production of antineutrophil cytoplasm antibodies derived from circulating B cells in patients with systemic vasculitis. Clin. Exp. Immunol. 132, 174.

Culton, D., Nicholas, M., Bunch, D., et al. 2007. Similar CD19 dysregulation in two autoantibody-associated autoimmune diseases suggests a shared mechanism of B-cell tolerance loss. J. Clin. Immunol. 27, 53.

Culton, D.A., O'Conner, B.P., Conway, K.L., et al. 2006. Early preplasma cells define a tolerance checkpoint for autoreactive B cells. J. Immunol. 176, 790.

Cupps, T.R., Edgar, L.C., Fauci, A.S. 1982. Suppression of human B lymphocyte function by cyclophosphamide. J. Immunol. 128, 2453.

Davies, D.J., Moran, J.E., Niall, J.F., et al. 1982. Segmental necrotising glomerulonephritis with antineutrophil antibody: possible arbovirus aetiology? Br. Med. J. (Clin. Res. Ed) 285, 606.

de Cerio, A.L.-D., Zabalegui, N., Rodriguez-Calvillo, M., et al. 2007. Anti-idiotype antibodies in cancer treatment. Oncogene 26, 3594.

de Lema, G.P., Maier, H., Franz, T.J., et al. 2005. Chemokine receptor Ccr2 deficiency reduces renal disease and prolongs survival in MRL/lpr lupus-prone mice. J. Am. Soc. Nephrol. 16, 3592.

Dembic, Z., Schenck, K., Bogen, B. 2000. Dendritic cells purified from myeloma are primed with tumor-specific antigen (idiotype) and activate CD4+ T cells. Proc. Natl. Acad. Sci. 97, 2697.

Demirkiran, A., Bosma, B.M., Kok, A., et al. 2007. Allosuppressive donor CD4+CD25+ regulatory T cells detach from the graft and circulate in recipients after liver transplantation. J. Immunol. 178, 6066.

Devitt, A., Parker, K.G., Ogden, C.A., et al. 2004. Persistence of apoptotic cells without autoimmune disease or inflammation in CD14−/− mice. J. Cell. Biol. 167, 1161.

Duffield, J.S., Forbes, S.J., Constandinou, C.M., et al. 2005a. Selective depletion of macrophages reveals distinct, opposing roles during liver injury and repair. J. Clin. Invest. 115, 56.

Duffield, J.S., Hong, S., Vaidya, V.S., et al. 2006. Resolvin D series and Protectin D1 mitigate acute kidney injury. J. Immunol. 177, 5902.

Duffield, J.S., Tipping, P.G., Kipari, T., et al. 2005b. Conditional ablation of macrophages halts progression of crescentic glomerulonephritis. Am. J. Pathol. 167, 1207.

Ehlers, M., Fukuyama, H., McGaha, T.L., et al. 2006. TLR9/MyD88 signaling is required for class switching to pathogenic IgG2a and 2b autoantibodies in SLE. J. Exp. Med. 203, 553.

Ehlers, M., Ravetch, J.V. 2007. Opposing effects of Toll-like receptor stimulation induce autoimmunity or tolerance. Trends Immunol. 28, 74.

Ettinger, R., Sims, G.P., Robbins, R., et al. 2007. IL-21 and BAFF/BLyS synergize in stimulating plasma cell differentiation from a unique population of human splenic memory B cells. J. Immunol. 178, 2872.

Fauci, A.S., Katz, P., Haynes, B.F., et al. 1979. Cyclophosphamide therapy of severe systemic necrotizing vasculitis. N. Engl. J. Med. 301, 235.

Ferenbach, D., Kluth, D., Hughes, J. 2007. Inflammatory cells in renal injury and repair. Semin. Nephrol. 27, 250.

Ferry, H., Leung, J.C., Lewis, G., et al. 2006. B-cell tolerance. Transplantation 81, 308.

Fukuyama, H., Nimmerjahn, F., Ravetch, J.V. 2005. The inhibitory Fc[gamma] receptor modulates autoimmunity by limiting the accumulation of immunoglobulin G+ anti-DNA plasma cells. Nat. Immunol. 6, 99.

Furuzawa-Carballeda, J., Vargas-Rojas, M.I., Cabral, A.R. 2007. Autoimmune inflammation from the Th17 perspective. Autoimmun. Rev. 6, 169.

Gocke, A.R., Cravens, P.D., Ben, L.-H., et al. 2007. T-bet regulates the fate of Th1 and Th17 lymphocytes in autoimmunity. J. Immunol. 178, 1341.

Gong, Q., Ou, Q., Ye, S., et al. 2005. Importance of cellular microenvironment and circulatory dynamics in B cell immunotherapy. J. Immunol. 174, 817.

Gordon, S., Taylor, P.R. 2005. Monocyte and macrophage heterogeneity. Nat. Rev. Immunol. 5, 953.

Grammer, A.C., Slota, R., Fischer, R., et al. 2003. Abnormal germinal center reactions in systemic lupus erythematosus demonstrated by blockade of CD154–CD40 interactions. J. Clin. Invest. 112, 1506.

Groom, J.R., Fletcher, C.A., Walters, S.N., et al. 2007. BAFF and MyD88 signals promote a lupuslike disease independent of T cells. J. Exp. Med. 204, 1959.

Gutcher, I., Becher, B. 2007. APC-derived cytokines and T cell polarization in autoimmune inflammation. J. Clin. Invest. 117, 1119.

Hahn, B.H., Singh, R.P., La Cava, A., et al. 2005. Tolerogenic treatment of lupus mice with consensus peptide induces Foxp3-expressing, apoptosis-resistant, TGFbeta-secreting CD8+ T cell suppressors. J. Immunol. 175, 7728.

Hargreaves, D.C., Hyman, P.L., Lu, T.T., et al. 2001. A coordinated change in chemokine responsiveness guides plasma cell movements. J. Exp. Med. 194, 45.

Harper, L., Cockwell, P., Adu, D., et al. 2001. Neutrophil priming and apoptosis in anti-neutrophil cytoplasmic autoantibody-associated vasculitis. Kidney Int. 59, 1729.

Harper, L., Ren, Y., Savill, J., et al. 2000. Antineutrophil cytoplasmic antibodies induce reactive oxygen-dependent dysregulation of primed neutrophil apoptosis and clearance by macrophages. Am. J. Pathol. 157, 211.

Harvey, B.P., Gee, R.J., Haberman, A.M., et al. 2007. Antigen presentation and transfer between B cells and macrophages. Eur. J. Immunol. 37, 1739.

Hauser, A.E., Debes, G.F., Arce, S., et al. 2002. Chemotactic responsiveness toward ligands for CXCR3 and CXCR4 is regulated on plasma blasts during the time course of a memory immune response. J. Immunol. 169, 1277.

Heal, J., Roberts, G., Raynes, J., et al. 2002. Specific interactions between sense and complementary peptides: the basis for the proteomic code. Chem. Bio. Chem. 3, 136.

Herve, M., Isnardi, I., Ng, Y.-S., et al. 2007. CD40 ligand and MHC class II expression are essential for human peripheral B cell tolerance. J. Exp. Med. 204, 1583.

Hirota, K., Hashimoto, M., Yoshitomi, H., et al. 2007. T cell self-reactivity forms a cytokine milieu for spontaneous development of IL-17+ Th cells that cause autoimmune arthritis. J. Exp. Med. 204, 41.

Hoeve, M.A., Savage, N.D., de Boer, T., et al. 2006. Divergent effects of IL-12 and IL-23 on the production of IL-17 by human T cells. Eur. J. Immunol. 36, 661.

Hoffman, G.S., Kerr, G.S., Leavitt, R.Y., et al. 1992. Wegener granulomatosis: an analysis of 158 patients. Ann. Intern. Med. 116, 488.

Hogan, S.L., Falk, R.J., Chin, H., et al. 2005. Predictors of relapse and treatment resistance in antineutrophil cytoplasmic antibody-associated small-vessel vasculitis. Ann. Intern. Med. 143, 621.

Hoyer, B.F., Moser, K., Hauser, A.E., et al. 2004. Short-lived plasmablasts and long-lived plasma cells contribute to chronic humoral autoimmunity in NZB/W mice. J. Exp. Med. 199, 1577.

Hutloff, A., Buchner, K., Reiter, K., et al. 2004. Involvement of inducible costimulator in the exaggerated memory B cell and plasma cell generation in systemic lupus erythematosus. Arthritis Rheum. 50, 3211.

Illei, G.G., Takada, K., Parkin, D., et al. 2002. Renal flares are common in patients with severe proliferative lupus nephritis treated with pulse immunosuppressive therapy: long-term followup of a cohort of 145 patients participating in randomized controlled studies. Arthritis Rheum. 46, 995.

Isenberg, D.A., Manson, J.J., Ehrenstein, M.R., et al. 2007. Fifty years of anti-ds DNA antibodies: are we approaching journey's end? Rheumatol. (Oxford) 46, 1052.

Ivanov, I.I., McKenzie, B.S., Zhou, L., et al. 2006. The orphan nuclear receptor ROR[gamma]t directs the differentiation program of proinflammatory IL-17+ T helper cells. Cell 126, 1121.

Jacob, C.O., Pricop, L., Putterman, C., et al. 2006. Paucity of clinical disease despite serological autoimmunity and kidney pathology in lupus-prone New Zealand mixed 2328 mice deficient in BAFF. J. Immunol. 177, 2671.

Jacobi, A.M., Odendahl, M., Reiter, K., et al. 2003. Correlation between circulating CD27high plasma cells and disease activity in patients with systemic lupus erythematosus. Arthritis Rheum. 48, 1332.

Jayne, D.R., Gaskin, G., Rasmussen, N., et al. 2007. Randomized trial of plasma exchange or high-dosage methylprednisolone as adjunctive therapy for severe renal vasculitis. J. Am. Soc. Nephrol. 18, 2180.

Jiang, S., Tsang, J., Lechler, R.I. 2006. Adoptive cell therapy using in vitro generated human CD4+CD25+ regulatory T cells with indirect allospecificity to promote donor-specific transplantation tolerance. Transplant. Proc. 38, 3199.

Joy, M.S., Hogan, S.L., Jennette, J.C., et al. 2005. A pilot study using mycophenolate mofetil in relapsing or resistant

ANCA small vessel vasculitis. Nephrol. Dial. Transplant. 20, 2725.

Kang, H.-K., Liu, M., Datta, S.K. 2007. Low-dose peptide tolerance therapy of lupus generates plasmacytoid dendritic cells that cause expansion of autoantigen-specific regulatory T cells and contraction of inflammatory Th17 cells. J. Immunol. 178, 7849.

Kim, J.M., Rasmussen, J.P., Rudensky, A.Y. 2007. Regulatory T cells prevent catastrophic autoimmunity throughout the lifespan of mice. Nat. Immunol. 8, 191.

Kimura, A., Naka, T., Kishimoto, T. 2007. IL-6-dependent and -independent pathways in the development of interleukin 17-producing T helper cells. Proc. Natl. Acad. Sci. 104, 12099.

Kluth, D.C., Ainslie, C.V., Pearce, W.P., et al. 2001. Macrophages transfected with adenovirus to express IL-4 reduce inflammation in experimental glomerulonephritis. J. Immunol. 166, 4728.

Koffler, D., Schur, P.H., Kunkel, H.G. 1967. Immunological studies concerning the nephritis of systemic lupus erythematosus. J. Exp. Med. 126, 607.

Krishnan, C., Kaplan, M.H. 1967. Immunopathologic studies of systemic lupus erythematosus. II. Antinuclear reaction of gamma-globulin eluted from homogenates and isolated glomeruli of kidneys from patients with lupus nephritis. J. Clin. Invest. 46, 569.

Lanzavecchia, A., Sallusto, F. 2007. Toll-like receptors and innate immunity in B-cell activation and antibody responses. Curr. Opin. Immunol. 19, 268.

Lau, C.M., Broughton, C., Tabor, A.S., et al. 2005. RNA-associated autoantigens activate B cells by combined B cell antigen receptor/Toll-like receptor 7 engagement. J. Exp. Med. 202, 1171.

Leandro, M., Cambridge, G., Ehrenstein, M., et al. 2006. Reconstitution of peripheral blood B cells after depletion with rituximab in patients with rheumatoid arthritis. Arthritis Rheum. 54, 613.

Lesley, R., Xu, Y., Kalled, S.L., et al. 2004. Reduced competitiveness of autoantigen-engaged B cells due to increased dependence on BAFF. Immunity 20, 441.

Lipsky, P.E. 2001. Systemic lupus erythematosus: an autoimmune disease of B cell hyperactivity. Nat. Immunol. 2, 764.

Little, M.A., Smyth, C.L., Yadav, R., et al. 2005. Antineutrophil cytoplasm antibodies directed against myeloperoxidase augment leukocyte–microvascular interactions in vivo. Blood 106, 2050.

Lucas, M., Stuart, L.M., Savill, J., et al. 2003. Apoptotic cells and innate immune stimuli combine to regulate macrophage cytokine secretion. J. Immunol. 171, 2610.

Mackay, F., Woodcock, S.A., Lawton, P., et al. 1999. Mice transgenic for BAFF develop lymphocytic disorders along with autoimmune manifestations. J. Exp. Med. 190, 1697.

Mackay, M., Stanevsky, A., Wang, T., et al. 2006. Selective dysregulation of the Fc{gamma}IIB receptor on memory B cells in SLE. J. Exp. Med. 203, 2157.

Maderna, P., Yona, S., Perretti, M., et al. 2005. Modulation of phagocytosis of apoptotic neutrophils by supernatant from dexamethasone-treated macrophages and annexin-derived peptide Ac2-26. J. Immunol. 174, 3727.

Mantovani, A., Sica, A., Locati, M. 2007. New vistas on macrophage differentiation and activation. Eur. J. Immunol. 37, 14.

Manz, R.A., Lohning, M., Cassese, G., et al. 1998. Survival of long-lived plasma cells is independent of antigen [in process citation]. Int. Immunol. 10, 1703.

Mathur, A.N., Chang, H.-C., Zisoulis, D.G., et al. 2006. T-bet is a critical determinant in the instability of the IL-17-secreting T-helper phenotype. Blood 108, 1595.

Medina, F., Segundo, C., Campos-Caro, A., et al. 2002. The heterogeneity shown by human plasma cells from tonsil, blood, and bone marrow reveals graded stages of increasing maturity, but local profiles of adhesion molecule expression. Blood 99, 2154.

Meffre, E., Catalan, N., Seltz, F., et al. 2001. Somatic hypermutation shapes the antibody repertoire of memory B cells in humans. J. Exp. Med. 194, 375.

Merrell, K.T., Benschop, R.J., Gauld, S.B., et al. 2006. Identification of anergic B cells within a wild-type repertoire. Immunity 25, 953.

Miller, J.J., III, Cole, L.J. 1967. Resistance of long lived lymphocytes and plasma cells in rat lymph nodes to treatment with prednisone, cyclophosphamide, 6-mercaptopurine and actinomycin D. J. Exp. Med. 126, 109.

Mok, C.C., Ying, K.Y., Tang, S., et al. 2004. Predictors and outcome of renal flares after successful cyclophosphamide treatment for diffuse proliferative lupus glomerulonephritis. Arthritis Rheum. 50, 2559.

Moosig, F., Csernok, E., Kumanovics, G., et al. 2000. Opsonization of apoptotic neutrophils by anti-neutrophil cytoplasmic antibodies (ANCA) leads to enhanced uptake by macrophages and increased release of tumour necrosis factor-alpha (TNF-alpha). Clin. Exp. Immunol. 122, 499.

Moser, K., Muehlinghaus, G., Manz, R., et al. 2006a. Long-lived plasma cells in immunity and immunopathology. Immunol. Lett. 103, 83.

Moser, K., Tokoyoda, K., Radbruch, A., et al. 2006b. Stromal niches, plasma cell differentiation and survival. Curr. Opin. Immunol. 18, 265.

Muehlinghaus, G., Cigliano, L., Huehn, S., et al. 2005. Regulation of CXCR3 and CXCR4 expression during terminal differentiation of memory B cells into plasma cells. Blood 105, 3965.

Munthe, L., Bogen, B. 1999. Resting small B cells present endogenous immunoglobulin variable-region determinants to idiotope-specific $CD^{4+}$ T cells in vivo. Eur. J. Immunol. 29, 4043.

Munthe, L.A., Os, A., Zangani, M., et al. 2004. MHC-restricted Ig V region-driven T–B lymphocyte collaboration: B cell receptor ligation facilitates switch to IgG production. J. Immunol. 172, 7476.

Olson, T.S., Bamias, G., Naganuma, M., et al. 2004. Expanded B cell population blocks regulatory T cells and exacerbates ileitis in a murine model of Crohn disease. J. Clin. Invest. 114, 389.

Papamattheou, M.G., Routsias, J.G., Karagouni, E.E., et al. 2004. T cell help is required to induce idiotypic–anti-idiotypic autoantibody network after immunization with complementary epitope 289–308aa of La/SSB autoantigen in non-autoimmune mice. Clin. Exp. Immunol. 135, 416.

Pascual, D.W., Blalock, J.E., Bost, K.L. 1989. Antipeptide antibodies that recognize a lymphocyte substance P receptor. J. Immunol. 143, 3697.

Pawar, R.D., Patole, P.S., Ellwart, A., et al. 2006. Ligands to nucleic acid-specific Toll-like receptors and the onset of lupus nephritis. J. Am. Soc. Nephrol. 17, 3365.

Pendergraft, W.F., III, Preston, G.A., Shah, R.R., et al. 2004. Autoimmunity is triggered by cPR-3(105-201), a protein complementary to human autoantigen proteinase-3. Nat. Med. 10, 72.

Peng, S.L., Szabo, S.J., Glimcher, L.H. 2002. T-bet regulates IgG class switching and pathogenic autoantibody production. Proc. Natl. Acad. Sci. 99, 5545.

Phan, T.G., Amesbury, M., Gardam, S., et al. 2003. B cell receptor-independent stimuli trigger immunoglobulin (Ig) class switch recombination and production of IgG autoantibodies by anergic self-reactive B cells. J. Exp. Med. 197, 845.

Pisitkun, P., Deane, J.A., Difilippantonio, M.J., et al. 2006. Autoreactive B cell responses to RNA-related antigens due to TLR7 gene duplication. Science 312, 1669.

Radbruch, A., Muehlinghaus, G., Luger, E.O., et al. 2006. Competence and competition: the challenge of becoming a long-lived plasma cell. Nat. Rev. Immunol. 6, 741.

Reynolds, J., Prodromidi, E.I., Juggapah, J.K., et al. 2005. Nasal administration of recombinant rat {alpha}3(IV)NC1 prevents the development of experimental autoimmune glomerulonephritis in the WKY rat. J. Am. Soc. Nephrol. 16, 1350.

Ripley, B.J.M., Goncalves, B., Isenberg, D.A., et al. 2005. Raised levels of interleukin 6 in systemic lupus erythematosus correlate with anaemia. Ann. Rheum. Dis. 64, 849.

Robson, M.G., Cook, H.T., Botto, M., et al. 2001. Accelerated nephrotoxic nephritis is exacerbated in C1q-deficient mice. J. Immunol. 166, 6820.

Romagnani, P., Lazzeri, E., Lasagni, L., et al. 2002. IP-10 and Mig production by glomerular cells in human proliferative glomerulonephritis and regulation by nitric oxide. J. Am. Soc. Nephrol. 13, 53.

Rossi, A.G., Sawatzky, D.A., Walker, A., et al. 2006. Cyclin-dependent kinase inhibitors enhance the resolution of inflammation by promoting inflammatory cell apoptosis. Nat. Med. 12, 1056.

Rui, L., Vinuesa, C.G., Blasioli, J., et al. 2003. Resistance to CpG DNA-induced autoimmunity through tolerogenic B cell antigen receptor ERK signaling. Nat. Immunol. 4, 594.

Sadanaga, A., Nakashima, H., Akahoshi, M., et al. 2007. Protection against autoimmune nephritis in MyD88-deficient MRL/lpr mice. Arthritis Rheum. 56, 1618.

Salama, A.D., Chaudhry, A.N., Holthaus, K.A., et al. 2003. Regulation by CD25+ lymphocytes of autoantigen-specific T-cell responses in Goodpasture's (anti-GBM) disease. Kidney Int. 64, 1685.

Sato, W., Aranami, T., Yamamura, T. 2007. Cutting edge: Human Th17 cells are identified as bearing CCR2+CCR5− phenotype. J. Immunol. 178, 7525.

Savill, J. 2001. Apoptosis in post-streptococcal glomerulonephritis. Kidney Int. 60, 1203.

Savill, J., Dransfield, I., Gregory, C., et al. 2002. A blast from the past: clearance of apoptotic cells regulates immune responses. Nat. Rev. Immunol. 2, 965.

Sawatzky, D.A., Willoughby, D.A., Colville-Nash, P.R., et al. 2006. The involvement of the apoptosis-modulating proteins ERK 1/2, Bcl-xL and Bax in the resolution of acute inflammation in vivo. Am. J. Pathol. 168, 33.

Scalapino, K.J., Tang, Q., Bluestone, J.A., et al. 2006. Suppression of disease in New Zealand Black/New Zealand White lupus-prone mice by adoptive transfer of ex vivo expanded regulatory T cells. J. Immunol. 177, 1451.

Scannell, M., Flanagan, M.B., deStefani, A., et al. 2007. Annexin-1 and peptide derivatives are released by apoptotic cells and stimulate phagocytosis of apoptotic neutrophils by macrophages. J. Immunol. 178, 4595.

Schwab, J.M., Chiang, N., Arita, M., et al. 2007. Resolvin E1 and protectin D1 activate inflammation-resolution programmes. Nature 447, 869.

Schwartz, M. 2006. The pathology of lupus nephritis. Semin. Nephrol. 27, 22.

Serhan, C.N., Brain, S.D., Buckley, C.D., et al. 2007. Resolution of inflammation: state of the art, definitions and terms. FASEB J. 21, 325.

Serhan, C.N., Savill, J. 2005. Resolution of inflammation: the beginning programs the end. Nat. Immunol. 6, 1191.

Shlomchik, M.J., Craft, J.E., Mamula, M.J. 2001. From T to B and back again: positive feedback in systemic autoimmune disease. Nat. Rev. Immunol. 1, 147.

Shlomchik, M.J., Madaio, M.P., Ni, D., et al. 1994. The role of B cells in lpr/lpr-induced autoimmunity. J. Exp. Med. 180, 1295.

Silverstein, A.M. 2000. Clemens Freiherr von Pirquet: explaining immune complex disease in 1906. Nat. Immunol. 1, 453.

Singh, R.P., La Cava, A., Wong, M., et al. 2007. CD8+ T cell-mediated suppression of autoimmunity in a murine lupus model of peptide-induced immune tolerance depends on Foxp3 expression. J. Immunol. 178, 7649.

Smith, K.G., Jones, R.B., Burns, S.M., et al. 2006. Long-term comparison of rituximab treatment for refractory systemic lupus erythematosus and vasculitis: remission, relapse, and re-treatment. Arthritis Rheum. 54, 2970.

Stassen, P.M., Cohen Tervaert, J.W., Stegeman, C.A. 2007. Induction of remission in active anti-neutrophil cytoplasmic antibody-associated vasculitis with mycophenolate mofetil in patients who cannot be treated with cyclophosphamide. Ann. Rheum. Dis. 66, 798.

Steinman, L. 2007. A brief history of TH17, the first major revision in the TH1/TH2 hypothesis of T cell-mediated tissue damage. Nat. Med. 13, 139.

Stohl, W., Looney, R.J. 2006. B cell depletion therapy in systemic rheumatic diseases: different strokes for different folks? Clin. Immunol. 121, 1.

Stohl, W., Metyas, S., Tan, S.M., et al. 2003. B lymphocyte stimulator overexpression in patients with systemic lupus erythematosus: longitudinal observations. Arthritis Rheum. 48, 3475.

Sze, D.M.Y., Toellner, K.-M., de Vinuesa, C.G., et al. 2000. Intrinsic constraint on plasmablast growth and extrinsic limits of plasma cell survival. J. Exp. Med. 192, 813.

Teague, B.N., Pan, Y., Mudd, P.A., et al. 2007. Cutting edge: transitional T3 B cells do not give rise to mature B cells, have undergone selection, and are reduced in murine lupus. J. Immunol. 178, 7511.

Thien, M., Phan, T.G., Gardam, S., et al. 2004. Excess BAFF rescues self-reactive B cells from peripheral deletion and allows them to enter forbidden follicular and marginal zone niches. Immunity 20, 785.

Tiller, T., Tsuiji, M., Yurasov, S., et al. 2007. Autoreactivity in human IgG+ memory B cells. Immunity 26, 205.

Tipping, P.G., Holdsworth, S.R. 2006. T cells in crescentic glomerulonephritis. J. Am. Soc. Nephrol. 17, 1253.

Townsend, S.E., Weintraub, B.C., Goodnow, C.C. 1999. Growing up on the streets: why B-cell development differs from T-cell development. Immunol. Today 20, 217.

Traynor, A.E., Schroeder, J., Rosa, R.M., et al. 2000. Treatment of severe systemic lupus erythematosus with high-dose chemotherapy and haemopoietic stem-cell transplantation: a phase I study. Lancet 356, 701.

Tsuiji, M., Yurasov, S., Velinzon, K., et al. 2006. A checkpoint for autoreactivity in human IgM+ memory B cell development. J. Exp. Med. 203, 393.

Uehara, A., Iwashiro, A., Sato, T., et al. 2007. Antibodies to proteinase 3 prime human monocytic cells via protease-activated receptor-2 and NF-[kappa]B for Toll-like receptor- and NOD-dependent activation. Mol. Immunol. 44, 3552.

Valencia, X., Yarboro, C., Illei, G., et al. 2007. Deficient CD4+CD25 high T regulatory cell function in patients with active systemic lupus erythematosus. J. Immunol. 178, 2579.

Voswinkel, J., Mueller, A., Kraemer, J.A., et al. 2006. B lymphocyte maturation in Wegener's granulomatosis: a comparative analysis of VH genes from endonasal lesions. Ann. Rheum. Dis. 65, 859.

Voswinkel, J., Muller, A., Lamprecht, P. 2005. Is PR3-ANCA formation initiated in Wegener's granulomatosis lesions? Granulomas as potential lymphoid tissue maintaining autoantibody production. Ann. N. Y. Acad. Sci. 1051, 12.

Walsh, M., James, M., Jayne, D., et al. 2007. Mycophenolate mofetil for induction therapy of lupus nephritis: a systematic review and meta-analysis. Clin. J. Am. Soc. Nephrol. 2, 968.

Walsh, M., Jayne, D. 2007. Rituximab in the treatment of antineutrophil cytoplasm antibody associated vasculitis and systemic lupus erythematosus: past, present and future. Kidney Int. 72, 676.

Wang, Y., Wang, Y.P., Zheng, G., et al. 2007. Ex vivo programmed macrophages ameliorate experimental chronic inflammatory renal disease. Kidney Int. 72, 290.

Wardemann, H., Yurasov, S., Schaefer, A., et al. 2003. Predominant autoantibody production by early human B cell precursors. Science 301, 1374.

Watson, S., Cailhier, J.F., Hughes, J., et al. 2006. Apoptosis and glomerulonephritis. Curr. Dir. Autoimmun. 9, 188.

Weber, M.S., Prod'homme, T., Youssef, S., et al. 2007. Type II monocytes modulate T cell-mediated central nervous system autoimmune disease. Nat. Med. 13, 935.

Wei, C., Anolik, J., Cappione, A., et al. 2007. A new population of cells lacking expression of CD27 represents a notable component of the B cell memory compartment in systemic lupus erythematosus. J. Immunol. 178, 6624.

Wellmann, U., Letz, M., Herrmann, M., et al. 2005. The evolution of human anti-double-stranded DNA autoantibodies. Proc. Natl. Acad. Sci. 102, 9258.

William, J., Euler, C., Christensen, S., et al. 2002. Evolution of autoantibody responses via somatic hypermutation outside of germinal centers. Science 297, 2066.

William, J., Euler, C., Shlomchik, M.J. 2005. Short-lived plasmablasts dominate the early spontaneous rheumatoid factor response: differentiation pathways, hypermutating cell types, and affinity maturation outside the germinal center. J. Immunol. 174, 6879.

Withers, D.R., Fiorini, C., Fischer, R.T., et al. 2007. T cell-dependent survival of CD20+ and CD20− plasma cells in human secondary lymphoid tissue. Blood 109, 4856.

Xiang, Z., Cutler, A.J., Brownlie, R.J., et al. 2007. Fc[gamma]RIIb controls bone marrow plasma cell persistence and apoptosis. Nat. Immunol. 8, 419.

Xiao, H., Heeringa, P., Hu, P., et al. 2002. Antineutrophil cytoplasmic autoantibodies specific for myeloperoxidase cause glomerulonephritis and vasculitis in mice. J. Clin. Invest. 110, 955.

Xu, L., Kitani, A., Fuss, I., et al. 2007. Cutting edge: regulatory T cells induce CD4+ CD25− Foxp3− T cells or are self-induced to become Th17 cells in the absence of exogenous TGF-beta. J. Immunol. 178, 6725.

Yan, J., Harvey, B.P., Gee, R.J., et al. 2006. B cells drive early T cell autoimmunity in vivo prior to dendritic cell-mediated autoantigen presentation. J. Immunol. 177, 4481.

Yurasov, S., Tiller, T., Tsuiji, M., et al. 2006. Persistent expression of autoantibodies in SLE patients in remission. J. Exp. Med. 203, 2255.

Yurasov, S., Wardemann, H., Hammersen, J., et al. 2005. Defective B cell tolerance checkpoints in systemic lupus erythematosus. J. Exp. Med. 201, 703.

Zheng, Y., Rudensky, A.Y. 2007. Foxp3 in control of the regulatory T cell lineage. Nat. Immunol. 8, 457.

# PART II:

# Pathogenic Mechanisms

CHAPTER 1

# Pathogenesis of Renal Diseases: Autoimmunity

Anikphe E. Imoagene-Oyedeji[a], Michael P. Madaio[b],*

[a]Renal-Electrolyte and Hypertension Division, Department of Medicine, University of Pennsylvania School of Medicine, Philadelphia, PA, USA
[b]Nephrology and Kidney Transplantation Section, Temple University School of Medicine, Philadelphia, PA, USA

## 1. Introduction

The human immune system is an integrated group of highly specialized defenses that limits invasion of foreign organisms and eliminates foreign cells, and through tightly regulated series of networks is able to distinguish self and non-self. This ability to recognize "self" and limit "auto"-immune responses against self-antigens is defined as tolerance. It was initially described by the forefathers of modern immunology, Burnet, Fenner, Medawar, and others as "indifference or non-reactivity" established to host tissue early in fetal life. However it is now known that tolerance is an active process that is regulated and maintained by the adaptive immune system throughout life. Nevertheless, tolerance may "break down" leading to undesirable immune responses directed against self-antigens and autoimmune disease.

Autoimmune responses resemble normal immune responses to pathogens in that they are specifically activated by antigens. In many cases, however, the targets are "self" or "auto"-antigens. In some instances, foreign antigens elicit an autoimmune response through molecular mimicry (e.g., through shared structures or epitopes with self-antigens), whereas in others the autoimmune response arises from epitope spreading (e.g., due to somatic mutations that encode autoantibodies that arise by chance during normal immune responses). Bystander activation, induction of co-stimulation, polyclonal activation, altered processing, and/or expression of cryptic antigens are other mechanisms through which autoimmune reactivity may be elicited by "foreign antigens". Alternatively, some foreign antigens induce a normal immune response, however, by nature of their physical properties, they enter the blood stream, localize within tissues, and complex with antibodies directed against them. In many situations, the mechanisms either inducing or maintaining tolerance are disrupted. This breakdown leads to activation of autoreactive cells which, in turn, may initiate overt autoimmune disease. The effectors of autoimmunity in the kidney are many, but most often disease is initiated either by antibody deposition or infiltration of immune cells. Once antibodies are deposited, their exposed Fc (fragment crystalline) regions activate and recruit inflammatory cells, and initiate complement activation. This process leads to further cellular infiltration, and secretion of inflammatory mediators by both infiltrating and endogenous cells. Infiltrating cells, which include neutrophils, T-cells and macrophages, and platelets also secrete soluble mediators and directly interact with renal cells and each other to perpetuate the disease process.

*Corresponding author.
Tel.: 215-707-3381; Fax: 215-707-4148
E-mail address: madaio@temple.edu

Within the kidney, the local response of resident cells plays an important role in determining the severity of inflammation. If severe and/or unlimited, these events may lead to fibrosis and organ failure. The intensity and severity of inflammation and fibrosis are influenced by genetic factors (e.g., that determine the fibrogenic response). In most situations, there is a complex interplay among immune and inflammatory cells and mediators, and their relative contributions often become difficult to distinguish, in part because the involved mediators overlap considerably, and in part because once the disease is established, the mediators may play multiple roles.

Over the past 50 plus years, many investigators have contributed to the understanding of the immune mechanisms leading to nephritis and the mediators involved in inflammation and fibrosis. In this chapter, we will focus on the *immune events that lead to autoimmunity and localization of immune reactants that initiate nephritis*. We will not describe the downstream events that lead to inflammation, fibrosis, or the clinical manifestations of autoimmune kidney diseases. The reader is referred to other chapters in this textbook for a comprehensive review of these subsequent events.

This chapter is designed to provide an overview of nephritogenic autoimmune responses, and to serve as a foundation for understanding the pathogenic mechanisms that lead to autoimmune renal diseases, in general. Our intent is to provide the background for a more comprehensive discussion of autoimmunity in individual renal diseases addressed in subsequent chapters of this text. In this context, the development and maintenance of immune tolerance, along with mechanisms by which tolerance is broken will be reviewed.

## 2. Mechanisms of tolerance

The ability of the immune system to generate a specific immune response after exposure to foreign antigen is defined as *adaptive immunity*. By contrast *innate immunity* comprises early "non-specific" defence mechanisms that combat a wide range of pathogens without prior exposure. The latter forms an early barrier to infection that does not rely on the clonal expansion of antigen-specific lymphocytes. Major differences between the innate and adaptive immunity are summarized in Table 1.

Table 1
Differences between the innate and adaptive immune systems

| Innate immune system | Adaptive immune system |
|---|---|
| Mostly accounts for the early phase of non-specific immune responses to infection that do not require prior antigenic exposure | Later immune responses against specific antigens |
| Involves phagocytosis and non-specific killing of pathogens by NK cells, monocytes, macrophages, dendritic cells, and the complement system | Involves clonal expansion of antigen-specific B- and T-lymphocytes |
| Antigen recognition is non-specific. Recognition is mainly via pattern recognition of pathogen associated molecular patterns (PAMPs) using toll-like receptors (TLRs) | Antigen recognition by specialized B- and T-cell receptors (BCR and TCR) |
| This system rapidly initiates immune responses by secretion of pro-inflammatory chemokines that serve as chemoattractants for other effector cells and guides the adaptive immune response | Involves more sophisticated mechanisms for pathogen destruction via antigen-specific B- and T-cells, that involve cell–cell contact and secreted factors |
| There is no residual memory to the antigen generated by the innate immune response | Emergence of long-lived memory cells directed against antigenic components with amnestic response on re-challenge with antigen |

The adaptive immune system is comprised of two broad subdivisions termed humoral and cell-mediated immunity. In the humoral arm, B lymphocytes recognize specific antigens via antibodies. Mature B-cells typically express membrane-bound immunoglobulins (Ig) that are coupled to transmembrane and intracellular proteins that modulate outside-in signaling (termed the B-cell receptor complex or BCR). Mature B-cells also secrete soluble immunoglobulins (i.e. antibodies; the same and only Ig expressed on the cell surface within the BCR). By contrast, in T-cell-mediated immune responses, T lymphocytes recognize "foreign" or "non-self antigen" via membrane-bound T-cell receptors (TCR), as presented to them by antigen presenting cells (APC). The APC phagocytize large proteins and break them down into small peptides; some of the peptides are coupled to major histocompatibility complex (MHC) molecules intracellularly, and then expressed on the cell surface bound to MHC I and MHC II molecules. Both B and T-cells have co-receptors that influence activation and signaling, and this activity is further modulated by soluble mediators (i.e. cytokines and chemokines secreted in an endocrine or autocrine fashion) through other, specific receptors expressed on their cell surfaces.

Dendritic cells (DCs), macrophages, and B-cells are examples of APC. While the former are more potent T-cell activators (thus termed "professional APC"), B-cells have the advantage of capturing antigen through antibody on the cell surface which, in turn, facilitates processing of specific Ag and presentation to T-cells. Typically, the epitopes, or regions of the antigen recognized by B and T-cells, differ, which facilitates interaction of antigen-specific B and T-cells (i.e. through the antigen) which, in turn, leads to further amplification of the immune response. T-cells generally exert their effects locally through both cell-to-cell contact and secretion of soluble mediators (e.g., cytokines, chemokines).

Since immune and autoimmune responses share similar pathways, the normal development and activation of B and T-cells will be reviewed to provide the foundation for discussion of general mechanisms leading to the emergence of autoimmunity. In this context, it has been observed that the majority of self-reactive immune cells are normally deleted or inactivated during development. This process has been termed central tolerance. There are also checkpoints that regulate the emergence of autoreactive cells during adult life (e.g., during immune responses versus foreign antigen); this process has been termed peripheral tolerance. Nevertheless, some cells escape both checkpoints, and their activation may lead to autoimmunity.

## 2.1. Development of B-cell tolerance

During both development in the bone marrow and on subsequent activation, the B-cell repertoire is regulated to limit autoantibody production. During these processes, a diverse range of Ig receptors (i.e. with different antigenic specificities) are generated through stochastic (e.g., gene rearrangements) and mutational (e.g., after antigenic stimulation) events. Prior to engaging antigen, variable (VH), diversity (DH), and joining (JH) heavy-chain genes rearrange to encode the Ig heavy-chain variable regions, whereas V and J genes encode the light-chain variable regions. This initial "germline" diversity is great; with $40+$ $V_H$ genes, $25+$ $D_H$ genes, 6 $J_H$ genes, $40+$ $V_\kappa$ genes, $5+$ $J_\kappa$ genes, $30+$ $V_\lambda$ genes, and 4 $J_\lambda$ genes, that result in many combinations. The diversity is amplified by random insertion of nucleotides during rearrangement at the $V_H$–$D_H$, $D_H$–$J_H$, $V_L$–$D_L$ junctions, and other recombinatory events. Although expression of a functional BCR and signaling during development of naive B-cells determines its survival, these early events are not dependent on antigen encounter. However, subsequently, signaling through the antigen receptor is required for B-cell maturation. Typically, this is delivered through the BCR complex following antigen binding, via the antibody expressed on the cell surface. Nevertheless, the ultimate fate of developing B-cells is dependent on both their maturation state when antigen encounter occurs, along with the presence of other factors that support the process (e.g., such as T-cell help through cell contact and cytokine stimulation).

B-cells deal with self-antigens differently. During the early stages of maturation in the bone marrow, when an immature B-cell encounters self-antigen (i.e. via the BCR complex), either *"clonal deletion" or "receptor editing"* occurs. In general, a highly avid ligation of a BCR by autoantigens results in receptor cross-linking and intense signaling through the BCR complex; this process activates cellular programs which lead to cell death (i.e. *clonal deletion*). Alternatively, encounter with an auto-antigen may lead to additional V gene rearrangements, so that the amino acid sequences of the antigen-binding region (of the antibody) are altered. This results in the production of an antibody with a different antigenic specificity, so that the membrane-bound antibodies no longer recognize the autoantigen. This process, termed receptor editing, requires reactivation of the recombinaces, so that antibody is encoded by different genetic elements. During receptor editing, either a different chain (light or heavy), or a secondary V gene rearrangement (e.g., on a previously rearranged gene) occurs, to encode a new antibody with a different antigenic specificity.

Another mechanism of B-cell tolerance is referred to as *ignorance/antigen segregation*. It has been postulated that some antigens in tissues, by nature of their location, never encounter B-cells, and therefore this tissue barrier regulates autoimmunity through ignorance. Whether this is the case, or whether low-level autoantigen exposure during normal physiology (i.e. in the context of lack of ongoing inflammation) leads to long-lived tolerance is uncertain. B-cells that do encounter autoantigens are not normally activated unless they receive help (i.e. via soluble mediators and/or T-cells).

For survival, emerging B-cells must receive survival signals (via the BCR). The first signal typically occurs after antigen binding by surface Ig. Secondary signals come through co-stimulatory molecules that facilitate B-cell interactions with T-cells (e.g., CD40L-CD40) and soluble mediators, e.g., cytokines and chemokines (e.g., IL-2, IL-4, IL10). Together these interactions facilitate B-cell maturation by promoting somatic hypermutation and affinity maturation in the germinal center of the lymphoid follicle (see below). Continual antigen binding by surface bound Ig leads to clonal expansion of B-cells and production of specific antibodies against the antigen. Some of these cells survive after the antigen is removed as long-lived antigen-specific B-cell clones, called memory B-cells. These cells mediate secondary immune responses and can be distinguished by the surface proteins they express.

It is emphasized that although many B-cells require co-stimulatory signals from T-cells (thymus-dependent), some antigens directly activate B-cells (thymus-independent). Typically, these direct stimulators are microbial antigens with repeating antigenic patterns that activate Toll-like receptors on B-cells directly.

Following antigen-induced activation and B-cell proliferation, mutations take place in complementary determining regions (CDRs, which are mutational hot spots), whereby B-cells that encode antibody with higher specificity are further selected through antigen binding and proliferate. B-cells that do not encounter antigen at this stage die. Despite these elaborate tolerogenic processes in the bone marrow, elimination of potentially autoreactive B-cells is incomplete and some autoreactive B-cells (normally of low affinity) exist in normal individuals. Furthermore, during antigen-driven immunity (e.g., to foreign antigens, bacteria), autoreactivity may emerge (e.g., with somatic mutations in CDR regions of new emerging antibody variable regions). These autoreactive cells are dealt with in peripheral lymphoid and other tissues.

The primary V gene rearrangements occur in the bone marrow, whereas the secondary, antigen dependent, maturing events occur in secondary lymphoid organs, mainly in the germinal centers of the spleen, lymph node and lymphoid follicles. As previously indicated, the extensive hypermutation of heavy-chain and light-chain genes is essential for the generation of a highly adaptive, diverse immune repertoire to eradicate potential pathogens, during affinity maturation. In the immune response against foreign antigen, maturing B-cells, upon exit from the bone marrow, acquire large numbers of point mutations in CDR regions in the germinal centers during affinity maturation reactions. During the process, autoreactive antibodies are generated. Typically these B-cells are short lived and undergo apoptotic cell death, unless rescued (positively selected) by appropriate recognition of antigen on follicular DCs. In this context, weak signals resulting from either low-affinity BCR–antigen interactions, or lack of co-stimulation and soluble mediators (e.g., cytokines and chemokines), will lead to either deletion or "*anergy*" (a state in which the receptor-positive B-cell persists, but is hyporesponsive to further stimulation by antigen). Nevertheless, despite all these checkpoints to eliminate autoreactive B-cells, some low-affinity cells may emerge during receptor editing or escape into the circulation. These autoreactive cells that escape into the periphery undergo class switching to IgG.

In recent work using a murine model of lupus nephritis, Ravetch et al. have demonstrated an essential peripheral tolerance checkpoint, mediated by the FcγRIIB receptor (i.e. an inhibitory murine FcR). They demonstrated that mice deficient in FcγRIIB, with normal central B-cell tolerance, developed IgG anti-DNA antibodies and nephritis, thus implicating that the balance of inhibitory and activating FcRs is essential to maintenance of peripheral tolerance.

Chronic exposure of B-cells to self-antigens in the absence of co-stimulation leads to the nuclear translocation of the calcium and calcineurin-dependent transcription factor, NFAT1, and anergy. Nevertheless, in some cases, the inflammatory milieu generated by normal immune responses to foreign antigens, the combination of T-cell help and soluble mediators, leads to activation of autoreactive B-cells. Nevertheless, other peripheral mechanisms such as *cytokine (immune) deviation* and *clonal exhaustion*, contribute to maintenance of tolerance. In the former, the maintenance of the immune response is influenced by cytokine secretion, and is therefore heavily influenced by the dominant T-cell phenotype (e.g., Th1, Th2, regulatory T-cells, and Th17). Classically, Th1 cells produce IFN-gamma and IL-2, and enhance production of autoreactive complement-fixing IgG2a antibodies. Th2 cells produce IL-4, IL-5, IL-10, and/or TGF β1, which enhance non-complement fixing antibodies. Cytokine (immune) deviation, is the process by which a switch to a particular phenotype occurs. Autoimmunity is prevented when the cytokines secreted limit further expansion of proliferating cells. The influence of T-cell phenotypes on autoimmunity is discussed below. These and previously discussed tolerance checkpoints in B-cell development and activation are illustrated in Fig. 1.

## 2.2. Development of T-cell tolerance

In contrast to B-cells which bind to soluble antigen, T-cells recognize antigens as small peptides that are displayed on the surface of APC in the context of MHC proteins. Other co-stimulatory molecules and soluble mediators are required for T-cell activation. Typically DCs and macrophages are the most potent stimulators of T-cells (especially naïve T-cells). However, B-cells can also be very effective, since endocytosis via surface Ig facilitates engagement of T-cells with TcR for that particular antigen, which leads to augmentation of antigen-specific immune responses.

T-cell-mediated immunity is essential for eradication of intracellular pathogens as occurs in viral infections, and to provide help for B-cells during the proliferative phase of B-cell antibody responses. T-cell activation occurs following an encounter with APC. In this process, antigenic peptide fragments are delivered to the APC surface by specialized host-cell glycoproteins encoded by a large gene complex called the MHC, of which there are two major classes, I and II. The expression of MHC class I and II molecules is different among tissues, and this influences whether antigens will be recognized. T-cell responses are dependent on the efficient and accurate processing of proteins by APC, through MHC molecules. MHC class I proteins are expressed on all nucleated cells, although they are most highly expressed in hematopoietic cells. MHC class II molecules are normally expressed only by a subset of hematopoietic cells and by thymic stromal cells, although they can be induced during inflammatory responses on parenchymal cells. Figure 2 shows a cognate T-cell–APC interaction. Noteworthy, the different

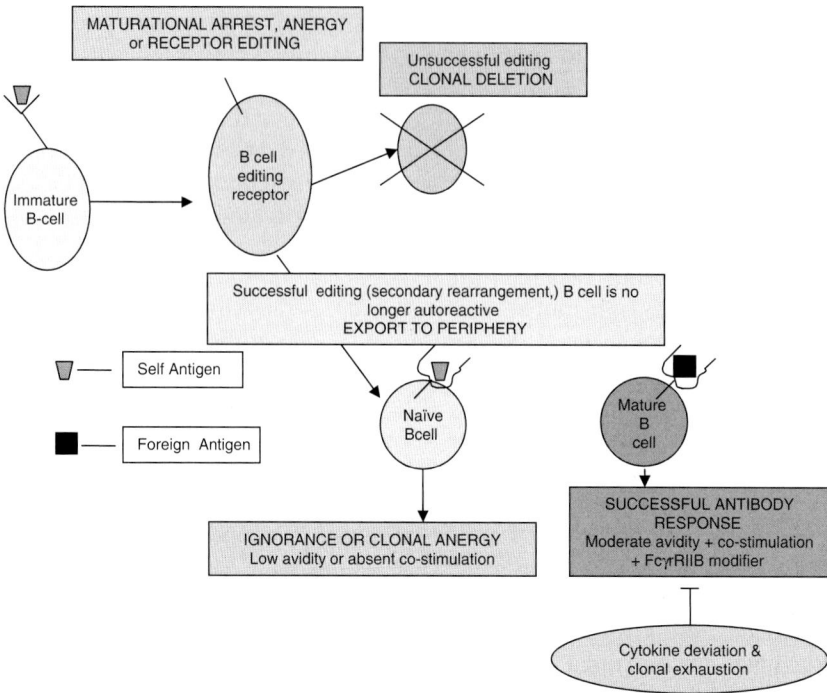

**Figure 1.** Central and peripheral tolerance checkpoints in B-cell development.

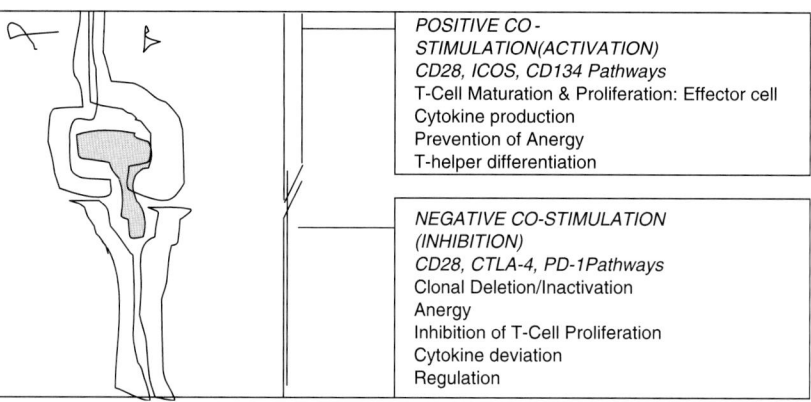

**Figure 2.** Tolerance checkpoints in T-cell activation.

responses are determined by the presence of competing costimulatory signals and cytokines.

Immunological tolerance, by T-cells, is maintained through diverse mechanisms, with multiple checkpoints. Autoreactive T-cells may be deleted centrally in the thymus on confrontation with autoantigen; this is especially evident for high-affinity TCR interactions. By contrast, outside the thymus (i.e. "periphery"), when T-cells encounter antigen (in the context of APC) and co-stimulatory signals from CD28 and CD134, enhanced T-cell proliferation and cytokine production occurs. However, lack of the appropriate co-stimulatory signals during this process results in T-cell anergy. When antigens are presented in a different context via the TCR (e.g., either by immature APC or autoreactive B-cells), negative signaling occurs via CTLA-4 and PD-1 pathways, which inhibit T-cell responsiveness. This negative signaling may result in apoptosis, inhibition of proliferation and/or cytokine deviation, and result in either the emergence of regulatory T-cells and/or T-cell anergy, with suppression of the immune response.

During T-cell development, the generation of autoreactivity is limited. In the thymus, lymphocytes that do not encounter antigen are eliminated. Furthermore strong TCR–Ag/MHC interactions in the thymus lead to deletion or inactivation of self-reactive lymphocytes through the processes of *clonal deletion* or *inactivation* (central tolerance). Thereafter, self-tolerance by T-cells is maintained in the periphery (i.e. outside the thymus), throughout adult life, by mechanisms similar to those discussed earlier for B-cells: these include hidden self-antigens (*ignorance/antigen segregation*) and absence of co-stimulation during antigen encounters. When the latter occurs it is termed "*peripheral anergy*," and it is important for maintenance of tolerance, since normally sequestered antigens may be exposed during life (e.g., inflammation). In this situation, lack of appropriate co-stimulation (e.g., cytokines and/or costimulatory cell–cell interactions; see below) limits autoreactivity.

Another less well-understood mechanism that contributes to immune regulation has been termed "*cytokine deviation.*" Naturally occurring and inducible regulatory T-cells (Tregs) have been recently characterized. Regulatory T-cells induce immune tolerance by suppressing host immune responses against self- or non-self-antigens by cytokine secretion and direct cell-to-cell contact. Although the mechanisms are incompletely understood, this involves pushing T-cell responses from Th1 to Th2 responses. In part the benefit is due to a switch from more pro-inflammatory cytokines (e.g., IL-1, IL-2, IFN-gamma, TNF and others), to cells that secrete IL-4, IL-6, IL-10, TGF-$\beta$, GM-CSF, and other more anti-inflammatory mediators. This process also limits maturation of DCs, so that they remain functionally immature and tolerogenic. More recently, another T-cell effector subset, Th17, which produces IL-17 and promotes autoimmune diseases, has been described, and it will be important to determine how it fits into the overall scheme. Summarized in Table 2 are some currently known mechanisms by which self-tolerance is established and maintained by the adaptive human immune system.

## 3. Mechanisms of tolerance maintenance

### 3.1. The innate immune system

The innate immune system plays an essential role in maintaining tolerance and preventing emergence of autoimmunity. The innate system consists of several powerful components that recognize and facilitate the elimination of pathogens and unwanted host materials following apoptosis and cell death. It forms an early barrier to pathogens, that does not rely on the clonal expansion of antigen-specific lymphocytes, but rather comprises multiple non-antigen-specific defence mechanisms that counteract a wide range of pathogens. The advantages of this immediate protection are obvious. The innate system may also act as a "*switch*" or an "*adaptor*" that helps to *turn-on* and *turn-off* the adaptive immune response. Nevertheless there is evidence that dysregulation of this system may result in autoimmunity.

The important cellular players of the innate immune system are macrophages, DCs (mature and immature), monocytes, and natural killer T-cells. These cells are essential for phagocytosis and lysis of foreign antigens. They act as "*scouts*" for the immune system, and play an important role in regulating both the sensor and effector arms of the adaptive response. Another powerful component of the innate immune system of effectors is the complement system. Over 30 effector and regulatory proteins act in concert to influence the strength of adaptive antigen-specific B-cell immune responses. Nevertheless these proteins must be controlled, as dysregulation in their activation leads to inflammation.

**Table 2**
Major mechanisms of induction and maintenance of tolerance

| Type of tolerance | Mechanism | Site of action |
| --- | --- | --- |
| B-cells | | |
| Central tolerance | Deletion | Bone marrow |
| | Editing | |
| Antigen segregation | Physical barrier to self-antigen access to lymphoid system | e.g., GBM, thyroid, pancreas, testes, lens; antigen inaccessible to B cells in peripheral organs |
| Peripheral anergy | Cellular inactivation by weak signaling without co-stimulus | B-cell anergy in lymphoid follicles/tissues |
| Clonal exhaustion | Apoptosis post-activation | Secondary lymphoid tissue and sites of inflammation |
| T-cells | | |
| Central tolerance | Deletion | Thymus |
| Antigen segregation | Physical barrier to access to lymphoid system | e.g., GBM, thyroid, self-antigen pancreas, testes, lens; antigen inaccessible to T-cells in peripheral organs |
| Peripheral anergy | Cellular inactivation by weak signaling without co-stimulus | T-cell anergy in lymphoid follicles/tissue |
| Cytokine deviation | Differentiation to Th 17, Th2 cells limiting inflammatory cytokine secretion | T-cells in secondary lymphoid tissues and sites of inflammation |
| Clonal exhaustion | Apoptosis post-activation | Secondary lymphoid tissue and sites of inflammation |
| Regulatory T-cells | Suppression by cytokines, intercellular signals | Secondary lymphoid tissue and sites of inflammation |

The following discussion focuses on the essential regulatory roles of various components of the innate immune system: including toll-like receptors (TLRs), APC and the complement system of proteins, and how they function together to limit the immune response against self-tissues.

## 3.2. Role of TLRs in regulating the innate immune response

Toll-like receptors (TLRs) are essential sensors of microbial infection that detect and respond specifically to a variety of conserved molecular patterns, including lipopolysaccharide, lipopeptides, and bacterial DNA from pathogens, termed pathogen-associated molecular patterns (PAMPS). These conserved molecular patterns serve as adjuvants. Upon recognition and engagement, these molecular patterns on pathogens are responsible for activating the immune/inflammatory response. Additionally, TLR activation often results in stimulation of the adaptive immune response through activation of DC, by upregulation of co-stimulatory molecules, and secretion of inflammatory cytokines. TLRs are expressed on many cell types including macrophages and DCs, and over ten different TLRs have now been shown to be involved in the recognition of molecular structures unique to bacterial and fungal cells. TLR ligation (e.g., by bacterial DNA) causes induction of pro-inflammatory cytokine and chemokine expression, and upregulation of co-stimulatory molecule expression by APC. Importantly, the distinction between foreign (e.g., bacterial DNA) and human substrates (e.g., mammalian DNA) is critical for maintenance of self-tolerance.

The expression of TLRs is compartmentalized within individual cells. Unique bacterial and fungal molecular structures are recognized by TLR-1, TLR-2, TLR-4, TLR-5, and TLR-6, localized in plasma membrane and then recruited into phagosomes. TLR-1/TLR-2 and TLR-2/TLR-6 exist functionally as heterodimers, and the existence of homodimers of TLR-2/TLR-2 has been suggested in the literature. TLR-3, TLR-7, TLR-8, and TLR-9 bind to nucleic acids localized in intracellular compartments and differentiate self from non-self. During viral infections, nucleic acid-binding TLRs are used in abrogating Treg suppression so that the activation threshold for viral-reactive T effectors is lowered and a vigorous T-cell response can be established. Table 3 summarizes the location of different TLRs described in humans and their exogenous and/or endogenous ligands, and function where currently known.

The distinctive recognition and response of TLR receptors to self-antigens (e.g., such as those derived from apoptotic cell death, including nucleoproteins) from TLRs that respond to invading pathogens, are essential for maintenance of immune tolerance. In this regard, in murine lupus, ligation of TLR-7 and TLR-8 on Tregs breaks peripheral tolerance, when ligated by apoptotic blebs containing RNP or other nucleic-binding autoantigens. The resulting dysregulation of suppressive activity by regulatory T-cell phenotypes leads to systemic autoimmunity.

**Table 3**
Human toll-like receptors: location and ligands

TLR-1
  *Location:* plasma membrane
  *Exogenous ligand:* dimerizes with TLR2 and binds triacyllipopeptides, lipoarbinomannan from mycobacterium, glycosylphosphatidyl inositol-linked proteins in parasites like *Trypanosoma cruzi*

TLR-2
  *Location:* plasma membrane
  *Exogenous ligand:* binds peptidoglycan and lipopeptides
  *Endogenous ligand:* HSP 60, HSP 70, gp96 HMG B1, hyaluronate, fibronectin, minimally modified LDL, heparin sulfate, HSPB8

TLR-3
  *Location:* intracellular
  *Exogenous ligand:* dsRNA from viruses
  *Endogenous ligand:* necrotic cells

TLR-4
  *Location:* intracellular
  *Exogenous ligand:* LPS
  *Endogenous ligand:* HSP 60, HSP 70, gp96 HMG B1, hyaluronate, fibronectin, minimally modified LDL, heparin sulfate, HSPB8. Abrogates regulatory T-cell function, independent of co-stimulation, mediated through DC expression of IL-6

TLR-5
  *Location:* intracellular
  *Ligand:* bacterial flagellin

TLR-6
  *Exogenous ligand:* dimerizes with TLR2 and binds diacyl lipopeptides, peptidoglycans found in yeast

TLR-7
  *Location:* intracellular constitutively expressed in ER, endosomes, and lysosomes of plasmacytoid DC
  *Ligand:* single stranded RNA (ssRNA), purified snRNPs; triggered by imiquimod, resiqimod

TLR-8
  *Ligand:* single-stranded RNA (ssRNA), imidazoquinolones

TLR-9
  *Location:* intracellular constitutively expressed in plasmacytoid DC
  *Ligand:* non-methylated cpG-containing DNA

TLR 10
  *Ligand:* unknown

## 3.3. Role of APC in determining: inflammation, tolerance, or autoimmunity?

Typically, a robust immune response occurs when foreign antigens are presented by professional APC (i.e. macrophages, B-cells, and mature DC (mDCs)). Such cells constitutively express ligands for T-cell signaling via CD 28/CTLA4/PD-1, and they elicit a robust immune response through upregulating expression of co-stimulatory molecules (e.g., B7.1, B7.2, B7-DC) and production of pro-inflammatory chemokines and cytokines (e.g., TNFα, IFNγ, IL-β, IL6 and IL-12). This process drives the adaptive immune response against the foreign antigen during cognate interactions with lymphocytes.

DCs act as sentinels and are the most potent antigen presenting cell involved in both the defence from pathogens and maintenance of immune tolerance. Regulation of their maturation, migration, and expression of stimulatory and costimulatory molecules has major consequences on the immune response. Under non-pathologic conditions, internalization of self-antigens (e.g., from apoptotic cells) by DC resident in peripheral tissue, leads to DC migration to secondary lymphoid organs, where presentation of self-peptides to T-cells occurs. However, the adaptive immune response against self-antigen is dampened in the absence of inflammation and usually results in tolerance. Additionally, presentation of self-antigens to immature DC (iDC) usually limits immune responsiveness, leading to preferential emergence of regulatory T-cell phenotypes. Thus DC play a significant role in the induction and maintenance of peripheral T-cell tolerance. During cognate interactions with T lymphocytes, tolerogenic DC exhibit decreased production and secretion of pro-inflammatory cytokines (e.g., IL-1, IL-6, IL-12 and TNF-α), demonstrate enhanced secretion of anti-inflammatory cytokines like IL-10, and receive tolerizing signals from complement receptors.

Furthermore, antigenic presentation to T-cells by non-professional APC, such as renal tubular epithelial cells, often limits immune responsiveness and promotes tolerance. Renal tubular epithelial cells (TECs) constitutively express MHC II molecules in low quantities and have the capacity to present peptides to T-cells. However, during inflammation, expression of MHC II molecules is upregulated and they assume an APC-like phenotype. Such non-professional APC participate in antigen presentation and activation of T-cells. Particularly noteworthy, this type of T-cell activation may not always be subject to usual regulatory mechanisms, so that TEC may perpetuate immune responsiveness.

### 3.3.1. Professional versus non-professional APC: the role of renal epithelial cells in emergence of autoimmunity

Renal tubular epithelial cells play an important role in inflammation in the kidneys. In addition to expressing MHC II molecules, they have been shown to express co-stimulatory ligands CD40, B7RP-1, and CD2, that interact with the receptors, CD154, ICOS, and LFA-3. It was previously thought that a second signal provided via this interaction might regulate T-cell function under pathologic conditions. More recently, however, a new member of the B7 family, B7-DC, was identified as a ligand for PD-1 (a homolog of CD28 and CTLA-4). It is expressed in renal tubular epithelial cells in various segments of the nephron in diseased kidneys, such as those with chronic nephritis, lupus nephritis, and tubulointerstitial nephritis. These observations raise the possibility that during inflammation, renal TEC upregulate expression of B7-DC, which in turn, plays a role in T-cell recruitment and local activation. There is some evidence that engagement of B7-DC with PD-1 causes inhibition of T-cell proliferation and cytokine production, similar to the overall *negative regulatory* function it exerts on professional APC. However there is also evidence that shows B7-DC acts as a co-stimulator to enhance production of IFN-γ and cellular proliferation. Although the precise role of B7-DC on renal tubular epithelial cells likely varies with the underlying pathology, these findings indicate that they can serve as APC. However, they may not be subject to usual control mechanisms and, therefore, could potentially perpetuate autoimmune activity in the kidney.

### 3.3.2. The role of immature versus mature DC as APC in the emergence of autoimmunity

Successful initiation of the adaptive immune response requires DC maturation, after signaling through the TLRs and CD40. DC play an important role in inducing and maintaining tolerance, in part, by promoting the generation of regulatory T-cells. mDC are potent APC, whereas immature APC promote tolerance. The distinction is related to secretion and expression of stimulatory and co-stimulatory molecules. During the immune response, mDC up-regulate their expression of B7.1 (CD80) and B7.2 (CD86), deliver strong stimulatory signals to T-cells, and this results in enhanced T-cell proliferation and Th1-type responses (T-cells that produce large amounts of IFN-$\gamma$ and IL-2 but no IL-4, IL-5, or IL10). In contrast, iDC with low expression of CD80 and CD86, promote tolerance as poor stimulators of T-cell proliferation and cytokine production. iDC promote preferential emergence of regulatory T-cell and Th2 phenotypes that promote peripheral tolerance. These T-cells produce high levels of IL-10 and TGF-$\beta$. IL10, in turn, arrests further maturation of iDC and prevents full expression of co-stimulatory molecules found on mDC.

Recently novel strategies using tolerogenic iDC have been employed to limit autoimmune diseases and graft-versus-host disease (i.e. after allogenic bone marrow transplantation), and to promote tolerance in solid organ transplantation. The role of various chemokines such as vasoactive intestinal peptide (VIP) for ex-vivo expansion of tolerizing iDC is currently being explored. However, since iDC are likely to mature in inflammatory conditions such as those seen in autoimmune diseases and solid organ transplantation, the major challenge of preventing maturation of iDC, after adoptive transfer from ex-vivo systems into animal models of human autoimmune diseases, will need to be overcome.

### 3.3.3. The role of the B-cell as an APC in emergence of autoimmunity

B-cells contribute to autoimmunity by production of pathogenic antibodies and by acting as APC. The latter conclusion is derived from experiments where autoimmune prone mice without B-cells do not develop disease. Furthermore, administration of autoantibodies alone is insufficient for severe disease. In murine lupus, it was observed that mice with surface Ig, but not secreted Ig, developed more severe disease than mice who received sufficient quantities of serum to maintain autoantibody levels for weeks. Similar findings in other forms of autoimmune diseases confirmed these results. Presumably, B-cells are crucial for antigen presentation and secretion of soluble mediators for T-cells. Furthermore, antigen capture is very efficient through surface Ig, and therefore, although not as potent as DC and macrophages in T-cell activation, B-cells are more efficient in directing antigen-specific responses. These investigations support an important role for B-cells in autoimmune diseases, and they provide the rationale for current therapy to eliminate them In this regard, therapeutic trials are underway in human lupus nephritis, membranous nephropathy, and other diseases.

### 3.4. Role of complement proteins and TLRs in immune regulation

In a later chapter of this handbook, complement proteins and the role of their dysregulation in the pathogenesis of autoimmune renal diseases is discussed in detail. This section emphasizes the role of complement pathways in immune regulation. Tight regulation of complement proteins is especially important for maintenance of tolerance in the innate immune response, and defects in the control of complement activation are associated with autoimmune diseases. As importantly, defective regulation of complement activity may also manifest in the uncontrolled activity of the innate immune response; this can result in defective clearance of apoptotic cell debris, impaired opsonization, or perturbed phagocytosis.

The regulatory roles played by the various cellular and non-cellular components of the innate immune system at the different levels that establish and maintain peripheral tolerance are summarized in Table 4. It is emphasized that interplay of these

**Table 4**
Regulatory role of the components of the innate immune system and examples of autoimmune kidney diseases in dysregulation

| Innate system activity | Cell players and function | Mode of regulation | Key proteins responsible for regulation | Examples of dysregulation/autoimmunity |
|---|---|---|---|---|
| Phagocytosis of microbes | Macrophage, NK cells monocytes, immature DC, neutrophils | TLR specificity | Ligands on microbes, phagocyte receptors, e.g., complement proteins, IgM, C-reactive protein | SLE |
| Phagocytosis of apoptotic cells; clearance of immune complexes | Clearance by receptors on RBC podocytes (platelets in rodents) Presentation of Ag by T-cells | Presence of cell surface receptors to clear waste on phagocytic cells e.g., FcγRs | Scavenger receptors, integrins, FcγR, collectin receptors | SLE |
| Regulation of immune response by signals from apoptotic cells | TLRs on macrophages, monocytes, and NK T-cells TRegs | Tolerogenic signals and anti-inflammatory cytokine secretion: for apoptotic cells usually expressing self-antigen Danger signals and pro-inflammatory cytokine secretion: for necrotic cells | TGF β, IL-10, IL-13 GM-CSF, TNFα, IFN-γ, IL-1 | AutoAg in apoptotic blebs (e.g., DNA, RNA, chromatin-delayed/ineffective clearance in SLE |
| Regulation by APC | Different outcome of Ag presentation by professional APC e.g., macrophages, mature DC vs. immature DC | Immune tolerance; anergizing CD4+, CD8+ T-cells by immature DC | Anti-inflammatory cytokines in micro-environment | Maturation of immature APC and upregulation of MHC II in inflammatory milieu results in AutoAb a autoreactive B and T-cells, e.g., RA |
| | Ag presentation by non-professional APC, e.g., renal epithelial cells | Induction of differentiation of naïve T-cells to TReg | Activating/inhibitory receptors expressed on surface of DC and T-cells | |
| Complement system: induction of antibody responses and opsonization and lysis of apoptotic cells and other cellular debris | Cell clearance; inactivation of C1q; covalently bound fragments of C3 and C4 | Focus activation of complement on microorganism surfaces; regulate complement activation and deposition on normal cells | Binding c1q, CRP, IgM to apoptotic cells Regulators of complement activation: factor H C4-binding protein, r CR1, CD35, decay accelerating factor, CD membrane cofactor protein (MCP, CD46) | Defective regulation of C3 causes MPGN C3 nephritic factor; (autoAb)-MPGN II in SLE end with MPGN. Factor H and I deficiencies lead to increased complement activation, in SLE, MPGN, HUS |

components of the innate immune response contribute to distinguishing self-antigen from non-self, and examples of how dysregulation of these proteins lead to autoimmunity are highlighted.

## 4. Emergence of autoimmune renal disease: breakdown of tolerance checkpoints

The generation, maintenance, and proliferation of autoreactive B and T-cells and emergence of autoimmune renal disease, involves the simultaneous breakdown of multiple central and peripheral checkpoints involved in the maintenance of tolerance. It is well established that the mere presence of autoreactive B or T-cells is insufficient. For example, in lupus patients autoantibodies have been detected long before the onset of clinical disease (e.g., nephritis). Although the precise sequence of events likely varies among individuals, the contributing factors will be reviewed.

of certain autoimmune diseases has been reportedly associated with individuals with particular genes. Nevertheless, serum autoantibodies have been found in individuals who never develop clinically overt disease, and autoantibodies may precede overt disease in some patients. These findings give credence to the notion that autoimmune disease likely requires several breakpoints in regulation of either adaptive and/or innate immune in genetically susceptible individuals. Furthermore, the particular inflammatory phenotype expressed in response to an injury, for example a Th1 versus Th2 response is likely also genetically determined. These observations help to explain why individuals with the same disease have different forms and severity of nephritis.

Table 5 lists autoimmune kidney diseases in which specific genes that have been implicated. Their precise role is discussed in detail in the respective chapters; we emphasize the associations here to illustrate the genetic contributions to pathogenesis.

### 4.1. Genetic and host factors in emergence of autoimmune kidney disease

Studies of genetic backgrounds in patients with autoimmune kidney diseases suggest linkage disequilibrium with some genes, and a preponderance

### 4.2. Environmental factors in emergence of autoimmune kidney disease

Various environmental factors may also contribute to elicit immune responses against antigens in the kidney. For example, in individuals who are

Table 5
Genetic factors in autoimmune kidney diseases

| Autoimmune kidney diseases with genetic susceptibility | | |
| --- | --- | --- |
| Disease | Genes linked | Relative risk |
| Goodpasture's disease | DR2(w15) | 10.5 |
| Membranous nephropathy | DR3, DR2 (w15) | 5–7 |
| IgA nephropathy | DR4 | 2.6 |
| Minimal change nephrotic syndrome | DR7, DR8 | 10.1 |
| Acute post-streptococcal GN | Ag-activates alternative | – |
| Systemic lupus erythematosus | DR3 ?DR2, complement genes def C1q, C2, C4 | – |
| ANCA-associated vasculitides | ?DR2, ?DR4, ?DR6 Alpha-1 antitrypsin locus abnormality | – |
| Membranous proliferative GN type II | Complement factor H deficiency | – |

genetically predisposed to develop autoimmune diseases such as SLE, factors that have been associated with initiation of symptoms and subsequent flares of disease include infectious agents, stress, toxins, and physical agents like sunlight. Similarly, in anti-GBM disease unmasking of the pathogenic epitopes in the kidney and the lung provides the nidus for deposition of circulating autoantibodies. Whether exposure stimulates immunity, however is not certain. Table 6 highlights some examples demonstrating how the complex interaction between various environmental factors in a susceptible host results in autoimmune kidney disease. It is emphasized that for disease expression, multiple events are required, including antigen exposure, access of the antigen to the immune cells, elicitation of an immune response against the exposed antigen, immune complex formation or T-cell infiltration, and downstream effector mechanisms that result in inflammation.

## 4.3. Role of nephritogenic autoantibodies in autoimmune kidney diseases

Nephritogenic autoantibodies form immune deposits in the kidney and induce injury. The major mechanisms of immune deposit formation include: direct binding to renal antigens, binding to exogenous antigens that localize in the kidney, and serve as planted antigens for circulating antibodies, or deposition of circulating immune complexes. In the latter situation the Ag may be endogenous (auto) or exogenous (foreign). In most situations, the location of the antigen determines the site of deposition. The ensuing inflammation

Table 6
Autoimmune kidney diseases and interplay of environmental factors, self-antigen, and immune response

| Example of autoimmune kidney disease | Environmental promoter resulting in kidney antigen exposure | Antigen; immune response |
| --- | --- | --- |
| Intrinsic antigens | | |
| Goodpasture's syndrome, anti-glomerular basement membrane disease | Exposure to organic solvents, cigarette smoke in the lungs expose lung basement membrane | GBM; humoral and cell-mediated immune response against NC1domain of $\alpha 3$ IV collagen (COL3A4) |
| Alport's syndrome, post kidney transplantation | Presence of transplanted kidney expressing NC1 domain of COL3A5 in GBM | GBM; Results in immune response against NC1domain of COL3A5 in GBM and autoantibody deposition |
| Tubulo-interstitial nephritis | Viruses, e.g., CMV, HIV, EBV lead to viral transformation of epithelial cells expressing new proteins | Neoantigen, TBM-; viral proteins expressed on epithelial cells, upregulation of MHC II and resultant cell-mediated immune responses |
| ANCA related vasculitides | Staphyloccocal infections, nasal carriers, viral lung infections, and inflammation | ANCA vs. intracellular PMN Ag; ANCA activate PMN which engage activated endothelia |
| Extrinsic antigens | | |
| Allergic interstitial nephritis | Penicillins, e.g., methicillin, nafcillin, cephalosporins, phenytoin, and inflammatory cytokines | Drug–hapten conjugates |
| APSGN | Ab vs. nephritogenic strain of streptococci | Nephritogenic Ag from strep localize in glomeruli; Ab bind to strep to form immune deposits |
| IgA nephropathy | Viral and bacterial infections | Immune complexes?; IgG? IgA? |
| Cryoglobinemia, MPGN | Viruses (Hepatitis C) | Cryoglobulins |

(or lack thereof) is dependent on the isotype and location of the deposited antibody. IgG containing immune deposits are generally more nephritogenic than IgM, since they have greater capacity to engage FcR on infiltrating cells. Persistence of immune deposits, due to either high-affinity glomerular Ag interactions, or stabilization of immune complexes within the capillary wall, also enhances pathogenicity. In the case of ANCA-associated vasculitis, although pathogenic, the antibodies do not deposit in the kidney. Instead they bind to activated neutrophils, which release enzymes and other contents on engaging activated glomerular endothelium to initiate local inflammation, in the absence of overt immune complexes in glomeruli. Some factors that enhance nephritogenic potential of an autoantibody are summarized in Table 7.

## 4.4. Other roles for B-cells in autoimmune kidney disease

In addition to producing autoantibodies, autoreactive B-cells have important roles in activating autoreactive, nephritogenic T-cells and infiltrating interstitial lesions. Locally they secrete cytokines and serve as APC for autoreactive T-cells. This latter function most likely contributes to disease progression independent of the underlying disease pathogenesis. Key roles for B-cells in emergence of autoimmunity are summarized in Table 8.

## 4.5. T-cells in autoimmune kidney disease

T-cells participate in nephritis in multiple ways. They infiltrate the kidney, interact with both professional APC and renal epithelia locally, and augment B-cell activity. Infiltration is most apparent in interstitial disease and vasculitis, however T-cells are also visualized during some forms of glomerulonephritis. In experimental models of Goodpasture's disease and ANCA-associated vasculitis, T-cells are present in inflammatory infiltrates suggesting that they help initiate disease. Furthermore, in experimental models of nephritis, lesions are significantly limited or absent in animals without T-cells, despite the presence of immune deposits. These observations support the notion that both T-cells and B-cells are required for full-blown expression of disease. Furthermore they provide the rationale to target either T-cells, B-cells, or molecules that modulate T–B interactions during the course of nephritis.

T-cells play a major role in initiating interstitial nephritis, and experimental rodent models provide insights into pathogenesis. For example, viral infection, with expression of new viral proteins, can trigger T-cell-mediated immunity leading to interstitial nephritis. Alternatively, tubular inflammation, per se, may lead to exposure of neoantigens and autoimmune nephritis. For example, cadmium exposure in mice leads to renal tubular

**Table 7**
Nephritogenic antibodies: factors that promote inflammation and injury

*FcR engagement*: Fc interaction with FcR provides positive and negative stimuli for both inflammatory and renal cells; Fc must be accessible to FcR on circulating cells

*Complement activation*: lytic and/or sublytic injury to renal cells; recruitment of cells to amplify inflammation

*Direct perturbations of local environment*: disruption of cell–cell or cell–basement membrane interactions; activation of renal cells via ligation of surface receptors

**Table 8**
The role of B-cells in autoimmune nephritis

Abnormal regulation of autoantibody production

Production of pathogenic antibodies that form immune deposits, e.g., SLE

Serve as APC for autoreactive T-cells, e.g., interstitial nephritis and vasculitis

Influence other autoantigen presenting cells by production of cytokines

Promote normal secondary lymphoid structure that in turn affects autoimmune responses

Therapies that target either pathogenic B-cells and/or molecules involved in B–T interactions have potential to alter the course of nephritis

**Table 9**
The role of T-cells in autoimmune nephritis

---
Abnormal regulation of T-cell activation; abnormal recognition of self

T-cell help for autoreactive B-cells

Abnormal regulatory T-cell activity

---

**Table 10**
The role of APC in autoimmune nephritis

---
Antigen presentation of self-antigens; abnormal TLR signaling

Loss of tolerogenic signals by maturation of immature DC

Abnormal co-stimulatory signaling and regulation resulting from MHC II upregulation and antigen presentation by renal epithelial cells

Inflammatory cytokine production enhancing autoimmune response: e.g., production of interferon by plasmacytoid DC

Upregulation of TLR 7 and TLR 9

Antigen presentation by renal epithelial cells and other non-professional APC causing propagation of inflammatory responses and escape from normal regulation

---

toxicity and necrosis, with exposure of heat shock proteins. In this context, the HSP elicit an inflammatory and autoimmune response; the latter leads to severe interstitial nephritis and renal failure.

In other situations the reasons for the breakdown in T-cell tolerance are not entirely known. In most circumstances *central* T-cell tolerance remains intact but the breakdown occurs in the periphery. An essential role for regulatory T-cells in maintaining peripheral tolerance by preventing long and sustained DC-effector T-cell cognate interactions has been observed in many autoimmune diseases and likely plays a critical role. Along these lines, a permissive role for dysfunctional Tregs in lupus has been observed. Table 9 summarizes the multiple roles for T-cells and their secretory products in the pathogenesis of autoimmune nephritis.

## *4.6. APC and their role in emergence of autoimmune kidney diseases*

In the foregoing sections of this chapter, a variety of mechanisms by which APC potentially promote autoimmune kidney diseases is discussed extensively. Table 10 summarizes these multiple roles. There is currently no known model of autoimmune kidney disease caused entirely by APC dysregulation. However, antigen presentation of self-antigens, loss of tolerogenic signals by maturation of iDC, abnormal TLR regulation and signaling, and inflammatory cytokine production enhancing the autoimmune response, are some of the roles played by APC in autoimmune nephritis. These are summarized in Table 10.

## 5. Conclusions

In the preceding sections of this chapter we have briefly introduced the concepts of central and peripheral tolerance, we have reviewed the development of T- and B-cells, and presented postulates on the roles of both the innate and adaptive immune systems in formation and maintenance of tolerance as currently understood. We have stressed the requirement for a breakdown in multiple tolerance checkpoints for the emergence of autoimmunity. An overview of the genetic and environmental factors leading to emergence of autoimmune kidney diseases is included. Table 11 briefly summarizes some of these concepts as currently understood, as they relate to autoimmune kidney diseases.

It is important to reiterate that clinically significant autoimmunity is a rarity, despite the prevalence of low-specificity, low-affinity autoantibodies in normal people. Before clinical presentation of an autoimmune disease, several breaks in checkpoints in both the innate and adaptive immune system have occurred. Autoreactive T- and B-cell clones must emerge, become activated, proliferate, and acquire the ability to sustain a self-directed immune response. The autoantibodies have to be present in sufficiently high quantities to bind antigen with necessary avidity and elicit appropriate co-stimulatory molecule expression to

**Table 11**
Pathogenic mechanisms for common autoimmune kidney diseases

Membranous nephropathy (subepithelial deposits)
  Human antigen(s) unknown
  Animal models: Heymann nephritis: antibodies bind to megalin and additional antigens present on renal epithelial cells. Proteinuria is complement dependent. Antibodies induce sublytic injury to cells. PMNs do not have access to Fc of deposited Ab on epithelial side of GBM
  Chronic serum sickness: foreign proteins lodge in the subepithelial space and serve as planted antigens for antibodies. Proteinuria is complement dependent

Post-streptococcal GN (mesangial, subepithelial, and subendothelial deposits)
  Cell-wall antigens from nephritogenic streptococci deposit within glomerular capillary wall before subsequent binding of anti-streptococcal antibodies. Ag-activated alternate pathway directly

Anti-GBM disease (human)
  Autoantibodies bind to alpha 3(IV) collagen
  Antigen normally sequestered. Antigen is expressed in glomerulus, lungs, and testes
  Needs two hits: antigen exposure and autoantibody production
  In patients with pre-existing lung disease, antibody deposition and pulmonary hemorrhage develop

IgA nephropathy/HSP
  Altered IgA lodges within the mesangium to initiate nephritis. Role of antigen unclear

Lupus nephritis
  Immune deposits form in situ by either cross-reactive autoantibodies binding to glomerular antigens or autoantibodies binding to soluble antigens that localize in the glomerulus. Nucleosomes may lodge in the basement membrane through charge-charge interactions to serve as planted antigens for anti-DNA antibodies. Nephritogenic lupus autoantibodies may bind directly to glomerular cells and matrix components
  It is postulated that the different specificities of lupus autoantibodies from immune deposits at different locations within the glomerulus, and that differences in the predominant antibody subtypes contributes to the diverse clinical and histologic presentations in lupus patients

Systemic vasculitis
  Patients with Wegener's granulomatosis or microscopic polyangiitis have circulating ANCAs, but lack glomerular immune deposits
  Postulate is that ANCAs react with cytokine-primed neutrophils during conditions in which the glomerular endothelium is activated to initiate nephritis

Membranoproliferative glomerulonephritis (primary: children)
  Congenital or acquired deficiency of complement regulatory proteins leads to nephritis. This clinical observation implies that inhibitors of complement activation (e.g., DAF) normally have a role in preventing complement activation within the glomerulus (and that low levels of complement activation may occur in normals). Spontaneous development of autoantibodies is a prominent feature of type I and type III MPGN

Membranoproliferative glomerulonephritis (secondary: adults)
  Associated with hepatitis C, hepatitis B, and malignancy
  Cryoglobulins have been detected in hepatitis variants with anti-hepatitis C Ab and hepatitis C Ag
  Deposited antibodies activate complement and engage FcR

propagate an inflammatory cytokine milieu, which often requires either Th1 or Th2 responses. In addition, components of the innate immune system must also be dysregulated, so that APC present autoantigen inappropriately and complement proteins escape multiple well-regulated control mechanisms. Thus, there must be a failure of multiple overlapping central and peripheral regulatory mechanisms to allow for propagation of an abnormal self-directed immune response, before there is emergence of autoimmune kidney disease.

> **Key points**
>
> - The autoimmune response is tightly regulated at multiple levels, during development and life.
> - B-cell tolerance occurs centrally in the bone marrow, through deletion and receptor editing, and peripherally through anergy, clonal exhaustion, and antigenic segregation.
> - T-cell tolerance occurs centrally in the thymus through deletion and peripherally through anergy, cytokine deviation, clonal exhaustion, and via regulatory T-cells.
> - The innate immune system, consisting of macrophages, DCs, monocytes, natural killer T-cells, and components of the complement system, provides an essential role in maintaining tolerance.
> - Toll-like receptors, key players in the innate immunity, serve as regulators of the adaptive immune response and maintaining tolerance.
> - DCs are key regulators of immunity with dual roles; immature cell types are tolerogenic, while mature cell types activate immunity and inflammation.
> - B-cells have multiple roles as producers of pathogenic autoantibodies and antigen presenting cells for autoreactive T-cells.
> - T-cells also have multiple roles, with subsets that are effectors of either immunity or/and inflammation, whereas others serve as regulators of the autoimmune response.
> - Deciphering the pathways leading to immune regulation, autoimmunity, and inflammation, provides the rationale for new therapeutic strategies to alter the course of immune mediated renal diseases.

# Further Reading

## 1. Introduction

Billingham, R.E., Brent, L., Medawar, F.R.S. 1953. 'Actively acquired tolerance' of foreign cells. Nature 172 (4379), 603–606.

## 2. Mechanisms of tolerance

Barrington, R.A., Borde, M., Rao, A., Carrol, M.C. 2006. Involvement of NFAT1 in B cell self-tolerance. J. Immunol. 177, 1510–1515.

Barrington, R.A., Zhang, M., Zhong, X., Jonsson, H., Holodick, N., Cherukuri, A., Ouerce, S.K., Rothstein, T.L., Carroll, M.C. 2005. CD21/CD19 coreceptor signaling promotes B cell survival during primary immune responses. J. Immunol. 175, 2859–2867.

Carroll, M.C. 2004a. The complement system in B cell regulation. Mol. Immunol. 41, 141–146.

Carroll, M.C. 2004b. The complement system in regulation of adaptive immunity. Nat. Immunol. 5, 981–986.

Carroll, M.C. 2004c. A protective role for innate immunity in systemic lupus erythermatosus. Nat. Rev. Immunol. 4, 825–831.

Carroll, M.C., Holers, V.M. 2005. Innate autoimmunity. Adv. Immunol. 86, 137–157.

Chan, O., Shlomchik, M.J. 1998. A new role for B cells in systemic autoimmunity: B cells promote spontaneous T cell activation in MRL-lpr/lpr mice. J. Immunol. 160, 51–59.

Janeway, C.A., Travers, P., Walport, M., Shlomchik, M.J., 2005. Immunobiology: The Immune System in Health and Disease, 6th ed., Garland Science Publishing, New York, NY.

Kukreja, A., Maclaren, N.K. 2000. Current cases in which epitope mimicry is considered as a component of autoimmune disease: immune-mediated (type I) diabetes. Cell. Mol. Life Sci. 57 (4), 534–541.

Richter, W., Mertens, T., Schoel, B., Muir, P., Ritzkowsky, A., Scherbaum, W.A., Boehm, B.O. 1994. Sequence homology of the diabetes-associated autoantigen glutamate decarboxylase with coxsackie B4-2C protein and heat shock 60 mediates no molecular mimicry of autoantibodies. J. Exp. Med. 180 (2), 721–726.

Shlomchik, M.J., Craft, J.E., Mamula, M.J. 2001. From T to B and back again: positive feedback in systemic autoimmune disease. Nat. Rev. Immunol. 1, 147–153.

Streilein, J.W., Takeuchi, M., Taylor, A.W. 1997. Immune privilege, T-cell tolerance and tissue-restricted autoimmunity. Hum. Immunol. 52 (2), 138–143.

Sonderegger, I., Rohn, T.A., Kurrer, M.O., Iezzi, G., Zou, Y., Kastelein, R.A.A., Bachmann, M.F., Kopf, M. 2006. Neutralization of LL-17 by active vaccination inhibits IL-23-dependent autoimmune myocarditis. Eur. J. Immunol. 36, 1–8.

von Boehmer, H. 1994. Positive selection of lymphocytes. Cell 76, 219–228.

## 3. Mechanisms of tolerance maintenance

Bagheri, N., Chintalacharuvu, S.R., Emancipator, S.N. 1997. Proinflammatory cytokines regulate Fc alphaR expression by human mesangial cells in vitro. Clin. Exp. Immunol. 107, 404–409.

Barton, G.M., Kagan, J.C., Medzhitov, R. 2006. Intracellular localization of Toll-like receptor 9 prevents recognition of self DNA but facilitates access to viral DNA. Nat. Immunol. 7 (1), 49–56.

Ben Chetrit, E., Dunsky, E.H., Wollner, S., Eilat, D. 1985. In vivo clearance and tissue uptake of an anti-DNA monoclonal antibody and its complexes with DNA. Clin. Exp. Immunol. 60, 159–168.

Chapoval, A.I., Hi, J., Lau, J.S., Wilcox, R.A., Flies, D.B., Liu, D., Dong, H., Sica, G.L., Zhu, G., Tamada, K., Chen, L. 2001. B7-H3: a costimulatory molecule for T cell activation and IFN-gamma production. Nat. Immunol. 2, 269–274.

Chorney, A., Gonzales-Rey, E., Delgado, M. 2006. Regulation of dendritic cell differentiation by vasoactive intestinal peptide: therapeutic applications on autoimmunity and transplantation. Ann. N.Y. Acad. Sci. 1088, 187–194.

Cravens, P.D., Lipsky, P.E. 2002. Dendritic cell, chemokine receptors and autoimmune inflammatory diseases. Immunol. Cell Biol. 80, 497–505.

De Haij, S., Woltman, A.M., Trouw, L.A., Bakker, A.C., Kamerling, S.W., van der Kooij, S.W., Chen, L., Kroczek, R.A., Daha, M.R., van Kooten, C. 2005. Renal tubular epithelial cells modulate T-cell responses via ICOS-1 and B7-H1. Kidney Int. 68 (5), 2091–2102.

Falcone, M., Bloom, B.R. 1997. A T helper cell 2 (Th2) immune response against non-self antigens modifies the cytokine profile of autoimmune T cells and protects against experimental allergic encephalomyelitis. J. Exp. Med. 185 (5), 901–907.

Frolich, A., Marsland, B.J., Sonderegger, I., Kurrer, M., Hodge, M.R., Harris, N.L., Kopf, M. 2007. IL-21 receptor signaling is integral to the development of Th2 effector responses in vivo. Blood 109, 2023–2031.

Fukuyama, H., Nimmerjahn, F., Ravetch, J. 2004. The inhibitory Fcγ receptor modulates autoimmunity by limiting the accumulation of immunoglobulin G+ anti-DNA plasma cells. Nat. Immunol. 6 (1), 99–106.

Gonzalez-Rey, C.A., Fernandez-Martin, A., Ganea, D., Delgado, M. 2006. Vasoactive intestinal peptide generates human tolerogenic dendritic cells that induce CD4 and CD8 regulatory T cells. Blood 107 (9), 3632–3638.

Kieber-Emmons, T., Monzavi-Karbassi, B., Wang, B., Luo, P., Weiner, D.B. 2000. Cutting edge: DNA immunization with minigenes of carbohydrate mimotopes induce functional anti-carbohydrate antibody response. J. Immunol. 165, 623–627.

Liu, H., Komai-Koma, M., Xu, D., Liew, F.Y. 2006. Toll-like receptor 2 signaling modulates the functions of CD4+ CD25+ regulatory T cells. Proc. Natl. Acad. Sci. U.S.A. 103 (18), 7048–7753.

Luo, P., Canziani, G., Cunto-Amesty, G., Kieber-Emmons, T. 2000. A molecular basis for functional peptide mimicry of a carbohydrate antigen. J. Biol. Chem. 275, 16146–16154.

Marshak-Rothstein, A. 2006. Toll-like receptors in systemic autoimmune disease. Nat. Rev. Immunol. 6, 823–835.

Morelli, A.E., Larregina, A.T., Shufesky, W.J., Zahorchak, A.F., Logar, A.J., Papworth, G.D., Wang, Z., Watkins, S.C., Falo, L.D., Jr. Thomson, A.W. 2003. Internalization of circulating apoptotic cells by splenic marginal zone dendritic cells: dependence on complement receptors and effect on cytokine production. Blood 101 (2), 611–620.

Su, S.B., Silver, P.B., Grajewki, R.S., Agarwal, R.K., Tang, J., Chan, C.C., Caspi, R.R. 2005. Essential role of the MyD88 pathway, but nonessential roles of TLRs 2, 4, and 9, in the adjuvant effect promoting Th1-mediated autoimmunity. J. Immunol. 175, 6303–6310.

Tseng, S.Y., Otsuji, M., Gorski, K., Huang, X., Slansky, J.E., Pai, S.I., Shalabi, A., Shin, T., Pardoll, D.M., Tsuchiya, H. 2001. B7-DC, a new dendritic molecule with potent co-stimulatory properties for T cells. J. Exp. Med. 193, 839–846.

Walport, M.J. 2001. Complement – first of two parts. N. Engl. J. Med. 344 (14), 1058–1066.

Walport, M.J. 2001. Complement – second of two parts. N. Engl. J. Med. 344 (15), 1140–1144.

Weis, K., Mattaj, I.W., Lamond, A.I. 1995. Identification of hSRP1 alpha as a functional receptor for nuclear localization sequences. Science 268, 1049–1053.

Zhang, J., Chen, Y., Li, J., Wu, Y., Zou, L., Zhao, T., Zhang, X., Han, J., Chen, A., Wu, Y. 2006. Renal tubular epithelial expression of the coinhibitory molecule B7-DC (programmed death-1 ligand). J. Nephrol. 19 (4), 429–438.

# 4. Emergence of autoimmune renal diseases: breakdown of tolerance checkpoints

Abrass, C. 2001. Mechanisms of immune complex formation and deposition in renal structures. In: E.G. Neilson, W.G. Couser (Eds.), Immunologic Renal Diseases. Lippincott, Williams & Williams, Philadelphia, pp. 277–296.

Abrera-Abeleda, M.A., Nishimura, C., Smith, J.L.H., Sethi, S., McRae, J.L., Murphy, B.F., Silvestri, G., Skerka, C., Jozsi, M., Zipfel, P.F., Hageman, G.S., Smith, R.J.H. 2006. Variations in the complementary regulatory genes factor H (CFH) and factor H related genes (CFHR5) are associated with membranoproliferative glomerulonephritis type II (dense deposit disease). J. Med. Genet. 43, 582–589.

Abrera-Abelada, M.A., Xu, Y., Pickering, M.C., Smith, R.J., Sethi, S. 2007. Mesangial immune complex glomerulonephritis due to complement factor D deficiency. Kidney Int. 71, 1142–1147.

Bagchus, W.M., Hoedmaeker, P.J., Rozing, J., Bakker, W.W. 1986. Glomerulonephritis induced by monoclonal anti-Thy1.1 antibodies. A sequential histological and ultrastructural study in the rat. Lab. Invest. 55, 680–687.

Bockenstedt, L.K., Gee, R.J., Mamula, M.J. 1995. Self peptides in the initiation of lupus autoimmunity. J. Immunol. 154 (7), 3516–3524.

Cameron, J.S. 1997. Systemic lupus erythematosus. In: E.G. Neilson, W.G. Couser (Eds.), Immunologic Renal Diseases. Lippincott-Williams, Philadelphia, pp. 1055–1098.

Carlson, J.A., Hodder, S.R., Ucci, A.A., Madaio, M.P. 1988. Glomerular localization of circulating single stranded DNA in mice. Dependence on the molecular weight of DNA. J. Autoimmunol. 1, 231–241.

Chan, O.T., Madaio, M.P., Shlomchik, M.J. 1999. B cells are required from lupus nephritis in the polygenic, FAs-intact MRL model of systemic autoimmunity. J. Immunol. 163, 3592–3596.

Christensen, S.R., Kashgarian, M., Alexpoulou, L., Flavell, R.A., Akira, S., Shlomchik, M.J. 2005. Toll-like receptor 9 controls anti-DNA autoantibody production in murine lupus. J. Exp. Med. 202 (2), 321–331.

Contreras, G., Tozman, E., Nahar, N., Metz, D. 2005. Maintenance therapies for proliferative lupus nephritis: mycophenolate mofetil, azathioprine and intravenous cyclophosphamide. Lupus 14 (Suppl. 1), s33–s38.

Couser, W.G. 1990. Medication of glomerular injury. J. Am. Soc. Nephrol. 1, 13–29.

D'Andrea, D.M., Coupaye-Gerard, B., Kleyman, T.R., Foster, M.H., Madaio, M.P. 1996. Lupus autoantibodies interact directly with distinct glomerular and vascular cell surface antigens. Kidney Int. 49, 1214–1221.

Dixon, F., Feldman, J., Vazquez, J. 1961. Experimental glomerulonephritis: the pathogenesis of a laboratory model resembling the spectrum of human glomerulonephritis. J. Exp. Med. 113, 899–921.

Dixon, F.J., Theofilopoulos, A.N., McConahey, P., Prud'homme, G.J. 1983. Murine systemic lupus erythematosus. Prog. Immunol. 5, 1115.

Grothaus, M.C., Srivastava, N., Smithson, S.L., Kieber-Emmons, T., Williams, D.B., Carlone, G.M., Westerink, M.A. 2000. Selection of an immunogenic peptide mimic of the capsular polysaccharide of Neisseria meningitidis serogroup A using a peptide display library. Vaccine 18, 1253–1263.

Hahn, B.H., 1980. Systemic lupus erythematosus. Clin. Immunol. 583–631.

Hahn, B.H. 2003. Systemic lupus erythematosus and accelerated atherosclerosis. N. Eng. J. Med. 349, 2379–2380.

Harlow, E., Lane, D. 1988. Antibodies: A Laboratory Manual. Cold Spring Harbor Laboratory, New York.

Houssiau, F.A. 2004. Management of lupus nephritis: an update. J. Am. Soc. Nephrol. 15, 2694–2704.

Kalluri, R., Meyers, K., Mogyorosi, A., Madaio, M.P., Neilson, E.G. 1997. Goodpasture's syndrome involving overlap with Wegener's granulomatosis and anti-glomerular basement membrane disease. J. Am Soc. Nephrol. 8, 1795–1800.

Kelley, V.R., Wuthrich, R.P. 1999. Cytokines in the pathogenesis of systemic lupus erythermatosus. Semin. Nephrol. 19, 57–66.

Kelly, K.M., Zhuang, H., Nacionales, D.C., Scumpia, P.O., Lyons, R., Akaogi, J., Lee, P., Williams, B., Yamamoto, M., Akira, S., Satoh, M., Reeves, W.H. 2006. "Endogenous adjuvant" activity of the RNA components of lupus autoantigens Sm/RNP and Ro 60. Arthritis Rheum. 5, 1557–1567.

Leadbetter, E.A., Rifkin, I.R., Hohlbaum, A.M., Beaudette, B.C., Shlomchik, M.J., Marshak-Rothstein, A. 2002. Chromatin-IgG complexes activate B cells by dual engagement of IgM and Toll-like receptors. Nature 416, 603–607.

Madaio, M.P., Foster, M.H. 2001. Molecular structure and expression of nephritogenic autoantibodies. In: Neilson, E.G., Couser, W.G. (Eds), Immunologic Renal Diseases, 2nd ed., Lippincott, Williams & Wilkins, Philadelphia, pp. 257–275.

Mudd, P.A., Teague, B.N., Farris, A.D. 2006. Regulatory T cells and systemic lupus erythematosus. Scand. J. Immunol. 64, 211–218.

Pawar, R.D., Patole, P.S., Zecher, D., Segerer, S., Kretzler, M., Schlondorff, D., Anders, H.J. 2006. Toll-like receptor-7 modulates immune complex glomerulonephritis. J. Am. Soc. Nephrol. 17 (1), 141–149.

Ring, G.H., Lakkis, F.G. 1999. Breakdown of self-tolerance and the pathogenesis of autoimmunity. Semin. Nephrol. 19 (1), 25–33.

Tahir, H., Isenberg, D.A. 2005. Novel therapies in lupus nephritis. Lupus 14, 77–82.

Tan, E.M. 1989. Antinuclear antibodies: diagnostic markers for autoimmune diseases and probes for cell biology. Adv. Immunol. 44, 93–151.

Theofilopoulos, A.N., Dixon, F.J. 1983. Murine models of systemic lupus erythematosus. In: F.J. Dixon (Ed.), Advances in Immunology. Academic Press, Inc., pp. 269–390.

Vlahakos, D.V., Foster, M.H., Ucci, A.A., Barrett, K.J., Datta, S.K., Madaio, M.P. 1992. Murine monoclonal anti-DNA antibodies penetrate cells, bind to nuclei and induce glomerular proliferation and proteinuria in vivo. J. Am. Soc. Nephrol. 2, 1345–1354.

Vlahakos, D.V., Foster, M.H., Adams, S., Katz, M., Ucci, A.A., Barrett, K.J., Datta, S.K., Madaio, M.P. 1992. Anti-DNA antibodies form immune deposits at distinct glomerular and vascular sites. Kidney Int. 41, 1690–1700.

Wallace, D. 2001. Current and emerging lupus treatments. Am. J. Mag. Care, 7, S490–S495.

Winfield, J.B., Faiferman, I., Koffler, D. 1977. Avidity of anti-DNA antibodies in serum and IgG glomerular eluates from patients with systemic lupus erythematosus. J. Clin. Invest. 59, 90–96.

Zimmerman, R., Radhakrishnan, J., Valeri, A., Appel, G. 2001. Advances in the treatment of lupus nephritis. Ann. Rev. Med. 52, 62–78.

# CHAPTER 2

# Pathogenesis of Renal Disease: Complement

Menaka Karmegam, Richard J. Quigg*

Section of Nephrology, Department of Medicine, The University of Chicago, 5841 S. Maryland Ave., MC5100, Chicago, IL 60637, USA

## 1. Introduction

The complement system is a collection of proteins that recognize and facilitate the removal of pathogens and unwanted host material (Walport, 2001a, b). In addition, certain members interface with the adaptive immune system to focus its response (Carroll and Holers, 2005; Carroll, 2004). Given the potency of complement activation products when generated either appropriately or inappropriately, the potential for inflammation and injury of self-tissue exists. Under certain circumstances, deficiencies or abnormalities in regulation of complement activation can also be relevant to disease pathogenesis.

In the two human kidneys, there are approximately three million glomeruli (Keller et al., 2003). To accomplish the sizable feat of creating nearly 170l of largely protein-free ultrafiltrate daily, glomeruli receive high blood flow under high pressure, and contain the specialized mesangium and highly negatively charged capillary wall comprised of a fenestrated endothelium, collagen IV-containing glomerular basement membrane (GBM), and the unique visceral epithelial cell (podocyte). These properties of the glomerulus favor its involvement in systemic autoimmune diseases, as well as account for the clinical findings of a decreased filtration rate and proteinuria. This normal physiology can also help explain certain disease features in the renal blood vessels and tubulointerstitium. For instance, in glomerular proteinuria, the response of tubular cells to plasma proteins normally absent in the ultrafiltrate underlies some of the subsequent pathology (Zoja et al., 2003).

Complement activation can contribute to systemic autoimmune diseases involving these three anatomic compartments (Quigg, 2003). Most commonly, the glomerulus is the primary site of involvement, while renal blood vessels and/or the tubulointerstitium can also be involved to a lesser or secondary extent, with particular patterns unique to the underlying disease process. For example, relevant to complement and systemic autoimmune diseases is acute allograft rejection and tubular necrosis, in which complement activation occurs on endothelia and renal tubules, respectively (Mauiyyedi and Colvin, 2002; Thurman et al., 2005).

Nearly every systemic autoimmune disease and its renal involvement is related to pathogenic antibodies (Abs) generated through abnormalities in the humoral immune system. Thus, nephritis in systemic lupus erythematosus (SLE) is characterized by immune complexes (ICs) bearing autoAbs directed towards a variety of autoantigens; anti-GBM Ab disease, anti-neutrophil cytoplasm Ab (ANCA)-associated small vessel vasculitis (AASV), and anti-phospholipid Ab syndrome (APS) each can be attributed to their respective autoAbs; and, cryoglobulinemic vasculitis and membranoproliferative

---

*Corresponding author.
Tel.: 1-773-702-0757; Fax: 1-773-702-4816
E-mail address: rquigg@uchicago.edu

© 2008 Elsevier B.V. All rights reserved.
DOI: 10.1016/S1571-5078(07)07002-X

glomerulonephritis (MPGN) occur from an aberrant humoral immune response towards hepatitis C. Even Henoch–Schönlein purpura (HSP) is related to the production and glomerular deposition of IgA immunoglobulins.

A variety of mechanisms exist for IC deposition in glomeruli, including passive trapping of preformed circulating ICs and the formation in situ in glomeruli, either with antigens intrinsic to the glomerulus or extrinsic antigens that arrive ahead of Ab. In some instances, the particular antigen reactivities may not be as important as the structural features of the Ab itself, such as appears to occur in HSP in which abnormal IgA molecules have a predilection for the mesangium (Barratt and Feehally, 2005; van der Boog et al., 2005). In the collection of diseases comprising post-infectious GN, the humoral immune response is directed appropriately to microorganisms; the resulting deposition of ICs and glomerular inflammation can be considered an "innocent bystander" reaction. Thus, these are not truly autoimmune diseases and will not be covered here.

Once in the glomerulus, pathophysiological effects of ICs containing IgG, IgM, and/or IgA can be attributed to the activation of complement and the particular effects of individual complement mediators. In addition, their location in specific anatomic sites within the glomerulus can affect disease expression. For instance, ICs in the mesangium are associated with proliferation of mesangial cells in HSP, on the endothelium with vessel injury and activation of coagulation pathways in APS, in a subendothelial location with exudative changes in proliferative lupus nephritis, and in a subepithelial location in lupus (and primary) membranous nephropathy. The latter is a non-inflammatory disease, which can be attributed to the lack of access of inflammatory cells to ICs and complement activation products in this location (Salant et al., 1985). The actions of ICs are due to complement activation and/or interactions with Fcγ receptors (R) on intrinsic glomerular and infiltrating inflammatory cells (Ravetch, 2002), which are often not easy to separate as they can be intertwined in some cases. Greater details of FcγR interactions are provided in later chapters.

## 2. Complement activation

The complement system contains the alternative, classical and lectin pathways along with regulators poised at key points throughout. All three activating pathways converge on C3 and then C5, after which they are equivalent (Fig. 1). The key difference among them concerns the initiator of activation. Typically, the classical pathway is activated when C1q binds to immunoglobulin in ICs, while the lectin pathway is activated when mannose-binding lectin (MBL) binds to terminal carbohydrate groups on certain microbes. Both MBL and C1q also may bind to apoptotic cells and aid in their clearance (Nauta et al., 2004). The activated serine esterases in each pathway (C1 s and MBL-associated serine proteases) share the capacity to cleave C4 and C2, thereby generating C4b, which covalently binds to neighboring carbohydrate and amino groups, and C2a, which is a serine esterase. The alternative pathway of complement activation relies upon hydrolysis of C3, which can bind factor B in a $Mg^{2+}$-dependent fashion. Factor B is then cleaved by factor D to generate the initial C3 convertase, C3($H_2O$)Bb. These events are unique and powerful as they occur spontaneously and independently in the fluid-phase (e.g., factor D is unusual in being produced as an active enzyme rather than a proenzyme). The fluid-phase C3 convertase generates C3b, which like C4b, binds covalently to nearby carbohydrate or amino groups. The alternative pathway C3 convertase can be stabilized by properdin or autoAbs. Reflecting the relevance to renal pathophysiology, these stabilizing autoAbs are referred to nephritic factors (Daha et al., 1976).

Thus, activation through each of the three pathways generates the structurally and functionally related C4bC2a and C3bBb C3 convertases. In these, C4b and C3b effectively anchor the growing complexes and also facilitate C3 cleavage by the serine esterases C2a and Bb. Cleavage of C3 leads to generation of the proinflammatory and regulatory fragments, C3a and C3b. The incorporation of C3b in the C3 convertases results in the formation of C4b2a3b of the classical and lectin pathways and C3bBbC3b in the alternative pathway. These are the C5 convertases, in which C2a and Bb cleave C5

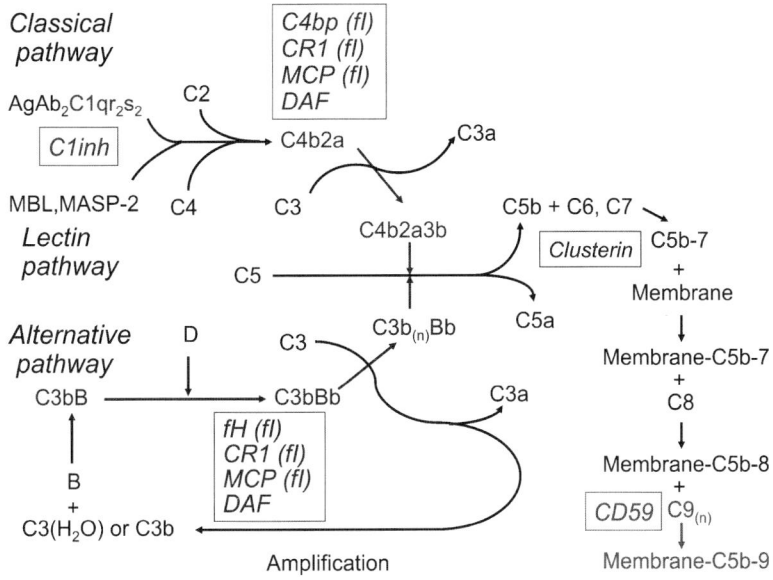

**Figure 1.** The complement system. Activation can occur through the classical, lectin, or alternative pathways. Proinflammatory mediators include anaphylatoxins C3a and C5a, C3b (and its cleavage fragments), which can interact with complement receptors, and the C5b-9 membrane attack complex (in boldface). Regulation occurs throughout the pathways by complement regulatory proteins, which are depicted in boxes adjacent to and matched in colored type for the complement proteins that they inhibit. Factor I (fI) can cleave and inactivate C4b and C3b by using C4-binding protein (C4bp), complement receptor 1 (CR1), membrane cofactor protein (MCP), and factor H (fH) as co-factors. CR1-related protein y (Crry) is found exclusively in rodents. Ag, antigen; Ab, antibody; C1inh, C1 inhibitor; DAF, decay-accelerating factor; MASP, MBL-associated serine protease; MBL, mannose-binding lectin.

to form the biologically active C5a and C5b products. The generation of C5b begins the non-enzymatic assembly of the C5b-9 membrane attack complex which can result in cellular death or activation following membrane insertion (Nicholson-Weller and Halperin, 1993).

Proteins of the complement activation pathways are all present in plasma. Although, traditional thinking has the liver as the major source of complement proteins, there is mounting evidence coming from the labs of Steve Sacks and Moh Daha that many of these proteins can be made outside the liver including the kidney (Morgan and Gasque, 1997; Fischer et al., 1998). Induction of glomerular cell production of C4 (Zhou et al., 1997), C3 (Sacks et al., 1993), and factor H (van den Dobbelsteen et al., 1994; Ren et al., 2003) by a variety of inflammatory mediators has the potential to influence the course of glomerular diseases (Daha and Van Kooten, 2000; Zhou et al., 2001). The tubules of the kidney, in particular the proximal tubule, can make functional complement proteins, most notably C3 which can influence allograft rejection (Brown et al., 2006; Pratt et al., 2002) and ischemia-reperfusion injury (Farrar et al., 2006).

## 3. Complement regulation

Complement activation ranges from the fairly discriminatory classical pathway, requiring specific Ab bound to cognate antigen, to the rather indiscriminate alternative pathway, which is constantly active. As noted above, fundamental to many systemic autoimmune diseases is the generation of autoreactive Abs. Thus, in these states the host is at a relative disadvantage in being required to defend against a self-directed immune response. There are naturally occurring proteins that can regulate complement activation from each of the three pathways, which are relevant in this defense from complement activation occurring in systemic autoimmune diseases (Nangaku, 2003). In plasma, C1 esterase inhibitor prevents C2 and C4 activation and S-protein and clusterin block C5b-9 from forming on cell membranes. CD59 is a widely distributed glycosylphosphatidyl inositol (GPI)-linked membrane protein which also restricts C5b-9 formation by interfering with the addition of C9 to the complex (Ratnoff et al., 1992; Morgan, 1992).

Undoubtedly because of the substantial biological properties of the anaphylatoxins C3a and C5a, the opsonic proteins derived from C3b, and the C5b-9 membrane attack complex, their generation through cleavage of C3 and C5 is heavily regulated. The human proteins that provide this regulation are the plasma proteins, factor H and C4-binding protein, and the intrinsic cellular proteins, complement receptor 1 (CR1, CD35), decay-accelerating factor (DAF, CD55), and membrane cofactor protein (MCP, CD46). These are all members of the regulators of complement activation gene family, with a high degree of structural and functional relatedness (Miwa and Song, 2001; Morgan and Harris, 1999; Hourcade et al., 1989). Key to their activities is their affinity for C4b and C3b, conferring upon them the ability to accelerate the intrinsic decay of C3/C5 convertases and/or act as a factor I cofactor for the cleavage and inactivation (I) of C3b and C4b. While CR2 (CD21) is also a member of this family, it has highest affinity for C3dg and does not inhibit C3 convertases. The $\beta_2$ integrins CR3 (*Itgam*, CD11b/CD18, Mac-1) and CR4 (*Itgax*, CD11c/CD18) also have binding affinity for C3b (and iC3b). Instead of inhibiting complement, these tend to be pro-inflammatory on blood cells which can infiltrate the kidney (Xia et al., 1999; Tang et al., 1997).

## 4. Human studies of complement and autoimmune renal disease

The ability to identify immunoglobulins and complement activation products in diseased kidney tissue obtained from percutaneous renal biopsies considerably advanced our understanding of renal pathophysiology (Coons and Kaplan, 1950; Dixon and Wilson, 1990). Of the systemic autoimmune diseases, those with readily identifiable complement activation products in glomeruli are lupus nephritis, cryoglobulinemic vasculitis, and HSP. In addition, the former two are characterized by systemic consumption of complement, leading to depressed levels of active complement proteins (Madaio and Harrington, 2001). In some settings, the particular pattern of complement depression in sera and deposition in glomeruli can be used to deduce which pathway of complement was activated. For instance the presence of depressed serum C3 and C4 levels, and IgG, IgM, IgA, C1q, C4, C3, and C5b-9 in a single biopsy specimen as in the "full-house" staining in lupus nephritis, can be taken as evidence for IC deposition and activation of the full classical pathway of complement (Biesecker et al., 1981; Lhotta et al., 1996).

Paradoxically, individuals with deficiencies of the early classical pathway components C1q, C1r, C1s and C4 actually are predisposed to develop SLE; this is not the case from C3 on, in which infectious complications are common (Pickering and Walport, 2000; Walport, 2001a). Interestingly, more data on abnormalities in the lectin pathway and SLE pathogenesis are starting to appear; for instance, genetic variants of MBL with lower functional activities have been associated with SLE, along with autoAbs to C1q (Seelen et al., 2005). It is now appreciated that almost a third of SLE patients have these autoAbs to C1q, which are potentially most relevant to lupus nephritis, given their apparent association, often as high-affinity Abs and rising titers with disease flares, as well as their presence in glomerular eluates from lupus nephritis kidney specimens (Horvath et al., 2001; Trouw and Daha, 2005).

Much of the protection against complement activation in the kidney is provided locally by intrinsic proteins CR1, DAF, MCP, and CD59. Each of these proteins tend to have their distinct localization patterns by immunohistochemical techniques. MCP and CD59 appear to be fairly uniformly distributed in all three intrinsic glomerular cells (Meri et al., 1991; Endoh et al., 1993; Ichida et al., 1994), while DAF is highly expressed in the juxtaglomerular apparatus (Cosio et al., 1989) and CR1 is strictly a podocyte protein (Kazatchkine et al., 1982). Functional DAF is also on cultured human podocytes (Quigg et al., 1989), which is relevant to studies with rodent podocyte DAF (discussed below). In disease states characterized by complement deposition in glomeruli, MCP, DAF, and CD59 all are present in increased intensity (Cosio et al., 1989; Endoh et al., 1993; Tamai et al., 1991) perhaps due to an "appropriate" protective response of glomerular cells to complement activation (Cosio et al., 1994). Interestingly, CR1 is considerably reduced in diseases such as lupus nephritis and MPGN; since similar reductions are found in diseases not considered autoimmune, such as focal and segmental glomerulosclerosis (Emancipator et al., 1983; Gelfand et al., 1976; Moran et al., 1977; Petterson et al., 1978; Kazatchkine et al., 1982), this may reflect damage of the podocyte from diverse etiologies (Pascual et al., 1994; Moll et al., 2001).

The complement system also appears relevant to renal diseases outside of the glomerulus. In tubules, MCP is present on the basolateral surfaces while CD59 is present in the brush border (Ichida et al., 1994). This relative lack of C3/C5 regulators may be attributable to the absence of the large C3 and C5 proteins (MW $\sim 200$ kDa) in the normal glomerular ultrafiltrate. Yet, in proteinuric diseases, particularly those in which large proteins escape the glomerular filter (i.e., poorly selective proteinuria), chronic C5b-9-mediated tubular damage may occur (Morita et al., 2000). Nath and Hostetter proposed several decades ago that ammonia-generated activation of C3 and persistent alternative pathway complement activation in the tubulointerstitium could lead to progressive tubular damage in chronic renal diseases (Nath et al., 1985, 1989), a hypothesis that continues to stand the test of time.

An extremely important exception to cell-based complement regulatory proteins as the kidney's primary defense concerns factor H. Abnormalities in this plasma complement regulator can underlie MPGN type II (dense deposit disease) and atypical hemolytic uremic syndrome (aHUS) (Saunders and Perkins, 2006; Zipfel et al., 2006a). Both "typical" HUS and aHUS are characterized by acute kidney injury together with consumptive anemia and thrombocytopenia, but are different by aHUS not being associated with diarrheal infections (as caused by Shiga toxin-producing *Escherichia coli*) and its propensity to recur (Zipfel et al., 2006b). A substantial proportion of aHUS cases are attributable to defects in complement regulation (Zipfel et al., 2006b; Bonnardeaux and Pichette, 2003; Stuhlinger et al., 1974), including genetic defects in factors H (Warwicker et al., 1998, 1999; Ying et al., 1999). Furthermore, aHUS is also associated with inherited defects of factor I and MCP, as well as inhibitory autoAbs to factor H (Kavanagh et al., 2005; Dragon-Durey et al., 2005; Fremeaux-Bacchi et al., 2004, 2006; Noris et al., 2003; Richards et al., 2003). As a general rule, MPGN type II is attributable to type I mutations in factor H leading to its altered appearance in plasma and the ensuing unrestricted systemic alternative pathway activation, while aHUS is attributable to type II mutations clustering in the terminal short consensus repeats. These lead to impaired ability of factor H to bind anionic sites such as on endothelium and provide local protection against complement activation (Rodriguez de Cordoba et al., 2004). Overall, aHUS occurs under the right genetic and environmental conditions, with excessive complement activation occurring on endothelia (Zipfel et al., 2006b). Exactly what initiates this complement activation has been elusive.

## 5. Animal studies of the role of complement in renal disease models

Studies of renal diseases modeled on animals can have a much broader scope allowing examination of mechanisms and manipulations that can alter disease, the latter of which might ultimately prove useful in a clinical setting. For instance, the use of corticosteroids, cyclophosphamide, and mycophenolate mofetil were all first applied in murine models of lupus nephritis before their now routine clinical use (Gelfand et al., 1972; Corna et al., 1997). These models include spontaneously occurring autoimmunity and tissue pathology in females of the $F_1$ cross between New Zealand black and white mice (NZB/W) and in both genders of MRL background mice with Fas deficiency due to the *lpr* mutation (MRL/MpJ-*Tnfrsf6$^{lpr/lpr}$* or simply

**Table 1**
Mouse models of systemic autoimmune diseases and beneficial effects of complement manipulations

| Human disease | Animal model | Inhibitor | Deficiency | References |
| --- | --- | --- | --- | --- |
| Lupus nephritis | MRL/*lpr*, NZB/W (spontaneously occurring) | Crry-Ig | Factors B and D | Bao et al. (2002a, 2003a), Elliott et al. (2004), Watanabe et al. (2000a) Wang et al. (1996) |
| | | anti-C5 | | |
| | | C3aRa, C5aRa | C5aR | Bao et al. (2005a, b), Wenderfer et al. (2005) |
| Anti-GBM GN | Passive anti-GBM IgG | Crry-Ig | C3, C4 | Quigg et al. (1998a), Sheerin et al. (1997) |
| APS (fetal loss) | Passive anti-phospholipid IgG | Crry-Ig | C3, C4 | Holers et al. (2002), Girardi et al. (2003) |
| | | anti-factor B | Factor B | |
| | | C5aRa | C5aR | |
| AASV | Passive anti-MPO IgG | | C3, factor B | Xiao et al. (2005) |
| aHUS | Passive anti-endothelial IgG | Crry | C6 | Hughes et al. (2000), Ren et al. (2002) |
| Cryoglobulinemic vasculitis | Passive IgG3 cryoglobulin | | C3, factor B | Trendelenburg et al. (2005) |
| | TSLP (spontaneously occurring) | Crry (negative) | | Muhlfeld et al. (2004) |

*Note*: Shown are systemic autoimmune diseases affecting the kidney which have been modeled in the mouse. The effects of complement in these models has been studied with the listed inhibitors or when disease was induced in mice with targeted or natural (C6) complement protein deficiencies. Abbreviations: a, antagonist; APS, anti-phospholipid antibody syndrome; AASV, anti-neutrophil cytoplasmic antibody-associated systemic vasculitis; aHUS, atypical hemolytic uremic syndrome; Crry, complement receptor 1-related gene/protein y; GBM, glomerular basement membrane; GN, glomerulonephritis; MPO, myeloperoxidase; R, receptor; TSLP, thymic stromal lymphopoeitin.

MRL/*lpr*). In addition to lupus nephritis, useful animal models for AASV, anti-GBM GN, APS, cryoglobulinemic vasculitis, and aHUS have been generated, which have allowed insightful studies into pathogenesis and the role for complement (Table 1).

Initial animal studies of the complement system were those in which complement was massively activated to deplete complement, such as by cobra venom factor. These showed a role for complement in models such as nephrotoxic serum nephritis (as a model for anti-GBM GN) (Kurtz and Donnell, 1962; Unanue and Dixon, 1964), mesangial proliferative GN (Yamamoto and Wilson, 1987), membranous nephropathy (Salant et al., 1980), and ICGN (Johnson et al., 1989). An elegant series of experiments by Boyce and Holdsworth in a rabbit model of anti-GBM GN (Boyce and Holdsworth, 1985) showed that the complement (and neutrophil) dependence of this model varied with the dose of passively transferred Ab. As the dose of Ab was raised the model was first complement and neutrophil-dependent, then complement-dependent but neutrophil-independent, and finally, complement- and neutrophil-independent. The latter might be attributable to direct reactivity of Ab with podocyte antigens (Chugh et al., 2001).

The use of rat and rabbit strains with spontaneous deficiencies of C6 has allowed assigning a role for C5b-9 in experimental mesangial proliferative GN (Brandt et al., 1996), membranous nephropathy (Groggel et al., 1983; Cybulsky et al., 1986), and a model of HUS induced by anti-glomerular endothelial cell antibodies (Hughes et al., 2000). In each of these models, antibody activation on the respective glomerular cell led to complement activation all the way to C5b-9. Although, this has the potential to lead to direct cell death, mounting experimental evidence in podocytes (Cybulsky et al., 1995; Shankland et al., 1999), mesangial cells (Couser et al., 2001; Nauta et al., 2002), and glomerular endothelial cells (Hughes et al., 2000) implicates other cellular effects induced by C5b-9 likely to be relevant to glomerular pathology, including production and release of cytokines, nitric oxide, activation of phospholipases, stimulation of DNA synthesis, and induction of the apotoptic machinery. Thus, complement activation in the vicinity of ICs or directed by Abs reactive with glomerular cell antigens can lead to C5b-9 generation which can affect a variety of cellular pathways.

More recently it has became possible to use natural protein and Ab inhibitors of complement to further dissect the role of complement in glomerular diseases. Extremely relevant to human disease therapy are the two protein inhibitors, soluble (s) recombinant CR1 (Weisman et al., 1990) and a monoclonal Ab to C5 (Wang et al., 1995). Couser et al. utilized models of membranous nephropathy, mesangial proliferative GN, and ICGN, previously shown to have a complement dependence, and showed that sCR1 was effective at reducing measures of disease in these short-term models (Couser et al., 1995). The availability of an inhibitory monoclonal Ab to mouse C5 made it possible to study chronic glomerular disease models in the mouse, as this monoclonal Ab was a natural mouse immunoglobulin to which an immune response would not be directed (unlike to cobra venom factor or to sCR1). Studies by Wang et al. in spontaneous lupus nephritis occurring in NZB/W mice showed that anti-C5 administration near the onset of autoimmune disease markedly prevented development of GN which translated into improved survival (Wang et al., 1996). Administration of anti-C5 Abs also significantly reduced proteinuria and podocyte foot process effacement in a model of lupus nephritis induced by monoclonal anti-double stranded DNA Abs, confirming the effects of products of C5 activation (C5a and C5b-9) in the pathogenesis of SLE (Ravirajan et al., 2004).

While the activating pathways in rodents and humans are largely conserved, there are some notable differences between the two species' regulators of complement activation cluster. These include the presence of a gene termed *Crry* for CR1-related gene *y* given its nucleotide similarity to human CR1 (Paul et al., 1989). The protein product is also known as Crry, and has widespread reactivity throughout the body in rats and mice, including all three glomerular cells (Quigg et al., 1995a, b). Unfortunately, Crry has no direct human homolog, so conclusions of human physiology are limited from studies of Crry function (Molina, 2002). Nonetheless, it is quite clear that Crry is a very important complement regulator, as shown by a series of studies by Seeichi Matsuo in which Crry function-neutralizing Abs exacerbated diseases of the mesangium (Nishikage et al., 1995), podocyte (Schiller et al., 1998), and tubulointerstitium (Nomura et al., 1995). Logically, Crry and CD59, which act sequentially in the activating pathway, have additive function (Quigg et al., 1995a, b; Watanabe et al., 2000b). A fascinating series of studies from Josh Thurman have shown that the normal polarization of Crry to the basolateral aspect of mouse tubules is lost in ischemia, which leads to unrestricted alternative pathway activation and acute kidney injury upon reperfusion (Thurman et al., 2003, 2006a, b). This appears to be relevant to acute kidney injury (tubular necrosis) in humans (Thurman et al., 2005).

To allow long-term studies in mouse disease models, together with Mike Holers we created a recombinant protein with two molecules of Crry linked to the Fc domain of mouse IgG1, termed Crry-Ig. This had complement inhibitory activity similar to native Crry and was effective in the short-term anti-GBM GN model (Quigg et al., 1998a). The true advantage to Crry-Ig came from studies in MRL/*lpr* mice given Crry-Ig from the onset of autoimmune disease at 12 weeks of age until it was well advanced at 24 weeks of age. Complement-inhibited mice were protected from renal functional injury as manifested by albuminuria and renal failure, and glomerular scarring determined by the extent of glomerulosclerosis and matrix accumulation in the kidney (Bao et al., 2003a, b). Comparable results occurred in transgenic MRL/*lpr* mice in which Crry was expressed as a soluble protein both systemically and locally in kidney (Bao et al., 2002a). These two studies in the accurate MRL/*lpr* model of lupus nephritis illustrated a clear role for products of C3 and C5 activation in this disease.

Another feature in mice that makes studies in this species confusing concerns the CR1 and CR2 proteins. In humans, these are encoded by separate genes, while in mice they are alternatively spliced products of the same *Cr2* gene (Kurtz et al., 1990; Molina et al., 1990). Thus, direct study of these individual proteins in rodents can be problematic. In humans, the CR1 protein in erythrocytes is key to the processing of ICs, as it binds to C3b/iC3b-bearing complexes and transports them to cells of the mononuclear phagocyte system in liver and spleen (Hebert, 1991). In contrast, factor H in platelets serves this function in rodents (Alexander et al., 2001). As with CR1 on human erythrocytes, platelet factor H has three essential features—it is on the membrane of a ubiquitous blood cell, it has binding affinity for C3b, and, it serves as a factor I-cofactor for the cleavage of C3b to iC3b. More recently, we have obtained evidence for a comparable exchange of CR1 for factor H in rodent podocytes (Ren et al., 2003).

The anaphylatoxins C3a and C5a have long been considered to play a role in leukocytic accumulation occurring in various inflammatory diseases, including GN (Wilson, 1996). The presence of their receptors, C3aR and C5aR, on inflammatory cells, such as neutrophils and monocytes, and alteration of several disease models in mice in which C3aR (Kildsgaard et al., 2000; Humbles et al., 2000) and C5aR (Hopken et al., 1997; Bozic et al., 1996) were deleted is further evidence for a role of these proteins in inflammatory diseases. Interestingly, both C3aR and C5aR are present in renal cells. C3aR is on podocytes (Bao et al., 2005a) and C5aR on mesangial cells (Wilmer et al., 1998; Braun and Davis, 1998), while both have been shown to be present on proximal tubular epithelial cells (Zahedi et al., 2000; Fayyazi et al., 2000; Bao et al., 2005a). The relevance of mesangial cell C5aR to conditions in vivo is unclear while accumulating evidence links proximal tubular epithelial cell C5aR to human diseases (Abe et al., 2001; Lhotta et al., 2000). Evidence for the latter also comes from a mouse model of IC-mediated glomerular disease and progressive tubulointerstitial damage with features comparable to lupus nephritis (Welch et al., 2002). In this study, C5aR deficiency did not affect the glomerular phenotype at all, while it ameliorated the tubulointerstitial disease. Their conclusions were that C5a, generated at least in part through local tubular complement synthesis, was chemoattractant to inflammatory cells bearing C5aR and also signaled tubular cell C5aR to result in apoptotic cellular death (Farkas et al., 1998).

In MRL/*lpr* mouse kidneys, C3aR and C5aR expression was significantly up-regulated at both the mRNA and protein levels and accompanied by a wider cellular distribution (Bao et al., 2005a, b). This upregulated expression started before the onset of kidney disease, supporting the fact that they may be involved in the development of disease, rather than simply a consequence. Chronic administration of a specific C3aR antagonist to MRL/*lpr* mice significantly reduced kidney disease prolonging their survival (Bao et al., 2005a). Similarly, when C5a signaling was blocked in our studies with a specific antagonist (Bao et al., 2005b), MRL/*lpr* mice displayed attenuated renal disease and prolonged viability. The effects of blocking C3aR and C5aR in lupus mice had certain features in common, including a reduction in renal neutrophil and macrophage infiltration, apoptosis, and interleukin (IL)-1$\beta$ expression (Bao et al., 2005a, b). Effects on chemokine expression were distinct, with C3aR- and C5aR-inhibited MRL/*lpr* mice having reduced CCL5 (RANTES) and CXCL2 (MIP-2) expression, respectively. C3aR-inhibited mice also had increased phosphorylation of protein kinase B (Akt), which we considered suggestive that C3aR signals renal cell apoptosis through an Akt pathway (Bao et al., 2005a).

The fetal loss that occurs following passive administration of human anti-phospholipid Abs into pregnant mice by Jane Salmon's group has provided considerable insights into the pathogenesis of APS (Salmon and Girardi, 2004). In this model, fetal loss can be blocked by Crry-Ig preventing C3 and C5 activation, an inhibitory Ab to factor B preventing alternative pathway activation, and with a specific C5aR antagonist blocking its activation by C5a. Placental infiltration with neutrophils was reduced in complement-inhibited animals and depletion of neutrophils prevented fetal loss, both providing evidence for complement-dependent neutrophil-mediated damage in this model (Girardi et al., 2003; Holers et al., 2002). Interestingly, the protective effects of heparin can also be attributed to its complement inhibitory effects rather than its anticoagulant actions (Girardi et al., 2004). Overall, these data can be interpreted to show that anti-phospholipid Abs bind endothelial cells on which they activate the classical pathway of complement, thereby recruiting the potent alternative pathway. The ultimate generation of C5a engages C5aR on neutrophils leading to inflammation in the placenta (Salmon and Girardi, 2004). It seems likely that at least some aspects of this pathophysiology are relevant to other organ systems such as the kidney.

There is no doubt that inhibiting complement at various levels is not without its potential problems, given the role of complement to process apoptotic material and ICs, and to fight infectious microorganisms (Wessels et al., 1995; Taylor et al., 2000; Bao et al., 2002a). A fascinating series of studies by Steve Tomlinson has shown that targeting complement inhibitors such as DAF, CD59, and Crry using Abs to target specific cell proteins or CR2 to target C3 activation products is a viable approach to deliver complement inhibitors locally (Song et al., 2003; Zhang et al., 2001, 1999). The validity of this appealing approach came from the ability of Ab-targeted Crry and CD59 to limit tubular damage in a rat glomerular proteinuria model (He et al., 2005) and in the MRL/*lpr* lupus nephritis model (Song et al., 2003).

## 6. Studies in mice with targeted deletion of complement proteins

Of the more than 30 proteins in the complement activation, receptor, and regulatory cascades, a growing number have been "knocked-out" in mice through the technique of homologous recombination. Combined with the use of complement inhibitors and animals with spontaneous complement deficiencies, these strains have been illustrative in our understanding of how the complement system affects the glomerulus (Table 2). Much like with genetic deficiencies of the homologous human protein, only deficiencies of C1q and factor H have led to spontaneous glomerular pathology. Other more subtle spontaneous defects relevant to the kidney have been observed in these mice, as will be discussed below.

Targeted deletion of *C1q* in mice with a mixed 129 and C57BL/6 genetic background led to development of GN with immune deposits and apoptotic bodies in diseased glomeruli (Botto et al., 1998). Yet, when bred into the C57BL/6 strain, this phenotype was lost. C1q deficiency accelerated development of the autoimmune renal disease normally seen as a late finding in the Fas-sufficient MRL strain, while it did not influence lupus nephritis in autoimmune MRL/*lpr* mice, nor did it bring out disease in autoimmune prone C57BL/6$^{lpr/lpr}$ mice (Mitchell et al., 2002). Overall, these data have been taken to suggest that the expression of autoimmunity in C1q-deficient mice reflects the altered processing of apoptotic material which is strongly influenced by other still undefined background genes (Botto and Walport, 2002).

As noted earlier, knockout of the *Cr2* gene leads to CR1 and CR2 protein deficiencies (Molina et al., 1996; Ahearn et al., 1996); therefore, any resulting phenotype can be ascribed either to the lack of CR1 and/or CR2. In C57BL/6$^{lpr/lpr}$ mice, deficiencies of C4 or CR1/CR2 led to autoimmune disease in this susceptible strain (Einav et al., 2002; Prodeus et al., 1998), while C4-deficient MRL/*lpr* mice developed accelerated disease features (Einav et al., 2002). Interestingly, *Cr2*-knockout MRL/*lpr* mice had significantly lower levels of complement-activating IgG3 autoAbs and reduced IgA glomerular deposition, although these proved to be of minor pathological significance (Boackle et al., 2004). Although almost certainly an oversimplification, these data have been interpreted to indicate that classical pathway activation on apoptotic debris, rich in nuclear components, is necessary for their appropriate clearance and maintenance of tolerance, as signaled through the B lymphocyte CR1/CR2 (Carroll, 2000; Pickering and Walport, 2000).

The generation of homologous mouse anti-mouse C1q Abs by the Daha group has provided a tool to study their role in lupus nephritis. When administered to wildtype mice, these led to glomerular deposition of C1q and granulocyte influx, yet no clinical expression of renal disease such as albuminuria (Trouw et al., 2004). However, when mice were pre-treated with a subnephritogenic dose of rabbit anti-GBM Abs, administration of mouse anti-C1q Abs resulted in increased deposition of immunoglobulins and complement as well as marked renal damage (Trouw et al., 2004). The

**Table 2**
Complement proteins that have undergone gene targeted deletions in mice

| Protein | Spontaneous phenotype | Effect of deficiency in renal disease models | References |
|---|---|---|---|
| C1q | Strain dependent GN in 25% | Exacerbated anti-GBM GN | Botto et al. (1998), Robson et al. (2001), Mitchell et al. (2002), Mitchell et al. (1999) |
| C2 | None | No effect in one spontaneous GN model | Mitchell et al. (1999), Taylor et al. (1998) |
| C3 | None | Impaired IC clearance, cryoglobulinemia | Quigg et al. (1998b) |
|  |  | Protection from anti-GBM GN | Sheerin et al. (1997) |
|  |  | No effect in lupus nephritis (see text) | Sekine et al. (2001) |
|  |  | Protection from cryoglobulinemic GN | Trendelenburg et al. (2005) |
|  |  | Protection from APS-mediated fetal loss | Holers et al. (2002) |
| C4 | ↑ autoAbs in C57Bl/6$^{lpr/lpr}$ mice | Impaired IC clearance | Prodeus et al. (1998), Quigg et al. (1998b) |
|  |  | Protection from anti-GBM GN | Sheerin et al. (1997) |
|  |  | Protection from APS-mediated fetal loss | Girardi et al. (2003) |
| Factor B | None | Protection from lupus nephritis | Watanabe et al. (2000a) |
|  |  | Protection from cryoglobulinemic GN | Trendelenburg et al. (2005) |
|  |  | Protection from APS-mediated fetal loss | Girardi et al. (2003) |
|  |  | Protection from anti-MPO GN | Xiao et al. (2005) |
| Factor D | None | Protection from lupus nephritis | Elliott et al. (2004) |
| C1INH | None | None reported | Han et al. (2002) |
| Factor H | MPGN | Exacerbated anti-GBM GN | Pickering et al. (2006), Pickering et al. (2002) |
|  |  | Exacerbated ICGN | Alexander et al. (2006), Alexander et al. (2005) |
| CR1/CR2 | ↑ autoAbs in C57Bl/6$^{lpr/lpr}$ mice | ↓ IgG3 autoAbs, ↓ glomerular IgA in lupus nephritis | Prodeus et al. (1998), Boackle et al. (2004) |
| DAF | None | Exacerbated anti-GBM GN | Sogabe et al. (2001), Lin et al. (2002) |
|  |  | ↑ autoAbs, dermatitis, not nephritis in SLE | Liu et al. (2005), Miwa et al. (2002) |
| MCP | None | None reported | Inoue et al. (2003) |
| Crry | Embryonic lethal[a] Tubulointerstitial nephritis[b] | Exacerbated ICGN | Xu et al. (2000), Mao et al. (2003) Bao et al. (2007) |
| CD59 | None | Exacerbated anti-GBM GN | Holt et al. (2001), Lin et al. (2004) |
| Clusterin | Mesangial ICGN[c] | Exacerbated mesangial ICGN | Rosenberg et al. (2002) |
| C3aR | None | None reported | Kildsgaard et al. (2000) |
| C5aR | None | Protection from lupus nephritis | Hopken et al. (1997), Wenderfer et al. (2005) |
|  |  | Protection from APS-mediated fetal loss | Girardi et al. (2003) |
| CR3 (CD11b) | None | Protection from anti-GBM GN | Tang et al. (1997) |

*Note*: Individual complement proteins that were subject to deletion through homologous recombination are listed above. Any spontaneous renal phenotype is provided, as well as the effect of the given protein deficiency in spontaneous or induced models of renal disease. In addition, the effect on anti-phospholipid antibody-mediated fetal loss as a model for APS in general is also provided. Abbreviations: Abs, antibodies; APS, anti-phospholipid antibody syndrome; C, complement; DAF, decay accelerating factor; GBM, glomerular basement membrane; GN, glomerulonephritis; IC, immune complex; INH, inhibitor; MCP, membrane cofactor protein; MPGN, membranoproliferative glomerulonephritis; MPO, myeloperoxidase; R, receptor.

[a] Animals died from 9.5–13.5 days post coitus (Xu et al., 2000); as such, no glomerular phenotype could be discerned.
[b] $Crry^{-/-}$ $C3^{-/-}$ kidneys transplanted into wildtype hosts.
[c] In aged animals.

application of this model to mice genetically deficient for C4, C3, or all three FcγRs demonstrated that anti-C1q-mediated renal damage was dependent both on complement activation and the contribution of FcγRs (Trouw et al., 2004).

Consistent with activation of the classical pathway being pathogenic in models of passively administered IgG Abs are the findings that disease features in anti-GBM GN and APS are reduced in C4 and C3 knockout mice (Sheerin et al., 1997; Girardi et al., 2003; Holers et al., 2002). As noted before, APS also appears to have an alternative pathway dependence, which was confirmed by studies with factor B-deficient mice (Girardi et al., 2003). A similar dependence on factor B has been observed in models of cryoglobulinemic GN (Trendelenburg et al., 2005) and anti-MPO SVV (Xiao et al., 2005). MRL/*lpr* mice with factor B or factor D deficiencies were also protected from lupus nephritis (Elliott et al., 2004; Watanabe et al., 2000a). Overall, these results can best be explained by the classical pathway providing sufficient C3b to the alternative pathway to overwhelm its normal regulation.

What is hard to reconcile with the various hypotheses is that C3 deficiency does not affect the development of lupus in MRL/*lpr* (Sekine et al., 2001) or C57BL/6$^{lpr/lpr}$ mice (with or without C4 deficiency) (Einav et al., 2002). Detailed serological studies illustrated the C3 deficiency did not affect the autoimmunity per se. Since C3 occupies the central portion of all three complement pathways (Fig. 1), these studies argued that complement activation is dispensable in glomerular pathology. However, C3 deficiency led to an increase in glomerular IgG deposition, reflecting IC processing abnormalities which clearly occurs in these C3-deficient mice (Quigg et al., 1998b; Sheerin et al., 1999). Glomerular deposited ICs interact with FcγRs on inflammatory cells, creating a complement-independent, but cell-dependent disease (Clynes et al., 1998; Sylvestre et al., 1996). Interestingly, lupus nephritis in the MRL/*lpr* model can also proceed independently from FcγRs (Matsumoto et al., 2003). Considering all available data, while lupus nephritis can proceed independently from FcγRs, when greater quantities of ICs are present in glomeruli, as in the case of C3-deficient animals, interactions with FcγRs on circulating leukocytes become more important, which is also consistent with results observed in the anti-GBM GN model (Clynes et al., 1998; Rosenkranz and Mayadas, 1999; Tarzi et al., 2002). Most likely in "native" lupus nephritis, a balance of complement and FcγR interactions exist.

Consistent with studies using a specific C5aR receptor antagonist (Bao et al., 2005b), studies by Michael Braun with C5aR-deficient MRL/*lpr* mice revealed attenuated renal disease and prolonged survival (Wenderfer et al., 2005). In these mice, there was a reduction in CD4$^+$ T cell renal infiltration, lower titers of anti-double stranded DNA Abs, and inhibition of IL-12 p20 and IFN-γ production, supporting that Th1 responses are important to link C5a signaling in lupus nephritis (Wenderfer et al., 2005).

As in humans, factor H is important to limit spontaneous complement activation in mice. Thus, factor H-deficient mice generated by the Pickering and Botto group have unrestricted activation of the alternative pathway of complement, with systemic complement consumption (Pickering et al., 2002). These mice developed factor B- and C5-dependent glomerular disease with features of MPGN type II later in life, which was fatal in some animals (Pickering et al., 2002, 2006). Complement deposition in the glomerular capillary wall (a feature of MPGN type II) preceded IC deposition (which is a feature of MPGN type I but not type II). In an accelerated model of anti-GBM GN using relatively low ("subnephritogenic") doses of Ab, factor H-deficient mice had a greater extent of disease compared to controls; similar to the spontaneous disease, this was factor B- and C5-dependent (Pickering et al., 2002, 2006). In a model of chronic serum sickness, C57BL/6 mice did not develop ICGN disease features unless deficient in factor H (Alexander et al., 2005).

In human SLE, erythrocyte levels of CR1 are reduced which potentially contributes to the excessive accumulation of ICs in glomeruli (and other renal and non-renal sites) (Iida et al., 1982; Ross et al., 1985). The direct study of this phenomenon in mice is problematic, given the rodent use of platelet factor H as the surrogate for primate erythrocyte CR1 (Alexander et al., 2001). Since platelet factor H is of intrinsic origin, we studied chronic serum sickness in bone marrow chimeric mice (Alexander et al., 2006). Consistent with the role of the platelet and its bound factor H to process ICs, mice with platelets lacking factor H had substantially greater amounts of complement-activating ICs in glomeruli compared to those with intact platelet factor H; yet, there were no phenotypic changes of GN in these mice, as their intact plasma factor H inactivated C3b (Alexander et al., 2006). In contrast, mice lacking plasma factor H uniformly developed GN even with limited glomerular deposition of ICs. In each of these disease models, classical pathway activating IgG Abs were present in the glomerular capillary wall. Since this is a site protected by factor H, disease proceeded only when factor H was absent, again implicating the alternative pathway as arguably the most potent mediator of Ab-dependent glomerular disease.

In rodent kidneys, DAF is primarily a podocyte and vascular endothelium protein (Lin et al., 2001; Bao et al., 2002b). Clearly podocyte DAF is important to restrict complement activation locally, such as can occur in anti-GBM GN (Lin et al., 2002, 2004; Sogabe et al., 2001) and recovery from puromycin aminonucleoside nephrosis, in which complement proteins are accessible to the apical portion of podocytes (Bao et al., 2002b). Studies by Ed Medof's group showed that CD59 deficiency alone had no effect on anti-GBM GN, yet worsened disease features (albuminuria and podocyte effacement) in DAF-deficient mice (Lin et al., 2004). These results suggest that DAF limits spontaneous and IgG-directed C3 activation on the podocyte, while CD59 limits consequent C5b-9 mediated cell damage. Consistent with this limited role, studies from Wenchao Song in MRL/*lpr* mice showed there was no effect of DAF-deficiency on the inflammatory lupus nephritis (Miwa et al., 2002).

Unlike in humans in which MCP has widespread distribution throughout the body, MCP expression in mice is limited to spermatozoa, making its absence in knockout mice of no consequence to renal disease models (Inoue et al., 2003). Overall, it is likely that the rodent uses Crry in place of MCP and/or DAF in many sites as its complement regulator. This is not that surprising, as Crry combines the functions of both (Kim et al., 1995). Given its widespread distribution in glomeruli and tubules (Quigg et al., 1995a, b; Li et al., 1993; Thurman et al., 2006a), Crry is likely to be very important in autoimmune renal diseases. This has proven to be difficult to study directly, as Crry deficiency is embryonically lethal due to unrestricted activation of maternal complement (Xu et al., 2000). Consistent with the previously mentioned studies of ischemia-reperfusion (Thurman et al., 2006a), studies by Lihua Bao and Ying Wang showed that transplantation of Crry-deficient kidneys into wild-type recipients led to massive complement activation in the tubulointerstitium, and the rapid development of scarring and failure of the kidney (Bao et al., 2007).

In the anti-GBM GN model, a CR3-dependence has been found (Wu et al., 1993; Tang et al., 1997). Although CR3 is present and functional in both neutrophils and monocyte/macrophages, the predominant cell affected in this model appears to be the neutrophil, as early glomerular accumulation of these cells was reduced (Lefkowith, 1997). The conclusions regarding CR3–iC3b interactions were limited in these studies, as CR3 has affinity for intercellular adhesion molecule (ICAM)-1, which is upregulated in anti-GBM GN (Mulligan et al., 1993), and CR3 also can function to facilitate Fc$\gamma$R effector functions (Krauss et al., 1994; Tang et al., 1997) which clearly can be important in this model (Suzuki et al., 1998). Thus, an effect of CR3 deficiency to limit glomerular injury could be ascribed to preventing leukocyte binding to iC3b or ICAM-1 or to impaired signaling through Fc$\gamma$R, or any combination thereof.

## 7. The future of complement and human systemic autoimmune diseases

Our increasing knowledge about the role of the complement system in the pathogenesis of various diseases has given us numerous options for the therapeutic manipulation of the complement system (Quigg, 2002; Holers and Thurman, 2004). Inhibiting at the level of the initiator of the complement system will allow specific blockade of one pathway without interfering with the functions of the other two pathways. Intervening at the level of C3 activation will inhibit the entire complement system with the possibility of high efficacy, but with the increased risk of infections (Figueroa and Densen, 1991). Inhibiting at the level of C5b-9 can prevent its specific tissue damage, yet comes at a risk of *Neisserial* infections (Figueroa and Densen, 1991). Additionally, receptors for the anaphylatoxins C3a and C5a can be blocked using small molecule selective inhibitors (Ames et al., 2001; Paczkowski et al., 1999). Providing normal proteins to replace those that are defective such as factor H in aHUS is a logical approach (Caprioli et al., 2006). Finally, the ability to selectively target complement inhibitors to sites of injury while sparing other uninvolved regions is clearly possible (Atkinson et al., 2005). Many of these possible approaches have been tested in animal models of renal disease as described here. Some are even in routine clinical use, such as providing C1-esterase inhibitor concentrates in hereditary angioedema (Kirschfink and Mollnes, 2001).

The future of how the complement system can be manipulated in systemic autoimmune diseases affecting the kidney is difficult to predict. There are certain approaches that seem likely, such as the use of recombinant C1-esterase inhibitor as treatment for hereditary angioedema (van Doorn et al., 2005), and some form to replace abnormal complement regulators when present in aHUS and MPGN (Caprioli et al., 2006). The clinical effectiveness of sCR1 and anti-C5 Abs is slowly growing with time (Lazar et al., 2004; Hill et al., 2005; Hillmen et al., 2004). So far, the only renal disease either of these has been applied to has been anti-C5 (eculizumab) in idiopathic membranous nephropathy. Disappointingly, this was a negative study, although the open label extension had promising features (Javaid and Quigg, 2005). Unfortunately, a multi-center phase II trial sponsored by the United States' National Institutes of Health using anti-C5 in proliferative lupus nephritis, supported by its beneficial effects in murine lupus nephritis (Wang et al., 1996), has been abandoned. The potential to block the alternative pathway with anti-factor B Abs (Holers and Thurman, 2004) and to target complement inhibitors is being advanced by Taligen Therapeutics, which seems to be the best hope for any of this work coming to fruition.

In summary, there is a great deal of evidence implicating the complement system as playing a pathogenic role in many systemic autoimmune diseases affecting the kidney. This includes the circumstantial evidence of complement activation products in glomeruli, plasma, and urine, and more direct evidence in experimental models of disease, principally carried out in rodents. Of the various diseases, it seems most likely complement is pathogenic in lupus nephritis, some or all forms of MPGN and aHUS, as well as postinfectious GN and membranous nephropathy. Thus far, the translational research includes early experiments implicating the complement system in these diseases, the development of rationale inhibitors, and testing of these in animal models. The end is testing them directly in human diseases.

## Key points

- The complement system is an integral part of the immune defense system, acting at the interface between innate and adaptive immunity.
- The complement system is like a double-edged sword. When activated appropriately, it can help to remove pathogens and unwanted host material; on the other hand, inappropriate activation can lead to inflammation and injury of self-tissue.
- Initial evidence supporting the role of complement activation in autoimmune diseases involving the kidney came from the presence of depressed complement levels in serum and the presence of complement activation products in the glomeruli, plasma, and urine. More direct evidence has come from experimental disease models, principally carried out in rodents.
- Of the various autoimmune diseases, complement is most likely pathogenic in lupus nephritis, MPGN, aHUS, postinfectious GN, and membranous nephropathy.
- Therapeutic manipulation of the complement system is now possible using disease-modifying biological agents. Those with promise in animal models are slowly making their way to clinical testing.

## Acknowledgments

Supported by National Institutes of Health grants R01DK41873 and R01D55357.

## References

Abe, K., Miyazaki, M., Koji, T., et al. 2001. Enhanced expression of complement C5a receptor mRNA in human diseased kidney assessed by in situ hybridization. Kidney Int. 60, 137.

Ahearn, J.M., Fischer, M.B., Croix, D., et al. 1996. Disruption of the Cr2 locus results in a reduction in B-1a cells and in an impaired B cell response to T-dependent antigen. Immunity 4, 251.

Alexander, J.J., Aneziokoro, O.G.B., Chang, A., et al. 2006. Distinct and separable roles of the complement system in factor H-deficient bone marrow chimeric mice with immune complex disease. J. Am. Soc. Nephrol. 17, 1354.

Alexander, J.J., Hack, B.K., Cunningham, P.N., et al. 2001. A protein with characteristics of factor H is present on rodent platelets and functions as the immune adherence receptor. J. Biol. Chem. 276, 32129.

Alexander, J.J., Pickering, M.C., Haas, M., et al. 2005. Complement factor H limits immune complex deposition and prevents inflammation and scarring in glomeruli of mice with chronic serum sickness. J. Am. Soc. Nephrol. 16, 52.

Ames, R.S., Lee, D., Foley, J.J., et al. 2001. Identification of a selective nonpeptide antagonist of the anaphylatoxin C3a receptor that demonstrates antiinflammatory activity in animal models. J. Immunol. 166, 6341.

Atkinson, C., Song, H., Lu, B., et al. 2005. Targeted complement inhibition by C3d recognition ameliorates tissue injury without apparent increase in susceptibility to infection. J. Clin. Invest. 115, 2444.

Bao, L., Haas, M., Boackle, S.A., et al. 2002a. Transgenic expression of a soluble complement inhibitor protects against renal disease and promotes survival in MRL/*lpr* mice. J. Immunol. 168, 3601.

Bao, L., Haas, M., Kraus, D.M., et al. 2003a. Administration of a soluble recombinant complement C3 inhibitor protects against renal disease in MRL/lpr mice. J. Am. Soc. Nephrol. 14, 670.

Bao, L., Osawe, I., Haas, M., et al. 2005a. Signaling through up-regulated C3a receptor is key to the development of experimental lupus nephritis. J. Immunol. 175, 1602.

Bao, L., Osawe, I., Puri, T., et al. 2005b. C5a promotes development of experimental lupus nephritis which can be blocked with a specific receptor antagonist. Eur. J. Immunol. 35, 3012.

Bao, L., Spiller, O.B., St, J.P., et al. 2002b. Decay-accelerating factor expression in the rat kidney is restricted to the apical surface of podocytes. Kidney Int. 62, 2010.

Bao, L., Wang, Y., Chang, A., et al. 2007. Unrestricted C3 activation occurs in Crry-deficient kidneys which rapidly leads to chronic renal failure. J. Am. Soc. Nephrol. 18, 811.

Bao, L., Zhou, J., Holers, V.M., et al. 2003b. Excessive matrix accumulation in the kidneys of MRL/*lpr* lupus mice is dependent on complement activation. J. Am. Soc. Nephrol. 14, 2516.

Barratt, J., Feehally, J. 2005. IgA nephropathy. J. Am. Soc. Nephrol. 16, 2088.

Biesecker, G., Katz, S., Koffler, D. 1981. Renal localization of the membrane attack complex in systemic lupus erythematosus nephritis. J. Exp. Med. 154, 1779.

Boackle, S.A., Culhane, K.K., Brown, J.M., et al. 2004. CR1/CR2 deficiency alters IgG3 autoantibody production and IgA glomerular deposition in the MRL/lpr model of SLE. Autoimmunity 37, 111.

Bonnardeaux, A., Pichette, V. 2003. Complement dysregulation in haemolytic uraemic syndrome. Lancet 362, 1514.

Botto, M., Dell'Agnola, C., Bygrave, A.E., et al. 1998. Homozygous C1q deficiency causes glomerulonephritis associated with multiple apoptotic bodies. Nat. Genet. 19, 56.

Botto, M., Walport, M.J. 2002. C1q, autoimmunity and apoptosis. Immunobiology 205, 395.

Boyce, N.W., Holdsworth, S.R. 1985. Anti-glomerular basement membrane antibody-induced experimental glomerulonephritis: evidence for dose-dependent direct antibody and complement-induced, cell-independent injury. J. Immunol. 135, 3918.

Bozic, C.R., Lu, B., Hopken, U.E., et al. 1996. Neurogenic amplification of immune complex inflammation. Science 273, 1722.

Brandt, J., Pippin, J., Schulze, M., et al. 1996. Role of the complement membrane attack complex (C5b-9) in mediating experimental mesangioproliferative glomerulonephritis. Kidney Int. 49, 335.

Braun, M., Davis, A.E., III 1998. Cultured human glomerular mesangial cells express the C5a receptor. Kidney Int. 54, 1542.

Brown, K.M., Kondeatis, E., Vaughan, R.W., et al. 2006. Influence of donor C3 allotype on late renal-transplantation outcome. N. Engl. J. Med. 354, 2014.

Caprioli, J., Noris, M., Brioschi, S., et al. 2006. Genetics of HUS: the impact of MCP, CFH and IF mutations on clinical presentation, response to treatment, and outcome. Blood 108, 1267.

Carroll, M.C. 2000. A protective role for innate immunity in autoimmune disease. Clin. Immunol. 95, S30–S38.

Carroll, M.C. 2004. The complement system in regulation of adaptive immunity. Nat. Immunol. 5, 981.

Carroll, M.C., Holers, V.M. 2005. Innate autoimmunity. Adv. Immunol. 86, 137.

Chugh, S., Yuan, H., Topham, P.S., et al. 2001. Aminopeptidase A: a nephritogenic target antigen of nephrotoxic serum. Kidney Int. 59, 601.

Clynes, R., Dumitru, C., Ravetch, J.V. 1998. Uncoupling of immune complex formation and kidney damage in autoimmune glomerulonephritis. Science 279, 1052.

Coons, A.H., Kaplan, M.H. 1950. Localization of antigen in tissue cells. II. Improvements in a method for the detection of antigen by means of fluorescent antibody. J. Exp. Med. 91, 1.

Corna, D., Morigi, M., Facchinetti, D., et al. 1997. Mycophenolate mofetil limits renal damage and prolongs life in murine lupus autoimmune disease. Kidney Int. 51, 1583.

Cosio, F.G., Sedmak, D.D., Mahan, J.D., et al. 1989. Localization of decay accelerating factor in normal and diseased kidneys. Kidney Int. 36, 100.

Cosio, F.G., Shibata, T., Rovin, B.H., et al. 1994. Effects of complement activation products on the synthesis of decay accelerating factor and membrane cofactor protein by human mesangial cells. Kidney. Int. 46, 986.

Couser, W.G., Johnson, R.J., Young, B.A., et al. 1995. The effects of soluble recombinant complement receptor 1 on complement-mediated experimental glomerulonephritis. J. Am. Soc. Nephrol. 5, 1888.

Couser, W.G., Pippin, J.W., Shankland, S.J. 2001. Complement (C5b-9) induces DNA synthesis in rat mesangial cells in vitro. Kidney Int. 59, 905.

Cybulsky, A.V., Monge, J.C., Papillon, J., et al. 1995. Complement C5b-9 activates cytosolic phospholipase A2 in glomerular epithelial cells. Am. J. Physiol. Renal Fluid Electrolyte Physiol. 269, F739–F749.

Cybulsky, A.V., Rennke, H.G., Feintzeig, I.D., et al. 1986. Complement-induced glomerular epithelial cell injury: role of the membrane attack complex in rat membranous nephropathy. J. Clin. Invest. 77, 1096.

Daha, M.R., Fearon, D.T., Austen, K.F. 1976. C3 nephritic factor (C3NeF) stabilization of fluid phase and cell-bound alternative pathway convertase. J. Immunol. 116, 1.

Daha, M.R., Van Kooten, C. 2000. Is there a role for locally produced complement in renal disease? Nephrol. Dial. Transplant. 15, 1506.

Dixon, F.J., Wilson, C.B. 1990. The development of immunopathologic investigation of kidney disease. Am. J. Kidney Dis. 16, 574.

Dragon-Durey, M.A., Loirat, C., Cloarec, S., et al. 2005. Anti-factor H autoantibodies associated with atypical hemolytic uremic syndrome. J. Am. Soc. Nephrol. 16, 555.

Einav, S., Pozdnyakova, O.O., Ma, M., et al. 2002. Complement C4 is protective for lupus disease independent of C3. J. Immunol. 168, 1036.

Elliott, M.K., Jarmi, T., Ruiz, P., et al. 2004. Effects of complement factor D deficiency on the renal disease of MRL/lpr mice. Kidney Int. 65, 129.

Emancipator, S.N., Iida, K., Nussenzweig, V., et al. 1983. Monoclonal antibodies to human complement receptor (CR1) detect defects in glomerular diseases. Clin. Immunol. Immunopathol. 27, 170.

Endoh, M., Yamashina, M., Ohi, H., et al. 1993. Immunohistochemical demonstration of membrane cofactor protein (MCP) of complement in normal and diseased kidney tissues. Clin. Exp. Immunol. 94, 182.

Farkas, I., Baranyi, L., Liposits, Z.S., et al. 1998. Complement C5a anaphylatoxin fragment causes apoptosis in TGW neuroblastoma cells. Neuroscience 86, 903.

Farrar, C.A., Zhou, W., Lin, T., et al. 2006. Local extravascular pool of C3 is a determinant of postischemic acute renal failure. FASEB J. 20, 217.

Fayyazi, A., Scheel, O., Werfel, T., et al. 2000. The C5a receptor is expressed in normal renal proximal tubular but not in normal pulmonary or hepatic epithelial cells. Immunology 99, 38.

Figueroa, J.E., Densen, P. 1991. Infectious diseases associated with complement deficiencies. Clin. Microbiol. Rev. 4, 359.

Fischer, M.B., Ma, M., Hsu, N.C., et al. 1998. Local synthesis of C3 within the splenic lymphoid compartment can reconstitute the impaired immune response in C3-deficient mice. J. Immunol. 160, 2619.

Fremeaux-Bacchi, V., Dragon-Durey, M.A., Blouin, J., et al. 2004. Complement factor I: a susceptibility gene for atypical haemolytic uraemic syndrome. J. Med. Genet. 41, e84.

Fremeaux-Bacchi, V., Moulton, E.A. and Kavanagh, D. et al. (2006). Genetic and functional analyses of membrane cofactor protein (CD46) mutations in atypical hemolytic uremic syndrome. J. Am. Soc. Nephrol. 17, 2017.

Gelfand, M.C., Shin, M.L., Nagle, R.B., et al. 1976. The glomerular complement receptor in immunologically mediated renal glomerular injury. N. Engl. J. Med. 295, 10.

Gelfand, M.C., Steinberg, A.D., Nagle, R., et al. 1972. Therapeutic studies in NZB-W mice. I. Synergy of azathioprine, cyclophosphamide and methylprednisolone in combination. Arthritis Rheum. 15, 239.

Girardi, G., Berman, J., Redecha, P., et al. 2003. Complement C5a receptors and neutrophils mediate fetal injury in the antiphospholipid syndrome. J. Clin. Invest. 112, 1644.

Girardi, G., Redecha, P., Salmon, J.E. 2004. Heparin prevents antiphospholipid antibody-induced fetal loss by inhibiting complement activation. Nat. Med. 10, 1222.

Groggel, G.C., Adler, S., Rennke, H.G., et al. 1983. Role of the terminal complement pathway in experimental membranous nephropathy in the rabbit. J. Clin. Invest. 72, 1948.

Han, E.D., MacFarlane, R.C., Mulligan, A.N., et al. 2002. Increased vascular permeability in C1 inhibitor-deficient mice mediated by the bradykinin type 2 receptor. J. Clin. Invest. 109, 1057.

He, C., Imai, M., Song, H., et al. 2005. Complement inhibitors targeted to the proximal tubule prevent injury in experimental nephrotic syndrome and demonstrate a key role for C5b-9. J. Immunol. 174, 5750.

Hebert, L.A. 1991. The clearance of immune complexes from the circulation of man and other primates. Am. J. Kidney Dis. 27, 352.

Hill, A., Hillmen, P., Richards, S.J., et al. 2005. Sustained response and long-term safety of eculizumab in paroxysmal nocturnal hemoglobinuria. Blood 106, 2559.

Hillmen, P., Hall, C., Marsh, J.C., et al. 2004. Effect of eculizumab on hemolysis and transfusion requirements in patients with paroxysmal nocturnal hemoglobinuria. N. Engl. J. Med. 350, 552.

Holers, V.M., Girardi, G., Mo, L., et al. 2002. Complement C3 activation is required for antiphospholipid antibody-induced fetal loss. J. Exp. Med. 195, 211.

Holers, V.M., Thurman, J.M. 2004. The alternative pathway of complement in disease: opportunities for therapeutic targeting. Mol. Immunol. 41, 147.

Holt, D.S., Botto, M., Bygrave, A.E., et al. 2001. Targeted deletion of the CD59 gene causes spontaneous intravascular hemolysis and hemoglobinuria. Blood 98, 442.

Hopken, U.E., Lu, B., Gerard, N.P., et al. 1997. Impaired inflammatory responses in the reverse arthus reaction through genetic deletion of the C5a receptor. J. Exp. Med. 186, 749.

Horvath, L., Czirjak, L., Fekete, B., et al. 2001. High levels of antibodies against C1q are associated with disease activity and nephritis but not with other organ manifestations in SLE patients. Clin. Exp. Rheumatol. 19, 667.

Hourcade, D., Holers, V.M., Atkinson, J.P. 1989. The regulators of complement activation (RCA) gene cluster. Adv. Immunol. 45, 381.

Hughes, J., Nangaku, M., Alpers, C.E., et al. 2000. C5b-9 membrane attack complex mediates endothelial cell apoptosis in experimental glomerulonephritis. Am. J. Physiol. Renal. Physiol. 278, F747.

Humbles, A.A., Lu, B., Nilsson, C.A., et al. 2000. A role for the C3a anaphylatoxin receptor in the effector phase of asthma. Nature 406, 998.

Ichida, S., Yuzawa, Y., Okada, H., et al. 1994. Localization of the complement regulatory proteins in the normal human kidney. Kidney Int. 46, 89.

Iida, K., Mornaghi, R., Nussenzweig, V. 1982. Complement receptor (CR1) deficiency in erythrocytes from patients with systemic lupus erythematosus. J. Exp. Med. 155, 1427.

Inoue, N., Ikawa, M., Nakanishi, T., et al. 2003. Disruption of mouse CD46 causes an accelerated spontaneous acrosome reaction in sperm. Mol. Cell Biol. 23, 2614.

Javaid, B., Quigg, R.J. 2005. Treatment of glomerulonephritis: will we ever have options other than steroids and cytotoxics? Kidney Int. 67, 1692.

Johnson, R.J., Alpers, C.E., Pruchno, C., et al. 1989. Mechanisms and kinetics for platelet and neutrophil localization in immune complex nephritis. Kidney Int. 36, 780.

Kavanagh, D., Kemp, E.J., Mayland, E., et al. 2005. Mutations in complement factor I predispose to development of a typical hemolytic uremic syndrome. J. Am. Soc. Nephrol. 16, 2150.

Kazatchkine, M.D., Fearon, D.T., Appay, M.D., et al. 1982. Immunohistochemical study of the human glomerular C3b receptor in normal kidney and in seventy-five cases of renal diseases. J. Clin. Invest. 69, 900.

Keller, G., Zimmer, G., Mall, G., et al. 2003. Nephron number in patients with primary hypertension. N. Engl. J. Med. 348, 101.

Kildsgaard, J., Hollmann, T.J., Matthews, K.W., et al. 2000. Targeted disruption of the C3a receptor gene demonstrates a novel protective anti-inflammatory role for C3a in endotoxin-shock. J. Immunol. 165, 5406.

Kim, Y.-U., Kinoshita, T., Molina, H., et al. 1995. Mouse complement regulatory protein Crry/p65 uses the specific mechanisms of both human decay-accelerating factor and membrane cofactor protein. J. Exp. Med. 181, 151.

Kirschfink, M., Mollnes, T.E. 2001. C1-inhibitor: an anti-inflammatory reagent with therapeutic potential. Expert. Opin. Pharmacother. 2, 1073.

Krauss, J.C., Poo, H., Xue, W., et al. 1994. Reconstitution of antibody-dependent phagocytosis in fibroblasts expressing Fc gamma receptor IIIB and the complement receptor type 3. J. Immunol. 153, 1769.

Kurtz, C.B., O'Toole, E., Christensen, S.M., et al. 1990. The murine complement receptor gene family. IV. Alternative splicing of Cr2 gene transcripts predicts two distinct gene products that share homologous domains with both human CR2 and CR1. J. Immunol. 144, 3581.

Kurtz, H.M., Donnell, G.N. 1962. The effect of depression of complement on nephrotoxic renal disease in rats. Bact. Proc. 62, 87.

Lazar, H.L., Bokesch, P.M., van, L.F., et al. 2004. Soluble human complement receptor 1 limits ischemic damage in cardiac surgery patients at high risk requiring cardiopulmonary bypass. Circulation 110, II274–II279.

Lefkowith, J.B. 1997. Leukocyte migration in immune complex glomerulonephritis: role of adhesion receptors. Kidney Int. 51, 1469.

Lhotta, K., Konig, P., Mayer, G., et al. 2000. Glomerular cells do not express the C5a receptor in human glomerulonephritis. Nephrol. Dial. Transplant. 15, 1888.

Lhotta, K., Schlogl, A., Kronenberg, F., et al. 1996. Glomerular deposition of the complement C4 isotypes C4A and C4B in glomeruonephritis. Nephrol. Dial. Transplant. 11, 1024.

Li, B., Sallee, C., Dehoff, M., et al. 1993. Mouse Crry/p65: characterization of monoclonal antibodies and the tissue distribution of a functional homologue of human MCP and DAF. J. Immunol. 151, 4295.

Lin, F., Emancipator, S.N., Salant, D.J., et al. 2002. Decay-accelerating factor confers protection against complement-mediated podocyte injury in acute nephrotoxic nephritis. Lab. Invest. 82, 563.

Lin, F., Fukuoka, Y., Spicer, A., et al. 2001. Tissue distribution of products of the mouse decay-accelerating factor (DAF) genes. Exploitation of a Daf1 knock-out mouse and site-specific monoclonal antibodies. Immunology 104, 215.

Lin, F., Salant, D.J., Meyerson, H., et al. 2004. Respective roles of decay-accelerating factor and CD59 in circumventing glomerular injury in acute nephrotoxic serum nephritis. J. Immunol. 172, 2636.

Liu, J., Miwa, T., Hilliard, B., et al. 2005. The complement inhibitory protein DAF (CD55) suppresses T cell immunity in vivo. J. Exp. Med. 201, 567.

Madaio, M.P., Harrington, J.T. 2001. The diagnosis of glomerular diseases: acute glomerulonephritis and the nephrotic syndrome. Arch. Intern. Med. 161, 25.

Mao, D., Wu, X., Deppong, C., et al. 2003. Negligible role of antibodies and C5 in pregnancy loss associated exclusively with C3-dependent mechanisms through complement alternative pathway. Immunity 19, 813.

Matsumoto, K., Watanabe, N., Akikusa, B., et al. 2003. Fc receptor-independent development of autoimmune glomerulonephritis in lupus-prone MRL/lpr mice. Arthritis Rheum. 48, 486.

Mauiyyedi, S., Colvin, R.B. 2002. Humoral rejection in kidney transplantation: new concepts in diagnosis and treatment. Curr. Opin. Nephrol. Hypertens. 11, 609.

Meri, S., Waldmann, H., Lachmann, P.J. 1991. Distribution of protectin (CD59), a complement membrane attack inhibitor, in normal human tissues. Lab. Invest. 65, 532.

Mitchell, D.A., Pickering, M.C., Warren, J., et al. 2002. C1q deficiency and autoimmunity: the effects of genetic background on disease expression. J. Immunol. 168, 2538.

Mitchell, D.A., Taylor, P.R., Cook, H.T., et al. 1999. C1q protects against the development of glomerulonephritis independently of C3 activation. J. Immunol. 162, 5676.

Miwa, T., Maldonado, M.A., Zhou, L., et al. 2002. Deletion of decay-accelerating factor (CD55) exacerbates autoimmune disease development in MRL/lpr mice. Am. J. Pathol. 161, 1077.

Miwa, T., Song, W.C. 2001. Membrane complement regulatory proteins: insight from animal studies and relevance to human diseases. Int. Immunopharmacol. 1, 445.

Molina, H. 2002. The murine complement regulator Crry: new insights into the immunobiology of complement regulation. Cell Mol. Life Sci. 59, 220.

Molina, H., Holers, V.M., Li, B., et al. 1996. Markedly impaired humoral immune response in mice deficient in complement receptors 1 and 2. Proc. Natl. Acad. Sci. USA 93, 3357.

Molina, H., Kinoshita, T., Inoue, K., et al. 1990. A molecular and immunochemical characterization of mouse CR2. Evidence for a single gene model of mouse complement receptors 1 and 2. J. Immunol. 145, 2974.

Moll, S., Miot, S., Sadallah, S., et al. 2001. No complement receptor 1 stumps on podocytes in human glomerulopathies. Kidney Int. 59, 160.

Moran, J., Colasanti, G., Amos, N., et al. 1977. C3b receptors in glomerular disease. Clin. Exp. Immunol. 28, 212.

Morgan, B.P. 1992. Isolation and characterization of the complement-inhibiting protein CD59 antigen from platelet membranes. Biochem. J. 282, 409.

Morgan, B.P., Gasque, P. 1997. Extrahepatic complement biosynthesis: where, when and why?. Clin. Exp. Immunol. 107, 1.

Morgan, B.P. and Harris, C.L. 1999. Regulation in the activation pathways. In: Complement Regulatory Proteins. Academic Press, San Diego, pp. 41–136.

Morita, Y., Ikeguchi, H., Nakamura, J., et al. 2000. Complement activation products in the urine from proteinuric patients. J. Am. Soc. Nephrol. 11, 700.

Muhlfeld, A.S., Segerer, S., Hudkins, K., et al. 2004. Overexpression of complement inhibitor Crry does not prevent cryoglobulin-associated membranoproliferative glomerulonephritis. Kidney Int. 65, 1214.

Mulligan, M.S., Johnson, K.J., Todd, R.F. III, et al. 1993. Requirements for leukocyte adhesion molecules in nephrotoxic nephritis. J. Clin. Invest. 91, 577.

Nangaku, M. 2003. Complement regulatory proteins: are they important in disease? J. Am. Soc. Nephrol. 14, 2411.

Nath, K.A., Hostetter, M.K., Hostetter, T.H. 1985. Pathophysiology of chronic tubulo-interstitial disease in rats. Interactions of dietary acid load, ammonia, and complement component C3. J. Clin. Invest. 76, 667.

Nath, K.A., Hostetter, M.K., Hostetter, T.H. 1989. Ammonia–complement interaction in the pathogenesis of progressive renal injury. Kidney Int. 36, S-52–S-54.

Nauta, A.J., Castellano, G., Xu, W., et al. 2004. Opsonization with C1q and mannose-binding lectin targets apoptotic cells to dendritic cells. J. Immunol. 173, 3044.

Nauta, A.J., Daha, M.R., Tijsma, O., et al. 2002. The membrane attack complex of complement induces caspase activation and apoptosis. Eur. J. Immunol. 32, 783.

Nicholson-Weller, A., Halperin, J.A. 1993. Membrane signaling by complement C5b-9, the membrane attack complex. Immunol. Res. 12, 244.

Nishikage, H., Baranyi, L., Okada, H., et al. 1995. Role of a complement regulatory protein in rat mesangial glomerulonephritis. J. Am. Soc. Nephrol. 6, 234.

Nomura, A., Nishikawa, K., Yuzawa, Y., et al. 1995. Tubulointerstitial injury induced in rats by a monoclonal antibody which inhibits function of a membrane inhibitor of complement. J. Clin. Invest. 96, 2348.

Noris, M., Brioschi, S., Caprioli, J., et al. 2003. Familial haemolytic uraemic syndrome and an MCP mutation. Lancet 362, 1542.

Paczkowski, N.J., Finch, A.M., Whitmore, J.B., et al. 1999. Pharmacological characterization of antagonists of the C5a receptor. Br. J. Pharmacol. 128, 1461.

Pascual, M., Steiger, G., Sadallah, S., et al. 1994. Identification of membrane-bound CR1 (CD35) in human urine: evidence for its release by glomerular podocytes. J. Exp. Med. 179, 889.

Paul, M.S., Aegerter, M., O'Brien, S.E., et al. 1989. The murine complement receptor gene family. I. Analysis of *mCRY* gene products and their homology to human CR1. J. Immunol. 142, 582.

Petterson, E.E., Bhan, A.K., Schneeberger, E.E., et al. 1978. Glomerular C3 receptors in human renal disease. Kidney Int. 13, 245.

Pickering, M.C., Cook, H.T., Warren, J., et al. 2002. Uncontrolled C3 activation causes membranoproliferative glomerulonephritis in mice deficient in complement factor H. Nat. Genet. 31, 424.

Pickering, M.C., Walport, M.J. 2000. Links between complement abnormalities and systemic lupus erythematosus. Rheumatology (Oxford) 39, 133.

Pickering, M.C., Warren, J., Rose, K.L., et al. 2006. Prevention of C5 activation ameliorates spontaneous and experimental glomerulonephritis in factor H-deficient mice. Proc. Natl. Acad. Sci. USA 103, 9649.

Pratt, J.R., Basheer, S.A., Sacks, S.H. 2002. Local synthesis of complement component C3 regulates acute renal transplant rejection. Nat. Med. 8, 582.

Prodeus, A.P., Goerg, S., Shen, L.M., et al. 1998. A critical role for complement in maintenance of self-tolerance. Immunity 9, 721.

Quigg, R.J. 2002. Use of complement inhibitors in tissue injury. Trends Mol. Med. 8, 430.

Quigg, R.J. 2003. Complement and the kidney. J. Immunol. 171, 3319.

Quigg, R.J., Holers, V.M., Morgan, B.P., et al. 1995a. Crry and CD59 regulate complement in rat glomerular epithelial cells and are inhibited by the nephritogenic antibody of passive Heymann nephritis. J. Immunol. 154, 3437.

Quigg, R.J., Kozono, Y., Berthiaume, D., et al. 1998a. Blockade of antibody-induced glomerulonephritis with Crry-Ig, a soluble murine complement inhibitor. J. Immunol. 160, 4553.

Quigg, R.J., Lim, A., Haas, M., et al. 1998b. Immune complex glomerulonephritis in C4- and C3-deficient mice. Kidney Int. 53, 320.

Quigg, R.J., Morgan, B.P., Holers, V.M., et al. 1995b. Complement regulation in the rat glomerulus: Crry and CD59 regulate complement in glomerular mesangial and endothelial cells. Kidney Int. 48, 412.

Quigg, R.J., Nicholson-Weller, A., Cybulsky, A.V., et al. 1989. Decay accelerating factor regulates complement activation on glomerular epithelial cells. J. Immunol. 142, 877.

Ratnoff, W.D., Knez, J.J., Prince, G.M., et al. 1992. Structural properties of the glycoplasmanylinositol anchor phospholipid of the complement membrane attack complex inhibitor CD59. Clin. Exp. Immunol. 87, 415.

Ravetch, J.V. 2002. A full complement of receptors in immune complex diseases. J. Clin. Invest. 110, 1759.

Ravirajan, C.T., Wang, Y., Matis, L.A., et al. 2004. Effect of neutralizing antibodies to IL-10 and C5 on the renal damage caused by a pathogenic human anti-dsDNA antibody. Rheumatology (Oxford) 43, 442.

Ren, G., Doshi, M., Hack, B.K., et al. 2003. Rat glomerular epithelial cells produce and bear factor H on their surface which is upregulated under complement attack. Kidney Int. 64, 914.

Ren, G., Hack, B.K., Minto, A.W., et al. 2002. A complement-dependent model of thrombotic thrombocytopenic purpura induced by antibodies reactive with endothelial cells. Clin. Immunol. 103, 43.

Richards, A., Kemp, E.J., Liszewski, M.K., et al. 2003. Mutations in human complement regulator, membrane cofactor protein (CD46), predispose to development of familial hemolytic uremic syndrome. Proc. Natl. Acad. Sci. USA 100, 12966.

Robson, M.G., Cook, H.T., Botto, M., et al. 2001. Accelerated nephrotoxic nephritis is exacerbated in C1q-deficient mice. J. Immunol. 166, 6820.

Rodriguez de Cordoba, S., Esparza-Gordillo, J., Goicoechea de, J.E., et al. 2004. The human complement factor H: functional roles, genetic variations and disease associations. Mol. Immunol. 41, 355.

Rosenberg, M.E., Girton, R., Finkel, D., et al. 2002. Apolipoprotein J/clusterin prevents a progressive glomerulopathy of aging. Mol. Cell. Biol. 22, 1893.

Rosenkranz, A.R., Mayadas, T.N. 1999. Leukocyte–endothelial cell interactions—lessons from knockout mice. Exp. Nephrol. 7, 125.

Ross, G.D., Yount, W.J., Walport, M.J., et al. 1985. Disease-associated loss of erythrocyte complement receptors (CR1, C3b receptors) in patients with systemic lupus erythematosus and other diseases involving autoantibodies and/or complement activation. J. Immunol. 135, 2005.

Sacks, S.H., Zhou, W., Andrews, P.A., et al. 1993. Endogenous complement C3 synthesis in immune complex nephritis. Lancet 342, 1273.

Salant, D.J., Adler, S., Darby, C., et al. 1985. Influence of antigen distribution on the mediation of immunological glomerular injury. Kidney Int. 27, 938.

Salant, D.J., Belok, S., Madaio, M.P., et al. 1980. A new role for complement in experimental membranous nephropathy in rats. J. Clin. Invest. 66, 1339.

Salmon, J.E., Girardi, G. 2004. The role of complement in the antiphospholipid syndrome. Curr. Dir. Autoimmun. 7, 133.

Saunders, R.E., Perkins, S.J. 2006. A user's guide to the interactive Web database of factor H-associated hemolytic uremic syndrome. Semin. Thromb. Hemost. 32, 160.

Schiller, B., He, C., Salant, D.J., et al. 1998. Inhibition of complement regulation is key to the pathogenesis of Heymann nephritis. J. Exp. Med. 188, 1353.

Seelen, M.A., van der Bijl, E.A., Trouw, L.A., et al. 2005. A role for mannose-binding lectin dysfunction in generation of autoantibodies in systemic lupus erythematosus. Rheumatology (Oxford) 44, 111.

Sekine, H., Reilly, C.M., Molano, I.D., et al. 2001. Complement component C3 is not required for full expression of immune complex glomerulonephritis in MRL/lpr mice. J. Immunol. 166, 6444.

Shankland, S.J., Pippin, J.W., Couser, W.G. 1999. Complement (C5b-9) induces glomerular epithelial cell DNA synthesis but not proliferation in vitro. Kidney Int. 56, 538.

Sheerin, N.S., Springall, T., Carroll, M., et al. 1999. Altered distribution of intraglomerular immune complexes in C3-deficient mice. Immunology 97, 393.

Sheerin, N.S., Springall, T., Carroll, M.C., et al. 1997. Protection against anti-glomerular basement membrane (GBM)-mediated nephritis in C3- and C4-deficient mice. Clin. Exp. Immunol. 110, 403.

Sogabe, H., Nangaku, M., Ishibashi, Y., et al. 2001. Increased susceptibility of decay-accelerating factor deficient mice to anti-glomerular basement membrane glomerulonephritis. J. Immunol. 167, 2791.

Song, H., He, C., Knaak, C., et al. 2003. Complement receptor 2-mediated targeting of complement inhibitors to sites of complement activation. J. Clin. Invest. 111, 1875.

Stuhlinger, W., Kourilsky, O., Kanfer, A., et al. 1974. Haemolytic–uraemic syndrome: evidence for intravascular C3 activation. Lancet 2, 788.

Suzuki, Y., Shirato, I., Okumura, K., et al. 1998. Distinct contributions of Fc receptors and angiotensin II-dependent pathways in anti-GBM glomerulonephritis. Kidney Int. 54, 1166.

Sylvestre, D., Clynes, R., Ma, M., et al. 1996. Immunoglobulin G-mediated inflammatory responses develop normally in complement-deficient mice. J. Exp. Med. 184, 2385.

Tamai, H., Matsuo, S., Fukatsu, A., et al. 1991. Localization of 20-kD homologous restriction factor (HRF20) in diseased human glomeruli. An immunofluorescence study. Clin. Exp. Immunol. 84, 256.

Tang, T., Rosenkranz, A., Assmann, K.M., et al. 1997. A role for Mac-1 (CDIIb/CD18) in immune complex-stimulated neutrophil function in vivo: Mac-1 deficiency abrogates sustained Fcgamma receptor-dependent neutrophil adhesion and complement-dependent proteinuria in acute glomerulonephritis. J. Exp. Med. 186, 1853.

Tarzi, R.M., Davies, K.A., Robson, M.G., et al. 2002. Nephrotoxic nephritis is mediated by Fcgamma receptors on circulating leukocytes and not intrinsic renal cells. Kidney Int. 62, 2087.

Taylor, P.R., Carugati, A., Fadok, V.A., et al. 2000. A hierarchical role for classical pathway complement proteins in the clearance of apoptotic cells in vivo. J. Exp. Med. 192, 359.

Taylor, P.R., Nash, J.T., Theodoridis, E., et al. 1998. A targeted disruption of the murine complement factor B gene resulting in loss of expression of three genes in close proximity, factor B, C2, and D17H6S45. J. Biol. Chem. 273, 1699.

Thurman, J.M., Ljubanovic, D., Edelstein, C.L., et al. 2003. Lack of a functional alternative complement pathway ameliorates ischemic acute renal failure in mice. J. Immunol. 170, 1517.

Thurman, J.M., Ljubanovic, D., Royer, P.A., et al. 2006a. Altered renal tubular expression of the complement inhibitor Crry permits complement activation after ischemia/reperfusion. J. Clin. Invest. 116, 357.

Thurman, J.M., Lucia, M.S., Ljubanovic, D., et al. 2005. Acute tubular necrosis is characterized by activation of the alternative pathway of complement. Kidney Int. 67, 524.

Thurman, J.M., Royer, P.A., Ljubanovic, D., et al. 2006b. Treatment with an inhibitory monoclonal antibody to mouse factor B protects mice from induction of apoptosis and renal ischemia/reperfusion injury. J. Am. Soc. Nephrol. 17, 707.

Trendelenburg, M., Fossati-Jimack, L., Cortes-Hernandez, J., et al. 2005. The role of complement in cryoglobulin-induced immune complex glomerulonephritis. J. Immunol. 175, 6909.

Trouw, L.A., Daha, M.R. 2005. Role of anti-C1q autoantibodies in the pathogenesis of lupus nephritis. Expert. Opin. Biol. Ther. 5, 243.

Trouw, L.A., Groeneveld, T.W., Seelen, M.A., et al. 2004. Anti-C1q autoantibodies deposit in glomeruli but are only pathogenic in combination with glomerular C1q-containing immune complexes. J. Clin. Invest. 114, 679.

Unanue, E., Dixon, F.J. 1964. Experimental glomerulonephritis. IV. Participation of complement in nephrotoxic nephritis. J. Exp. Med. 119, 965.

van den Dobbelsteen, M.E., Verhasselt, V., Kaashoek, J.G., et al. 1994. Regulation of C3 and factor H synthesis of human glomerular mesangial cells by IL-1 and interferon-gamma. Clin. Exp. Immunol. 95, 173.

van der Boog, P.J., Van, K.C., de Fijter, J.W., et al. 2005. Role of macromolecular IgA in IgA nephropathy. Kidney Int. 67, 813.

van Doorn, M.B., Burggraaf, J., van, D.T., et al. 2005. A phase I study of recombinant human C1 inhibitor in asymptomatic patients with hereditary angioedema. J. Allergy Clin. Immunol. 116, 876.

Walport, M.J. 2001a. Advances in immunology: complement (first of two parts). N. Engl. J. Med. 344, 1058.

Walport, M.J. 2001b. Advances in immunology: complement (second of two parts). N. Engl. J. Med. 344, 1140.

Wang, Y., Hu, Q., Madri, J.A., et al. 1996. Amelioration of lupus-like autoimmune disease in NZB/W $F_1$ mice after treatment with a blocking monoclonal antibody specific for complement component C5. Proc. Natl. Acad. Sci. USA 93, 8563.

Wang, Y., Rollins, S.A., Madri, J.A., et al. 1995. Anti-C5 monoclonal antibody therapy prevents collagen-induced arthritis and ameliorates established disease. Proc. Natl. Acad. Sci. USA 92, 8955.

Warwicker, P., Donne, R.L., Goodship, J.A., et al. 1999. Familial relapsing haemolytic uraemic syndrome and complement factor H deficiency. Nephrol. Dial. Transplant. 14, 1229.

Warwicker, P., Goodship, T.H., Donne, R.L., et al. 1998. Genetic studies into inherited and sporadic hemolytic uremic syndrome. Kidney Int. 53, 836.

Watanabe, H., Garnier, G., Circolo, A., et al. 2000a. Modulation of renal disease in MRL/lpr mice genetically deficient in the alternative complement pathway factor B. J. Immunol. 164, 786.

Watanabe, M., Morita, Y., Mizuno, M., et al. 2000b. CD59 protects rat kidney from complement mediated injury in collaboration with Crry. Kidney Int. 58, 1569.

Weisman, H.F., Bartow, T., Leppo, M.K., et al. 1990. Soluble human complement receptor type 1: In vivo inhibitor of complement suppressing post-ischemic myocardial inflammation and necrosis. Science 249, 146.

Welch, T.R., Frenzke, M., Witte, D., et al. 2002. C5a is important in the tubulointerstitial component of experimental immune complex glomerulonephritis. Clin. Exp. Immunol. 13, 43.

Wenderfer, S.E., Ke, B., Hollmann, T.J., et al. 2005. C5a receptor deficiency attenuates T cell function and renal disease in MRLlpr mice. J. Am. Soc. Nephrol. 16, 3572.

Wessels, M.R., Butko, P., Ma, M., et al. 1995. Studies of group B streptococcal infection in mice deficient in complement component C3 or C4 demonstrate an essential role for complement in both innate and acquired immunity. Proc. Natl. Acad. Sci. USA 92, 11490.

Wilmer, W.A., Kaumaya, P.T., Ember, J.A., et al. 1998. Receptors for the anaphylatoxin C5a (CD88) on human mesangial cells. J. Immunol. 160, 5646.

Wilson, C.B. 1996. Renal response to immunologic glomerular injury. In: B.M. Brenner (Ed.), The Kidney, W.B. Saunders, Philadelphia, pp. 1253–1391.

Wu, X., Pippin, J., Lefkowith, J.B. 1993. Attenuation of immune-mediated glomerulonephritis with an anti-CD11b monoclonal antibody. Am. J. Physiol. Renal, Fluid Electrolyte Physiol. 264, F715.

Xia, Y., Vetvicka, V., Yan, J., et al. 1999. The beta-glucan-binding lectin site of mouse CR3 (CD11b/CD18) and its function in generating a primed state of the receptor that mediates cytotoxic activation in response to iC3b-opsonized target cells. J. Immunol. 162, 2281.

Xiao, H., et al. 2005. A pathogenic role for alternative pathway complement activation in anti-MPO induced necrotizing and crescentic glomerulonephritis. Kidney Blood Press. Res. 28, 159.

Xu, C., Mao, D., Holers, V.M., et al. 2000. A critical role for murine complement regulator Crry in fetomaternal tolerance. Science 287, 498.

Yamamoto, T., Wilson, C.B. 1987. Complement dependence of antibody-induced mesangial cell injury in the rat. J. Immunol. 138, 3758.

Ying, L., Katz, Y., Schlesinger, M., et al. 1999. Complement factor H gene mutation associated with autosomal recessive atypical hemolytic uremic syndrome. Am. J. Hum. Genet. 65, 1538.

Zahedi, R., Braun, M., Wetsel, R.A., et al. 2000. The C5a receptor is expressed by human renal proximal tubular epithelial cells. Clin. Exp. Immunol. 121, 226.

Zhang, H., Lu, S., Morrison, S.L., et al. 2001. Targeting of functional antibody-decay-accelerating factor fusion proteins to a cell surface. J. Biol. Chem. 276, 27290.

Zhang, H., Yu, J., Bajwa, E., et al. 1999. Targeting of functional antibody-CD59 fusion proteins to a cell surface. J. Clin. Invest. 103, 55.

Zhou, W., Andrews, P.A., Wang, Y., et al. 1997. Evidence for increased synthesis of complement C4 in the renal epithelium of rats with passive Heymann nephritis. J. Am. Soc. Nephrol. 8, 214.

Zhou, W., Marsh, J.E., Sacks, S.H. 2001. Intrarenal synthesis of complement. Kidney Int. 59, 1227.

Zipfel, P.F., Heinen, S., Jozsi, M., et al. 2006a. Complement and diseases: defective alternative pathway control results in kidney and eye diseases. Mol. Immunol. 43, 97.

Zipfel, P.F., Misselwitz, J., Licht, C., et al. 2006b. The role of defective complement control in hemolytic uremic syndrome. Semin. Thromb. Hemost. 32, 146.

Zoja, C., Morigi, M., Remuzzi, G. 2003. Proteinuria and phenotypic change of proximal tubular cells. J. Am. Soc. Nephrol. 14 (Suppl. 1), S36–S41.

CHAPTER 3

# Pathogenesis of Renal Disease: Cytokines and Other Soluble Factors

Stephen R. Holdsworth*, A. Richard Kitching

*Centre for Inflammatory Diseases, Monash University Department of Medicine and Monash Institute of Medical Research, Monash Medical Centre, 246 Clayton Rd, Clayton, Vic. 3168, Australia*

## 1. Introduction

Autoimmunity resulting in renal injury occurs as a systemic disturbance of immunity with the central feature being loss of tolerance to normal cellular and/or extracellular proteins. In autoimmune diseases where tissue injury includes the kidney, some of the target autoantigens are now identified, although the molecular characterization of the relevant epitopes remains to be clarified. Inflammatory renal disease in the context of autoimmunity occurs because the kidney is targeted by effector responses. In most cases, the autoantigens are non-renal and become renal targets because of the physiological properties of the high flow, high-pressure permselective filtration function of the glomerulus. Circulating autoantigens can deposit in glomeruli as part of circulating immune complexes or become a "planted" target antigen by their physico-chemical properties that predispose to their glomerular fixation. A potentially unique model of deposition of a non-renal antigen in the kidney is seen in anti-neutrophil cytoplasmic antibody (ANCA)-associated small vessel vasculitis, where target autoantigens originating in neutrophil cytoplasmic granules and expressed in the cell membrane (including proteinase-3 [PR3] and myeloperoxidase [MPO]) are targeted by ANCA. These ANCA-activated neutrophils have altered flow characteristics resulting in their lodging in small vessels, particularly glomeruli, resulting in renal injury. An additional consequence of this recruitment is the deposition of the autoantigen in the target organ, which becomes available to attract autoimmune effectors. Other planted antigens may themselves be biologically inert and initiate injury only as targets of auto-immune effector responses. In this context, renal cells are complicit in the resulting injury by participating in the recognition of these antigens by effector/memory T-cells by their expression of MHC Class II and CD40 (Li et al., 1998; Ruth et al., 2003).

The origins of autoimmune responses affecting the kidney, involving loss of either central and or peripheral tolerance, are examined elsewhere in this text. CD4+ T cells play a central role in tolerance and autoimmunity. Dendritic cells and other leukocytes help initiate and moderate their responses. The development of the immune system and the initiation, amplification, mediation, and regulation of immunity involves numerous soluble protein products of the immune system called cytokines. While cytokines are proteins best known as originating in immune cells and locally directing their organized interactions, it is now recognized that tissue cells can both produce cytokines and be actively involved in the organization of immunity. Moreover, it is clear that some

*Corresponding author.
Tel.: +61-3-9594-5525; Fax: +61-3-9594-6437
E-mail address: Stephen.Holdsworth@med.monash.edu.au
(S. R. Holdsworth).

© 2008 Elsevier B.V. All rights reserved.
DOI: 10.1016/S1571-5078(07)07003-1

cytokines circulate and may induce their effects at distant sites, the acute phase response being the best characterized example of a systemic cytokine organized response. Cytokines have considerable promiscuity in their involvement in both adaptive and innate immunity. They are involved in the initiation, amplification, and regulation of defensive and autoreactive immunity, as well as promoting or limiting inflammatory responses in target tissues. Furthermore there is a degree of overlap, in that some cytokines can play roles in both the initiation and polarization of immune responses and more local roles in target tissues. Understanding the complex regulatory and amplification cytokine networks underpinning these responses offers hope for the definition of critical intermediaries that may be therapeutic targets. Evidence for the merit of this concept is provided by the successful biological immunoneutralization of tumor necrosis factor (TNF) with anti-TNF antibodies, most notably in the treatment of rheumatoid arthritis (Feldmann and Maini, 2001). The clinical success of this therapy provides proof of concept that other effective therapeutics may be developed from improved knowledge of the molecular regulation of injurious cytokine-mediated autoimmune responses. Such therapies offer hope for effective, more targeted biologically based therapies without the predictable toxicities of the older drugs that are still the mainstays of current therapy.

The cytokine super-family comprises several groups of molecular families which are now regarded as separate entities, either because of their structural commonalities or their similar functional roles. These will be the focus of this review and include immune cytokines, inflammatory cytokines, and chemokines. A recent focus of attention that will also be included is a largely but not exclusively exogenous group of cell bound and soluble proteins, predominantly microbial in origin, that have powerful effects on defensive and autoimmunity by acting as ligands of toll-like receptors (TLRs).

The best recognized systemic autoimmune diseases involving the kidney are anti-glomerular basement membrane (GBM) antibody-associated glomerulonephritis (GN), ANCA-associated vasculitis, and systemic lupus erythematosus (SLE). These diseases will be the focus of this review. In each of these three diseases, the target groups of autoantigens are known. One autoantigen is extracellular (the non-collagenous domain of the α3 chain of type IV collagen [α3(IV)NC1]) in anti-GBM disease and two are intracellular. One intracellular grouping is cytoplasmic intragranular molecules, a large group but with two predominant enzymes as autoantigens—MPO and proteinase-3 (PR3) in the case of small vessel vasculitis. The other intracellular group is intranuclear (nuclear and nucleosomal) antigens in the case of SLE. Severe or persistent inflammation may result in renal fibrosis. While cytokines are also relevant to the development of renal fibrosis, consideration of their role in this process is beyond the scope of this chapter.

## 2. Cytokine regulation and differentiation of adaptive immunity

While protective immunity is activated and regulated by cytokines, dysregulated cytokine responses are involved in the generation, differentiation, and effector pathways of autoimmune responses. The central role of CD4+ T cells in adaptive immunity is initiated by the recognition of peptide antigens presented in the context of major histocompatibility complex (MHC) Class II expression by appropriately activated antigen presenting cells (APCs). These events initiate regulated clonal proliferation of CD4+ cells through T cell receptors (TcRs) recognizing antigen. Subsequent differentiation of these cells into effector and memory cells normally facilitates host defence by recruiting and activating innate immune effector cells (for example, macrophages) and directs the development of humoral immunity that also recruits innate effectors such as complement. These effectors can eliminate infection or wreak damage on essential organs in the context of autoimmunity. Perhaps the best example is found in crescentic forms of GN where functional glomeruli can undergo irreversible damage within 1 to 2 weeks. Following antigen recognition, CD4+ cells differentiate along at least two well-established pathways, Th1 and Th2 (Holdsworth et al., 1999). Recent evidence strongly suggests the presence of a third pathway, Th17 (reviewed in Weaver et al., 2007). The factors determining the particular differentiation pathways include the nature, dose, TcR affinity, and antigenic context (for example, the presence of danger signals and sepsis) as well as, in autoimmunity, the competence of tolerogenic systems (central and peripheral).

Subsets of CD4+ cells were defined by the profile of cytokines they produce and the nature of the response they directed (Mosmann and Coffman, 1989). Th1 cell polarization occurs if interleukin (IL)-12 predominates in the cytokine milieu at the time of antigen recognition. Strongly TLR-activated APCs presenting antigen with high TCR affinity, and expressing costimulatory molecules CD80, CD86, and CD40, favor Th1 differentiation (Koch et al., 1996). The Th1 subset produces interferon-$\gamma$ (IFN-$\gamma$), IL-2, and TNF, and expresses chemokine receptors CXCR3, CCR1, and CCR5. Th1 cells recruit and activate macrophages that effect injury, this response being termed delayed type hypersensitivity (DTH). Th1 cells provide help to B cells, directing (in mice) switching to the complement fixing and opsonising IgG subclasses IgG1, IgG2a, and IgG3. It has been suggested that so-called "organ specific" autoimmune diseases in man, such as Type I diabetes mellitus and multiple sclerosis, are predominantly Th1 polarized, though recent data, predominantly in animals, implicate the emerging Th17 subset as a potential culprit.

Th2 polarization is strongly influenced by IL-4 and low antigen/TcR affinity as well as TcR independent dose effects (Grakoui et al., 1999). Expression of the costimulatory molecules OX40 and ICOS by APCs favors Th2 polarization (Jankovic et al., 2001). Th2 cells produce IL-4, IL-5, IL-10 (in mice), and IL-13, directing non-complement fixing immunoglobulin subclasses and IgE. They are important in directing allergic responses. Th2 cell production of IL-4 and IL-10 inhibits Th1 differentiation, while IFN-$\gamma$ and IL-12 from Th1 cells inhibit Th2 differentiation.

Th1 cells are induced by dual antigen triggered TcR and cytokine gene signaling (IFN I & II and IL-27) through signal transducer and activation of transcription (STAT)-1 (Hibbert et al., 2003). T-bet is upregulated which inhibits Th2 signaling pathways and causes the expression of the inducible IL-12R$\beta$2 chain (Mullen et al., 2001), IL-12 signaling through STAT-4 leads to production of IL-18 and IFN-$\gamma$. Th2 differentiation is signaled by the IL-4 receptor inducing STAT-6 that induces GATA-3 (Zheng and Flavell, 1997) the master regulator of Th2 differentiation, which suppresses signaling of Th1 pathways and directs the expression of the genes encoding the Th2 cytokines IL-4, IL-5, and IL-13.

Recent evidence confirms a third pathway of CD4 differentiation, Th17 (Weaver et al., 2007), that seems to be relevant to organ-specific autoimmune disease. The discovery of this subset came from advances in the biology of the IL-12 family. IL-12 is a heterodimer composed of an IL-12p40 and an IL-12p35 chain. Studies in IL-12p40−/− and IFN-$\gamma$−/− mice in organ-specific autoimmunity, including experimental autoimmune encephalomyelitis and autoimmune anti-GBM GN (Kitching et al., 2004a), showed a pathogenetic role for IL-12p40, but either no role or a protective role for IFN-$\gamma$. This paradox may be explained by the cloning of IL-23, another heterodimer composed of the IL-12p40 chain and the IL-23p19 chain. Studies using IL-23 suggest a role for this cytokine in the development and/or maintenance of Th17 cells (Tato and O'Shea, 2006), characterized by the production of IL-17. They may have evolved to enhance host immunity to specific extracellular pathogens, e.g. *Klebsiella* pneumonia (Happel et al., 2005). IL-17 is involved in autoimmune injury (Lubberts et al., 2001) and Th17 cells may perform some of the effector functions previously attributed to Th1 cells. Unlike Th1 cells, Th17 cells do not express high levels of IFN-$\gamma$. The differentiation of these cells occurs under the direction of TGF-$\beta$ and IL-6 (Bettelli et al., 2006; Weaver et al., 2007). Recent publications are reciprocally linking the Th17 subset with regulatory T cells, important in the development of peripheral tolerance. Gene profiling shows that Th1 cells preferentially express genes associated with cytotoxicity (IFN-$\gamma$, granzyme B) while Th17 cells express genes associated with chronic inflammation

(IL-17, IL-6, and TNF) as well as proinflammatory chemokines (Langrish et al., 2005). The potential role of Th17 CD4+ cells or IL-17 itself in renal inflammation, and in particular autoimmune responses, is yet to be defined.

The polarization of T cell subsets is relevant to autoimmune renal disease. It is now recognized that a major determinant of injury and outcome results from the strength and direction of the nephritogenic CD4+ responses (reviewed in Holdsworth et al., 1999). Accumulating evidence from human observations and experimental models supports the view that strong Th1 polarized responses to nephritogenic antigens, defined by the associated antigen-specific immunoglobulin isotypes, cytokines produced by CD4+ antigen responding cells, and the pattern of effectors in nephritic glomeruli, induce proliferative/crescentic forms of GN. In this setting, (human) IgG1 and IgG3 predominate systemically and are found in affected kidneys, together with CD4 cells producing IFN-$\gamma$, DTH effector T cells, macrophages, and fibrin. Membranous GN (idiopathic or secondary to SLE) is the best example of a form of GN associated with Th2 polarized immunity. Glomerular DTH effectors are absent and the Th2 associated subclass IgG4 is present in affected glomeruli.

Several autoimmune diseases associated with glomerular injury have well accepted and characterized experimental animal models. The most widely studied are models of SLE, where strains of mice spontaneously developing immune complex disease and nephritis have been identified. The best studied of these are MRL/lpr and NZB/W mice. Experimental mercuric chloride induced GN also involves the production of multiple autoantibodies, Th2 responses, and renal lesions akin to human membranous GN. Human anti-GBM GN has stimulated the development of relevant models. These include experimental anti-GBM GN (nephrotoxic nephritis) and autoimmune anti-GBM GN (experimental autoimmune glomerulonephritis). Although in much earlier stages of development and characterization, models of injury resulting from or amplified by immunity to MPO (Heeringa et al., 1996; Xiao et al., 2002; Little et al., 2005; Ruth et al., 2006) and PR3 (Pfister et al., 2004) are becoming available and have confirmed the capacity of immunity to MPO to induce crescentic GN.

Manipulation of experimental models by cytokine gene deletion, the administration of individual cytokines, or their specific neutralization in these in vivo animal models, has helped define the roles of cytokines in GN. Cytokines play key roles in systemic autoimmune disease, affecting the kidney at the level of the generation and regulation of systemic nephritogenic immunity and in the effector responses injuring glomeruli. Analyses of the role of Th1 and Th2 polarized systemic nephritogenic immunity suggests that severe proliferative crescentic GN results from Th1 polarized responses, while milder, more slowly progressing forms of GN arise in the context of Th2 polarized nephritogenic immunity (Holdsworth et al., 1999). In general, cytokine manipulation aimed at selectively affecting the Th1 response may offer therapeutic benefits. A key challenge will be defining the potential role of Th17 cells and dissecting the relative roles of Th1, Th2, and Th17 cells in future studies of autoimmune GN in the context of rapidly evolving understanding of how Th cell subsets direct loss of tolerance and the resultant patterns of injury in autoimmune disease.

## 3. Cytokine regulation of renal inflammation in specific autoimmune diseases and their animal models

### 3.1. Human autoimmune anti-GBM GN

This uncommon but devastating disease usually presents with severe destructive crescentic glomerulonephritis due to autoimmunity to $\alpha3(IV)NC1$ (Hudson et al., 2003). Because the disease is rare, there are few studies enabling comprehensive understanding of the cytokine regulation of the systemic autoimmune response, the cytokines present in the affected organs, or the cytokine profile associated with the injurious effector responses. Immunohistological studies show disease is characterized by the accumulation of macrophages, fibrin deposition, and T cells, characteristic effectors of Th1 polarized immunity (Holdsworth et al., 1999). IFN-$\gamma$ production by antigen-stimulated T cells ex vivo during disease activity and IL-10 production in remission implicate Th1 responses in active disease (Cairns et al., 2003; Salama et al., 2003).

## 3.2. Lessons from experimental anti-GBM GN

The most widely studied model of this disease is nephrotoxic nephritis or experimental anti-GBM GN, induced by injecting foreign (heterologous) polyclonal anti-GBM antibodies. It is a robust model that has been established in different species, commonly resulting in crescentic GN. A similar pattern of injury occurs in man, with crescentic GN and linear antibody GBM staining. Human antibodies eluted from kidneys of patients with anti-GBM GN induce similar injury when administered to primates (Lerner et al., 1967). However, nephrotoxic nephritis is not a true autoimmune disease. In most reports, crescentic GN results from the host animal's immune response to the heterologous antibody, which becomes a planted antigen. Nonetheless, this model has enabled studies of the cytokine regulation of the systemic and local effector nephritogenic immune responses that are relevant to human anti-GBM GN and other autoimmune diseases that cause crescentic GN. Autoimmunity to GBM components can be induced in susceptible mouse strains (Kalluri et al., 1997) and especially WKY rats (Reynolds et al., 2002).

To determine the effects of Th1 or Th2 predominance on anti-GBM GN, disease was compared between the more Th1 prone C57BL/6 mouse strain and the more Th2 prone BALB/c strain (Huang et al., 1997a, b). C57BL/6 mice developed Th1 predominant systemic responses to the nephritogenic antigen, with glomerular crescent formation and DTH effectors in glomeruli. The lesion was dependent on effector CD4+ cells (Huang et al., 1997b; Li et al., 1997), but not autologous antibody (Li et al., 1997) and could be ameliorated by antibody neutralization or genetic deletion of IL-12p40 or IFN-$\gamma$ (Huang et al., 1997b; Kitching et al., 1999a, b, 2005; Timoshanko et al., 2001, 2002). Crescentic disease, and Th1 responses, could be accelerated by IL-12 administration, or deletion of IL-4 or IL-10 (Kitching et al., 1998, 2000b), but not IL-13 (Kitching et al., 2004b). Further evidence supporting Th1 and Th2 cytokine manipulation in a therapeutic context was provided by administration of Th2 polarizing IL-4 and/or the Th1 attenuating cytokine IL-10 to Th1 prone mice at the time of, or after induction of anti-GBM GN. These cytokines attenuate crescentic GN and diminish Th1 nephritogenic immune responses (Kitching et al., 1997; Tipping et al., 1997; Cook et al., 1999). In contrast, BALB/c mice developed Th2 predominant systemic immune responses to the nephritogenic antigens and the resulting GN was complement-dependent, but not effector CD4+ cell dependent and showed less severe renal injury with modest accumulation of DTH effectors in the kidney (Huang et al., 1997a, b). While IL-12 administration could establish Th1 responses and crescentic GN, IL-4 deletion did not result in a default to a Th1 crescentic lesion (Kitching et al., 1999b).

Renal injury is also directed by inflammatory cytokines produced in the kidney induced by recognition of the nephritogenic antigen by CD4 effectors. MHC class II and co-stimulatory molecule-dependent interactions between intrinsic renal cells and infiltrating cells are necessary for severe disease (Li et al., 1998; Ruth et al., 2003). The influence of intrinsic renal cell derived IL-12p40 (Timoshanko et al., 2001), IFN-$\gamma$ (Timoshanko et al., 2002), and TNF (Timoshanko et al., 2003) in experimental crescentic GN has also been demonstrated. In anti-GBM GN, a number of inflammatory cytokines are required for the development of severe renal injury, including TNF, IL-1, and macrophage inhibitory factor (MIF) (Tomosugi et al., 1989; Lan et al., 1993, 1997; Karkar et al., 2001; Khan et al., 2005).

IL-18 is a pro-inflammatory cytokine which was originally described as a potent inducer of IFN-$\gamma$, but also has broader proinflammatory roles and is expressed in glomeruli in experimental anti-GBM GN (Kitching et al., 2005). Administration of

IL-18 enhanced immune responses and glomerular injury in murine anti-GBM GN and was able to partially restore injury, independent of IFN-γ when given to IL-12p40−/− mice (Kitching et al., 2000a). IL-18−/− mice exhibited decreased injury, associated with reduced leukocyte infiltration and chemokine expression (Kitching et al., 2005).

TGF-β, although best known for its injurious profibrotic role in renal scarring, also has the potential to attenuate acute glomerular inflammation (Zhou et al., 2003). In addition to IL-4 and IL-10, a number of other cytokines have anti-inflammatory potential. IL-11 is one such cytokine. Therapeutic IL-11 administration in anti-GBM GN attenuated inflammation (Lai et al., 2001), in part due to suppression of NF-κb (Lai et al., 2005). While IL-6 is generally regarded as being pro-inflammatory, infusion of IL-6 into rats developing anti-GBM GN had anti-proliferative effects (Karkar et al., 1997). Leptin deficient mice were protected from crescentic anti-GBM antibody induced injury suggesting a pro-inflammatory role for this cytokine (Tarzi et al., 2004).

In addition to its effects on antigen presentation and T cells, IL-10 is known for its anti-inflammatory effects and has been shown to attenuate inflammatory glomerular injury in a macrophage-dependent passive transfer model of anti-GBM GN in which it reduced macrophage influx and injury (Huang et al., 2000). IL-15 is another traditionally pro-inflammatory cytokine that when deleted in mice which were then subjected to anti-GBM GN, was associated with more severe injury suggesting a normal immuno-regulatory role (Shinozaki et al., 2002).

The cytokine induction of inflammatory injury in nephritic glomeruli requires a series of interactions between infiltrating effector leukocytes and intrinsic glomerular cells. Studies of anti-GBM GN in cytokine chimeric mice has allowed dissection of these interactions. These chimeric mice, created by bone marrow irradiation and donor marrow reconstitution, represent mice with a particular cytokine expressed either exclusively by bone marrow cells or by peripheral non-marrow derived intrinsic renal cells. These studies demonstrate a leukocyte/intrinsic renal cell effector cytokine network with injury resulting from sequential cytokine interactions. IFN-γ production by intrinsic renal cells (Timoshanko et al., 2002) directs infiltrating leukocyte production of IL-1 (Timoshanko et al., 2004). This cytokine engages the IL-1R on intrinsic renal cells (Timoshanko et al., 2004) that stimulates renal cell derived TNF (Timoshanko et al., 2003). TNF appears to be the final step in the injurious effector response. It is of note that it is renal not leukocyte-derived TNF that induces injury (Timoshanko et al., 2003). This is consistent with reports demonstrating the capacity of intrinsic renal cells to produce TNF in vivo and in vitro (Neale et al., 1995). TNF is also a major effector of injury in experimental autoimmune anti-GBM GN (Huugen et al., 2005; Little et al., 2006).

## 4. ANCA-associated autoimmune vasculitis

Evidence from human studies suggests a prominent role for cytokines in the immunopathogenesis of this form of vasculitis. These diseases are characterized by systemic inflammation which has been shown to be associated with elevated serum levels of TNF (Arimura et al., 1993). In experimental models induced by passive transfer of ANCA, including both anti-PR3 (Pfister et al., 2004) and anti-MPO (Huugen et al., 2005; Little et al., 2006), TNF enhances neutrophil margination to endothelia and augments injury. The mechanisms involved are likely to include TNF-induced endothelial activation, subsequent augmentation of adhesion molecule expression and cytokine production, facilitating ANCA binding to neutrophils, by inducing MPO and PR3 translocation from cytoplasmic granules to the cell surface (Falk et al., 1990).

Patients with active disease have peripheral blood mononuclear cells (PBMCs) with high IL-12 and IFN-γ production and low IL-4 and IL-10 production (Ludviksson et al., 1998; Masutani et al., 2003). In remission, the IFN-γ:IL-4 ratio falls (Masutani et al., 2003) and cytokine profiles show a predominant IL-10 production in response to PR3 (Popa et al., 2002). Other studies have confirmed the Th1 predominant cytokine profile of circulating leukocytes (Csernok et al., 1999). Studies of diseased tissue, both kidney (Masutani et al., 2003) and upper airway (Komocsi et al., 2002), demonstrate Th1-dependent immune and inflammatory cytokines. The Th1 associated cytokine IL-18 has also recently been described in glomeruli of patients with acute disease (Hewins et al., 2006). IL-18 acts like TNF to prime neutrophils via p38 mitogen-activated protein (MAP) kinase to release reactive oxygen species. These findings confirm Th1 polarization and IFN-$\gamma$ predominance in the progress of ANCA-associated vasculitis. This, together with the prominence of Th1 effectors of DTH (T-cells, macrophages and fibrin) in the glomeruli of most patients with ANCA-associated crescent GN (Cunningham et al., 1999), suggests that this disease is driven systemically and locally at sites of injury by Th1 effectors, and is mediated by their cytokines. The shift to IL-10 in remission is also suggestive of a role for Th2 cytokines in maintaining remission by its role in peripheral tolerance (Abdulahad et al., 2006). The capacity of IL-10, at least in vitro, to attenuate vasculitis patients' leukocyte IFN$\gamma$/IL-12 production suggests a possible therapeutic role in active disease (Ludviksson et al., 1998).

## 5. Lupus nephritis

### 5.1. Observations in human lupus nephritis

A spectrum of histological features characterizes lupus nephritis. Similarly, patterns of cytokines in the blood, made by PBMCs, expressed in diseased kidneys and measured in the urine show heterogenous profiles. Further complicating concepts surrounding the pathogenesis of renal injury in SLE are paradoxical reports from animal models and humans that implicate IL-10 (traditionally considered an anti-inflammatory cytokine) in induction of autoimmunity and TNF, a prototypic pro-inflammatory cytokine, in protection from disease induction. It is possible that these cytokines (especially TNF) may play differential roles in the induction of autoimmunity and in effector responses. Alternately, SLE may represent a spectrum of a number of diseases with, at times, similar development of autoantibodies.

In general, in more severe proliferative WHO Class IV lupus nephritis, Th1 patterns of cytokines (IL-18, IL-12, and IFN-$\gamma$, with low IL-4) are found in PBMCs and in renal tissues from patients (Masutani et al., 2001; Uhm et al., 2003; Calvani et al., 2004), and are associated with DTH effectors in the kidney. These features are associated with pro-inflammatory cytokine expression, including TNF, shown to be up-regulated in these kidneys (Aringer and Smolen, 2005). In membranous lupus nephritis, expression of IL-4 and IL-10 without IFN-$\gamma$ in glomeruli has been reported (Uhm et al., 2003; Kawasaki et al., 2004). This, together with lack of leukocyte infiltration and proliferation, and the presence of the Th2 associated subclass IgG4 (Haas, 1994), suggests Th2 predominant autoimmunity. Thus, membranous lupus nephritis appears to be similar to idiopathic membranous where the association between Th2 immunoglobulin isotypes is also found (Haas, 1994). IL-4 has been found in Class II and IV lupus nephritis by immunohistochemistry (Okada et al., 1994), and by mRNA analysis in the context of oligoclonal T cells (Murata et al., 2002), with IL-4 mRNA expression inversely correlating with glomerular injury (Furusu et al., 1997). IL-10 has also been detected in kidneys of patients with lupus nephritis; IFN-$\gamma$/IL-10 ratios were elevated in active class IV disease but low in non-proliferative lupus nephritis (Uhm et al., 2003).

TNF is a prominent participant in lupus nephritis. Raised serum levels of TNF correlate with disease activity (Studnicka-Benke et al., 1996). In lupus kidneys, TNF participation and renal cell expression of TNF receptors has been confirmed (Schlondorff, 1996). Immunolocalization of TNF has been shown on infiltrating mononuclear leukocytes (Herreraesparza et al., 1998), but also on mesangial cells (Malide et al., 1995) and glomerular epithelial cells in WHO class V lupus nephritis (Neale et al., 1995). TNF participation has been demonstrated in all classes of lupus nephritis but it correlates most strongly with activity rather than histological class (Aringer and Smolen, 2005). IL-6, IL-1, IFN-$\gamma$, and IL-18 have also been demonstrated in human lupus nephritis. IL-6 and IL-1 are most closely associated with infiltrating mononuclear cells, although IL-1 could also be demonstrated in association with epithelial and mesangial cells (Fukatsu et al., 1991; Takemura et al., 1994). In proliferative lupus nephritis, IL-18 is expressed in glomeruli, and IL-18R expressing DCs infiltrate glomeruli (Tucci et al., 2005).

## 5.2. Role of cytokines in experimental models of SLE

A number of inbred mouse strains has been developed that spontaneously develop autoimmunity to a variety of nuclear antigens, including anti-dsDNA antibodies, and severe lupus-like GN. Evidence for a significant role in autoimmune nephritis has been provided for several proinflammatory cytokines. Blockade of TNF attenuates disease (Segal et al., 2001). Administration of IL-6 augments and accelerates disease (Finck et al., 1994), while immunoneutralization of IL-6 attenuates disease (Kiberd, 1993; Finck et al., 1994). IL-18 inhibition (by cDNA vaccination) attenuates (Bossu et al., 2003), while IL-18 injection increases disease (Esfandiari et al., 2001). IFN-$\gamma$ is a potential therapeutic target, as evidenced by augmentation of disease by its administration and attenuation of disease observed by its neutralization (Jacob et al., 1987) or genetic deletion (Balomenos et al., 1998; Schwarting et al., 1998). IL-1 administration augments disease (Brennan et al., 1989), but IL-1RA did not alter established disease (Kiberd and Stadnyk, 1995). CSF-1 and MIF are both likely to play an adverse role in the outcome of autoimmune GN as deletion of either cytokine in MRL/lpr mice protected them from renal inflammatory injury (Lenda et al., 2004; Hoi et al., 2006).

Amongst the "immune" cytokines, IL-12 is a potential therapeutic target. Exogenous IL-12 accelerates disease (Huang et al., 1996) while genetic deletion attenuates autoimmunity and renal injury (Kikawada et al., 2003). BlyS (also known as BAFF) is a cytokine member of the TNF family that stimulates and improves survival of B cells. Over-expression of BlyS induces a lupus like syndrome (Mackay et al., 1999), while treatment of lupus mice with a fusion protein that binds BlyS attenuates diseases (Gross et al., 2000). The demonstration of enhanced levels of IL-4 and IL-10 (Vasoo and Hughes, 2005) has led many to suggest SLE is a Th2-dependent disease, with autoantibody driven immune complex formation. In MRL/lpr mice genetic deletion of IL-4 reduces disease (Peng et al., 1997). However, other experimental observations suggest IL-4 may act as an immunomodulator (Theofilopoulos and Lawson, 1999) and an inverse correlation between renal IL-4 mRNA and disease activity has been reported (Furusu et al., 1997). Type I interferons may be immunomodulatory as their administration to MRL/lpr mice attenuated nephritis (Schwarting et al., 2005). However, other human and experimental studies suggest that Type I interferons may be harmful. Patients treated with IFN-$\alpha$ can develop autoimmune disease, including SLE (Ioannou and Isenberg, 2000), but Type I IFN receptor deficient lupus prone mice are variably protected (Santiago-Raber et al., 2003; Hron and Peng, 2004).

## 6. Targeting cytokines in human autoimmune GN

A number of anti-cytokine therapies have been or are being trialled in human autoimmune renal disease. In human lupus, an open label Phase 1 study of anti-IL-6 therapy in active SLE is underway (Tackey et al., 2004). Six months therapy with an anti-IL-10 neutralizing antibody has shown reduction in indices of activity (Mex-SLEDAI scores) and reduction in prednisolone dose (Llorente et al., 2000). A study of the efficacy of humanized monoclonal anti-BLyS antibody in SLE showed decreased circulating B cells but no clinical or serological changes (Stohl, 2004; Vasoo and Hughes, 2005). While lupus nephritis is a disease where inhibition of TNF would also seem worthy of consideration, a significant side effect of anti-TNF therapy in rheumatoid arthritis is the development of anti-nuclear antibodies, raising potential risks in a disease characterized by the presence of these autoantibodies. One open label study has been performed involving six patients (four with nephritis) with refractory SLE (Aringer et al.,

2004). Treatment for 6 months reduced proteinuria and lupus activity, despite transient elevations in anti-DNA antibodies. Given studies in experimental crescentic glomerulonephritis, including models of ANCA-associated glomerulonephritis (Huugen et al., 2005; Little et al., 2006), showing a pathogenetic role for TNF, anti-TNF therapies have been trialled in human ANCA-associated vasculitis. One study in Wegener's granulomatosis suggested a soluble TNF receptor compared with conventional therapy produced greater adverse effects without increased efficacy (The Wegener's Granulomatosis Etanercept Trial (WGET) Research Group, 2005). The other, a smaller study in renal predominant ANCA-associated GN used anti-TNF antibody and showed low toxicity and evidence of clinical efficacy (Booth et al., 2004).

## 7. Chemokines in autoimmune renal disease

Chemokines comprise a large family of at least 23 cytokine-like molecules sharing common chemical structures and involvement in leukocyte migration and activation. They play an important role in immune development, T cell activation and differentiation, leukocyte homeostasis, and host immune responses. Four broad families are recognized according to structural similarities principally based on the disposition of their cysteine residues. Different groups have broad similarities in function, particularly the leukocyte sub-populations with which they interact. However, promiscuity of chemokine receptor affinity (with 12 known receptors) is a feature confirming considerable functional overlap.

In inflammation, chemokines play critical roles in the molecular regulation of leukocyte emigration from the circulation. The sequential engagement of receptors between leukocyte and endothelium is dependent on chemokine-mediated activation and sequential expression of ligands, culminating in firm adhesion, diapedesis, and movement down a chemotactic gradient. Within the kidney, while leukocyte recruitment to the interstitial compartment is likely to involve the usual post-capillary venular processes, the glomerulus is a specialized capillary bed, where usual paradigms of leukocyte accumulation seem not to apply (Kuligowski et al., 2006). However, the prominence of leukocytes in glomeruli in the most severe forms of GN clearly indicates that leukocyte recruitment occurs. In vitro culture studies show most renal cells, including endothelial cells, mesangial cells, epithelial cells, interstitial cells, and tubular cells, can produce a range of chemokines in response to immune inflammatory stimuli (Panzer et al., 2006). Renal inflammation clearly involves chemokine regulation of leukocyte participation (reviewed in Anders et al., 2004c; Panzer et al., 2006). Immunohistochemical studies demonstrate the presence of chemokines in human autoimmune renal disease. In animal models, chemokines are significant participants and their manipulation has both confirmed their role in directing leukocyte-mediated renal disease and suggested that they may be therapeutic targets.

A number of studies have documented chemokine expression in human autoimmune renal disease. MCP-1/CCL2 and its receptor CCR2, MIP-1$\alpha$/CCL3, MIP-1$\beta$/CCL4, and RANTES/CCL5 are expressed in glomeruli and the tubulointerstitium of humans with anti-GBM GN, lupus nephritis, and ANCA-associated vasculitis (Cockwell et al., 1998; Wada et al., 1999; Segerer et al., 2000; Liu et al., 2003). Chemokine expression was particularly prominent in severe lesions and in anti-GBM GN (Cockwell et al., 1998; Liu et al., 2003). CCR5 has been detected in the interstitium (Segerer et al., 1999, 2000; Wada et al., 1999) and, at least in one study, in glomeruli (Wada et al., 1999). IL-8/CXCL8 is relevant to ANCA-associated GN, both by virtue of its potential effects on neutrophils and by its presence in glomeruli of affected patients (Cockwell et al., 1999). Flow chamber studies using human ANCA and neutrophils reveal a potential role for CXCR2 in neutrophil transmigration (Calderwood et al., 2005). Fractalkine is present in ANCA-associated renal disease, with mRNA concentrated at sites of significant injury (Chakravorty et al., 2002).

While a number of chemokines and their receptors are potential therapeutic targets, arguably the most convincing data exists for MCP-1/CCL2 and its receptor, CCR2. This work has been derived from studies of rodent models of monocyte/macrophage associated glomerular injury. A variety of approaches have confirmed the importance of this chemokine/chemokine receptor pair in the pathogenesis of macrophage recruitment and injury, including immunoneutralization in murine anti-GBM GN (Lloyd et al., 1997), studies using CCL2−/− (Tesch et al., 1999) or CCR2−/− (Perez de Lema et al., 2005) MRL/lpr mice, and studies using truncated CCL2 (Hasegawa et al., 2003) or virally derived antagonists (Chen et al., 1998). Other chemokines and their receptors have also been targeted, confirming their functional roles in experimental models (predominantly in experimental anti-GBM GN, but also in murine lupus nephritis). These include neutralization/antagonism of MIP-1α/CCL3 (Wu et al., 1997), MIP-2/CXCL1 (Feng et al., 1995), MDC/CCL22 (Garcia et al., 2003), fractalkine/CX3CLI (Feng et al., 1999), and RANTES (Lloyd et al., 1997).

However, some studies using chemokine or chemokine receptor gene deletion showed worsening of renal diseases. Experimental anti-GBM GN is significantly worse in CCR1 (Topham et al., 1999) or CCR2 (Bird et al., 2000) deficient mice. There seems to be the potential for reduced expression or function of at least some chemokines/chemokine receptors to result in altered regulatory or homeostatic immune or non-immune effects that counteract or override any therapeutic benefit. For example, while CXCR3 and its ligands, due to their effects on effector CD4+ cells, may be attractive targets, they may play a role in maintaining podocyte function and integrity (Han et al., 2003).

## 8. Soluble microbial products

It is generally accepted that infections are associated with the initiation and exacerbation of autoimmune renal disease. Many experimental immune models of renal injury require the administration of microbial products to induce inflammation. These products also exacerbate established glomerular inflammation. The effects of microbial products are mediated through toll-like receptors (TLRs) that are expressed on leukocytes and resident tissue cells (Anders et al., 2004a). At least 11 different TLRs have so far been recognized and a large number of ligands have been defined. In general, these are microbial products with highly conserved pathogen-associated molecular patterns (PAMPs). TLRs thus recognize infectious agents and demonstrate that the innate immune system is "hard wired" to recognize and respond to microbial invasion (Germain, 2004). PAMPs, as well as being commonly expressed by many different microorganisms have molecular signatures quite different from mammalian cellular constitution so that under normal circumstances they also signal "non-self".

TLRs are likely to play a role in the induction of autoimmunity. Antigen uptake by APCs/DCs in the absence of inflammation (and therefore APC/DC activation and licensing) is often insufficient to induce costimulatory molecule expression to fully activate CD4+ cells. Such presentation can induce anergy and maintain peripheral tolerance to self antigens. In contrast, APCs that have responded to infection-induced TLR-mediated stimulation exhibit enhanced costimulatory molecule and MHC class II expression, which induces strong CD4+ cell proliferation, activation, and differentiation. Thus, TLRs not only facilitate recognition of microbial invasion by the innate immune system, but also signal "danger" to the adaptive immune system and thus recruit strong cognate responses. TLR ligation of innate leukocytes recruited by CD4+ cells greatly enhances inflammation induced by adaptive CD4+ effector responses. TLRs are likely to mediate the effects of infection on the enhancement and induction of autoimmune renal inflammation. They help explain the mechanism of adjuvants, which are a key requirement in many experimental models to induce injury. These long used (but not widely discussed) technical maneuvers were described as "the immunologists, dirty little secret" by Charles Janeway, pioneer in defining the role of TLRs (Germain, 2004). Microbial products are likely to enhance immune injury and lower the threshold for immune stimuli to induce nephritogenic immunity and effector cell-mediated injury. PAMP/TLR interactions are likely to favor loss of tolerance and autoimmunity. Studies in animal models of renal inflammation have, in general, confirmed expectations that TLR ligand binding would enhance injury. This occurs both by augmentation of systemic nephritogenic adaptive immunity and by enhancing innate effector cell-mediated renal inflammation. Given the potential complexity of PAMP/TLR interactions, involving many microbial products and a number of TLRs, it is not surprising that different expression profiles of inflammation have been observed with different patterns of disease outcome.

A role for TLRs in autoimmunity, including renal disease, has been suggested by studies in lupus prone mice, that develop autoantibodies to DNA and RNA. Several TLRs have RNA or DNA components as their ligands, including virally derived ligands or potentially endogenous DNA. It is relevant that patients with SLE have increased levels of hypomethylated self-DNA, a potential TLR9 ligand (Richardson et al., 1990). A role for TLR7 has been demonstrated by the acceleration of disease in MRL/lpr mice injected repeatedly with a TLR7 ligand, which bound to infiltrating macrophages and DCs (Pawar et al., 2006). Exogenous TLR3 ligand (polyI:C RNA) given to the same strain also worsened disease (Patole et al., 2005), but TLR3 deficient lupus prone mice did not develop reduced autoantibodies or glomerular injury (Christensen et al., 2005). The role of TLR9 remains controversial, with variable results from studies of its relevance. Exogenous CpG DNA (TLR9 ligand) bound to leukocytes and increased autoantibodies and crescentic GN in MRL/lpr mice (Anders et al., 2004b), while inhibition of TLR9 via the administration of synthetic G rich DNA effectively reduced autoantibodies and renal disease (Patole et al., 2005). However, studies in TLR9−/− lupus prone mice have shown variable reduction in some autoantibodies, but paradoxical elevation in others, with either little alteration in disease or enhanced nephritis (Christensen et al., 2005; Lartigue et al., 2006; Yu et al., 2006).

Studies in experimental anti-GBM GN support a role for TLRs in immune renal injury. TLR2 binds a number of bacterial cell membrane and soluble ligands. TLR2 on both leukocytes and resident tissue cells plays a pathogenetic role in experimental anti-GBM GN (Brown et al., 2006). Fu et al. (2006) explored the effects of multiple TLRs and their ligands (TLR2/peptidoglycan, TLR3/polyI:C, TLR4/LPS, TLR5/flagellin) in mice with anti-GBM antibody initiated disease. All of these ligands augmented disease although the TLR9 ligand CpG showed no capacity to enhance this disease. The relevance of these studies becomes more cogent when it is recognized that a variety of normal mammalian proteins can act as ligands of TLRs, including heat shock proteins/TLR4 (Ohashi et al., 2000), products of necrotic cells/TLR2 (Li et al., 2001) and in the kidney, Tamm-Horsfall proteins/TLR4 (Saemann et al., 2005). Whether these (and other yet to be discovered TLR ligands) play roles in autoimmune renal disease awaits further studies.

### Key points

- Pathological renal inflammation is organized by several families of small molecules including cytokines, chemokines, and TLR ligands. Inhibition of their actions offers new therapeutic opportunities.
- Cytokines have diverse and sometimes pleotrophic effects at multiple stages of the autoimmune response, from loss of tolerance through determination of T-cell subset polarization to mediating effector responses.
- Cytokine/anti-cytokine therapies are being used in autoimmune diseases and may prove to be therapeutic in autoimmune diseases affecting the kidney.
- Chemokine and their receptors, particularly CCL2 (MCP-1)/CCR2 are important in leukocyte mediated experimental (and probably human) renal autoimmunity. Neutralizing/antagonizing chemokines have therapeutic potential, but redundancy and adverse effects may limit these approaches.
- TLRs bind endogenous and exogenous small molecular ligands that activate leukocytes and enhance injurious autoimmune responses resulting in renal injury.

## Acknowledgments

The authors acknowledge the grant support of the National Health and Medical Research Council of Australia, and acknowledge the work of many researchers that could not be discussed or cited in this review due to space limitations.

## References

Abdulahad, W.H., van der Geld, Y.M., et al. 2006. Persistent expansion of CD4+ effector memory T cells in Wegener's granulomatosis. Kidney Int. 70 (5), 938–947.

Anders, H.J., Banas, B., et al. 2004a. Signaling danger: toll-like receptors and their potential roles in kidney disease. J. Am. Soc. Nephrol. 15 (4), 854–867.

Anders, H.J., Vielhauer, V., et al. 2004b. Activation of toll-like receptor-9 induces progression of renal disease in MRL-Fas(lpr) mice. FASEB J 18 (3), 534–536.

Anders, H.J., Vielhauer, V., et al. 2004c. Current paradigms about chemokines as therapeutic targets. Nephrol. Dial. Transplant. 19 (12), 2948–2951.

Arimura, Y., Minoshima, S., et al. 1993. Serum myeloperoxidase and serum cytokines in anti-myeloperoxidase antibody-associated glomerulonephritis. Clin. Nephrol. 40 (5), 256–264.

Aringer, M., Graninger, W.B., et al. 2004. Safety and efficacy of tumor necrosis factor alpha blockade in systemic lupus erythematosus: an open-label study. Arthritis Rheum. 50 (10), 3161–3169.

Aringer, M., Smolen, J.S. 2005. Cytokine expression in lupus kidneys. Lupus 14 (1), 13–18.

Balomenos, D., Rumold, R., et al. 1998. Interferon-$\gamma$ is required for lupus-like disease and lymphoaccumulation in MRL-$lpr$ mice. J. Clin. Invest. 101 (2), 364–371.

Bettelli, E., Carrier, Y., et al. 2006. Reciprocal developmental pathways for the generation of pathogenic effector TH17 and regulatory T cells. Nature 441 (7090), 235–238.

Bird, J.E., Giancarli, M.R., et al. 2000. Increased severity of glomerulonephritis in C–C chemokine receptor 2 knockout mice. Kidney Int. 57 (1), 129–136.

Booth, A., Harper, L., et al. 2004. Prospective study of TNFalpha blockade with infliximab in anti-neutrophil cytoplasmic antibody-associated systemic vasculitis. J. Am. Soc. Nephrol. 15 (3), 717–721.

Bossu, P., Neumann, D., et al. 2003. IL-18 cDNA vaccination protects mice from spontaneous lupus-like autoimmune disease. Proc. Natl. Acad. Sci. USA 100 (24), 14181–14186.

Brennan, D.C., Yui, M.A., et al., 1989. Tumor necrosis factor and IL-1 in New Zealand Black/White mice. Enhanced gene expression and acceleration of renal injury. J. Immunol. 143, 3470–3475.

Brown, H.J., Lock, H.R., et al. 2006. TLR2 stimulation of intrinsic renal cells in the induction of immune-mediated glomerulonephritis. J. Immunol. 177 (3), 1925–1931.

Cairns, L.S., Phelps, R.G., et al. 2003. The fine specificity and cytokine profile of T-helper cells responsive to the alpha3 chain of type IV collagen in Goodpasture's disease. J. Am. Soc. Nephrol. 14 (11), 2801–2812.

Calderwood, J.W., Williams, J.M., et al. 2005. ANCA induces beta2 integrin and CXC chemokine-dependent neutrophil-endothelial cell interactions that mimic those of highly cytokine-activated endothelium. J. Leukoc. Biol. 77 (1), 33–43.

Calvani, N., Richards, H.B., et al. 2004. Up-regulation of IL-18 and predominance of a Th1 immune response is a hallmark of lupus nephritis. Clin. Exp. Immunol. 138 (1), 171–178.

Chakravorty, S.J., Cockwell, P., et al. 2002. Fractalkine expression on human renal tubular epithelial cells: potential role in mononuclear cell adhesion. Clin. Exp. Immunol. 129 (1), 150–159.

Chen, S.H., Bacon, K.B., et al. 1998. In vivo inhibition of CC and $CX_3C$ chemokine-induced leukocyte infiltration and attenuation of glomerulonephritis in Wistar-Kyoto (WKY) rats by vMIP-ii. J. Exp. Med. 188 (1), 193–198.

Christensen, S.R., Kashgarian, M., et al. 2005. Toll-like receptor 9 controls anti-DNA autoantibody production in murine lupus. J. Exp. Med. 202 (2), 321–331.

Cockwell, P., Brooks, C.J., et al. 1999. Interleukin-8: A pathogenetic role in antineutrophil cytoplasmic autoantibody-associated glomerulonephritis. Kidney Int. 55 (3), 852–863.

Cockwell, P., Howie, A.J., et al. 1998. In situ analysis of C-C chemokine mRNA in human glomerulonephritis. Kidney Int. 54 (3), 827–836.

Cook, H.T., Singh, S.J., et al. 1999. Interleukin-4 ameliorates crescentic glomerulonephritis in Wistar Kyoto rats. Kidney Int. 55 (4), 1319–1326.

Csernok, E., Trabandt, A., et al. 1999. Cytokine profiles in Wegener's granulomatosis: predominance of type 1 (Th1) in the granulomatous inflammation. Arthritis Rheum. 42 (4), 742–750.

Cunningham, M.A., Huang, X.R., et al. 1999. Prominence of cell-mediated immunity effectors in "pauci-immune" glomerulonephritis. J. Am. Soc. Nephrol. 10 (3), 499–506.

de Lema, G.P., Maier, H., et al. 2005. Chemokine receptor Ccr2 deficiency reduces renal disease and prolongs survival in MRL/lpr lupus-prone mice. J. Am. Soc. Nephrol. 16 (12), 3592–3601.

Dean, E.G., Wilson, G.R., et al. 2005. Experimental autoimmune Goodpasture's disease: a pathogenetic role for both effector cells and antibody in injury. Kidney Int. 67 (2), 566–575.

Dweik, R.A., Arroliga, A.C., et al. 1997. Alveolar hemorrhage in patients with rheumatic disease. Rheum. Dis. Clin. N. Am. 23 (2), 395–410.

Esfandiari, E., McInnes, I.B., et al. 2001. A proinflammatory role of IL-18 in the development of spontaneous autoimmune disease. J. Immunol. 167 (9), 5338–5347.

Falk, R.J., Terrell, R.S., et al. 1990. Anti-neutrophil cytoplasmic autoantibodies induce neutrophils to degranulate and produce oxygen radicals in vitro. Proc. Natl. Acad. Sci. U. S. A. 87 (11), 4115–4119.

Feldmann, M., Maini, R.N. 2001. Anti-TNFα therapy of rheumatoid arthritis: what have we learned? Annu. Rev. Immunol. 19, 163–196.

Feng, L., Chen, S., et al. 1999. Prevention of crescentic glomerulonephritis by immunoneutralization of the fractalkine receptor CX3CR1 rapid communication. Kidney Int. 56 (2), 612–620.

Feng, L., Xia, Y., et al. 1995. Modulation of neutrophil influx in glomerulonephritis in the rat with anti-macrophage inflammatory protein-2 (MIP-2) antibody. J. Clin. Invest. 95, 1009–1017.

Finck, B.K., Chan, B., et al. 1994. Interleukin 6 promotes murine lupus in NZB/NZW F1 mice. J. Clin. Invest. 94 (2), 585–591.

Fu, Y., Xie, C., et al. 2006. Innate stimuli accentuate end-organ damage by nephrotoxic antibodies via Fc receptor and TLR stimulation and IL-1/TNF-alpha production. J. Immunol. 176 (1), 632–639.

Fujii, A., Tomizawa, K., et al. 2000. Epitope analysis of myeloperoxidase (MPO) specific anti-neutrophil cytoplasmic autoantibodies (ANCA) in MPO-ANCA-associated glomerulonephritis. Clin. Nephrol. 53 (4), 242–252.

Fukatsu, A., Matsuo, S., et al., 1991. Distribution of interleukin-6 in normal and diseased human kidney. Lab Invest. 65, 61–66.

Furusu, A., Miyazaki, M., et al. 1997. Involvement of IL-4 in human glomerulonephritis—an in situ hybridization study of IL-4 mRNA and IL-4 receptor mRNA. J. Am. Soc. Nephrol. 8 (5), 730–741.

Garcia, G.E., Xia, Y., et al. 2003. Mononuclear cell-infiltrate inhibition by blocking macrophage-derived chemokine results in attenuation of developing crescentic glomerulonephritis. Am. J. Pathol. 162 (4), 1061–1073.

Germain, R.N. 2004. An innately interesting decade of research in immunology. Nat. Med. 10 (12), 1307–1320.

Grakoui, A., Donermeyer, D.L., et al. 1999. TCR-independent pathways mediate the effects of antigen dose and altered peptide ligands on Th cell polarization. J. Immunol. 162 (4), 1923–1930.

Gross, J.A., Johnston, J., et al. 2000. TACI and BCMA are receptors for a TNF homologue implicated in B-cell autoimmune disease. Nature 404 (6781), 995–999.

Haas, M. 1994. IgG subclass deposits in glomeruli of lupus and nonlupus membranous nephropathies. Am. J. Kidney Dis. 23 (3), 358–364.

Han, G.D., Koike, H., et al. 2003. IFN-inducible protein-10 has a differential role in podocyte during Thy 1.1 glomerulonephritis. J. Am. Soc. Nephrol. 14 (12), 3111–3126.

Hansen, T., Brockmann, H., et al. 2002. Fulminant course of diffuse alveolar hemorrhage in systemic lupus erythematosus—a case report. Z. Rheumatol. 61 (2), 175–179.

Happel, K.I., Dubin, P.J., et al. 2005. Divergent roles of IL-23 and IL-12 in host defense against Klebsiella pneumoniae. J. Exp. Med. 202 (6), 761–769.

Harper, L., Cockwell, P., et al. 1998. Case of propylthiouracil-induced ANCA associated small vessel vasculitis. Nephrol. Dial. Transpl. 13 (2), 455–458.

Hasegawa, H., Kohno, M., et al. 2003. Antagonist of monocyte chemoattractant protein 1 ameliorates the initiation and progression of lupus nephritis and renal vasculitis in MRL/lpr mice. Arthritis Rheum. 48 (9), 2555–2566.

Heeringa, P., Brouwer, E., et al. 1996. Autoantibodies to myeloperoxidase aggravate mild anti-glomerular-basement-membrane-mediated glomerular injury in the rat. Am. J. Pathol. 149 (5), 1695–1706.

Herreraesparza, R., Barbosacisneros, O., et al. 1998. Renal expression of IL-6 and TNF-α genes in lupus nephritis. Lupus 7 (3), 154–158.

Hewins, P., Morgan, M.D., et al. 2006. IL-18 is upregulated in the kidney and primes neutrophil responsiveness in ANCA-associated vasculitis. Kidney Int. 69 (3), 605–615.

Hibbert, L., Pflanz, S., et al. 2003. IL-27 and IFN-alpha signal via Stat1 and Stat3 and induce T-Bet and IL-12Rbeta2 in naive T cells. J. Interferon Cytokine Res. 23 (9), 513–522.

Hoi, A.Y., Hickey, M.J., et al. 2006. Macrophage migration inhibitory factor deficiency attenuates macrophage recruitment, glomerulonephritis, and lethality in MRL/lpr mice. J. Immunol. 177 (8), 5687–5696.

Holdsworth, S.R., Kitching, A.R., et al. 1999. Th1 and Th2 T helper cell subsets affect patterns of injury and outcomes in glomerulonephritis. Kidney Int. 55 (4), 1198–1216.

Hron, J.D., Peng, S.L. 2004. Type I IFN protects against murine lupus. J. Immunol. 173 (3), 2134–2142.

Huang, F.P., Feng, G.J., et al. 1996. The role of interleukin 12 and nitric oxide in the development of spontaneous autoimmune disease in MRL/mp-lpr/lpr mice. J. Exp. Med. 183 (4), 1447–1459.

Huang, X.R., Holdsworth, S.R., et al. 1997a. Th2 responses induce humorally mediated injury in experimental anti-glomerular basement membrane glomerulonephritis. J. Am. Soc. Nephrol. 8 (7), 1101–1108.

Huang, X.R., Kitching, A.R., et al. 2000. Interleukin-10 inhibits macrophage-induced glomerular injury. J. Am. Soc. Nephrol. 11 (2), 262–269.

Huang, X.R., Tipping, P.G., et al. 1997b. Th1 responsiveness to nephritogenic antigens determines susceptibility to crescentic glomerulonephritis in mice. Kidney Int. 51 (1), 94–103.

Hudson, B.G., Tryggvason, K., et al. 2003. Alport's syndrome, Goodpasture's syndrome, and type IV collagen. N. Engl. J. Med. 348 (25), 2543–2556.

Huugen, D., Xiao, H., et al. 2005. Aggravation of anti-myeloperoxidase antibody-induced glomerulonephritis by bacterial lipopolysaccharide: role of tumor necrosis factor-alpha. Am. J. Pathol. 167 (1), 47–58.

Ioannou, Y., Isenberg, D.A. 2000. Current evidence for the induction of autoimmune rheumatic manifestations by cytokine therapy. Arthritis Rheum. 43 (7), 1431–1442.

Jacob, C.O., Van Der Meide, P.H., et al. 1987. *In vivo* treatment of (NZB X NZW) F1 lupus-like nephritis with monoclonal antibody to interferon. J. Exp. Med. 166, 798–803.

Jankovic, D., Liu, Z., et al. 2001. Th1- and Th2-cell commitment during infectious disease: asymmetry in divergent pathways. Trends Immunol. 22 (8), 450–457.

Jennette, J.C., Falk, R.J. 1990. Antineutrophil cytoplasmic autoantibodies and associated diseases: a review. Am. J. Kidney Dis. 15 (6), 517–529.

Jennette, J.C., Xiao, H., et al. 2006. Pathogenesis of vascular inflammation by anti-neutrophil cytoplasmic antibodies. J. Am. Soc. Nephrol. 17 (5), 1235–1242.

Kalluri, R., Danoff, T.M., et al. 1997. Susceptibility to antiglomerular basement membrane disease and Goodpasture syndrome is linked to MHC class II genes and the emergence of T cell-mediated immunity in mice. J. Clin. Invest. 100 (9), 2263–2275.

Karkar, A.M., Smith, J., et al. 1997. Abrogation of glomerular injury in nephrotoxic nephritis by continuous infusion of interleukin-6. Kidney Int. 52 (5), 1313–1320.

Karkar, A.M., Smith, J., et al. 2001. Prevention and treatment of experimental crescentic glomerulonephritis by blocking tumour necrosis factor-alpha. Nephrol. Dial. Transpl. 16 (3), 518–524.

Kawasaki, Y., Suzuki, J., et al. 2004. Evaluation of T helper-1/-2 balance on the basis of IgG subclasses and serum cytokines in children with glomerulonephritis. Am. J. Kidney Dis. 44 (1), 42–49.

Khan, S.B., Cook, H.T., et al. 2005. Antibody blockade of TNF-alpha reduces inflammation and scarring in experimental crescentic glomerulonephritis. Kidney Int. 67 (5), 1812–1820.

Kiberd, B.A. 1993. Interleukin-6 receptor blockage ameliorates murine lupus nephritis. J. Am. Soc. Nephrol. 4 (1), 58–61.

Kiberd, B.A., Stadnyk, A.W. 1995. Established murine lupus nephritis does not respond to exogenous interleukin-1 receptor antagonist; a role for the endogenous molecule? Immunopharmacology 30 (2), 131–137.

Kikawada, E., Lenda, D.M., et al. 2003. IL-12 deficiency in MRL-Fas(lpr) mice delays nephritis and intrarenal IFN-gamma expression, and diminishes systemic pathology. J. Immunol. 170 (7), 3915–3925.

Kitching, A.R., Holdsworth, S.R., et al. 1999a. IFN- mediates crescent formation and cell-mediated immune injury in murine glomerulonephritis. J. Am. Soc. Nephrol. 10 (4), 752–759.

Kitching, A.R., Tipping, P.G., et al. 1999b. IL-12 directs severe renal injury, crescent formation and Th1 responses in murine glomerulonephritis. Eur. J. Immunol. 29 (1), 1–10.

Kitching, A.R., Tipping, P.G., et al. 1997. Interleukin-4 and interleukin-10 attenuate established crescentic glomerulonephritis in mice. Kidney Int. 52 (1), 52–59.

Kitching, A.R., Tipping, P.G., et al. 1998. Interleukin-4 deficiency enhances Th1 responses and crescentic glomerulonephritis in mice. Kidney Int. 53 (1), 112–118.

Kitching, A.R., Tipping, P.G., et al. 2000a. IL-18 has IL-12-independent effects in delayed-type hypersensitivity: studies in cell-mediated crescentic glomerulonephritis. J. Immunol. 165 (8), 4649–4657.

Kitching, A.R., Tipping, P.G., et al. 2000b. Endogenous interleukin-10 regulates Th1 responses that induce crescentic glomerulonephritis. Kidney Int. 57 (2), 518–525.

Kitching, A.R., Turner, A.L., et al. 2004a. Experimental autoimmune anti-glomerular basement membrane glomerulonephritis: a protective role for IFN-gamma. J. Am. Soc. Nephrol. 15 (7), 1764–1774.

Kitching, A.R., Turner, A.L., et al. 2004b. Endogenous IL-13 limits humoral responses and injury in experimental glomerulonephritis but does not regulate Th1 cell-mediated crescentic glomerulonephritis. J. Am. Soc. Nephrol. 15 (9), 2373–2382.

Kitching, A.R., Turner, A.L., et al. 2005. IL-12p40 and IL-18 in crescentic glomerulonephritis: IL-12p40 is the key Th1-defining cytokine chain, whereas IL-18 promotes local inflammation and leukocyte recruitment. J. Am. Soc. Nephrol. 16, 2023–2033.

Koch, F., Stanzl, U., et al. 1996. High level IL-12 production by murine dendritic cells: upregulation via MHC class II and CD40 molecules and downregulation by IL-4 and IL-10. J. Exp. Med. 184 (2), 741–746.

Komocsi, A., Lamprecht, P., et al. 2002. Peripheral blood and granuloma CD4(+)CD28(−) T cells are a major source of interferon-gamma and tumor necrosis factor-alpha in Wegener's granulomatosis. Am. J. Pathol. 160 (5), 1717–1724.

Kuligowski, M.P., Kitching, A.R., et al. 2006. Leukocyte recruitment to the inflamed glomerulus: a critical role for platelet-derived P-selectin in the absence of rolling. J. Immunol. 176 (11), 6991–6999.

Lai, P.C., Cook, H.T., et al. 2001. Interleukin-11 attenuates nephrotoxic nephritis in Wistar Kyoto rats. J. Am. Soc. Nephrol. 12 (11), 2310–2320.

Lai, P.C., Smith, J., et al. 2005. Interleukin-11 reduces renal injury and glomerular NF-kappa B activity in murine experimental glomerulonephritis. Nephron Exp. Nephrol. 101 (4), e146–154.

Lan, H.Y., Bacher, M., et al. 1997. The pathogenic role of macrophage migration inhibitory factor in immunologically induced kidney disease in the rat. J. Exp. Med. 185 (8), 1455–1465.

Lan, H.Y., Nikolic-Paterson, D.J., et al. 1993. Suppression of experimental crescentic glomerulonephritis by the interleukin-1 receptor antagonist. Kidney Int. 43, 479–485.

Langrish, C.L., Chen, Y., et al. 2005. IL-23 drives a pathogenic T cell population that induces autoimmune inflammation. J. Exp. Med. 201 (2), 233–240.

Lartigue, A., Courville, P., et al. 2006. Role of TLR9 in anti-nucleosome and anti-DNA antibody production in lpr mutation-induced murine lupus. J. Immunol. 177 (2), 1349–1354.

Lenda, D.M., Stanley, E.R., et al. 2004. Negative role of colony-stimulating factor-1 in macrophage, T cell, and B cell mediated autoimmune disease in MRL-Fas(lpr) mice. J. Immunol. 173 (7), 4744–4754.

Lerner, R.A., Glassock, R.J., et al. 1967. The role of anti-glomerular basement membrane antibody in the pathogenesis of human glomerulonephritis. J. Exp. Med. 126 (6), 989–1004.

Li, M., Carpio, D.F., et al. 2001. An essential role of the NF-kappa B/Toll-like receptor pathway in induction of inflammatory and tissue-repair gene expression by necrotic cells. J. Immunol. 166 (12), 7128–7135.

Li, S., Holdsworth, S.R., et al. 1997. Antibody independent crescentic glomerulonephritis in chain deficient mice. Kidney Int. 51 (3), 672–678.

Li, S., Kurts, C., et al. 1998. Major histocompatibility complex class II expression by intrinsic renal cells is required for crescentic glomerulonephritis. J. Exp. Med. 188 (3), 597–602.

Little, M.A., Bhangal, G., et al. 2006. Therapeutic effect of anti-TNF-alpha antibodies in an experimental model of anti-neutrophil cytoplasm antibody-associated systemic vasculitis. J. Am. Soc. Nephrol. 17 (1), 160–169.

Little, M.A., Smyth, C.L., et al. 2005. Antineutrophil cytoplasm antibodies directed against myeloperoxidase augment leukocyte-microvascular interactions in vivo. Blood 106 (6), 2050–2058.

Liu, Z.H., Chen, S.F., et al. 2003. Glomerular expression of C–C chemokines in different types of human crescentic glomerulonephritis. Nephrol. Dial. Transpl. 18 (8), 1526–1534.

Llorente, L., Richaud-Patin, Y., et al. 2000. Clinical and biologic effects of anti-interleukin-10 monoclonal antibody administration in systemic lupus erythematosus. Arthritis Rheum. 43 (8), 1790–1800.

Lloyd, C.M., Minto, A.W., et al. 1997. RANTES and monocyte chemoattractant protein-1 (MCP-1) play an important role in the inflammatory phase of crescentic nephritis, but only MCP-1 is involved in crescent formation and interstitial fibrosis. J. Exp. Med. 185 (7), 1371–1380.

Lubberts, E., Joosten, L.A., et al. 2001. IL-1-independent role of IL-17 in synovial inflammation and joint destruction during collagen-induced arthritis. J. Immunol. 167 (2), 1004–1013.

Ludviksson, B.R., Sneller, M.C., et al. 1998. Active Wegener's granulomatosis is associated with HLA-DR+ CD4+ T cells exhibiting an unbalanced Th1-type T cell cytokine pattern: reversal with IL-10. J. Immunol. 160 (7), 3602–3609.

Mackay, F., Woodcock, S.A., et al. 1999. Mice transgenic for BAFF develop lymphocytic disorders along with autoimmune manifestations. J. Exp. Med. 190 (11), 1697–1710.

Malide, D., Russo, P., et al. 1995. Presence of tumor necrosis factor alpha and interleukin-6 in renal mesangial cells of lupus nephritis patients. Hum. Pathol. 26 (5), 558–564.

Manzoor, K., Khan, S., et al. 2005. Crescentic glomerulonephritis associated with bacterial endocarditis—antibiotics alone may be sufficient. A case report. J. Pak. Med. Assoc. 55 (8), 352–354.

Masutani, K., Akahoshi, M., et al. 2001. Predominance of Th1 immune response in diffuse proliferative lupus nephritis. Arthritis Rheum. 44 (9), 2097–2106.

Masutani, K., Tokumoto, M., et al. 2003. Strong polarization toward Th1 immune response in ANCA-associated glomerulonephritis. Clin. Nephrol. 59 (6), 395–405.

Merkel, P.A., Lo, G.H., et al. 2005. Brief communication: high incidence of venous thrombotic events among patients with Wegener granulomatosis: the Wegener's Clinical Occurrence of Thrombosis (WeCLOT) Study. Ann. Intern. Med. 142 (8), 620–626.

Mitsui, I., Ichihara, H., et al. 1996. Interstitial pneumonia complicated by rapidly progressive glomerulonephritis associated with anti-myeloperoxidase antibody. Nihon Kyobu Shikkan Gakkai Zasshi 34 (9), 1015–1020.

Mosmann, T.R., Coffman, R.L. 1989. Heterogeneity of cytokine secretion patterns and functions of helper T cells. Adv. Immunol. 46, 111–147.

Mullen, A.C., High, F.A., et al. 2001. Role of T-bet in commitment of TH1 cells before IL-12-dependent selection. Science 292 (5523), 1907–1910.

Murata, H., Matsumura, R., et al. 2002. T cell receptor repertoire of T cells in the kidneys of patients with lupus nephritis. Arthritis Rheum. 46 (8), 2141–2147.

Neale, T.J., Ruger, B.M., et al. 1995. Tumor necrosis factor-alpha is expressed by glomerular visceral epithelial cells in human membranous nephropathy. Am. J. Pathol. 146 (6), 1444–1454.

Ohashi, K., Burkart, V., et al. 2000. Cutting edge: heat shock protein 60 is a putative endogenous ligand of the toll-like receptor-4 complex. J. Immunol. 164 (2), 558–561.

Okada, H., Konishi, K., et al. 1994. Interleukin-4 expression in mesangial proliferative glomerulonephritis. Am. J. Kidney Dis. 23 (2), 242–246.

Panzer, U., Steinmetz, O.M., et al. 2006. Kidney diseases and chemokines. Curr. Drug Targets 7 (1), 65–80.

Patole, P.S., Zecher, D., et al. 2005. G-rich DNA suppresses systemic lupus. J. Am. Soc. Nephrol. 16 (11), 3273–3280.

Pawar, R.D., Patole, P.S., et al. 2006. Toll-like receptor-7 modulates immune complex glomerulonephritis. J. Am. Soc. Nephrol. 17 (1), 141–149.

Peng, S.L., Moslehi, J., et al. 1997. Roles of interferon-$\gamma$ and interleukin-4 in murine lupus. J. Clin. Invest. 99 (8), 1936–1946.

Perez de Lema, G., Maier, H., et al. 2005. Chemokine receptor Ccr2 deficiency reduces renal disease and prolongs survival in MRL/lpr lupus-prone mice. J. Am. Soc. Nephrol. 16 (12), 3592–3601.

Pfister, H., Ollert, M., et al. 2004. Antineutrophil cytoplasmic autoantibodies against the murine homolog of proteinase 3 (Wegener autoantigen) are pathogenic in vivo. Blood 104 (5), 1411–1418.

Popa, E.R., Franssen, C.F., et al. 2002. In vitro cytokine production and proliferation of T cells from patients with anti-proteinase 3- and antimyeloperoxidase-associated vasculitis, in response to proteinase 3 and myeloperoxidase. Arthritis Rheum. 46 (7), 1894–1904.

Reynolds, J., Norgan, V.A., et al. 2002. Anti-CD8 monoclonal antibody therapy is effective in the prevention and treatment of experimental autoimmune glomerulonephritis. J. Am. Soc. Nephrol. 13 (2), 359–369.

Richardson, B., Scheinbart, L., et al. 1990. Evidence for impaired T cell DNA methylation in systemic lupus erythematosus and rheumatoid arthritis. Arthritis Rheum. 33 (11), 1665–1673.

Ruth, A.J., Kitching, A.R., et al. 2006. Anti-neutrophil cytoplasmic antibodies and effector CD4+ cells play nonredundant roles in anti-myeloperoxidase crescentic glomerulonephritis. J. Am. Soc. Nephrol. 17 (7), 1940–1949.

Ruth, A.J., Kitching, A.R., et al. 2003. Intrinsic renal cell expression of CD40 directs Th1 effectors inducing experimental crescentic glomerulonephritis. J. Am. Soc. Nephrol. 14 (11), 2813–2822.

Salama, A.D., Chaudhry, A.N., et al. 2003. Regulation by CD25+ lymphocytes of autoantigen-specific T cell responses in Goodpasture's (anti-GBM) disease. Kidney Int. 64 (5), 1685–1694.

Salama, A.D., Dougan, T., et al. 2002. Goodpasture's disease in the absence of circulating anti-glomerular basement membrane antibodies as detected by standard techniques. Am. J. Kidney Dis. 39 (6), 1162–1167.

Santiago-Raber, M.L., Baccala, R., et al. 2003. Type-I interferon receptor deficiency reduces lupus-like disease in NZB mice. J. Exp. Med. 197 (6), 777–788.

Schlondorff, D. 1996. Roles of the mesangium in glomerular function. Kidney Int. 49 (6), 1583–1585.

Schwarting, A., Paul, K., et al. 2005. Interferon-beta: a therapeutic for autoimmune lupus in MRL-Faslpr mice. J. Am. Soc. Nephrol. 16 (11), 3264–3272.

Schwarting, A., Wada, T., et al. 1998. IFN-γ receptor signaling is essential for the initiation, acceleration, and destruction of autoimmune kidney disease in MRL-$Fas^{lpr}$ Mice. J. Immunol. 161 (1), 494–503.

Segal, R., Dayan, M., et al. 2001. Suppression of experimental systemic lupus erythematosus (SLE) in mice via TNF inhibition by an anti-TNFalpha monoclonal antibody and by pentoxiphylline. Lupus 10 (1), 23–31.

Segerer, S., Cui, Y., et al. 2000. Expression of the chemokine monocyte chemoattractant protein-1 and its receptor chemokine receptor 2 in human crescentic glomerulonephritis. J. Am. Soc. Nephrol. 11 (12), 2231–2242.

Segerer, S., Mac, K.M., et al. 1999. Expression of the C–C chemokine receptor 5 in human kidney diseases. Kidney Int. 56 (1), 52–64.

Shinozaki, M., Hirahashi, J., et al. 2002. IL-15, a survival factor for kidney epithelial cells, counteracts apoptosis and inflammation during nephritis. J. Clin. Invest. 109 (7), 951–960.

Stohl, W. 2004. A therapeutic role for BLyS antagonists. Lupus 13 (5), 317–322.

Studnicka-Benke, A., Steiner, G., et al. 1996. Tumour necrosis factor alpha and its soluble receptors parallel clinical disease and autoimmune activity in systemic lupus erythematosus. Br. J. Rheumatol. 35 (11), 1067–1074.

Tackey, E., Lipsky, P.E., et al. 2004. Rationale for interleukin-6 blockade in systemic lupus erythematosus. Lupus 13 (5), 339–343.

Takemura, T., Yoshioka, K., et al. 1994. Cellular localization of inflammatory cytokines in human glomerulonephritis. Virchows Arch. 424 (5), 459–464.

Tarzi, R.M., Cook, H.T., et al. 2004. Leptin-deficient mice are protected from accelerated nephrotoxic nephritis. Am. J. Pathol. 164 (2), 385–390.

Tato, C.M., O'Shea, J.J. 2006. Immunology: what does it mean to be just 17? Nature 441 (7090), 166–168.

Tesch, G.H., Maifert, S., et al. 1999. Monocyte chemoattractant protein 1-dependent leukocytic infiltrates are responsible for autoimmune disease in MRL-Fas(lpr) mice. J. Exp. Med. 190 (12), 1813–1824.

The Wegener's Granulomatosis Etanercept Trial (WGET) Research Group. 2005. Etanercept plus standard therapy for Wegener's granulomatosis. N. Engl. J. Med. 352 (4), 351–361.

Theofilopoulos, A.N., Lawson, B.R. 1999. Tumour necrosis factor and other cytokines in murine lupus. Ann. Rheum. Dis. 58 (Suppl. 1), I49–I55.

Timoshanko, J.R., Holdsworth, S.R., et al. 2002. IFN-gamma production by intrinsic renal cells and bone marrow-derived cells is required for full expression of crescentic glomerulonephritis in mice. J. Immunol. 168 (8), 4135–4141.

Timoshanko, J.R., Kitching, A.R., et al. 2001. Interleukin-12 from intrinsic cells is an effector of renal injury in crescentic glomerulonephritis. J. Am. Soc. Nephrol. 12 (3), 464–471.

Timoshanko, J.R., Kitching, A.R., et al. 2004. Leukocyte-derived interleukin-1beta interacts with renal interleukin-1 receptor I to promote renal tumor necrosis factor and glomerular injury in murine crescentic glomerulonephritis. Am. J. Pathol. 164 (6), 1967–1977.

Timoshanko, J.R., Sedgwick, J.D., et al. 2003. Intrinsic renal cells are the major source of tumor necrosis factor contributing to renal injury in murine crescentic glomerulonephritis. J. Am. Soc. Nephrol. 14 (7), 1785–1793.

Tipping, P.G., Kitching, A.R., et al. 1997. Immune modulation with interleukin-4 and interleukin-10 prevents crescent formation and glomerular injury in experimental glomerulonephritis. Eur. J. Immunol. 27 (2), 530–537.

Tomosugi, N.I., Cashman, S.J., et al. 1989. Modulation of antibody-mediated glomerular injury in vivo by bacterial lipopolysaccharide, tumor necrosis factor, and IL-1. J. Immunol. 142 (9), 3083–3090.

Topham, P.S., Csizmadia, V., et al. 1999. Lack of chemokine receptor CCR1 enhances Th1 responses and glomerular injury during nephrotoxic nephritis. J. Clin. Invest. 104, 1549–1557.

Tucci, M., Calvani, N., et al. 2005. The interplay of chemokines and dendritic cells in the pathogenesis of lupus nephritis. Ann. N. Y. Acad. Sci. 1051, 421–432.

Uhm, W.S., Na, K., et al. 2003. Cytokine balance in kidney tissue from lupus nephritis patients. Rheumatology (Oxford) 42 (8), 935–938.

Vacher-Coponat, H., Pache, X., et al. 1997. Pulmonary–renal syndrome responding to corticosteroids: consider cholesterol embolization. Nephrol. Dial. Transpl. 12 (9), 1977–1979.

Vasoo, S., Hughes, G.R. 2005. Theory, targets and therapy in systemic lupus erythematosus. Lupus 14 (3), 181–188.

Wada, T., Furuichi, K., et al. 1999. MIP-1alpha and MCP-1 contribute to crescents and interstitial lesions in human crescentic glomerulonephritis. Kidney Int. 56 (3), 995–1003.

Weaver, C.T., Hatton, R.D., et al., 2007. IL-17 family cytokines and the expanding diversity of effector T cell lineages. Annu. Rev. Immunol. 25, 821–852.

Wu, X., Dolecki, G.J., et al. 1997. Chemokines are expressed in a myeloid cell-dependent fashion and mediate distinct functions in immune complex glomerulonephritis in rat. J. Immunol. 158 (8), 3917–3924.

Yu, P., Wellmann, U., et al. 2006. Toll-like receptor 9-independent aggravation of glomerulonephritis in a novel model of SLE. Int. Immunol. 18 (8), 1211–1219.

Zheng, W., Flavell, R.A. 1997. The transcription factor GATA-3 is necessary and sufficient for Th2 cytokine gene expression in CD4 T cells. Cell 89 (4), 587–596.

Zhou, A., Ueno, H., et al. 2003. Blockade of TGF-beta action ameliorates renal dysfunction and histologic progression in anti-GBM nephritis. Kidney Int. 64 (1), 92–101.

# CHAPTER 4

# Pathogenesis of Renal Disease: Cellular Mechanisms

Lars-Peter Erwig*, Heather Wilson, Andrew J. Rees

*Department of Medicine and Therapeutics, Institute of Medical Sciences, University of Aberdeen, Aberdeen AB25 2ZD, Scotland, UK*

## 1. Introduction

Renal disease has a wide spectrum of histological patterns and clinical outcomes, indicating that a variety of immunopathogenic mechanisms of injury are involved. Not all renal inflammatory processes lead to end-stage renal failure but those that do are characterized by progressive renal fibrosis. Over the last two decades it has become apparent that all types of renal injury are associated with migration of immunologically competent cells into the affected area (Kluth et al., 2004; Erwig et al., 2003; Tipping and Kitching, 2005). Macrophages and T-cells are the most extensively studied but there is increasing evidence that other cells of the innate and the acquired immune system are intricately involved in renal inflammation. This review focuses on recent advances in understanding of these immunocompetent cells and their role in experimental models of nephritis and human disease. It is beyond the scope of this review to include resident renal cells, which nonetheless play an important role in creating the microenvironment that determines subsequent function of the infiltrating cells (reviewed in Tipping and Timoshanko, 2005; Gómez-Guerrero et al., 2005).

It would be intuitive to discuss the individual cell types involved in renal inflammation separately but, despite their distinctiveness, we felt that the common underlying principles that govern their activation, subsequent function, and consequences for renal injury are best illustrated when discussed collectively.

## 2. Overview of immune inflammation

Knowledge about cell-mediated immune responses is expanding at a bewildering rate. Established paradigms such as the separation of Th1 and Th2 responses are no longer adequate to explain T-cell-mediated inflammation. Two themes dominate recent advances in understanding immune-mediated inflammation: the ever more intimate links between the innate and adaptive immune systems; and the dual pro- and anti-inflammatory roles of the myeloid cells and lymphocytes that comprise the innate and adaptive immune system respectively.

Despite the wealth of new information it remains clear that antigen is presented to T-cells by antigen presenting cells. This is done most effectively by dendritic cells (DCs) but also by macrophages, B-cells, and mast cells and probably by other cell types as well. The new insight is that depending on the context even (or especially) DCs can induce either T helper responses or immune tolerance. Similarly, T-cells can be activated to become helper (Th) cells or regulatory (Treg) cells depending on the cytokine environment or the co-stimulating molecules engaged.

The T-cells in turn activate macrophages and here again the traditional separation into

*Corresponding author.
Tel.: +44 1224 550526; Fax: +44 1224 555766
E-mail address: L.P.Erwig@abdn.ac.uk

© 2008 Published by Elsevier B.V.
DOI: 10.1016/S1571-5078(07)07004-3

classically activated (histotoxic) and alternatively activated (reparative or pro-fibrotic) macrophages has proved inadequate. It is now clear that macrophages have the ability to develop many different properties, but as yet there are few data about the molecular cues responsible.

## 3. Activation

The inflammatory response to injury should be viewed as an effort designed to restore normal function with as little residual tissue damage as possible. This requires activation of the infiltrating cells of the immune system to adopt functions appropriate for the injury encountered.

Classical macrophage activation was first described in the 1960s in studies by North and Mackaness (Hamilton, 2002; North and Mackaness, 1973). It requires priming by IFN-$\gamma$ together with a second activating signal such as a microbial product ligating Toll-like receptors (LPS, CpG), or a pro-inflammatory cytokine (IL-1, TNF-$\alpha$). Classically activated macrophages kill and degrade bacteria by production of toxic oxygen species and nitric oxide (NO). They express high levels of MHC class II, co-stimulatory molecules (e.g., CD86) and cytokines (e.g., IL-12) that support Th1-driven immune responses (Wilson et al., 2005). Th1 and Th2 cells are the classical subsets of primed CD4+ T helper cells that can be distinguished functionally by their cytokine profile and their ability to generate different types of immune effector responses. More recently Th17 cells have been described which are generated in the presence of IL-6 combined with TGF-$\beta$ and secrete IL-17 abundantly. These Th17 cells play an essential role in injury in some rodent models of autoimmune disease, such as EAE and collagen-induced arthritis but have yet to be investigated in renal injury.

Th1 cells produce IFN-$\gamma$, IL-2, and TNF-$\alpha$ and are therefore directly linked with classical macrophage activation but also activate B-cells to produce complement fixing antibodies that mediate opsonization and phagocytosis. Th2 cells produce IL-4, IL-5, and IL-13 that promote production of non-complement fixing IgG isotypes and IgE. This links Th2 cells with the more recently described alternatively activated macrophages (Gordon, 2003) (induced by IL-4, IL-13, and glucocorticoids). These macrophages are not cytotoxic but are primarily involved in tissue repair, and provoke increased deposition of extracellular matrix (Gordon, 2003). Their characteristics are increased expression of mannose receptor together with other scavenger receptors, galactose-like receptors, and the IL-1 receptor antagonist. Alternatively activated mouse macrophages express increased arginase and the transcription factors FIZZ1 and Ym1 (Raes et al., 2002). They deal poorly with intracellular pathogens because of their inability to produce nitrogen radicals.

Another more recently described macrophage activation state, the so-called Type II activation, develops after exposure to LPS or CD40 ligand in cells primed by the presence of IgG immune complexes (Mosser, 2003). These cells are anti-inflammatory because of enhanced IL-10 and decreased IL-12 production (Wilson et al., 2005; Mosser, 2003). IL-10 was viewed as a cytokine that merely de-activates macrophages but more recent data suggest that it activates expression of sets of genes that control resolution of inflammation, matrix synthesis, and tissue remodeling (Mantovani et al., 2004; Williams et al., 2004). Furthermore, IL-10 is essential for the generation, and one of the main products, of regulatory CD4+ CD25+ Treg cells and appears to be more active in inhibiting Th1 differentiation than promoting Th2 responses (Constant and Bottomly, 1997). Treg cells develop when T-cells are activated in the presence of TGF-$\beta$, IL-10, or possibly IL-9. Again Treg are heterogeneous with two broad categories that have been identified: "natural Tregs" that appear to suppress T-cell responses non-specifically and antigen specific Treg cells that are the product of specific immune responses. The exact relationship between these two types of Treg cells has not been elucidated and it is highly likely that studies to clarify the issue will also reveal additional types of Treg cells. DCs play a dominant role in activation of naïve T-cells and various subsets have been identified with a bias toward stimulating T-cells to either produce IFN-$\gamma$ or IL-4, -5, and -10, respectively, in vitro (Moser and Murphy, 2000).

Thus, over the last decade an increasing number of activation states for cells of the innate and acquired immune system have been described with a remarkable symmetry for the distinct cell lineages. However, much remains to be learned about the different activation states of immune-competent cells in vitro and vivo. A few basic principles are beginning to emerge: (i) activation requires a priming stimulus to confer specificity (such as IFN-$\gamma$, FcR ligation, or ingestion of a dying cell) followed by an amplification stimulus, most commonly TLR ligation; (ii) activation occurs early either during localization or shortly thereafter and renders cells at least temporarily unresponsive to other activation signals; and (iii) as outlined above, specific activation of one of the cell types involved is likely to bias the activation of others leading to an injury specific response.

Systems biology will be at the heart of future approaches to understanding complex systems with "emergent properties" (properties that cannot be predicted even with full understanding of the parts alone) (reviewed in Aderem, 2005). Macrophage or T-cell activation and even more so the immune response to injury are such systems. Reductionist approaches will not be sufficient and genuine understanding will only be achievable using high-throughput approaches (microarray, proteomics, etc.) combined with advanced bioinformatics and subsequent visualization programs. The results of comprehensive gene and protein expression studies are just beginning to emerge (Williams et al., 2004; Ravasi et al., 2002) but already they illustrate the limitations of the traditional nomenclature for macrophage activation (Wilson et al., 2005).

## 4. Regulation of immune cell activation

Immune cell activation is regulated at multiple levels: (i) outside the cell, through the release of inhibitors and decoy receptors into the microenvironment (Mantovani et al., 2001); (ii) at the cell surface, where a large number of pattern recognition receptors including Toll-like receptors, scavenger receptors, complement receptors, C-type lectin receptors, and integrins, recognize conserved motifs on pathogens that are not found on higher eukaryotes. Cytokine receptors are important for innate immune cell activation and the differentiation of T-cells, together with co-stimulatory receptors that enhance or inhibit the adaptive immune response; (iii) inside the cell, a vast number of signaling pathways regulate immune cell activation. They can be separated into signaling modules such as IFN-$\gamma$ or Toll-like receptor signaling. Many of these modules are engaged simultaneously on immune cell activation and the cross talk and integration of information required for an appropriate immune response is astonishing.

A robust immune response requires feedback loops to prevent unrestrained and damaging immune cell activation. These include negative regulators of intracellular signaling, such as inhibitory Smads and SOCS proteins that inhibit cytokine signaling (Gómez-Guerrero, 2004; Takahashi et al., 2005). Paired activating and inhibitory receptors have been described (i.e., Fc receptor signaling) where the inhibitory receptor possesses an ITIM motif in the intracellular portion instead of the ITAM motif found on activating receptors. The interaction of two opposing receptors will set a threshold for stimulation and the ratio of activating to inhibitory receptor will modulate immune cell activation. Increasing numbers of non-paired inhibitory receptors been described which include CD200, SIRP-$\alpha$, and MSP/RON (Wright et al., 2000; Gardai et al., 2003; Wang et al., 2002).

### 4.1. Manipulation of immune cell activation by tumors

Manipulation of immune-competent cells to induce properties that contribute to inhibition of inflammation is becoming the "Holy Grail" of immunological research and not unattainable because tumors and microorganisms have already evolved to achieve this goal. Hematopoetic cells are recruited to most tumors, and tumor-associated macrophages (TAMs) can constitute a large portion of tumor mass (Pollard. 2004). A high density of TAMs correlates with poor prognosis (Bingle et al., 2002). Macrophage depleted mice homozygous for a null mutation in the CSF-1 gene showed a markedly reduced rate of tumor progression and ablation of metastasis formation in a mouse model of breast cancer (Lin et al., 2001). Tumor macrophages have a rather immature phenotype characterized by low expression of carboxypeptidase M and CD51 and low production of TNF-α. They have a markedly reduced ability to present tumor-associated antigens to T-cells and to stimulate the proliferation of T-cells and natural killer cells. Moreover, Mantovani et al. (2006) proposed that exposure to IL-4 in tumors induces TAMs to develop into alternatively activated macrophages that promote angiogenesis and growth factor production supporting stromal invasion. The ability of tumors to subvert macrophage function and subsequent T-cell and NK-cell activation provides a clear precedent to altering immune cell activation to control inflammation and favor angiogenesis and resolution of tissue injury.

## 5. Immune cells and clinical renal disease

Renal macrophages were first identified using electron microscopy in biopsies from patients with severe proliferative glomerulonephritis (GN, Churg, 1973) and these observations were extended by Atkins and colleagues using glomerular culture (Nikolic-Paterson et al., 1997). It is now apparent that macrophage infiltration is a hallmark feature of all types of acute injury and chronic progressive renal disease. This is true for primarily inflammatory diseases such as GN and renal transplant rejection, as well as for diseases with secondary inflammation such as ureteric obstruction, and also for diseases such as diabetes in which an inflammatory component has only been recently appreciated (Schreiner, 1991; Furuta et al., 1993). Careful quantitative studies in each of these settings have correlated the number of infiltrating macrophages with the severity of the disease and they have been used to assess prognosis. Indeed, Hill et al. (2001) showed that estimating macrophage numbers was the best prognostic marker in follow-up biopsies of patients treated for lupus nephritis.

CD4+ T-cells are invariably present in crescentic nephritis even in uncommon causes of crescents such as membranous GN (Arrizabalaga et al., 1998). In ANCA-associated GN, T-cells and macrophages are present in glomerular lesions (Cunningham et al., 1999) and biopsies show high IFN-γ and low IL-4 glomerular mRNA expression indicating a Th1 and classical macrophage activation dominant effector response (Masutani et al., 2003). These macrophages express high levels of MHC class II and TNF-α whereas less than 30% of macrophages in cryoglobulinaemic nephritis express these proteins. Peripheral blood T-cells in ANCA-associated GN showed a high IFN:IL-4 ratio compared to non-proliferative GN and IgA disease (Masutani et al., 2003). Wegeners granulomatosis patients in remission demonstrate a persistent expansion of Th2 effector memory T-cells with a concomitant decrease of naive CD4+ T-cells in their peripheral blood which may contribute to the frequent relapses in this disease (Abdulahad et al., 2006).

Goodpasture's disease provides the clearest example yet of the evolution of autoimmune responses to a renal antigen: the NC1 domain of the α3 chain of Type IV collagen (α3(IV)NC1). Rees and colleagues mapped the α3(IV)NC1 epitopes recognized by patients' T-cells and showed that they resulted in a Th1 response in the acute phase of the disease but this evolved into IL-10 dominated Tr cell responses over time even in the absence of immunosuppressive therapy (Cairns et al., 2003) This is consistent with findings in Goodpasture's disease where a population of regulatory CD25+ T-cells appear in the peripheral blood approximately 3 months after the acute presentation and may play a critical role in preventing relapses, which are rare in this condition in comparison to other human autoimmune diseases (Salama et al., 2003).

Not surprisingly human lupus nephritis displays heterogeneity of Th1 and Th2 responses, given the diverse underlying glomerular lesions ranging from severe crescentic disease to the less proliferative membranous GN, to minimal or no glomerular changes. Overall the data support the hypothesis that severe proliferative GN results from a Th1-predominant response with increased renal CD3+ cells and macrophages accompanied by Th1 cytokines IL-2 and IFN-γ in the urine (Chan et al., 2003), whereas less severe disease is associated with cytokines and IgG subclasses in keeping with a Th2 immune response (Masutani et al., 2001). B-cell depletion in patients with refractory nephritis using Rituximab, a monoclonal anti-CD20 antibody, is a promising new treatment alternative. Interestingly, the published data show that, following B-cell depletion, remission of lupus nephritis is associated with a decrease in helper T-cell activation (Sfikakis et al., 2005) and, in another study, increased numbers of CD4+ regulatory cells (Treg, Th3, Tr1) but not CD8+ cells (Vigna-Perez et al., 2006). This suggests an additional role for B-cells, independent of autoantibody production in promoting disease.

Non-proliferative forms of GN, such as membranous GN and minimal change nephropathy, are associated with an incomplete Th2 response, with lack of a substantial leukocytic infiltrate and/or deposition of IgG4 in glomeruli (Imai et al., 1997; Doi et al., 1984). In IgA nephropathy MCP-1 expression was associated with more severe disease and a number of studies have corelated urinary MCP-1 levels with severity of injury (Eardley et al., 2006). Furthermore, the presence of γ/δ T-cells in renal biopsies is associated with progressive renal deterioration possibly due to a marked production of TGF-β by these cells and associated IgA subclass switching in B-cells (Falk et al., 1995; Toyabe et al., 2001). Kooten and colleagues show that DCs of IgA patients have an impaired capacity to induce IgA production in naive B-cells (Eijgenraam et al., 2005). Thus, severe disease appears to be associated with a Th1-predominant response whereas the onset of the disease may be related to a Th2 predominant environment that promotes dysregulated IgA production.

It is important to keep in mind that immune cell activation in nephritis is critically dependent on location. Interstitial but not glomerular macrophages express the chemokine receptor CCR5 in both proliferative GN (Segerer et al., 1999) and transplant rejection (Segerer et al., 2001) whereas macrophages in both locations express the fractalkine receptor (CX3CR1) (Segerer et al., 2002). Similarly, glomerular macrophages in renal biopsies from patients with severe nephritis have abundant myeloid related protein (MRP)-8 and MRP-14 complexes that are associated with inflammatory macrophages, whereas interstitial macrophages show lower levels (Frosch et al., 2004). In Wegener's granulomatosis, increased levels of IL-4 and CCR3 expression were reported in nasal tissue, suggesting Th2 bias, whereas both IL-2 and CCR5+ (Th1) and IL-4 and CCR2+ cells (Th2) were present in renal tissue with no Th2 bias (Balding et al., 2001).

Although fragmentary, these data already demonstrate the heterogeneity of immune cells in renal biopsies, and provide compelling evidence that immune cell activation and function vary depending on the type of injury.

## 6. Immune cells in experimental models of nephritis

Initial depletion studies in nephrotoxic nephritis (NTN) in rabbits using an anti-macrophage antibody reduced the severity of inflammation, while induction of leucopenia by nitrogen mustard protected from development of disease which could be reconstituted by injection of peritoneal macrophages (Holdsworth et al., 1981; Holdsworth and Neale, 1984). More recent studies in which leukopenia was induced by cyclophosphamide showed that disease could be reconstituted by injection of either bone-marrow derived macrophages or a macrophage cell line (Ikezumi et al., 2003b). Stimulation of macrophages with IFN-γ prior to injection increased the severity of proteinuria (Ikezumi et al., 2003a), while inhibiting the JNK signaling pathway before adoptive transfer reduced proteinuria and cell proliferation, showing that the state of macrophage activation is critical in determining outcome (Ikezumi et al., 2004). Administration of clodronate liposomes selectively kills macrophages and has been used to deplete macrophages in rodent models. This approach attenuates inflammatory injury in NTN in WKY rats (Isome et al., 2004), and renal transplant rejection in rats (Jose et al., 2003). Macrophage depletion by the same method also reduces mesangial matrix expansion but not proteinuria in Thy 1.1 nephritis (Westerhuis et al., 2000). Conditional ablation of macrophages in transgenic mice by minute injections of diphtheria toxin reduced the number of glomerular crescents, improved renal function, and reduced proteinuria in established NTN and this was associated with a reduced number of CD4 positive T-cells in the kidney (Duffield et al., 2005b).

Mice with genetic deficiency of mast cells exhibit increased mortality in NTN compared to wildtype littermates. The mast cell-deficient mice showed thick subendothelial deposits enriched in fibrin and collagen, expanded glomerular matrix, a marked increase in glomerular macrophages and a small but significant rise in CD4+ T-cells (Kanamaru et al., 2006). Thus, mast cells have protective properties in immune complex-mediated GN, most likely through their ability to secrete proteases that prevent fibrin and collagen deposition. Mast cells are best known as primary responders in allergic reactions such as asthma and anaphylaxis, but recent data establish that they are functionally diverse and can function as immunoregulatory cells that influence both innate and adaptive immunity. This is beautifully illustrated by the work of Noelle and colleagues, which shows their essential role in regulatory T-cell allograft tolerance (Lu et al., 2006).

## 7. Immune cell function in nephritis

Appropriately activated macrophages produce a wide range of potentially cytotoxic products including proteolytic enzymes, reactive oxygen, and nitrogen species, eicosanoids, pro-inflammatory cytokines and chemokines. Macrophages isolated from nephritic glomeruli in rats and rabbits generate reactive oxygen species (Cook et al., 1989; Boyce et al., 1989; Cattell et al., 1990) and similarly nephritic glomeruli from rats produce large amounts of NO. In both NTN and Heymann's nephritis macrophages are the principal source of NO (Cattell et al., 1991). It remains unclear, however, whether NO itself causes glomerular injury as inhibition experiments have produced conflicting results (Waddington et al., 1996; Ogawa et al., 2002; Duffield et al., 2000).

Direct evidence that renal macrophages can attenuate injury and facilitate repair has been difficult to obtain, but the increasing amount of data from other tissues such as lung and skin (Teder et al., 2002; Nagaoka et al., 2000), provides a compelling reason to believe they do. In vitro studies show the vast range of reparative properties of macrophages including secretion of anti-inflammatory cytokines, matrix repair proteins and angiogenic factors, and their ability to phagocytose apoptotic cells, immune complexes and fibrin. Likewise, infusing anti-inflammatory cytokines, including IL-4, IL-6, IL-10, and TGF-$\beta$ reduces injury without a change in the number of renal macrophages (Kluth et al., 2004). More recently, a study in liver injury by Duffield et al. (2005a) verifies that functionally distinct subpopulations of macrophages exist in the same tissue, favoring ECM accumulation during ongoing injury but enhancing matrix degradation during recovery, highlighting their role in both injury and recovery phases of inflammatory scarring. Nishida et al. (2001) have shown that infiltrating macrophages in the kidney may play a beneficial anti-fibrotic role that, surprisingly, requires the action of angiotensin II.

A population of CD11C+ DCs has been described in normal mouse kidney and cell numbers are upregulated in the tubulointerstitium but not within glomeruli in NTN (Kruger et al., 2004). Nelson and colleagues have shown that within the renal parenchyma, there exists little immunological privilege from the surveillance provided by renal CX3CR1+ DCs, a major constituent of the heterogeneous mononuclear phagocyte system populating normal kidney (Soos et al., 2006). Activation of multiple TLRs has been shown to aggravate the immune complex GN induced by apoferritin as well as the lupus like GN in MRLlpr/lpr mice (Anders et al., 2004; Pawar et al., 2006). In both disease models aggravation was associated with enhanced autoantibody production and intrarenal activation of antigen presenting cells, which secreted increased amounts of IFN-α, IL-12p70, and CCL2.

T-cell function in experimental nephritis is influenced by multiple stimuli including cytokines, co-stimulatory molecules, and inhibitors of signaling pathways. Genetic deletion or blocking of Th1 cytokines with inhibitory antibodies attenuates T-cell and macrophage accumulation and crescentic injury. Administration of IL-12 augments Th1 responses and crescentic GN. Interleukin-18 (which contributes to Th1 responses and is produced by macrophages and DCs) augmented cutaneous DTH responses and exacerbated crescentic GN (Kitching et al., 2000), and inhibition of IL-18 reduced lymphoproliferation, IFN-γ production, and improved survival in murine lupus (Bossu et al., 2003).

Studies in murine NTN, in which co-stimulatory molecules were inhibited by antibody or genetically deficient, showed augmentation of injury in CD86 deficiency and reduction of crescent formation in CD80 deficiency. CD28 deficiency in mice or administration of CTLA4-Ig ameliorated murine NTN without an observable Th1/Th2 shift (Li et al., 2000). Numerous signaling and transcription factors have been implicated in T-cell activation in experimental nephritis, these include members of almost all relevant cytokine signaling pathways. These can influence Th1/Th2 differentiation, for example activation of STAT signaling can promote Th1 responses through STAT1 and the transcription factor T-bet (Singh et al., 2003) or promote Th2 responses following activation of STAT6 and GATA-3 by IL-4 (Yoh et al., 2003).

## 8. Characterization of immune cells within inflamed glomeruli

The characterization of immune cells within inflamed tissue at a single cell level is lacking due to a relative paucity of markers that clearly delineate different states of activation, although this is being addressed by gene chip analysis of macrophage expression under specific conditions (Ragno et al., 2001).

Macrophages both respond to and produce pro-inflammatory cytokines within foci of renal inflammation, and a recent series of studies has attempted to dissect their relative contributions. Using bone marrow chimeras in knockout mice, Tipping and colleagues have shown that TNF-α and IL-12 production during NTN in mice is mainly dependent on intrinsic renal cells rather than infiltrating leukocytes (Timoshanko et al., 2001, 2003), while IFN-γ production requires contributions from both (Timoshanko et al., 2002), with macrophage production potentially as significant as the T-cell contribution (Carvalho-Pinto et al., 2002).

Work by Erwig and colleagues has shown that potent activating signals, such as IFN-γ and TNF-α, commit macrophages to distinct sets of properties in vitro, and commitment to one set of properties is accompanied by unresponsiveness to other activating stimuli (Erwig et al., 1998). Macrophages infiltrating acutely inflamed glomeruli of rats with NTN behave as though activated by IFN-γ (Erwig et al., 2000), and maintain these characteristics during the acute phase of injury despite systemic administration of alternatively activating cytokines such as IL-4 (Erwig et al., 2000; Robertson et al., 2002). Subsequent observations in anti-Thy1.1 nephritis have shown: first, that macrophage localization itself does not induce specific activation states; second, that all macrophages infiltrating an appropriate environment become specifically activated shortly after localization; and third, macrophages infiltrating glomeruli at the same time can be activated in different ways (Minto et al., 2003). These observations raise questions about the factors that induce macrophage activation at early stages of the inflammatory disease and its consequences for the outcome of the inflammatory process. It provides an important mechanistic insight into how macrophage functional development is influenced by the underlying disease process.

## 8.1. Immune cell fate during progressive inflammation

Macrophages contain high levels of lysosomal proteases and rapidly degrade internalized proteins, while DCs and B lymphocytes are protease-poor, resulting in a limited capacity for lysosomal degradation (Delamarre et al., 2005; Erwig et al., 2006). Consistent with these findings, DCs in vivo emigrate from inflamed tissue and retain antigen in lymphoid organs for extended periods, which favors antigen presentation (Delamarre et al., 2005). The fate of macrophages that proliferate within or enter a focus of renal inflammation remains less clear. The two possibilities are death within the glomerulus or interstitium or emigration to regional lymph nodes. Widespread macrophage apoptosis is rarely seen within inflamed kidney but professional and non-professional phagocytes rapidly remove dying cells and it is therefore, to date, impossible to define the degree of local cell death. Macrophage migration to regional lymph nodes has been demonstrated in rats with NTN (Lan et al., 1993). Furthermore, in a mouse model of resolving peritonitis, fluorescently labeled macrophages could be tracked to draining lymph nodes and emigrated with a half-life of 48 h (Bellingan et al., 1996). This process has recently been shown to be actively mediated and partially dependent on VLA-4 and -5 (Bellingan et al., 2002). In our own studies where we have injected labeled adenoviral transduced macrophages into rats with NTN these cells disappear from inflamed glomeruli again with a half-life of approximately 48 h (Kluth et al., 2000; Kluth et al., 2001). These data imply that macrophages and DCs continually traffic through a site of inflammation where they sense injury and instruct the subsequent immune response.

## 9. Immune modulation of renal inflammatory disease

Tumors and microorganisms have evolved ways to manipulate macrophage function to protect them from immune attack while simultaneously enhancing their growth (Rosenberger and Finlay, 2003; Bingle et al., 2002). An important challenge for nephrologists is to develop equally effective strategies for manipulating macrophage function therapeutically. Three experimental strategies have been used to achieve this: modulation of cytokine activity systemically; modifying macrophage activation ex vivo before re-infusion; and genetic manipulation of macrophages. Numerous agents have been administered systemically to modulate renal inflammation, including antibodies and other antagonists of IL-1 and TNF-$\alpha$, anti-inflammatory cytokines such as IL-4, IL-6, IL-10, and IL-11 (reviewed in Kluth et al., 2004). An alternative approach is manipulating intracellular signaling pathways such as the transcription factor NF-$\kappa$B (Lopez-Franco et al., 2002) or PPAR-$\gamma$ (Haraguchi et al., 2003).

Infusion of macrophages genetically modified by transducing them with adenovirus expressing IL-4 (Kluth et al., 2001), IL-10 (Wilson et al., 2002) or IL-1RA (Yokoo et al., 1999) into rats with NTN, or IL-1RA into mice with unilateral ureteric obstruction (Yamagishi et al., 2001), reduces macrophage infiltration and injury. Interestingly, infusion of IL-4 and IL-10 expressing macrophages into the left renal artery also reduces injury in the non-injected contra-lateral kidney, even though negligible numbers of injected macrophages localize there and circulating IL-4 or IL-10 is undetectable (Kluth et al., 2001; Wilson et al., 2002). The most likely explanation is that high concentrations of locally secreted cytokine modify the inflammatory cells trafficking through the glomerulus to regional lymph nodes where they down-modulate the immune response.

Yokoo et al. (2001) have recently developed a system of regulated trans-gene expression so that macrophages release IL-1RA only after localization to inflamed glomeruli. This was achieved using double transduced macrophages with an adenovirus containing Cre recombinase under the control of the IL-1$\beta$ promoter and a second adenovirus carrying a floxed reporter gene under the control of strong viral promoter. However, gene expression by transduced macrophages is short term. One way to overcome this is integration of genes into bone marrow cells that differentiate into macrophages, which has been achieved using retroviral transformation. More recently, successful gene delivery using retrovirally transduced cord blood-derived CD34+ cells into inflamed glomeruli in NOD/SCID mice has been demonstrated indicating that human stem cells can mature into macrophages in vivo (Yokoo et al., 2003). These approaches offer promise for the future.

## 10. Summary

In this chapter, we have tried to summarize the current knowledge about cellular mechanisms in immune-mediated renal injury. Clearly there is much yet to be learned, especially as the recently acquired knowledge emphasizes the ever increasing subtlety of the mechanisms that control immune-mediated inflammation. Old views that immune-mediated injury could be treated effectively by preventing lymphocytes and macrophages from infiltrating the kidney have proven simplistic and the current emphasis is to use emerging knowledge to develop strategies for deviating infiltrating inflammatory cells, whether lymphocytes or macrophages, toward an anti-inflammatory and reparative type. Currently, macrophages provide the most promising opportunities to achieve this. Indeed the precedent of how effectively microorganisms and tumors manipulate immune cell function provides a challenge for physicians to do the same.

**Key points**

- All types of renal injury are associated with infiltration of immune-competent cells
- The same basic principles govern the activation and subsequent function of immune-competent cells of different lineages
- These cells become activated and depending on the microenvironment either facilitate repair or promote injury
- Manipulation of activation and subsequent function rather than preventing infiltration is a promising avenue for therapeutic gain

## References

Abdulahad, W.H., van der Geld, Y.M., Stegeman, C.A., et al. 2006. Persistent expansion of CD4+ effector memory T cells in Wegener's granulomatosis. Kidney Int. 70, 938.

Aderem, A. 2005. Systems biology: its practice and challenges. Cell 121, 511.

Anders, H.J., Vielhauer, V., Eis, V., et al. 2004. Activation of toll-like receptor-9 induces progression of renal disease in MRL-Fas(lpr) mice. FASEB J. 18, 534.

Arrizabalaga, P., Sans Boix, A., Torras Rabassa, A., et al. 1998. Monoclonal antibody analysis of crescentic membranous glomerulonephropathy. Am. J. Nephrol. 18, 77.

Balding, C.E., Howie, A.J., Drake-Lee, A.B., et al. 2001. Th2 dominance in nasal mucosa in patients with Wegener's granulomatosis. Clin. Exp. Immunol. 125, 332.

Bellingans, G.J., Caldwell, H., Howie, S.E., et al. 1996. In vivo fate of the inflammatory macrophage during the resolution of inflammation: inflammatory macrophages do not die locally, but emigrate to the draining lymph nodes. J. Immunol. 157, 2577.

Bellingan, G.J., Xu, P., Cooksley, H. 2002. Adhesion molecule-dependent mechanisms regulate the rate of macrophage clearance during the resolution of peritoneal inflammation. J. Exp. Med. 196, 1515.

Bingle, L., Brown, N.J., Lewis, C.E. 2002. The role of tumour-associated macrophages in tumour progression: implications for new anticancer therapies. J. Pathol. 196, 254.

Bossu, P., Neumann, D., Del Giudice, E., et al. 2003. IL-18 cDNA vaccination protects mice from spontaneous lupus-like autoimmune disease. Proc. Natl. Acad. Sci. U.S.A. 100, 14181.

Boyce, N.W., Tipping, P.G., Holdsworth, S.R. 1989. Glomerular macrophages produce reactive oxygen species in experimental glomerulonephritis. Kidney Int. 35, 778.

Cairns, L.S., Phelps, R.G., Bowie, L., et al. 2003. The fine specificity and cytokine profile of T-helper cells responsive to the alpha3 chain of type IV collagen in Goodpasture's disease. J. Am. Soc. Nephrol. 14, 2801.

Carvalho-Pinto, C.E., Garcia, M.I., Mellado, M., et al. 2002. Autocrine production of IFN-gamma by macrophages controls their recruitment to kidney and the development of glomerulonephritis in MRL/lpr mice. J. Immunol. 169, 1058.

Cattell, V., Cook, T., Moncada, S. 1990. Glomeruli synthesize nitrite in experimental nephrotoxic nephritis. Kidney Int. 38, 1056.

Cattell, V., Largen, P., de Heer, E., et al. 1991. Glomeruli synthesize nitrite in active Heymann nephritis; the source is infiltrating macrophages. Kidney Int. 40, 847.

Chan, R.W., Tam, L.S., Li, E.K., et al. 2003. Inflammatory cytokine gene expression in the urinary sediment of patients with lupus nephritis. Arthritis. Rheum. 48, 1326.

Churg, J. 1973. Structure and development of the gomerular crescent. Am. J. Pathol. 72, 349.

Constant, S.L., Bottomly, K. 1997. Induction of Th1 and Th2 CD4+ T cell responses: the alternative approaches. Ann. Rev. Immunol. 15, 297.

Cook, H.T., Smith, J., Salmon, J.A., et al. 1989. Functional characteristics of macrophages in glomerulonephritis in the rat. NO- generation, MHC class II expression and eicosanoid synthesis. Am. J. Pathol. 134, 431.

Cunningham, M.A., Huang, X.R., Dowling, J.P., et al. 1999. Prominence of cell-mediated immunity effectors in "pauci-immune" glomerulonephritis. J. Am. Soc. Nephrol. 10, 499.

Delamarre, L., Pack, M., Chang, H., et al. 2005. Differential lysosomal proteolysis in antigen-presenting cells determines antigen fate. Science. 307, 1630.

Doi, T., Mayumi, M., Kanatsu, K., et al. 1984. Distribution of IgG subclasses in membranous nephropathy. Clin. Exp. Immunol. 58, 57.

Duffield, J.S., Erwig, L-P., Wei, X., et al. 2000. Activated macrophages direct apoptosis and suppress mitosis of mesangial cells. J. Immunol. 164, 2110.

Duffield, J.S., Forbes, S.J., Constandinou, C.M., et al. 2005a. Selective depletion of macrophages reveals distinct, opposing roles during liver injury and repair. J. Clin. Invest. 111, 56.

Duffield, J.S., Tipping, P.G., Kipari, T., et al. 2005b. Conditional ablation of macrophages halts progression of crescentic glomerulonephritis. Am. J. Pathol. 167, 1207.

Eardley, K.S., Zehnder, D., Quinkler, M., et al. 2006. The relationship between albuminuria, MCP-1/CCL2, and interstitial macrophages in chronic kidney disease. Kidney Int. 69, 1189.

Eijgenraam, J.W., Woltman, A.M., Kamerling, S.W., et al. 2005. Dendritic cells of IgA nephropathy patients have an impaired capacity to induce IgA production in naive B cells. Kidney Int. 68, 1604.

Erwig, L.-P., Kluth, D.C., Rees, A.J. 2003. Macrophage heterogeneity in renal inflammation. Nephrol. Dial.Transplant. 18, 1962.

Erwig, L.-P., Kluth, D.C., Walsh, G.M., et al. 1998. Initial cytokine exposure determines macrophage function and renders them unresponsive to other cytokines. J. Immunol. 161, 1983.

Erwig, L.-P., McPhilips, K.A., Wynes, M., et al. 2006. Differential regulation of phagosome maturation in macrophages and dendritic cells mediated by Rho GTPases and ezrin-radixin-moesin (ERM) proteins. Proc. Natl. Acad. Sci. U.S.A. 103, 12825.

Erwig, L.-P., Stewart, K., Rees, A.J. 2000. Macrophages from inflamed but not normal glomeruli are unresponsive to anti-inflammatory cytokines. Am. J. Pathol. 156, 295.

Falk, M.C., Ng, G., Zhang, G.Y., et al. 1995. Infiltration of the kidney by alpha beta and gamma delta T cells: effect on progression in IgA nephropathy. Kidney Int. 47, 177.

Frosch, M., Vogl, T., Waldherr, R., et al. 2004. Expression of MRP8 and MRP14 by macrophages is a marker for severe forms of glomerulonephritis. J. Leukoc. Biol. 75, 198.

Furuta, T., Saito, T., Ootaka, T., et al. 1993. The role of macrophages in diabetic glomerulosclerosis. Am. J. Kidney. Dis. 5, 480.

Gardai, S.J., Xiao, Y.Q., Dickinson, M., et al. 2003. By binding SIRPalpha or calreticulin/CD91, lung collectins act as dual function surveillance molecules to suppress or enhance inflammation. Cell. 1, 13.

Gómez-Guerrero, C., Hernandez-Vargas, P., Lopez-Franco, O., et al. 2005. Mesangial cells and glomerular inflammation: from the pathogenesis to novel therapeutic approaches. Curr. Drug. Targets. Inflamm. Allergy. 4, 341.

Gómez-Guerrero, C., Lopez-Franco, O., Sanjuan, G. 2004. Suppressors of cytokine signaling regulate Fc receptor signaling and cell activation during immune renal injury. J. Immunol. 72 (11), 6969.

Gordon, S. 2003. Alternative activation of macrophages. Nat. Rev. Immunol. 3, 23.

Hamilton, T.A. 2002. Molecular basis of macrophage activation: from gene expression to phenotypic diversity. In: B. Burke, C.E. Lewis (Eds.), The Macrophage. Oxford University Press, Oxford, UK, p. 91.

Haraguchi, K., Shimura, H., Onaya, T. 2003. Suppression of experimental crescentic glomerulonephritis by peroxisome proliferator-activated receptor (PPAR)gamma activators. Clin. Exp. Nephrol. 7, 27.

Hill, G.S., Delahousse, M., Nochy, D., et al. 2001. Predictive power of the second renal biopsy in lupus nephritis: significance of macrophages. Kidney Int. 1, 304.

Holdsworth, S.R., Neale, T.J. 1984. Macrophage-induced glomerular injury. Cell transfer studies in passive autologous antiglomerular basement membrane antibody-initiated experimental glomerulonephritis. Lab. Invest. 51, 172.

Holdsworth, S.R., Neale, T.J., Wilson, C.B. 1981. Abrogation of macrophage-dependent injury in experimental glomerulonephritis in the rabbit. Use of an antimacrophage serum. J. Clin. Invest. 68, 686.

Ikezumi, Y., Atkins, R.C., Nikolic-Paterson, D.J. 2003a. Interferon-gamma Augments Acute Macrophage-Mediated Renal Injury Via a Glucocorticoid-Sensitive Mechanism. J. Am. Soc. Nephrol. 14, 888.

Ikezumi, Y., Hurst, L.A., Masaki, T., et al. 2003b. Adoptive transfer studies demonstrate that macrophages can induce proteinuria and mesangial cell proliferation. Kidney Int. 63, 83.

Ikezumi, Y., Hurst, L., Atkins, R.C., et al. 2004. Macrophage-mediated renal injury is dependent on signaling via the JNK pathway. J. Am. Soc. Nephrol. 7, 1775.

Imai, H., Hamai, K., Komatsuda, A., et al. 1997. IgG subclasses in patients with membranoproliferative glomerulonephritis, membranous nephropathy, and lupus nephritis. Kidney Int 51, 270.

Isome, M., Fujinaka, H., Adhikary, L.P., et al. 2004. Important role for macrophages in induction of crescentic anti-GBM glomerulonephritis in WKY rats. Nephrol. Dial. Transplant. 12, 2997.

Jose, M.D., Ikezumi, Y., van Rooijen, N., et al. 2003. Macrophages act as effectors of tissue damage in acute renal allograft rejection. Transplantation. 7, 1015.

Kanamaru, Y., Scandiuzzi, L., Essig, M., et al. 2006. Mast cell-mediated remodeling and fibrinolytic activity protect against fatal glomerulonephritis. J. Immunol. 176, 5607.

Kitching, A.R., Tipping, P.G., Kurimoto, M., et al. 2000. IL-18 has IL-12-independent effects in delayed-type hypersensitivity: studies in cell-mediated crescentic glomerulonephritis. J Immunol. 165 (8), 4649.

Kluth, D.C., Ainslie, C.V., Pearce, W.P., et al. 2001. Macrophages transfected with adenovirus to express IL-4 reduce inflammation in experimental glomerulonephritis. J. Immunol. 166, 4728.

Kluth, D.C., Erwig, L.-P., Rees, A.J. 2000. Gene transfer into inflamed glomeruli using macrophages transfected with adenovirus. Gene Ther. 7, 263.

Kluth, D.C., Erwig, L.-P., Rees, A.J. 2004. Multiple facets of macrophages in renal injury. Kidney Int 2, 542.

Kruger, T., Benke, D., Eitner, F., et al. 2004. Identification and functional characterization of dendritic cells in the healthy murine kidney and in experimental glomerulonephritis. J. Am. Soc. Nephrol. 15, 613.

Lan, H.Y., Nikolic-Paterson, D.J., Atkins, R.C. 1993. Trafficking of inflammatory macrophages from the kidney to draining lymph nodes during experimental glomerulonephritis. Clin. Exp. Immunol. 92, 336.

Li, S., Holdsworth, S.R., Tipping, P.G. 2000. B7.1 and B7.2 costimulatory molecules regulate crescentic glomerulonephritis. Eur. J. Immunol. 30, 1394.

Lin, E.Y., Nguyen, A.V., Russell, R.G., et al. 2001. Colony-stimulating factor 1 promotes progression of mammary tumors to malignancy. J. Exp. Med. 193, 727.

Lopez-Franco, O., Suzuki, Y., Sanjuan, G., et al. 2002. Nuclear factor-kappa B inhibitors as potential novel anti-inflammatory agents for the treatment of immune glomerulonephritis. Am. J. Pathol. 4, 1497.

Lu, L.F., Lind, E.F., Gondek, D.C., et al. 2006. Mast cells are essential intermediaries in regulatory T-cell tolerance. Nature 442, 997.

Mantovani, A., Locati, M., Vecchi, A., et al. 2001. Decoy receptors: a strategy to regulate inflammatory cytokines and chemokines. Trends. Immunol. 22 (6), 328.

Mantovani, A., Schioppa, T., Porta, C., et al. 2006. Role of tumor-associated macrophages in tumor progression and invasion. Cancer Metastasis Rev. Sep 25 (3), 315.

Mantovani, A., Sica, A., Sozzani, S., et al. 2004. The chemokine system in diverse forms of macrophage activation and polarization. Trends. Immunol. 12, 677.

Masutani, K., Akahoshi, M., Tsuruya, K., et al. 2001. Predominance of Th1 immune response in diffuse proliferative lupus nephritis. Arthritis Rheum. 44, 2097.

Masutani, K., Tokumoto, M., Nakashima, H., et al. 2003. Strong polarization toward Th1 immune response in ANCA-associated glomerulonephritis. Clin. Nephrol. 59, 395.

Minto, A.W., Erwig, L.-P., Rees, A.J. 2003. Heterogeneity of macrophage activation in Anti-Thy-1.1 nephritis. Am. J. Pathol. 163, 2033.

Moser, M., Murphy, K.M. 2000. Dendritic cell regulation of TH1-TH2 development. Nat. Immunol. 1 (3), 199.

Mosser, D.M. 2003. The many faces of macrophage activation. J. Leukoc. Biol. 73, 209.

Nagaoka, T., Kaburagi, Y., Hamaguchi, Y., et al. 2000. Delayed wound healing in the absence of intercellular adhesion molecule-1 or L-selectin expression. Am. J. Pathol. 157, 237.

Nikolic-Paterson, D. J., Lan, H. Y., Atkins, R.C., 1997. Macrophages in immune renal injury, in Neilson EG, Couser WG (eds) Immunologic Renal Diseases, Philadelphia, Lippincott-Raven, 592.

Nishida, M., Fujinaka, H., Matsusaka, T., et al. 2001. Absence of angiotensin II type 1 receptor in bone marrow derived cells is detrimental in the evolution of renal fibrosis. J. Clin. Invest. 110, 1859.

North, R.J., Mackaness, G.B. 1973. Immunological control of macrophage proliferation in vivo. Infect. Immun. 8, 68.

Ogawa, D., Shikata, K., Matsuda, M., et al. 2002. Protective effect of a novel and selective inhibitor of inducible nitric oxide synthase on experimental crescentic glomerulonephritis in WKY rats. Nephrol. Dial. Transplant. 17, 2117.

Pawar, R.D., Patole, P.S., Zecher, D., et al. 2006. Toll-like receptor-7 modulates immune complex glomerulonephritis. J. Am. Soc. Nephrol. 17, 141.

Pollard, J.W. 2004. Tumour-educated macrophages promote tumour progression and metastasis. Nat. Rev. Cancer. 4, 71.

Raes, G., De Baetselier, P., Noel, W., et al. 2002. Differential expression of FIZZ1 and Ym1 in alternatively versus classically activated macrophages. J. Leukoc. Biol. 71, 597.

Ragno, S., Romano, M., Howell, S., et al. 2001. Changes in gene expression in macrophages infected with Mycobacterium tuberculosis: A combined transcriptomic and proteomic approach. Immunology. 104, 99.

Ravasi, T., Wells, C., Forest, A., et al. 2002. Generation of diversity in the innate immune system: macrophage heterogeneity arises from gene-autonomous transcriptional probability of individual inducible genes. J. Immunol. 1, 44.

Robertson, M.J., Erwig, L.-P., Liversidge, J., et al. 2002. Retinal microenvironment controls resident and infiltrating macrophage function during uveoretinitis. Invest. Ophthalmol. Vis. Sci. 43, 2250.

Rosenberger, C.M., Finlay, B.B. 2003. Phagocyte sabotage: disruption of macrophage signalling by bacterial pathogens. Nat. Rev. Mol. Cell. Biol. 5, 385.

Salama, A.D., Chaudhry, A.N., Holthaus, K.A., et al. 2003. Regulation by CD25+ lymphocytes of autoantigen-specific T-cell responses in Goodpasture's (anti-GBM) disease. Kidney Int. 64, 1685.

Schreiner, G.F. 1991. The role of the macrophage in glomerular injury. Semin. Nephrol. 11, 268.

Segerer, S., Cui, Y., Eitner, F., et al. 2001. Expression of chemokines and chemokine receptors during human renal transplant rejection. Am. J. Kidney Dis. 3, 518.

Segerer, S., Hughes, E., Hudkins, K., L., et. al. 2002. Expression of the fractalkine receptor (CX3CR1) in human kidney diseases. Kidney Int. 2, 488.

Segerer, S., MacK, M., Regele, H., et al. 1999. Expression of the C-C chemokine receptor 5 in human kidney diseases. Kidney Int. 1, 52.

Sfikakis, P.P., Boletis, J.N., Lionaki, S., et al. 2005. Remission of proliferative lupus nephritis following B cell depletion therapy is preceded by down-regulation of the T cell costimulatory molecule CD40 ligand: an open-label trial. Arthritis Rheum. 52 (2), 50.

Singh, R.R., Saxena, V., Zang, S., et al. 2003. Differential contribution of IL-4 and STAT6 vs STAT4 to the development of lupus nephritis. J. Immunol. 170, 4818.

Takahashi, T., Abe, H., Arai, H., et al. 2005. Activation of STAT3/Smad1 is a key signaling pathway for progression to glomerulosclerosis in experimental glomerulonephritis. J. Biol. Chem. 280 (8), 7100.

Teder, P., Vandivier, R.W., Jiang, D., et al. 2002. Resolution of lung inflammation by CD44. Science 296, 155.

Timoshanko, J.R., Holdsworth, S.R., Kitching, A., et al. 2002. IFN-gamma production by intrinsic renal cells and bone marrow-derived cells is required for full expression of crescentic glomerulonephritis in mice. J. Immunol. 168, 4135.

Timoshanko, J.R., Kitching, A.R., Holdsworth, S.R., et al. 2001. Interleukin-12 from intrinsic cells is an effector of renal injury in crescentic glomerulonephritis. J Am. Soc. Nephrol. 12, 464.

Timoshanko, J.R., Sedgwick, J.D., Holdsworth, S.R., et al. 2003. Intrinsic renal cells are the major source of tumor necrosis factor contributing to renal injury in murine crescentic glomerulonephritis. J. Am. Soc. Nephrol. 14, 1785.

Tipping, P.G., Kitching, A.R. 2005. Glomerulonephritis, Th1 and Th2: what's new? Clin. Exp. Immunol. 142, 207.

Tipping, P.G., Timoshanko, J. 2005. Contributions of intrinsic renal cells to crescentic glomerulonephritis. Nephron. Exp. Nephrol. 101, 173.

Toyabe, S., Harada, W., Uchiyama, M. 2001. Oligoclonally expanding gammadelta T lymphocytes induce IgA switching in IgA nephropathy. Clin. Exp. Immunol. 124, 110.

Vigna-Perez, M., Hernandez-Castro, B., Paredes-Saharopulos, O., et al. 2006. Clinical and immunological effects of Rituximab in patients with lupus nephritis refractory to conventional therapy: a pilot study. Arthritis Res. Ther. 8, R83.

Waddington, S., Cook, H.T., Reaveley, D., et al. 1996. L-arginine depletion inhibits glomerular nitric oxide synthesis and exacerbates rat nephrotoxic nephritis. Kidney Int. 49, 1090.

Wang, M.H., Zhou, Y.Q., Chen, Y.Q. 2002. Macrophage-stimulating protein and RON receptor tyrosine kinase: potential regulators of macrophage inflammatory activities. Scan. J. Immunol. 56, 545.

Westerhuis, R., van Straaten, S.C., van Dixhoorn, M.G., et al. 2000. Distinctive roles of neutrophils and monocytes in anti-thy-1 nephritis. Am. J. Pathol. 156, 303.

Williams, L.M., Ricchetti, G., Sarma, U., et al. 2004. Interleukin-10 suppression of myeloid cell activation—a continuing puzzle. Immunology. 3, 281.

Wilson, H.M., Kluth, D.C., Erwig, L.P., et al., 2005. Macrophages and Renal Disease. Actualties Nephrologiques. Medecine Sciences, Flammarion 37.

Wilson, H.M., Stewart, K., Brown, P.A., et al. 2002. Bone marrow derived macrophages (BMDM) genetically modified to produce IL-10 reduce injury in experimental glomerulonephritis. Mol. Ther. 6, 710.

Wright, G.J., Puklavec, M.J., Willis, A.C., et al. 2000. Lymphoid/neuronal cell surface OX2 glycoprotein recognizes a novel receptor on macrophages implicated in the control of their function. Immunity. 13, 233.

Yamagishi, H., Yokoo, T., Imasawa, T., et al. 2001. Genetically modified bone marrow-derived vehicle cells site specifically deliver an anti-inflammatory cytokine to inflamed interstitium of obstructive nephropathy. J. Immunol. 166, 609.

Yoh, K., Shibuya, K., Morito, N., et al. 2003. Transgenic overexpression of GATA-3 in T lymphocytes improves autoimmune glomerulonephritis in mice with a BXSB/MpJ-Yaa genetic background. J. Am. Soc. Nephrol. 14, 2494.

Yokoo, T., Ohashi, T., Utsunomiya, Y., et al. 1999. Prophylaxis of antibody-induced acute glomerulonephritis with genetically modified bone marrow-derived vehicle cells. Hum. Gene. Ther. 16, 2673.

Yokoo, T., Ohashi, T., Utsunomiya, Y., et al. 2001. Inflamed glomeruli-specific gene activation that uses recombinant adenovirus with the Cre/loxP system. J. Am. Soc. Nephrol. 12, 2330.

Yokoo, T., Ohashi, T., Utsunomiya, Y., et al. 2003. Gene delivery using human cord blood-derived CD34+ cells into inflamed glomeruli in NOD/SCID mice. Kidney Int. 1, 102.

# CHAPTER 5

# Pathogenesis of Renal Diseases: Renal Cell Response to Injury

Josef Pfeilschifter*, Heiko Mühl, Liliana Schaefer

*Pharmazentrum Frankfurt/ZAFES, Klinikum der Johann Wolfgang Goethe-Universität Frankfurt am Main, Germany*

## 1. Introduction

In the following chapter, pathophysiological principles of renal cell injury are discussed in their clinical context. Renal cell injury is often caused by renal manifestations of more generalized syndromes, such as infectious disease, autoimmunity, diabetes, metabolic disturbance, or hypertension. Key pathophysiological mechanisms that may finally culminate in tissue damage and kidney failure will be described. These include formation of immune complexes and their detection by Fcγ receptors, activation of the complement system, activation of the *toll-like receptor* (TLR) system, overt action of growth factors such as insulin and transforming growth factor-β (TGFβ), as well as renal consequences of dyslipidemia and mechanical stimulation.

## 2. Formation of reactive oxygen species and nitric oxide are key determinants of renal tissue damage

Free radical production is supposed to play a decisive role in renal diseases (Pfeilschifter et al., 1993; Baud and Ardaillou, 1993). Specifically, nitric oxide (NO) and reactive oxygen species (ROS), mainly superoxide anion ($O_2^-$) and hydrogen peroxide ($H_2O_2$), have been identified as key compounds that are involved in widespread cellular damage to macromolecules, including DNA, proteins, and lipids. Besides, in the context of pro-inflammatory cytokines and TLR activation, ROS production can be observed to be under the influence of angiotensin II, bradykinin, arachidonic acid, thrombin, and growth factors such as epidermal growth factor, fibroblast growth factor, platelet-derived growth factor, and insulin-like growth factor (Wardle, 2005). In addition, mechanical pressure as seen in hypertensive patients is able to activate production of ROS (Sowers, 2002). Under those conditions ROS generation may contribute to endothelial cell dysfunction by scavenging NO and thereby impairing endothelium-dependent vasorelaxation. In fact, parameters of oxidative stress are increased in patients with essential hypertension (Russo et al., 1998).

Deleterious actions of oxidative stress are to a certain degree held in check by cellular antioxidant capacity, which can be increased in response to a particular insult. Examples of such protective mechanisms are induction of heme oxygenase-1 (HO-1) (Wardle, 2005), superoxide dismutase (SOD) (Pfeilschifter et al., 2002), upregulation of cellular GSH status (Wardle, 2005), and the activation of the Nrf2-dependent antioxidant response program (Sozzani et al., 2005). Obviously, uncontrolled oxidative stress resulting from an imbalanced redox-state is inevitably associated with cellular hyperactivation, subsequent damage, and finally tissue injury and loss of function.

---

*Corresponding author.
Tel.: +49-69-6301 6951; Fax: +49-69-6301 7942
E-mail address: Pfeilschifter@em.uni-frankfurt.de

© 2008 Elsevier B.V. All rights reserved.
DOI: 10.1016/S1571-5078(07)07005-5

ROS are generated as accidental by-products of aerobic energy metabolism or deliberately as signaling compounds and effector molecules during immune defense. Enzymes with critical functions in ROS production include xanthine oxidase, cyclooxygenases, lipoxygenases, cytochrome P450 oxidases, nitric oxide synthases (NOS), and nicotinamide adenine dinucleotide phosphate (NADPH) oxidases. The latter family of ROS producing enzymes, recently renamed as Nox enzymes, appear to be of prime relevance in pathophysiology. Among family members, Nox1 and Nox4 can be detected in renal resident cells such as glomerular mesangial cells. Notably, Nox2, formerly known as gp91phox, is primarily expressed in phagocytes but not detectable in resident cells such as mesangial cells. Besides these specific differences in cellular distribution, it is generally assumed that all Nox isoenzymes have the potential to contribute to renal tissue damage, particularly in the context of acute and chronic inflammation. Overproduction of NO is established by gene activation of inducible nitric oxide synthase (iNOS), which is able to produce large amounts of the volatile radical NO for extended periods of time. Through the action of iNOS, L-arginine and $O_2$ are converted to citrulline and NO. Enhanced expression of iNOS is a chief characteristic of inflammatory conditions that can be observed in a variety of human diseases and their respective animal models. Specifically, pro-inflammatory cytokines like interleukin (IL)-1, tumor necrosis factor-α, and interferons are of prime importance in establishing high-output production of NO via this enzyme. Induction of iNOS is achieved by action of transcription factors such as nuclear factor (NF)-κB, signal transducer and activator of transcription (STAT) proteins, and interferon regulatory factor (IRF)-1 on regulatory elements in the iNOS promoter. Interestingly, iNOS is a significant source of ROS in the setting of substrate (L-arginine) deficiency (Wardle, 2005; Pfeilschifter et al., 2002; Pleskova et al., 2006, Kleinert et al., 2004). Both principles, ROS and NO are able to induce tissue damage via a similar spectrum of mechanisms that include inhibition of mitochondrial enzymes and glyceraldehyde-3-phosphate dehydrogenase, activation of lipid peroxidation, induction of DNA damage, activation of poly-ADP ribose polymerase (PARP), and apoptotic as well as necrotic cell death (Wardle, 2005; Brüne et al., 1999). Formation of peroxynitrite ($ONOO^-$) by the instant reaction of NO with $O_2^-$ is of particular relevance in this context. In fact, peroxynitrite is an outstandingly powerful oxidant and nitrating agent that is assumed to play a key role in the pathophysiology of cellular injury and tissue damage under conditions of ROS and NO overproduction (Szabo, 1996).

Evidence that production of ROS contributes to the pathogenesis of kidney diseases is manifold and appears to be based on several mechanisms of action. In fact, studies on rat anti-Thy 1 glomerulonephritis revealed that ROS production is key to cell proliferation, matrix accumulation, and fibrosis. Addition of antioxidants was actually curative in this model of immune-mediated glomerular injury (Budisavljevic et al., 2003). ROS may also be involved in formation of neoepitopes, thereby perpetuating core mechanisms of autoimmunity associated with kidney diseases. Induction of tumor necrosis factor-α (TNFα) production is proposed to be a further crucial mechanism of ROS driven inflammatory diseases. This assumption concurs with $H_2O_2$-mediated production of this cytokine, as observed in nephrotoxic nephritis. Here, ROS production is a consequence of Fc receptor (FcR) activation on infiltrating neutrophils (Suzuki et al., 2003). Under conditions of proteinuria, albumin uptake by tubular cells leads to NF-κB activation via protein kinase C and thereby to ROS production and subsequent amplification of inflammation (Tang et al., 2003). ROS production has been connected in particular to apoptotic cell death. For example, ROS mediate angiotensin II-induced apoptosis in proximal tubular epithelial cells (Bhaskaran et al., 2003). Taken together, current data strongly emphasize the view that imbalanced ROS production by infiltrating leukocytes and/or local resident cells plays a key role in renal inflammation and subsequent tissue injury.

## 3. Immune-mediated renal injury and the TLR system of innate immunity

Renal immune complexes, either formed in the circulation or in situ, play a key role in the pathogenesis of kidney diseases and renal injury associated with autoimmunity and/or infection. Interestingly, recent data also suggest that a complex interplay between different components of the adaptive and the innate immune systems determines the pathogenesis and outcome of immune-mediated kidney diseases. In the following section, we will review related novel aspects of kidney immunopathology. Moreover, therapeutic strategies that may evolve from those recent insights will be discussed.

## 3.1. Immune complexes contribute to immune-mediated renal injury

Immune complexes are dynamic structures consisting of antibodies and their respective antigens. It is a widely accepted concept that the formation of immune complexes and their renal deposition is a key event in the pathogenesis of many immune-mediated kidney diseases (Nangaku and Couser, 2005). These immune complexes may be formed in the circulation, as in the case of systemic lupus erythematosus, or may be formed in situ, as seen in Heymann nephritis. Besides this class of diseases with an autoimmune etiology, the renal manifestations of infectious diseases also appear to be mediated at least in part by renal deposition of immune complexes. In this context, hepatitis C (Philipneri and Bastani, 2001) and human immunodeficiency virus (HIV) (Weiner et al., 2003) infections are of particular relevance. A prominent and well-characterized animal model of immune-complex mediated kidney disease is acute serum sickness. This disease is induced by injection of bovine serum albumin (BSA) into rabbits. As a consequence, anti-BSA/BSA immune complexes accumulate in renal glomeruli and thereafter result in an acute glomerulonephritis (Nangaku and Couser, 2005). Immune complexes are able to mediate activation of infiltrating leukocytes as well as resident renal cells by two major mechanisms. First, they activate a class of specific receptors for antibodies. These receptors recognize the Fc portion of immunglobulins and are known as FcRs. In addition, immune complexes induce proinflammatory effects by activating the complement system via the classical pathway. Notably, the role of immune complexes in pathophysiology is determined by their size. Small immune complexes are biologically inert because they neither efficiently activate FcRs nor the complement system. In contrast, large immune complexes are potent activators of both systems and are therefore efficiently removed by phagocytosis. Thus, medium-sized complexes are regarded as pathophysiologically most relevant.

## 3.2. Fcγ receptors: major sensors of immune complexes

FcRs located in the membrane of leukocytes and certain resident kidney cells are a major means by which the immune system senses the formation and deposition of immune complexes. Among the family of FcR, those specific for immunoglobulin G (IgG), classified as FcγR, appear to be of pivotal relevance for the development of inflammatory kidney diseases. These receptors specifically recognize Fc regions of IgG coupled to antigen. As a consequence immune complexes may be removed and/or cellular activation is achieved. Three different classes of Fcγ receptors can be distinguished: FcγRI, FcγRII, and FcγRIII. Whereas FcγRI is a high-affinity receptor that is capable of binding even monomeric IgG, FcγRII and FcγRIII bind to immune complexes with low affinity. FcγRI and FcγRIII are activating receptors. These receptors associate with homodimers of the common γ-chain (FcRγ) containing cytoplasmatic ITAM (immunotyrosine activatory motif) sequences, which are responsible for signal transduction. FcγRIIa and FcγRIIc are activating receptors furnished with their own ITAM motifs. In contrast to the aforementioned family members, FcγRIIb is an inhibitory receptor equipped with an intracellular amino acid motif called ITIM (immunotyrosine inhibitory motif). Docking of immune complexes to activating FcγR leads to the phosphorylation of ITAM motifs with subsequent activation of key signal transduction components, namely phospholipase Cγ, cytosolic phospholipase $A_2$, and mitogen-activated protein kinases. Activation of these signaling pathways by immune complexes is linked to expression of pro-inflammatory molecules such as iNOS and TNFα (Tarzi and Cook, 2003; Ravetch and Bolland, 2001; Jancar and Sanchez Crespo, 2005). Murine renal mesangial cells are able to express both FcγRII and FcγRIII receptors. Interestingly, activation of FcγRIII on these cells induces expression of pro-inflammatory chemokines such as monocyte chemoattractant protein-1 (MCP-1) (Radeke et al., 2002). In fact, animal models reveal that this chemokine may play an important role in murine lupus nephritis (Hasegawa et al., 2003).

The relevance of the FcR system for immune-mediated kidney diseases has been underscored by use of suitable animal models. The absence of FcγRIIb in lupus-prone Fas (lpr/lpr) mice resulted in fatal nephritis confirming the protective character of this inhibitory FcR. In contrast, lack of FcγRI and FcγRIII biological functions in FcRγ knockout animals was protective against severe lupus-like nephritis that spontaneously develops in mice with a genetic NZB/NZW background (Tarzi and Cook, 2003; Oates and Gilkeson, 2002).

## 3.3. Activation of complement amplifies renal inflammation and injury

Through the classical activation pathway, immune complexes efficiently activate the complement system and thus represent an important arm of innate immunity. Activation of complement is able to potently enhance inflammatory reactions by different mechanisms, including production of the anaphylatoxins C3a and C5a and the generation of the membrane attack complex C5b-9 (Tarzi and Cook, 2003; Oates and Gilkeson, 2002; Seelen et al., 2005; Berger et al., 2005). By stimulating their respective receptors on leukocytes and resident mesangial cells, these anaphylatoxins synergize with cytokines and/or FcγR-derived signals for production of pro-inflammatory mediators. This interaction can be regarded as one hallmark of immune-mediated renal injury. Accordingly, administration of a C3a receptor antagonist to MRL/lpr mice significantly ameliorated development of lupus nephritis (Bao et al., 2005a). Similar results were obtained by administration of a C5a receptor antagonist (Bao et al., 2005b). Notably, urinary C3d, a degradation product of C3, has been identified as a valuable disease marker in human lupus nephritis (Negi et al., 2000).

The other pathogenic component of the complement system is the membrane attack complex. Sublytic quantities of C5b-9 inserted into target cell membranes mediate cellular activation and a pro-inflammatory cellular program that favors tissue injury. This process is well characterized in rat Heymann nephritis, a model of membranous nephropathy. Podocyte injury in this disease is dependent on C5b-9 and involves subsequent production of prostaglandins, proteases, and ROS. In addition, C5b-9 has been related to endoplasmic reticulum stress and DNA damage. Besides podocytes, other renal cell types can be affected by C5b-9, including glomerular epithelial and mesangial cells. For example, activation of glomerular mesangial cells in models of IgA nephropathy depends on C5b-9 activity. Notably, uncontrolled activation of the complement pathway has been associated with severity of disease in human IgA nephropathy. At this point, it should however be recognized that complement has a dual role in the context of immune complex diseases. Whereas excessive complement activation must certainly be considered as a pathogenic factor, complement also has the potential to achieve distinct beneficial functions based on the role of the complement system in immune complex disaggregation and clearance (Tarzi and Cook, 2003; Oates and Gilkeson, 2002; Seelen et al., 2005; Berger et al., 2005).

## 3.4. The toll-like receptor dependent arm of innate immunity

The TLR system provides an inherent cellular recognition device for pathogen-associated molecular patterns (PAMP) that are encoded by a myriad of infectious agents. This phylogenetically ancient system of immune recognition is of paramount importance for the development and function of innate as well as adaptive immunity. Distinct TLR expression profiles have been identified on key players of the immune system such as dendritic cells, B and T lymphocytes, natural killer cells, and monocytes/macrophages. In addition,

**Table 1**
Overview on the human TLR system

| TLR | Location | Exogenous ligands |
|---|---|---|
| TLR-1, -2, -6 | Membrane | Microbial lipoproteins, peptidoglycans, zymosan |
| TLR-4 | Membrane | Lipopolysaccharide |
| TLR-5 | Membrane | Flagellin |
| TLR-10 | Membrane | ? |
| TLR-3 | Endosome | dsRNA |
| TLR-7,-8 | Endosome | ssRNA |
| TLR-9 | Endosome | Hypomethylated CpG DNA |

strong TLR expression is characteristic for cells of epithelial origin. At least ten different human TLR can be discriminated. These TLR and their exogenous ligands are shown in Table 1. In particular, activation of transcription factor NF-$\kappa$B and of the p38 MAP kinase pathway are regarded as culmination points of TLR-mediated pro-inflammatory cellular responses. Subsequent activation of pro-inflammatory genes such as TNF$\alpha$, IL-1$\beta$, and IL-8 as well as production of interferons, are hallmarks of immune defense mechanisms initiated by activation of the TLR system. Functionally, this innate component of the immune system is supposed to be the first line of defense against infectious agents of viral, bacterial, or fungal origin. However, the TLR system is not only a basic initial gate keeper of immunity but also shapes and amplifies the subsequently evolving adaptive arm of the immune response (Takeda and Akira, 2005; Anders et al., 2004a; Czyzyk, 2006; Pawar et al., 2006). In recent years, knowledge of TLR biology has developed at an impressive pace. These studies have also demonstrated that unwanted activation of the TLR system by exogenous or endogenous ligands could contribute to or even establish processes that finally lead to the development of autoimmune diseases.

## 3.5. Activation of the TLR system: a link between innate immunity and immune mediated glomerular injury

Receptors of the TLR system are expressed in the diseased human kidney not only in infiltrating leukocytes but also in certain populations of local resident cells. Specifically, expression of TLR3 was observed on activated human mesangial cells. Stimulation of mesangial TLR3 results in expression of pro-inflammatory genes like ICAM-1, IL-1$\beta$, IL-6, and IL-8. In addition, TLR3 has been identified on collecting duct cells (Wornle et al., 2006). Expression of TLR4 by human mesangial cells is uncertain. In contrast, TLR4 has been detected on human tubular epithelial cells (Samuelsson et al., 2004). Concerning the murine system, expression of TLR1-4/6 has been reported on tubular epithelial cells, whereas only TLR3/4 appears to be present on mesangial cells (Anders et al., 2004a, b).

Activation of the TLR system on either leukocytes or intrinsic renal cells is inevitably linked to an increased pro-inflammatory activation status of the affected tissue. Consequently, exposure to infectious agents has been associated with increased disease activity and flares of common kidney diseases such as IgA nephropathy or lupus nephritis. Further examples of infections driving renal disease include viral infections (e.g., hepatitis C virus or HIV) and acute renal failure (ARF) observed in sepsis patients. Interestingly, murine models revealed that activation of systemic but not renal TLR4 mediates ARF in endotoxemia, indicating that influx of activated leukocytes into the kidney is key to the pathogenic mechanism in this condition of acute systemic inflammation (Anders et al., 2004a; Czyzyk, 2006; Pawar et al., 2006). However, in the context of chronic inflammation, increasing evidence points to a pathophysiological role of local renal TLR expression (see below).

Renal deposition of immune complexes is regarded as a key mechanism in the pathogenesis of postinfectious glomerulonephritis mediated by the aforementioned viral infections. However, activation of TLR by viral products may play a key role in amplifying underlying inflammatory processes in the renal compartment. In this context, detection of viral RNA by TLR3 appears to be of particular interest. Activation of this TLR is generally accomplished by dsRNA, but potentially as well by double-stranded sections of ssRNA (e.g., achieved by formation of hairpin-loops). It is remarkable that renal TLR3 is upregulated in hepatitis C patients with glomerulonephritis and that TLR3 expression is enhanced by stimulation of cultured mesangial cells with pro-inflammatory cytokines. As already pointed out, TLR3 expressed on mesangial cells is able to amplify inflammatory responses of this cell type (Wornle et al., 2006). Moreover, experiments in the murine system proved that injected viral RNA accumulates in vivo in the renal glomerulus and can be detected in the endosomal "TLR3 compartment" of mesangial cells (Pawar et al., 2006; Patole et al., 2005). The present data therefore strongly suggest that activation of TLR3 in the renal glomerulus may play an important role in the pathogenesis of glomerulonephritis associated with viral infections.

## 3.6. The role of the TLR system in renal autoimmunity

Activation of the TLR pathway may amplify autoimmune processes by two principal mechanisms. First, by providing signals that generally increase the pro-inflammatory activation state of cell populations, either infiltrating leukocytes or resident cells, which are involved in the local tissue response and show a suitable TLR expression pattern. Second, distinct TLR ligands are able to efficiently activate B cells and may dramatically upregulate antibody production (Krieg, 2002). In this context, TLR9 is of particular relevance since it is highly expressed on B cells. Studies on MRL$^{lpr/lpr}$ mice, a model for systemic lupus erythematosus (SLE) and associated lupus nephritis, recently provided further insights into the potential role of TLR ligands in autoimmunity. Notably, application of the TLR3 ligand, pI:C-RNA, aggravated nephritis in MRL$^{lpr/lpr}$ mice. pI:C-RNA administration was not associated with B cell activation or changes in anti-DNA autoantibody levels, an observation consistent with the notion that B cells do not express TLR3. Data from these experiments suggest that pI:C-RNA worsens the outcome of nephritis by pro-inflammatory activation of local TLR3 expressing cells (intrarenal macrophages, mesangial cells) followed by induction of mesangiolysis (Patole et al., 2005).

Similar to pI:C-RNA, treatment of MRL$^{lpr/lpr}$ mice with TLR9 activating CpG motifs significantly aggravated nephritis. However, the mechanisms of action of TLR3 and TLR9 show significant differences. Direct activation of intrinsic renal cells, such as mesangial cells, was not observed in response to TLR9 activation. This is in accordance with a lack of this receptor on those cells. However, glomerular and tubulointerstitial injury, after CpG application was associated with a marked upregulation of anti-DNA antibody production and increased presence of glomerular IgG deposits. These observations indicate that, in contrast to pI:C-RNA, stimulatory CpG motifs are able to amplify experimental autoimmune nephritis by mechanisms that include TLR9-dependent activation of B cell functions (Anders et al., 2004b) (see below).

TLR are designed to recognize exogenous ligands derived from microbial pathogens. However, recent developments in this field reveal the presence of endogenous ligands for certain TLR, further strengthening the hypothesis of a link between this arm of innate immunity and autoimmune diseases. In fact these ligands may be released, for example, by dying cells during development of autoimmunity. By stimulating their specific TLR they may enhance or even establish pathological processes finally leading to autoimmune diseases. These endogenous ligands are best characterized for TLR3, TLR4, and TLR9. U1 small nuclear RNA (Hoffman et al., 2004) and hypomethylated CpG self-DNA (Czyzyk, 2006; Krieg, 2002) are able to activate TLR3 and TLR9, respectively. Notably, SLE patients show lower methyltransferase activity and higher serum levels of hypomethylated CpG-DNA (Krieg, 2002). A whole panel of endogenous ligands for TLR4 has been identified, among others heat-shock proteins, fibronectin, $\beta$-defensin-2 (Anders et al., 2004a), and biglycan (Schaefer et al., 2005). Uncontrolled release of these ligands will, similarly to bacterial lipopolysaccharide, enhance TLR4-driven inflammation.

Importantly, activation of TLR9 by hypomethylated self-CpG-DNA has the potential to efficiently activate B cells, leading to subsequent initiation of autoantibody production. Hypomethylated self-CpG-DNA is over-represented in SLE immune complexes and can be regarded as a pathogenic factor in this disease. In particular, promoter sequences involved in gene regulation represent areas in mammalian genomes with a high degree of hypomethylated CpG-DNA (Krieg, 2002). In the context of autoimmunity, production of anti-chromatin antibodies and of antibodies directed against Fc portions of IgG (rheumatoid factors) are of special clinical interest. The presence of these antibodies is characteristic of several autoimmune diseases, and often associated with the generation and renal deposition of pathogenic immune complexes. Current understanding of the underlying mechanism by which TLR9 may facilitate autoantibody production is shown in Fig. 1. B cells recognizing self-chromatin/DNA structures (left panel) or IgG2a/chromatin complexes (right panel) are activated by stimulation of their respective B cell receptors (BCR) at the cell membrane. This interaction provides the first signal for B cell activation. The BCR/antigen complex is endocytosed and, during subsequent maturation of the endosome, TLR9 is activated by the incorporated chromatin material. TLR9-mediated activation of specific B cells by this pathway, or alternatively by microbial infection, provides the essential second signal that finally leads to B cell differentiation, proliferation, and production of anti-chromatin antibodies or rheumatoid factors, respectively. Notably, this pathway provides a means of T helper cell-independent B cell activation that has

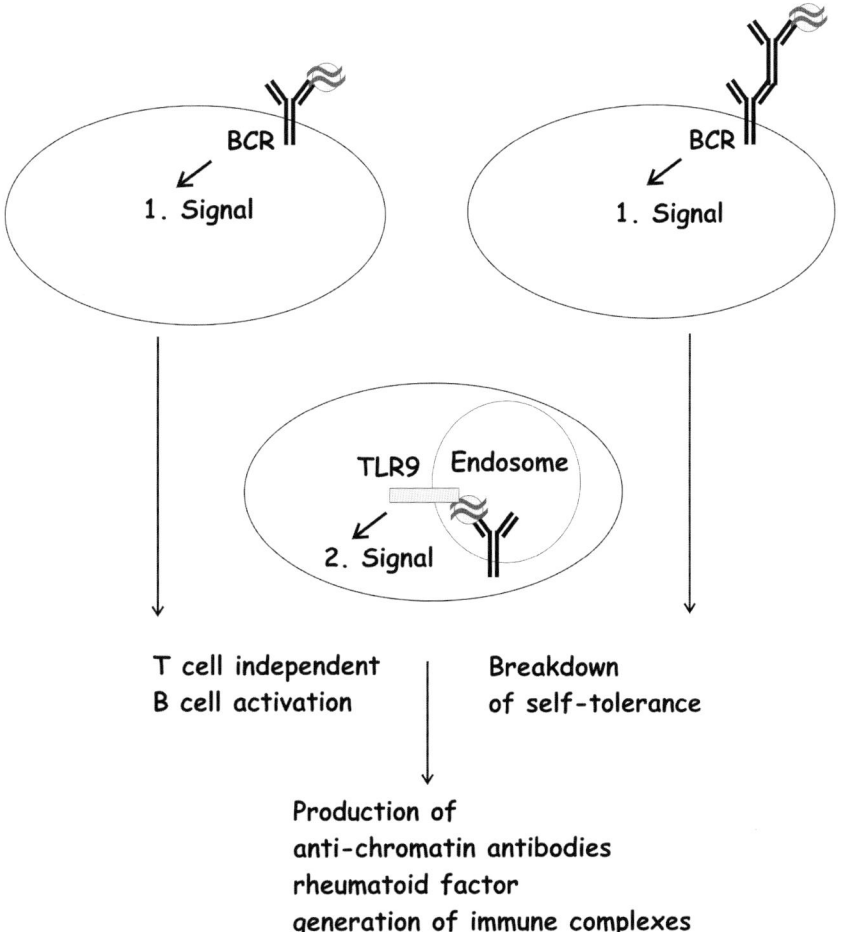

**Figure 1.** Current concept by which TLR9 activation provides a 2nd stimulus for autoantibody production.

the potential to break self-tolerance. Recent data indicate that TLR9-dependent production of IFNα by plasmacytoid dendritic cells is an important cofactor for this process. In fact, flares of disease correlate with high levels of IFNα in SLE patients (Oates and Gilkeson, 2002).

As discussed above, current data suggest that TLR activation, particularly TLR9, by endogenous ligands may be involved in the etiology of certain forms of autoimmune disease, including lupus nephritis (Christensen et al., 2005). This knowledge may open the avenue to innovative therapeutic strategies that are based on the biology of the TLR system. Blockade of TLR9 can be achieved by several strategies. First, TLR9 belongs to the group of TLR molecules that are located at the cellular endosomal compartment. Endosome maturation is associated with a drop in the local pH-value, which is a prerequisite for TLR9 function. Therefore, pharmacological agents that have the capability to inhibit endosomal acidification should interfere with TLR9 activation. Clinical data support this concept. The drug hydroxychloroquine is widely used with some success in the therapy of rheumatoid arthritis and SLE patients. Interestingly, hydroxychloroquine is an inhibitor of endosomal acidification. It might thus be speculated that novel and therapeutically more efficient compounds may evolve from the recently gained knowledge on the function of hydroxychloroquine concerning endosomal acidification and TLR9 activation (Krieg, 2002). Additionally, it became apparent that TLR9 activation can be suppressed by use of so-called inhibitory oligodeoxyribonucleotides (iODN). Particularly active iODNs are 15 mers with the motifs CCT and GGG, as in 5′-TCCTGGAGGGGAAGT-3′. Cellular activation achieved by TLR9 ligands can be significantly suppressed by coincubation with iODN. Recent data suggest that these molecules may be effective in vivo, and application of iODN molecules delayed the development of lupus nephritis in NZB/NZW mice (Lenert, 2005). Regardless of whether the target is the TLR9 molecule itself, or acidification of the endosomal compartment, the present data imply that weakening the function of this arm of innate immunity may open the avenue toward novel therapeutic strategies for the treatment of autoimmune diseases with renal manifestations.

## 4. Renal cell response to metabolic injury

### 4.1. Diabetes mellitus

The response of the various renal cell types to hyperglycemia ultimately defines the evolution of diabetic nephropathy. Initial stages, characterized by hyperfiltration, microalbuminuria, and later by declining renal function, are reflected morphologically by marked cellular and extracellular changes in the glomerulus and the tubulointerstitium. The glomerular changes include thickening of the GBM, expansion of the mesangial matrix, hypertrophy of mesangial cells, and alterations in podocytes. Comparable changes occur in the tubulointerstitium, including thickening of the tubular basement membrane, epithelial-mesenchymal transition of tubular cells, and interstitial fibrosis (Mason and Wahab, 2003).

#### 4.1.1. Effects of insulin on renal cell growth

The stimulation of cell growth by insulin was first described more than 30 years ago in a study performed by Stout et al. (1975), in which insulin was shown to stimulate the proliferation of vascular smooth muscle cells. However, it was only after the discovery of insulin-like growth factors (IGF) that the mitogenic effects of insulin were understood. Insulin is able to signal through the IGF-1 receptor, as there is a 40–50% homology between IGF-1 and insulin. Even though the affinity of insulin for the IGF-1 receptor is lower than that of IGF-1, elevated insulin levels are likely to signal through the IGF-1 receptor (Aron et al., 1989). In glomeruli from diabetic animals both IGF-1 and its receptor levels are increased, suggesting that this factor might be involved in growth processes in diabetic nephropathy (Conti et al., 1988).

Insulin may further contribute to the progression of kidney disease via modulation of the production or action of TGF-$\beta$, a cytokine playing a key role in renal injury in diabetic patients. In vitro insulin increases TGF-β1 expression in mesangial and tubular epithelial cells, which is associated with type IV collagen gene expression and its accumulation in the extracellular matrix (Anderson et al., 1996). Moreover, IGF-1 has been shown to increase the activity of CTGF (connective tissue growth factor), which has profibrogenic actions on tubular epithelial cells and interstitial fibroblasts (Wang et al., 2001).

### 4.1.2. Glucose flux through various intracellular pathways

Glucose entry into renal cells is regulated by specific transporters such as GLUT-1 and -4, as well as by sodium co-transporters such as SGLT-1 and -2. These transporters are transmembrane proteins that translocate glucose into cells. Elevated glucose levels appear to upregulate the expression of these receptors, thereby enhancing the flux of glucose through various intracellular metabolic pathways. GLUT-1 appears to be the most relevant transporter in diabetic nephropathy, as there is excessive production of ECM by GLUT-1-overexpressing mesangial cells in normoglycemia. Also, since GLUT-1 antisense treatment decreases the glucose-induced production of fibronectin in mesangial cells, it seems that these transport molecules exert biologically relevant influences on downstream cellular and extracellular events (Heilig et al., 1997).

### 4.1.3. Hyperglycemia and protein kinase C (PKC) signaling

PKC, which has dozens of isoforms, has been reported to be activated in glomerular cells under hyperglycemic conditions. PKC is activated by diacylglycerol (DAG) and through ROS generated by increased activity of the polyol pathway, as well as by AGE–RAGE interactions (Inoguchi et al., 2003). The activation of PKC by hyperglycemia induces pathophysiological changes in a number of ways, including decreased expression of endothelial NO synthase with reduced production of NO, and increased expression of vascular endothelial growth factor (VEGF). In addition, ECM components accumulate due to increased synthesis of type IV collagen and fibronectin under the influence of TGF-β1. PKC-induced activation of NF-κB generates an inflammatory response. These deleterious effects are further amplified by the generation of ROS secondary to the PKC-activated membrane-associated NADPH oxidase (Inoguchi et al., 2003). These events underline the central role of PKC in the pathogenesis of diabetic nephropathy. This concept is further supported by studies in which the administration of ruboxistaurin, a PKC inhibitor, at least partially improved glomerular pathophysiology in experimental diabetes.

### 4.1.4. TGF-β signaling in the diabetic kidney

TGF-β appears to play a central role in the evolution of diabetic nephropathy. TGF-β-induced signaling and subsequent transcriptional events have been extensively studied in mesangial cells. The TGF-β1, 2 and 3 isoforms inhibit proliferation in most cells and apoptosis in epithelial cells, but stimulate mesenchymal cells, like those of the glomerular mesangium. All isoforms are present as latent propeptides, which are complexed by the latent TGF-β-binding protein. The latter is cross-linked with matrix proteins and is cleaved by metalloproteinases and thrombospondin-1 to generate active TGF-β. TGF-β may also be activated by the integrin αvβ6 (Leask and Abraham, 2004).

The effects of activated TGF-β are mediated by interactions with its heterodimeric type-I and -II receptors. The type-I and -II receptors are co-expressed in most cells, including mesangial cells, where TGF-β first binds to the constitutively active type-II receptor, which phosphorylates the type I receptor to produce a heterodimer. The receptor complex then signals through the Smad, MAPK, and PKA pathways. More than nine distinct vertebrate Smad proteins (homolog of Drosophila protein MAD: *Mothers against decapentaplegic*) have been described. The activated TGF-β type-I receptor interacts with Smad2 and 3, which in turn form a heterodimeric complex with Co-Smad4. This complex translocates into the nucleus and regulates transcription by binding to the promoters of specific TGF-β target genes, for example, collagen α1(I), PAI-1, Jun B, c-Jun, and fibronectin (Schiffer et al., 2000).

In addition to Smad signaling, three major subgroups of MAPK superfamily members, such as extracellular signal-regulated kinases 1 and 2 (ERK1 and 2, p44/p42 MAPKs), c-Jun N-terminal kinase/stress-activated protein kinase (JNK/SAPK) and p38 MAPK appear to be involved in TGF-$\beta$ signaling in mesangial cells. These kinases are activated by hyperglycemia and modulate the transcriptional regulation of pro-$\alpha$1(I) procollagen and fibronectin mRNA through formation of the activated protein-1 (AP-1). There is some evidence for cross-talk between MAPK and Smad pathways since c-Fos and c-Jun, regulated by ERK and JNK, can bind directly to Smad3 while the Smad3/Smad4 heterodimer can bind to the AP-1-binding site of various promoters of TGF-$\beta$ target genes, suggesting that TGF-$\beta$ signaling is central to the excessive matrix formation in diabetic nephropathy (Ziyadeh, 2004).

These TGF-$\beta$-induced effects were initially observed in mesangial cell culture systems, but have also been corroborated by in vivo studies. The initial evidence implicating TGF-$\beta$ in diabetic nephropathy came from various murine models of diabetes. Subsequently, increased bioactivity of TGF-$\beta$ and expression of its receptor were observed in kidneys from diabetic patients. The direct role of TGF-$\beta$ was shown in studies with neutralizing anti-TGF-$\beta$ antibodies, where renal hypertrophy, mesangial matrix expansion, increase in $\alpha$1(IV) collagen and fibronectin mRNA, and a decline in renal function could be prevented. Moreover, upregulated tissue expression and enhanced urinary excretion of TGF-$\beta$ in patients with diabetic nephropathy have been described. Interestingly, ACE inhibitors which protect the kidney from diabetic injury also lower TGF-$\beta$ production (Ziyadeh, 2004).

### 4.1.5. GTP-binding proteins in diabetes mellitus

The relevance of GTP-binding proteins in diabetes mellitus was originally described more than a decade ago, and subsequently a number of these proteins including Rad, Gem, and Rho were shown to be activated by hyperglycemia. The small GTP-binding proteins belong to a superfamily with over 100 small GTPases (Takai et al., 2001). They are involved in the regulation of cell growth, motility and morphogenesis. In insulin deficiency, Rap1 is activated by its association with Raf-1. DAG can directly or through PKC activate the Rap/Raf/MAPK pathway. Enhanced expression of Rap1b was observed in kidneys of diabetic mice, thus implicating small GTP-binding proteins in intracellular signaling events induced by diabetes (Lin et al., 2001). Recently, the Rho family of GTPases has been reported to influence the biology of ECM proteins such as fibronectin in glomerular and tubulointerstitial cells, where it was found to modulate the TGF-$\beta$-induced upregulation of CTGF, a powerful pro-fibrogenic cytokine. Similarly, Rho-dependent pathways have been shown to be activated by other known pro-fibrogenic molecules, including angiotensin II, platelet-derived growth factor and endothelin-1 (Kim et al., 2000).

### 4.1.6. Reactive oxygen species (ROS) and apoptosis

ROS seem to be essential in the pathogenesis of many diabetic complications. Once generated, they are capable of self-perpetuating renal injury, and thus play an important role in the initiation and progression of diabetic injury to renal cells. Several species of ROS are known, including the superoxide radical, hydrogen peroxide, and the hydroxyl radical. In addition, ROS may react with other radicals including NO, giving rise to peroxynitrite which is considered a very powerful oxidant (Li and Shah, 2003). There is a critical balance between ROS production and neutralization that is maintained by antioxidant enzymes, including catalase, glutathione peroxidase and superoxide dismutase, as well as by several stress-response genes, such as HO-1. The levels of several constitutively expressed antioxidants may be increased, but the most remarkable change is seen in the expression of the inducible form of HO-1 in glomeruli derived from STZ-diabetic rats (Lee et al., 2003).

ROS are generated intracellularly through the NADPH oxidase system and by mitochondrial metabolism. NADPH oxidase was originally observed in phagocytic cells and subsequently described in numerous nonphagocytic cells, including renal cells. It is a flavocytochrome made up of a heterodimer of p22 phox and gp91 phox, and serves as a plasma membrane-bound electron transport chain. Nox1 and Nox4, which are homologs of the neutrophil gp91 phox, are expressed in the kidney (Pleskova et al., 2006). NADPH oxidase is activated on its association with cytosolic phox proteins, p47 phox, p67 phox, and p40 phox and a GTP-binding protein, p21rac. High glucose levels may, via AGE, free fatty acids, PKC and TGF-$\beta$, activate NADPH oxidase in renal cells (Li and Shah, 2003).

The glucose-induced generation of ROS in mesangial and tubular epithelial cells, and increased fibronectin expression, are significantly reduced by inhibitors of NADPH oxidase. The amount of ROS generated via the nonphagocytic NADPH oxidase system is normally relatively low, even under high-glucose ambience or in the hyperglycemic state, but may still exert significant effects on redox-sensitive signaling cellular processes (i.e., cell growth, apoptosis, and matrix turn-over). ROS may also activate various transcription factors (i.e., NF-$\kappa$B, AP-1, and Sp1), which in turn affect the expression of MCP-1, TGF-$\beta$, and PAI-1 (Lee et al., 2003).

Taken together, it seems that all cellular elements of the kidney are affected by hyperglycemia. On glucose entry the subsequent intracellular signaling events in all these cells might be similar, with variations depending on the expression of a given molecule in a particular cell, for example, aldose reductase in the tubular epithelium and PKC in the glomerulus. A large number of intracellular events occur in the presence of high glucose, including increased flux of polyols and hexosamines, formation of AGE and ROS, activation of PKC, TGF-$\beta$, and G-protein signaling, and altered expression of cyclin kinases, of matrix proteins, metalloproteinases, and their inhibitors. These events are connected at various levels of different signaling pathways, all leading to a defined end-point, that is, increased extracellular matrix deposition, a typical finding in diabetic nephropathy.

## 4.2. Dyslipidemia

Dyslipidemia is thought to cause renal damage and to play an important role in the progression of chronic kidney disease. It is a common feature in many chronic kidney disorders, is characterized by high triglyceride and low high-density lipoprotein (HDL) cholesterol levels, accumulation of remnant particles, a predominance of small dense low-density lipoprotein (LDL) particles, and increased levels of lipoprotein A. LDL may undergo oxidative modification, resulting in the formation of oxidized LDL (Moorhead et al., 1982).

In experimental models hyperlipidemic diets worsen renal cell injury, and lipid-lowering strategies improve renal cell function. Dyslipidemia may damage glomerular capillary endothelial and mesangial cells as well as podocytes. Mesangial cells have receptors for LDL and oxidized LDL, which upon activation induce mesangial cell proliferation, increase mesangial matrix deposition, and enhance the production of chemokines (i.e., MCP-1), cytokines (i.e., IL-6), and growth factors. Macrophages phagocytose oxidized lipids and thereby turn into foam cells. These macrophage-derived foam cells release cytokines that recruit more macrophages to the lesion, increase lipid deposition, impair endothelial cell function, and enhance proliferation of vascular smooth muscle cells. These events typically take place in the atherosclerotic vessel wall, but to a certain degree are believed to occur within the glomerulus as well. Therefore, similar pathogenetic mechanisms may contribute to the progression of atherosclerosis and glomerulosclerosis (Joles et al., 2000).

Hypercholesterolemia is also associated with podocyte injury. Oxidized LDL induces apoptosis of podocytes and a loss of the slit membrane protein nephrin, and in vitro increases the diffusion of albumin through podocytes (Bussolati et al., 2005). There is also evidence that circulating lipids bind to and become sequestered in the extracellular matrix, where they undergo oxidation by ROS. The resultant reduction in the actions of endothelium-derived vasodilators, such as prostacyclin and NO, with increased formation of endothelium-derived vasoconstrictors/growth promoters, such as angiotensin II, endothelin-1, and PAI-1, may have significant pathophysiologic consequences (Joles et al., 2000).

---

**Key points**

- The balance between ROS production and the protective cellular antioxidant response program determines the pathogenesis of kidney diseases associated with renal cell injury.
- Immune complexes are key parameters of immune-mediated renal injury that act via mechanisms involving Fc$\gamma$ receptors and the complement system.
- Activation of TLRs by infection or endogenous ligands aggravates immune mediated glomerular injury.
- There are a number of intracellular events that occur in the presence of high glucose, which include increased flux of polyols and hexosamines, formation of AGE and ROS, activation of PKC and TGF-$\beta$.
- In the hyperglycemic state ROS are generated by renal cells and exert significant effects on various redox-sensitive signaling processes (i.e., cell growth, apoptosis, and matrix turnover).
- All three TGF-$\beta$ isoforms are upregulated in the diabetic kidney and these cytokines signal through the Smad, MAPK, and PKA pathways in renal cells, which is essential for the excessive matrix formation in diabetic nephropathy.

---

# References

Anders, H.J., Banas, B., Schlondorff, D. 2004a. Signaling danger: toll-like receptors and their potential roles in kidney disease. J. Am. Soc. Nephrol. 15, 854.

Anders, H.J., Vielhauer, V., Eis, V., et al. 2004b. Activation of toll-like receptor-9 induces progression of renal disease in MRL-Fas(lpr) mice. FASEB J. 18, 534.

Anderson, P.W., Zhang, X.Y., Tian, J., et al. 1996. Insulin and angiotensin II are additive in stimulating TGF-beta 1 and matrix mRNAs in mesangial cells. Kidney Int. 50, 745.

Aron, D.C., Rosenzweig, J.L., Abboud, H.E. 1989. Synthesis and binding of insulin-like growth factor I by human glomerular mesangial cells. J. Clin. Endocrinol. Metab. 68, 585.

Bao, L., Osawe, I., Haas, M., et al. 2005a. Signaling through up-regulated C3a receptor is key to the development of experimental lupus nephritis. J. Immunol. 175, 1947.

Bao, L., Osawe, I., Puri, T., et al. 2005b. C5a promotes development of experimental lupus nephritis which can be blocked with a specific receptor antagonist. Eur. J. Immunol. 35, 2496.

Baud, L., Ardaillou, R. 1993. Involvement of reactive oxygen species in kidney damage. Br. Med. Bull. 49, 621.

Berger, S.P., Roos, A., Daha, M.R. 2005. Complement and the kidney: what the nephrologist needs to know in 2006? Nephrol. Dial. Transplant. 20, 2613.

Bhaskaran, M., Reddy, K., Radhakrishanan, N., et al. 2003. Angiotensin II induces apoptosis in renal proximal tubular cells. Am. J. Physiol. Renal Physiol. 284, F955.

Brüne, B., von Knethen, A., Sandau, K.B. 1999. Nitric oxide (NO): an effector of apoptosis. Cell Death Differ. 6, 969.

Budisavljevic, M.N., Hodge, L., Barber, K., et al. 2003. Oxidative stress in the pathogenesis of experimental mesangial proliferative glomerulonephritis. Am. J. Physiol. Renal Physiol. 285, F1138.

Bussolati, B., Deregibus, M.C., Fonsanto, V., et al. 2005. Statins prevent oxidized LDL-induced injury of glomerular podocytes by activating phosphatidylinositol 3-kinase/AKT-signaling pathway. J. Am. Soc. Nephrol. 16, 1936.

Christensen, S.R., Kashgarian, M., Alexopoulou, L., et al. 2005. Toll-like receptor 9 controls anti-DNA autoantibody production in murine lupus. J. Exp. Med. 202, 321.

Conti, F.G., Striker, L.J., Lesniak, M.A., et al. 1988. Studies on binding and mitogenic effect of insulin and insulin-like growth factor I in glomerular mesangial cells. Endocrinology 122, 2788.

Czyzyk, J. 2006. The role of Toll-like receptors in the pathogenesis of renal disease. Semin. Nephrol. 26, 167.

Hasegawa, H., Kohno, M., Sasaki, M., et al. 2003. Antagonist of monocyte chemoattractant protein 1 ameliorates the initiation and progression of lupus nephritis and renal vasculitis in MRL/lpr mice. Arthritis Rheum. 48, 2555.

Heilig, C.W., Brosius, F.C., Henry, D.N. 1997. Glucose transporters of the glomerulus and the implications for diabetic nephropathy. Kidney Int. 60, S91.

Hoffman, R.W., Gazitt, T., Foecking, M.F., et al. 2004. U1 RNA induces innate immunity signaling. Arthritis Rheum. 50, 2891.

Inoguchi, T., Sonta, T., Tsubouchi, H., et al. 2003. Protein kinase C-dependent increase in reactive oxygen species (ROS) production in vascular tissues of diabetes: role of vascular NADPH oxidase. J. Am. Soc. Nephrol. 14, S227.

Jancar, S., Sanchez Crespo, M. 2005. Immune complex-mediated tissue injury: a multistep paradigm. Trends Immunol. 26, 48.

Joles, J.A., Kunter, U., Janssen, U., et al. 2000. Early mechanisms of renal injury in hypercholesterolemic or hypertriglyceridemic rats. J. Am. Soc. Nephrol. 11, 669.

Kim, S.I., Kim, H.J., Han, D.C., et al. 2000. Effect of lovastatin on small GTPbinding proteins and TGF-ß1 and fibronectin expression. Kidney Int. 58, S88.

Kleinert, H., Pautz, A., Linker, K., et al. 2004. Regulation of the expression of inducible nitric oxide synthase. Eur. J. Pharmacol. 500, 255.

Krieg, A.M. 2002. A role for Toll in autoimmunity. Nat. Immunol. 3, 423.

Leask, A., Abraham, D.J. 2004. TGF-ß signaling and the fibrotic response. FASEB J. 18, 816.

Lee, H.B., Yu, M.R., Yang, Y., et al. 2003. Reactive oxygen species-regulated signaling pathways in diabetic nephropathy. J. Am. Soc. Nephrol. 14, S241.

Lenert, P. 2005. Inhibitory oligodeoxynucleotides-therapeutic promise for systemic autoimmune diseases? Clin. Exp. Immunol. 140, 1.

Li, J.M., Shah, A.M. 2003. ROS generation by non-phagocytic NADPH oxidase: potential relevance in diabetic nephropathy. J. Am. Soc. Nephrol. 14, S221.

Lin, S., Chugh, S.S., Pan, X., et al. 2001. Identification of up-regulated Ras-like GTPase, Rap1b, by suppression substractive hybridization. Kidney Int. 60, 2129.

Mason, R.M., Wahab, N.A. 2003. Extracellular matrix metabolism in diabetic nephropathy. J. Am. Soc. Nephrol. 14, 1358.

Moorhead, J.F., Chan, M.K., El-Nahas, M., et al. 1982. Lipid nephrotoxicity in chronic progressive glomerular and tubulointerstitial disease. Lancet 2, 1309.

Nangaku, M., Couser, W.G. 2005. Mechanisms of immune-deposit formation and the mediation of immune renal injury. Clin. Exp. Nephrol. 9, 183–191.

Negi, V.S., Aggarwal, A., Dayal, R., Naik, S., Misra, R. 2000. Complement degradation product C3d in urine: marker of lupus nephritis. J. Rheumatol. 27, 380–383.

Oates, J.C., Gilkeson, G.S. 2002. Mediators of injury in lupus nephritis. Curr. Opin. Rheumatol. 14, 498–503.

Patole, P.S., Grone, H.J., Segerer, S., et al. 2005. Viral double-stranded RNA aggravates lupus nephritis through Toll-like receptor 3 on glomerular mesangial cells and antigen-presenting cells. J. Am. Soc. Nephrol. 16, 1326.

Pawar, R.D., Patole, P.S., Wornle, M., Anders, H.J. 2006. Microbial nucleic acids pay a toll in kidney disease. Am. J. Physiol. Renal Physiol. 291, F509.

Pfeilschifter, J., Beck, K.F., Eberhardt, W., Huwiler, A. 2002. Changing gears in the course of glomerulonephritis by shifting superoxide to nitric oxide-dominated chemistry. Kidney Int. 61, 809.

Pfeilschifter, J., Kunz, D., Mühl, H. 1993. Nitric oxide: an inflammatory mediator of glomerular mesangial cells. Nephron 64, 518.

Philipneri, M., Bastani, B. 2001. Kidney disease in patients with chronic hepatitis C. Curr. Gastroenterol. Rep. 3, 79.

Pleskova, M., Beck, K.F., Behrens, M.H., et al. 2006. Nitric oxide down-regulates the expression of the catalytic NADPH oxidase subunit Nox1 in rat renal mesangial cells. FASEB J. 20, 139.

Radeke, H.H., Janssen-Graalfs, I., Sowa, E.N., et al. 2002. Opposite regulation of type II and III receptors for immunoglobulin G in mouse glomerular mesangial cells and in the induction of anti-glomerular basement membrane (GBM) nephritis. J. Biol. Chem. 277, 27535.

Ravetch, J.V., Bolland, S. 2001. IgG Fc receptors. Annu. Rev. Immunol. 19, 275–290.

Russo, C., Olivieri, O., Girelli, D., et al. 1998. Anti-oxidant status and lipid peroxidation in patients with essential hypertension. J. Hypertens. 16, 1267.

Samuelsson, P., Hang, L., Wullt, B., et al. 2004. Toll-like receptor 4 expression and cytokine responses in the human urinary tract mucosa. Infect. Immun. 72, 3179.

Schaefer, L., Babelova, A., Kiss, E., et al. 2005. The matrix component biglycan is proinflammatory and signals through Toll-like receptors 4 and 2 in macrophages. J. Clin. Invest. 115, 2223.

Schiffer, M., von Gersdorf, G., Bitzer, M., et al. 2000. Smad proteins and transforming growth factor-ß signaling. Kidney Int. 58, S45.

Seelen, M.A., Roos, A., Daha, M.R. 2005. Role of complement in innate and autoimmunity. J. Nephrol. 18, 642.

Sowers, J.R. 2002. Hypertension, angiotensin II, and oxidative stress. N. Engl. J. Med. 346, 1999.

Sozzani, S., Bosisio, D., Mantovani, A., Ghezzi, P. 2005. Linking stress, oxidation and the chemokine system. Eur. J. Immunol. 35, 3095.

Stout, R.W., Bierman, E.L., Ross, R. 1975. Effect of insulin on the proliferation of cultured primate arterial smooth muscle cells. Circ. Res. 36, 319.

Suzuki, Y., Gomez-Guerrero, C., Shirato, I., et al. 2003. Pre-existing glomerular immune complexes induce polymorphonuclear cell recruitment through an Fc receptor-dependent respiratory burst: potential role in the perpetuation of immune nephritis. J. Immunol. 70, 3243.

Szabo, C. 1996. The pathophysiological role of peroxynitrite in shock, inflammation, and ischemia-reperfusion injury. Shock 6, 79.

Takai, Y., Sasaki, T., Matozaki, T. 2001. Small GTPbinding proteins. Physiol. Rev. 81, 153.

Takeda, K., Akira, S. 2005. Toll-like receptors in innate immunity. Int. Immunol. 17, 1.

Tang, S., Leung, J.C., Abe, K., et al. 2003. Albumin stimulates interleukin-8 expression in proximal tubular epithelial cells in vitro and in vivo. Clin. Invest. 111, 515.

Tarzi, R.M., Cook, H.T. 2003. Role of Fcgamma receptors in glomerulonephritis. Nephron Exp. Nephrol. 95, e7.

Wang, S., Denichilo, M., Brubaker, C., et al. 2001. Connective tissue growth factor in tubulointerstitial injury of diabetic nephropathy. Kidney Int. 60, 96.

Wardle, E.N. 2005. Cellular oxidative processes in relation to renal disease. Am. J. Nephrol. 25, 13.

Weiner, N.J., Goodman, J.W., Kimmel, P.L. 2003. The HIV-associated renal diseases: current insight into pathogenesis and treatment. Kidney Int. 63, 1618.

Wornle, M., Schmid, H., Banas, B., et al. 2006. Novel role of toll-like receptor 3 in hepatitis C-associated glomerulonephritis. Am. J. Pathol. 168, 370.

Ziyadeh, F.N. 2004. Mediators of diabetic renal disease: the case for TGF-ß as the major mediator. J. Am. Soc. Nephrol. 15, S55.

CHAPTER 6

# Renal Toxicities Associated with Immunomodulatory Drugs

Alan D. Salama*

*Renal Section, Division of Medicine, Imperial College London, Hammersmith Hospital, London W12 ONN, United Kingdom*

## 1. Introduction

Immunosuppressive drug therapy remains an essential cornerstone of treatment in autoimmunity. Re-establishing immunological tolerance to particular autoantigens, although highly desirable, is not yet achievable in a reproducible manner (Salama and Sayegh, 2007). As such we are left with the need to use non-specific immunosuppressants in order to modulate autoimmune processes. By doing so, we suppress the autoimmune-mediated damage, but also hamper beneficial immune responses to foreign antigens and the immunological feedback mechanisms, which normally act as natural regulators of immune reactivity. The net effect is that although the autoimmune disease is treated, the patients may experience to adverse effects related to their loss of defensive immunity to pathogens and to malignantly transformed cells. In some circumstances, treatment might also prevent the development of tolerance to autoantigens.

In addition, each particular immunosuppressant has a specific adverse effect profile, which adds to iatrogenic morbidity. In all cases, attempts to balance the risks of the autoimmune disease manifestations and the potential adverse drug effects are made. Thus, a hierarchy of immunosuppressive agents has evolved, which is used in particular autoimmune settings to provide disease control, with side effects that are in proportion to disease severity. The more severe the disease, the greater is the risk that is considered acceptable. For example we reserve cyclophosphamide, in limited courses, for organ or life-threatening disease since it is associated with significant pro-malignant potential, risk of bone marrow suppression and bladder toxicity. Conversely, we rely on azathioprine to act as a steroid-sparing maintenance agent in a number of conditions, since it is generally well tolerated with few serious, irreversible adverse effects. It is therefore critical to be aware of the risks of particular agents, so that an informed decision regarding their use can be made.

Traditionally, we have been limited by the number of available efficacious agents, however, with many newer drugs being developed, some imported from the field of transplantation, we are adopting an increasingly large number of immunomodulatory tools that can be applied to the autoimmune setting. Moreover, with the introduction of newer biological agents the potential for different drug combinations has expanded considerably. With these comes a new series of potential adverse effects, which we will have to remain vigilant to identify. Hopefully, with increasing understanding of the immunobiology of certain autoimmune diseases, we may be able to apply a more logical strategy for therapy, that while suppressing the autoimmune process, will also allow the development of more stringent regulatory pathways, ultimately even re-establishing immune tolerance.

---

*Corresponding author.
Tel.: +44 20 8383 3980; Fax: +44 20 8383 3980
E-mail address: A.Salama@imperial.ac.uk

© 2008 Elsevier B.V. All rights reserved.
DOI: 10.1016/S1571-5078(07)07006-7

In this chapter, I will review the renal toxicity associated with currently used immunosuppressants, immune modulators, and some adjuvant therapies frequently utilized with these agents. Where possible, the explanation for these effects will be highlighted. I will further discuss some of the novel agents that are becoming available and what we may expect in the future regarding their use and their adverse effects on the kidney. I will discuss the effects according to the renal compartments affected, as well as according to the agent used. There should be a note of caution, since establishing a causal effect for an agent used in the treatment of multisystem diseases is not always easy. A number of pathologies may be associated with the underlying disease and it may not be always possible to fulfill Koch's postulate with respect to the adverse effect and drug exposure. Additionally, it should be borne in mind that patients with one form of autoimmune disease may have a propensity to develop other (auto)-immune conditions, which may present with renal pathology. It is therefore critical to maintain a high index of suspicion that unexpected clinical features may be related to the use of novel or established drugs (or their combinations) in a new setting.

## 2. Drug effects and renal pathology

The kidney can be effectively divided into three compartments, the glomeruli, the tubulointerstitium, and the vasculature. Although drugs may affect one or all of these compartments, many agents are associated with particular adverse renal effects. In many cases, the common signs of toxicity include abnormal renal function and the development of abnormal urinary sediment. This highlights the need for monitoring any urinary abnormalities that develop in patients with autoimmune disease and, as will be seen, often creates a challenge to understand whether the effects are due to the therapy or to the disease itself. It should be emphasized that monitoring changes in serum creatinine may not allow for early detection of toxicity, while estimations of glomerular filtration rate (GFR), using one of the available equations, may be a more sensitive measure in patients with renal impairment. This topic is reviewed in Lamb et al. (2005).

### 2.1. The glomerular compartment

The glomerulus may be affected by a number of agents with the subsequent development of a nephrotic syndrome, due to membranous glomerulonephritis (secondary to penicillamine or gold therapy), a focal and segmental collapsing glomerulopathy (following biphosphonate therapy using pamidronate), or crescentic glomerulonephritis such as an anti-GBM or pauci-immune ANCA-associated disease (following penicillamine). Establishing a causal link with the responsible agent is often difficult, as patients may have been treated with the drug for a considerable period of time before developing the complication (Bindi et al., 1997). Moreover, in order to treat the glomerular lesion, it may be insufficient to simply withdraw the drug, rather additional therapy may be needed (Derk and Jimenez, 2003), making it more difficult to fulfill Koch's postulate to link drug and disease. Glomerular abnormalities present with abnormal urinalysis, urinary sediment, or impairment of renal function. Estimation of urinary proteinuria does not require cumbersome 24 h urine collections, but can be accurately estimated with spot urinary protein:creatinine ratios (Newman et al., 2000).

### 2.2. The tubulointerstitium

The tubulointerstitium is a frequent target of drug toxicity. Direct toxic damage to the tubular cells from drugs which may be concentrated in the urine, or immune-mediated reactions to drug-related antigens, are common. Tubulointerstitial nephritis (TIN) can result from exposure to almost any drug and can only be diagnosed on renal biopsy (see Fig. 1). Drug-related causes of TIN now predominate in the etiology of this condition (Baker and Pusey, 2004). Particular tubular pathologies may result following certain drug exposure (such as isometric vacuolization

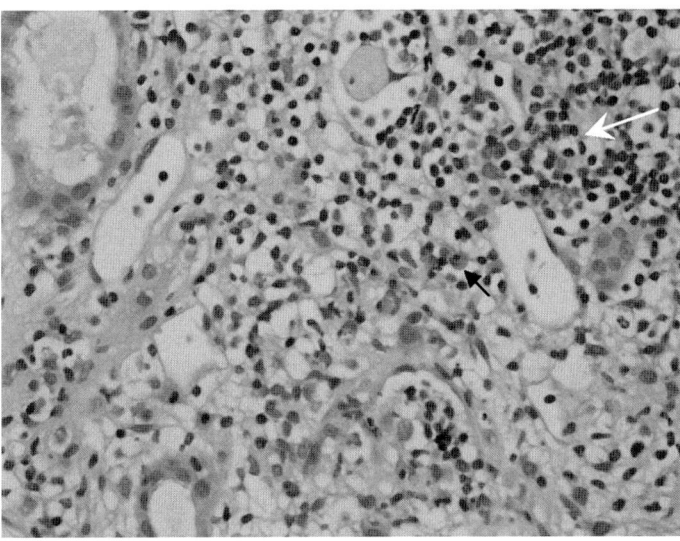

**Figure 1.** Photomicrograph of a renal biopsy section (Hematoxylin and Eosin × 400) demonstrating tubulointerstitial nephritis with marked leukocyte infiltration of the interstitium and tubular epithelium (tubulitis) (white arrow). Eosinophils are marked by the small black arrow.

following ciclosporin or intravenous immunoglobulin (IVIG)) and although these are not pathognomonic, a knowledge of drug exposure and potential toxicities helps establish the diagnosis. Tubular dysfunction manifests with urinary abnormalities or abnormal renal function. Urine testing may reveal the presence of blood, protein, or other substances usually reabsorbed in the tubules such as glucose and amino acids (in rare cases a complete Fanconi syndrome may occur). Urinary pH may therefore be abnormally high due a renal tubular disorder of bicarbonate or hydrogen ion regulation. More specific proteins expressed, secreted, or reabsorbed by the tubules may be measured in the urine as indicators of tubular disease (tubular proteinuria) and these include retinal binding protein (RBP), $N$-acetyl B glucosaminidase (NAG), or kidney injury molecule-1 (KIM-1). However, these are not routinely performed in clinical practice.

## 2.3. The vasculature

Damage to the renal vasculature can result in a rapid deterioration of renal function (e.g., acute thrombotic microangiopathy (TMA) associated with calcineurin inhibitors (CNIs)), or may follow a more protracted chronic course due to progressive renal ischemia (hyalinosis lesions associated with CNIs). Clues as the etiology may come from associated clinical or laboratory findings, such as thrombocytopenia, red cell fragmentation, and hemolysis in the case of TMA, but more often are lacking and establishment of a diagnosis requires a confirmatory renal biopsy.

Drugs may affect one or more renal compartments and pattern recognition enables pathologists to suggest likely drug-mediated etiologies when reviewing renal biopsy lesions. It is therefore of paramount importance to have good dialogue between the clinicians and pathologists to enable an accurate conclusion to be made regarding potential adverse drug reactions.

## 3. Individual drugs

The mainstay of therapy for most autoimmune diseases remains corticosteroids, which are not associated with renal dysfunction except indirectly by induction of diabetes mellitus. I have highlighted

**Table 1**
Immunomodulatory drugs used to treat autoimmune disorders, their common indications and renal toxicities

| Drug | Condition | Renal adverse effect | Risk factors |
| --- | --- | --- | --- |
| Azathioprine | RA, AAV, SLE | Tubulointerstitial nephritis, allergic reaction | |
| Calcineurin inhibitors | MG, membranous GN, psoriasis, RA | Acute renal dysfunction, TMA, Chronic interstitial fibrosis, glomerulosclerosis, arteriolar hyalinosis | Older age, doses >5 mg/kg/day, renal impairment |
| D-Penicillamine | RA, SS, PBC | Membranous GN, minimal change disease, crescentic GN (immune complex, pauci immune and anti-GBM antibody associated). Development of ANCA | Certain HLA-DQ/DR alleles |
| Gold salts | RA | Membranous GN, minimal change disease, immune complex GN | |
| Intravenous immunoglobulin | SLE, AAV, dermatomyositis, Guillain–Barre syndrome, ITP, Kawasaki's disease | Acute renal failure (osmotic nephropathy) | Older age, renal impairment, volume depletion |
| Sirolimus | FSGS, dermatomyositis, IPEX, AIHA | TMA, proteinuria, acute renal failure | |
| Sulfasalazine and 5-ASA compounds | RA, IBD | Tubulointerstitial nephritis, minimal change disease | |
| TNF antagonists | RA, AS, IBD, AAV | Lupus nephritis, membranous, pauci immune GN | |

AAV, ANCA associated vasculitis; RA, rheumatoid arthritis; SS, systemic sclerosis; PBC, primary biliray cirrhosis; MG, myaesthenia gravis; GN, glomerulonephritis; ITP, immune thrombocytopaenic purpura; TMA, thrombotic microangiopathy; FSGS, focal and segmental glomerulosclerosis; IPEX, immunodysregulation polyendocrinopathy enteropathy X-linked syndrome; AIHA, autoimmune hemolytic anemia; IBD, inflammatory bowel disease; AS, Ankylosing spondylitis.

the more commonly used drugs which have been reported to cause renal complications (Table 1). Those that are not cited have not had such reports made to date.

## 3.1. Azathioprine

Azathioprine is metabolized in the liver to become an active drug, through its conversion to 6-mercaptopurine. It inhibits de novo purine synthesis and hence DNA and RNA synthesis. Its metabolites are excreted via the kidneys but in an inactive form. It remains a popular drug for the treatment of numerous autoimmune conditions, and is commonly used as a steroid-sparing agent.

Its predominant toxicities are related to bone marrow suppression, megaloblastic anemia, and hepatic dysfunction. The risk of marrow suppression is increased in patients with low thiopurine methyltransferase (TPMT) activity, the enzyme responsible for drug metabolism. Rarely, its use has been associated with the development of interstitial nephritis, complicating Wegener's granulomatosis (Parnham et al., 1996; Bir et al., 2006), classical polyarteritis nodosa (Parnham et al., 1996), and rheumatoid arthritis (Meys et al., 1992) (Table 1). In addition, allergic reactions marked by fevers, arthralgias, and generalized malaise have been reported in patients with mixed essential cryoglobulinaemia and leukocytoclastic vasculitis, as well as ANCA associated vasculitis (Stratton and Farrington, 1998). These complications may appear at anytime from 1 week to over a year following the introduction of the drug (Stratton and Farrington, 1998). In contrast, resolution occurs rapidly after cessation of the drug, generally within a week, and re-exposure to azathioprine results in a more rapid recurrence of allergic symptoms and decline in renal function (Parnham et al., 1996; Stratton and Farrington, 1998). In one patient with anti-GBM disease allergic symptoms, which included pulmonary infiltrates associated with hemoptysis, mimicking the pulmonary-renal syndrome, occurred shortly after azathioprine initiation and promptly resolved following cessation of the drug (Stetter et al., 1994). Overall, the incidence of these reactions appears to be low, occurring in both acute and convalescent disease, and not associated with any particular patient phenotype.

## 3.2. Intravenous immunoglobulin

IVIG, in the form of a pooled polyclonal preparation, has been increasingly used for the treatment of a variety of autoimmune and rheumatic conditions (Roifman, 1995; Jayne et al., 2000; Zandman-Goddard et al., 2005). Originally utilized and licensed for replacement therapy in primary and secondary immunoglobulin deficiency, it was also licensed for the treatment of Kawasaki's disease, immune thrombocytopaenic purpura, bone marrow transplantation, B-cell lymphocytic leukemia and pediatric HIV disease. However, it has been increasingly utilized off-label at high doses (up to 5 g/kg) for several autoimmune conditions, including systemic lupus erythematosus, ANCA-associated vasculitis (AAV), Guillain–Barre syndrome, and dermatomyositis. Its mechanism of action remains incompletely understood, although proposals include modulation of antibody effector functions through anti-idiotype networks (Shoenfeld and Katz, 2005), an influence on cytokine production or lymphocyte activation, or more recently upregulation of inhibitory FcReceptors on macrophages (Kaneko et al., 2006).

A number of different IVIG preparations exist in which the immunoglobulin molecules are stabilized in a carbohydrate rich solution (to prevent aggregation of the IgG) (see Table 2). The adverse renal effects of IVIG appear to be related to the stabilizers rather than the immunoglobulin fraction per se, with 70–90% of patients who developed IVIG nephropathy having received a sucrose-based preparation (Orbach et al., 2004). However, a lower proportion of other sugar-based and non-sugar-based preparations have been implicated (Table 2), and so it appears that all IVIG preparations require vigilance with relation to renal dysfunction. In some studies, patient-related

Table 2
Different preparations of IVIG, their stabilizers content of sucrose and reported role in renal failure

| IVIG preparation | Stabilizer (concentration of sucrose g/g IgG) | Reported to cause renal impairment |
| --- | --- | --- |
| Flebogamma | Sorbital | NK |
| Gammagard S/D | Glucose, albumin, and glycine | Yes |
| Gammagard liquid | Glycine only | Yes |
| Gammar | Sucrose (1.0) | Yes |
| Gamimune | Maltose or glycine | Yes |
| Intragam | Maltose | Yes |
| Iveegam | Glucose | NK |
| Octagam | Maltose | NK |
| Panglobulin | Sucrose (1.7) | Yes |
| Polygam | Glucose, albumin, or glycine | NK |
| Sandoglobulin | Sucrose (1.7) | Yes |
| Venoglobulin | Sorbitol or aluminum | NK |
| Vigam | Sucrose (0.5), albumin, and glycine | Yes |

NK, not known.

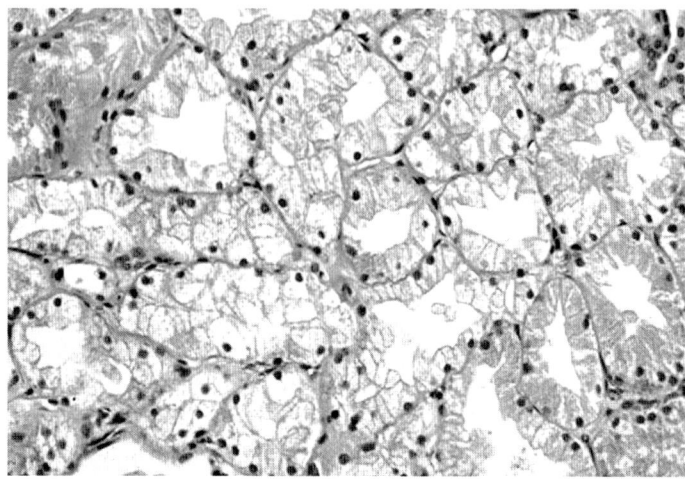

**Figure 2.** Photomicrograph of a renal biopsy section (Hematoxylin and Eosin × 400) demonstrating tubular vacuolation and some degeneration of the tubular epithelium, in this case secondary to ciclosporin toxicity. Similar lesions are found in IVIG nephrotoxicity.

characteristics predisposing to the development of the IVIG-related nephrotoxicity included diabetes, pre-existing renal impairment, volume depletion, and older age (Table 1) although this was not a uniform finding (Levy and Pusey, 2000; Sati et al., 2001; Orbach et al., 2004).

The characteristics of the nephropathy are typical of osmotic injury, with vacuolation of proximal tubular cells (Fig. 2) and evidence of tubular dysfunction with acute tubular necrosis (Soares and Sethi, 2006). The incidence of the condition is low, with approximately 7% of patients treated for a variety of conditions developing renal dysfunction (Levy and Pusey, 2000; Sati et al., 2001). In a significant proportion of patients, acute renal failure requiring dialysis support occurs, generally within 8 days from the onset of treatment. In a 13-year period from 1985 to 1999, 120 cases of IVIG nephropathy were reported to the Food and Drug Administration (FDA), 88 within the USA, and these had a high rate of acute renal failure with 40% requiring dialysis (MMWR, 1999). For the most part this is temporary and the lesion resolves on withdrawal of the offending IVIG preparation. However, in some series up to 2% develop established renal failure (Levy and Pusey, 2000), and a mortality rate of up to 15% was reported in the FDA series, although many patients had significant co-morbid conditions which undoubtedly contributed (MMWR, 1999).

## 3.3. Calcineurin inhibitors (ciclosporin and tacrolimus)

Ciclosporin and more recently tacrolimus were originally introduced as immunosuppressants in the field of transplantation. Ciclosporin revolutionized the outcome of solid organ transplantation, but due to its perceived erratic bioavailability and difficult pharmacokinetics, it has been largely superseded by tacrolimus. Both agents have been used, at lower doses than in transplantation, for the treatment of autoimmune conditions, including hepatic (Aqel et al., 2004), renal (Cattran et al., 2001; Duncan et al., 2004), rheumatological (Salvarani et al., 2001), dermatological (Griffiths et al., 2006; Hengge et al., 2006), endocrine, ocular, and neuromuscular disorders (Schneider-Gold et al., 2006). However, CNIs are associated with both short-term and long-term renal toxicities, which have limited their more widespread use. Major toxicities appear to be similar for both agents, while some adverse effects predominate for each, such as diabetes for tacrolimus and hirsuitism for ciclosporin. Reports of patients changing from one agent to the other to reverse major toxicities have been made, suggesting that there is also an idiosyncratic element. The principle acute problems relate to hypertension and vasoconstriction of the afferent renal arterioles resulting in a decline in GFR. In parallel, there are increases in serum potassium, uric acid, and evidence of sodium retention. These generally respond to a reduction in drug dose, although hypertension may persist. Tubular toxicity may be the result of ischemic injury or a direct effect of the drug, and manifests as acute tubular necrosis with evidence of isometric vacuolation (see Fig. 2).

Another form of acute CNI toxicity, though much rarer, is the development of a TMA. It generally occurs soon after the introduction of the CNI, although delayed and chronic forms of TMA have been reported. TMA presents with a sudden decline in GFR and is due to endothelial damage and activation, leading to the formation of microthrombi with subsequent vessel occlusion. The occurrence of TMA is not clearly related to drug dose, and although it generally responds to drug discontinuation, permanent damage may result.

More important in the context of relapsing–remitting autoimmune diseases is the chronic nephropathy that occurs from prolonged treatment with CNIs. This is characterized by a "striped" interstitial fibrosis, arteriolar thickening with nodular hyalinosis, and segmental glomerular sclerosis (Fig. 3). Evidence of early chronic damage (within 3 months) has been reported from some transplant series based on protocol biopsies, although a period of 6 months of treatment is generally required (Nankivell et al., 2004). This renal lesion may not be reversible; however, cessation of the drug may prevent further sclerosis and organ damage. The diagnosis is a histological one requiring renal biopsy (Fig. 3). It is this more indolent damage that has made treatment of autoimmune disease with CNIs less appealing, although they have the advantage of not being bone marrow suppressive, unlike many other agents used in autoimmunity. Risk factors for development of CNI toxicity appear to be older age, co-administration of non-steroidal anti-inflammatory agents, use of doses in excess of 5 mg/kg/day, and pre-existing renal impairment (Table 1). Encouragingly, two small series of patients with rheumatoid arthritis, treated using doses of less than 5 mg/kg/day for 6 months

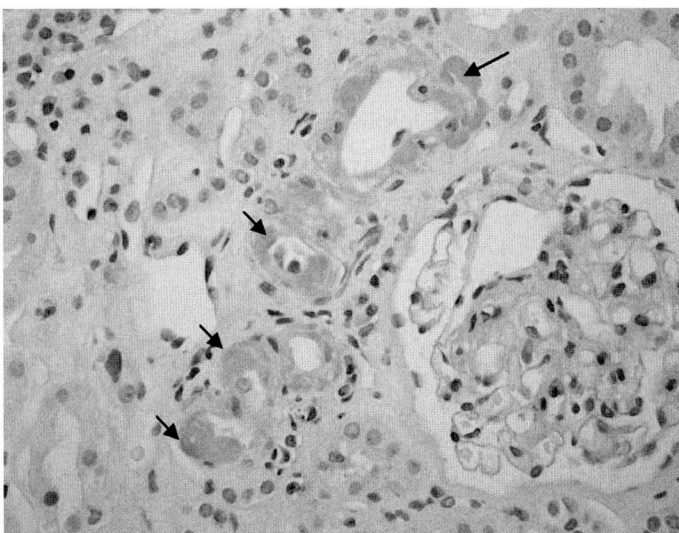

**Figure 3.** Photomicrograph of a renal biopsy section (Hematoxylin and Eosin × 400) demonstrating nodular hyaline material in renal arterioles (arrows) secondary to chronic calcineurin toxicity.

(Ludwin et al., 1994), or more than 7 years (Rodriguez et al., 1996), reported a low overall incidence of CNI-related toxicity based on renal biopsy findings.

## 3.4. D-Penicillamine

This agent is used in the treatment of rheumatoid arthritis and systemic sclerosis, although less frequently than before, as a result of the introduction of more effective novel second line agents. Its mode of action is unclear, but it is cleared through an oxidative process forming disulfides with circulating proteins. Altered metabolic processing through this pathway of sulfoxidation may lead to increased adverse effects. An association with certain HLA-DR alleles has also been found in those with renal adverse effects (Hall, 1989). Numerous side effects occur in a dose-dependent manner with this agent, and a number of renal lesions have also been described. These include membranous glomerulonephritis, minimal change disease (Falck et al., 1979; Hall, 1989), focal and segmental necrotizing glomerulonephritis with or without ANCA (Harper et al., 1997; Karpinski et al., 1997; Nanke et al., 2000), crescentic glomerulonephritis in association with anti-glomerular basement membrane (GBM) antibodies (Bindi et al., 1997; Derk and Jimenez, 2003), immune complex nephritis (and a lupus-like disease) (Chalmers et al., 1982; Nanke et al., 2000), and less commonly interstitial nephritis (Feehally et al., 1987). In some cases, the drug had been administered for over 10 years before the renal lesion developed (Bindi et al., 1997), although most cases present within the first 2 years. A number of similarities appear to exist between patients susceptible to adverse effects from penicillamine and gold therapy (see below) (Table 1). In many cases, the renal lesions resolve on cessation of the drug, but in the more aggressive lesions additional immunotherapy has been required; despite that the outcome may be poor. Interestingly, in a number of a patients, co-administration of iron appears to have adequately chelated the penicillamine in the gut, and on discontinuation of the iron, renal complications related to penicillamine therapy were diagnosed (Harkness and Blake, 1982).

## 3.5. Gold salts

Gold salts remain a useful therapy in the treatment of an increasingly small group of patients with resistant rheumatoid arthritis. Like penicillamine, treatment with gold salts is associated with the development of a membranous glomerulonephropathy in up to 10% of patients in some series, with a clinical nephrotic syndrome in a third of cases. The renal lesion does not appear to be dependent on the dose of gold administered or its duration, although the formulation (oral or parenteral) may make a difference. Typically, the lesion occurs within the first 2 years of therapy (Hall, 1989). Generally, the proteinuria remits following cessation of the gold, although this may take up to 3 years. Gold may be implicated as the etiological agent in membranous glomerulonephropathy, as it may be found within the tubular and glomerular epithelial cells, as well as within mesangial cells. There may be an HLA susceptibility for gold-related toxicity, with certain DR and DQ alleles being implicated (Sakkas et al., 1993). Other lesions reported in patients treated with gold include immune complex mesangial glomerulonephritis and minimal change disease (Hall, 1989).

## 3.6. Sulfasalazine and related 5-ASA compounds

Sulfasalazine is commonly used in the treatment of rheumatoid arthritis and, along with other 5-aminosalicylic acid (5-ASA) compounds, in the treatment of inflammatory bowel disease. Sulfasalazine is poorly soluble and is, for the major part, not absorbed in the gut, rather it is cleaved in the colon by gut bacteria to produce 5-ASA and sulfapyridine. The latter appears to be responsible for its beneficial effects in rheumatoid arthritis, while 5-ASA compounds are beneficial in inflammatory bowel disease. Adverse effects with sulfasalzine more commonly relate to hepatic and bone marrow toxicity, while renal toxicity is rarer (with an incidence of less than 0.2 per 100 patients) (Van Staa et al., 2004). The renal toxicity of sulfasalazine appears similar to that of other 5-ASA compounds (Riley et al., 1992), although it is of interest to note that patients with inflammatory bowel disease not treated with 5-ASA compounds are also at increased risk of developing renal impairment, suggesting that there may be some effect of the underlying disease as well. Many cases of 5-ASA-induced TIN have been reported (Calvino et al., 1998; Gisbert et al., 2007), which may be acute or chronic (Dwarakanath et al., 1992). In addition, cases of nephrotic syndrome secondary to minimal change disease have been reported in patients taking sulfasalazine and 5-ASA compounds (Barbour and Williams, 1990; Fornaciari et al., 1997) (Table 1). There appears to be no correlation between renal toxicity and total dose of drug. It therefore remains important to carefully monitor renal function in all patients treated with 5-ASA compounds.

### 3.7. Anti-tumor necrosis factor (TNF)α therapy and other biologics

Targeting specific cytokines or particular cell subtypes known to be intimately involved in autoimmune disease pathogenesis is a novel direction and has proven to be successful for a number of disorders. New agents, including soluble cytokine receptors, monoclonal blocking or depleting antibodies, or fusion proteins containing a receptor or ligand linked to an immunoglobulin molecule, are rapidly being developed. The anti-TNF agents have proven to be highly successful in the treatment of rheumatoid arthritis, ankylosing spondylitis, psoriatic arthropathy, and inflammatory bowel disease (Atzeni et al., 2005). Moreover, some formulations appear to be a useful adjunct in AAV (Booth et al., 2004; Feldmann and Pusey, 2006).

Generally, the biologic agents are most often associated with immediate infusion related adverse effects, followed infrequency by infectious complications. For all the different formulations of anti-TNF therapy (infliximab, etanercept, and adalimumab), anti-nuclear autoantibodies, antibodies to ds-DNA, and anti-phospholipid antibodies are reported to be induced (Ferraro-Peyret et al., 2004; Atzeni et al., 2005), and a drug-induced systemic lupus erythematosus syndrome can rarely develop (Favalli et al., 2002; De Bandt et al., 2005). More recently, cases of glomerulonephritis and cutaneous vasculitis following TNF blockade have been reported (Roux et al., 2004; Stokes et al., 2005). The glomerular lesions reported have included membranous nephropathy, pauci-immune glomerulonephritis (in association with an anti-myeloperoxidase ANCA), and lupus nephritis (Table 1) (Mor et al., 2005; Stokes et al., 2005). Other biologics used to treat autoimmune diseases, such as rituximab (anti-CD20) (Salama and Pusey, 2006) and anakinra (interleukin-1 receptor antagonist), have not been associated with renal dysfunction so far.

### 3.8. Sirolimus

Sirolimus (rapamycin) is a lipophilic macrolide antibiotic, which binds to FK-binding protein (like tacrolimus), but has a completely different mode of action and associated adverse effects. Sirolimus is currently used primarily in transplantation, but has been used occasionally for autoimmune diseases (Bindl et al., 2005; Nadiminti and Arbiser, 2005; Fernandez et al., 2006), and may be increasingly used in the future as a novel agent finding a niche. It has been associated with a rapid decline in renal function and increasing proteinuria, in a group of patients with resistant focal and segmental glomerulosclerosis (Cho et al., 2007). Additionally, conversion of renal transplant recipients from CNIs to sirolimus has been associated with development of de novo proteinuria in up to 30% of cases (Sennesael et al., 2005), which is generally reversible. Moreover, sirolimus has been reported to be associated with the development of TMA (Barone et al., 2003; Pelle et al., 2005) and may predispose to myoglobin cast

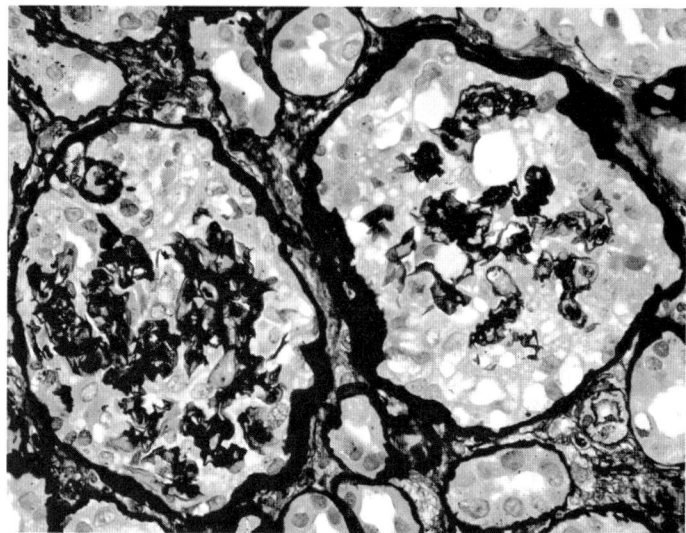

Figure 4. Photomicrograph of a renal biopsy section (Hematoxylin and Eosin ×400) demonstrating collapsing glomerulopathy secondary to pamidronate therapy. The glomerular tuft is shrunken and Bowman's space is occupied by proliferating epithelial cells.

formation and acute renal failure (Pelletier et al., 2006) (Table 1).

## 3.9. Miscellaneous drugs used in the treatment of autoimmunity

*Methotrexate* can rarely be nephrotoxic as a result of precipitation of the drug in the renal tubules, leading to tubulointerstitial damage, but this seems to occur at doses used in the context of cancer therapy, which are in excess of those used in the treatment of autoimmune diseases. Therapy with carboxypeptidase G2, which catabolizes methotrexate, appears to be effective in preventing ongoing toxicity (Widemann and Adamson, 2006).

*Allopurinol*, a xanthine oxidase inhibitor, which decreases uric acid formation, is used as prophylaxis to prevent gout and has rarely been associated with the development of interstitial nephritis (Handa, 1986; Baker and Pusey, 2004).

*Pamidronate*, a bisphosphonate used for the treatment of malignant hypercalcemia, as well as prophylaxis for pulsed steroid-induced osteoporosis, has been associated in a small number of patients with tubular damage and a glomerular sclerotic lesion. Following prolonged therapy (up to 2 years) with high-dose pamidronate, a nephrotic syndrome developed as the result of a collapsing variant of focal and segmental glomerulosclerosis (see Fig. 4) (Markowitz et al., 2001; Kunin et al., 2004). The doses required to induce the lesion are highly variable, suggesting that other factors are critically important in determining the susceptibility to this complication. Used at the recommended doses, renal toxicity is infrequent and other oral preparations commonly used for prophylaxis have not been associated with this condition.

## 4. Conclusions

Renal toxicities are found with many agents used to treat autoimmune disease. Individual drugs may produce particular patterns of dysfunction, which are now well recognized. Newer agents or novel combinations of drugs may yet produce renal complications, which we must remain vigilant to identify.

> **Key points**
>
> Renal toxicity from immunomodulatory agents
> - Many standard agents used to treat autoimmunity are associated with renal toxicity
> - Newer agents or combinations of agents may also lead to renal toxicity but are yet to be recognized
> - Regular monitoring of renal function and urine dipstick testing should be carried out in patients treated with immunomodulatory agents
> - Specific pathologies can only be confirmed on renal biopsy
> - Renal dysfunction or persistent unexplained urinary abnormalities should prompt referral to a nephrologist

# Acknowledgments

I am most grateful to Professor Terry Cook, Imperial College London, for providing the renal biopsy images.

# References

Aqel, B.A., Machicao, V., Rosser, B., et al. 2004. Efficacy of tacrolimus in the treatment of steroid refractory autoimmune hepatitis. J. Clin. Gastroenterol. 38 (9), 805–809.

Atzeni, F., Turiel, M., Capsoni, F., et al. 2005. Autoimmunity and anti-TNF-alpha agents. Ann. N Y Acad. Sci. 1051, 559–569.

Baker, R.J., Pusey, C.D. 2004. The changing profile of acute tubulointerstitial nephritis. Nephrol. Dial. Transplant. 19 (1), 8–11.

Barbour, V.M., Williams, P.F. 1990. Nephrotic syndrome associated with sulphasalazine. BMJ 301 (6755), 818.

Barone, G.W., Gurley, B.J., Abul-Ezz, S.R., et al. 2003. Sirolimus-induced thrombotic microangiopathy in a renal transplant recipient. Am. J. Kidney Dis. 42 (1), 202–206.

Bindi, P., Gilson, B., Aymard, B., et al. 1997. Antiglomerular basement membrane glomerulonephritis following D-penicillamine-associated nephrotic syndrome. Nephrol. Dial. Transplant. 12 (2), 325–327.

Bindl, L., Torgerson, T., Perroni, L., et al. 2005. Successful use of the new immune-suppressor sirolimus in IPEX (immune dysregulation, polyendocrinopathy, enteropathy, X-linked syndrome). J. Pediatr. 147 (2), 256–259.

Bir, K., Herzenberg, A.M., Carette, S. 2006. Azathioprine induced acute interstitial nephritis as the cause of rapidly progressive renal failure in a patient with Wegener's granulomatosis. J. Rheumatol. 33 (1), 185–187.

Booth, A., Harper, L., Hammad, T., et al. 2004. Prospective study of TNFalpha blockade with infliximab in anti-neutrophil cytoplasmic antibody-associated systemic vasculitis. J. Am. Soc. Nephrol. 15 (3), 717–721.

Calvino, J., Romero, R., Pintos, E., et al. 1998. Mesalazine-associated tubulo-interstitial nephritis in inflammatory bowel disease. Clin. Nephrol. 49 (4), 265–267.

Cattran, D.C., Appel, G.B., Hebert, L.A., et al. 2001. Cyclosporine in patients with steroid-resistant membranous nephropathy: a randomized trial. Kidney Int. 59 (4), 1484–1490.

Chalmers, A., Thompson, D., Stein, H.E., et al. 1982. Systemic lupus erythematosus during penicillamine therapy for rheumatoid arthritis. Ann. Intern. Med. 97 (5), 659–663.

Cho, M.E., Hurley, J.K., Kopp, J.B. 2007. Sirolimus therapy of focal segmental glomerulosclerosis is associated with nephrotoxicity. Am. J. Kidney Dis. 49 (2), 310–317.

De Bandt, M., Sibilia, J., Le Loet, X., et al. 2005. Systemic lupus erythematosus induced by anti-tumour necrosis factor alpha therapy: a French national survey. Arthritis Res. Ther. 7 (3), R545–R551.

Derk, C.T., Jimenez, S.A. 2003. Goodpasture-like syndrome induced by D-penicillamine in a patient with systemic sclerosis: report and review of the literature. J. Rheumatol. 30 (7), 1616–1620.

Duncan, N., Dhaygude, A., Owen, J., et al. 2004. Treatment of focal and segmental glomerulosclerosis in adults with tacrolimus monotherapy. Nephrol. Dial. Transplant. 19 (12), 3062–3067.

Dwarakanath, A.D., Michael, J., Allan, R.N. 1992. Sulphasalazine induced renal failure. Gut 33 (7), 1006–1007.

Falck, H.M., Tornroth, T., Kock, B., et al. 1979. Fatal renal vasculitis and minimal change glomerulonephritis complicating treatment with penicillamine. Report on two cases. Acta Med. Scand 205 (1–2), 133–138.

Favalli, E.G., Sinigaglia, L., Varenna, M., et al. 2002. Drug-induced lupus following treatment with infliximab in rheumatoid arthritis. Lupus 11 (11), 753–755.

Feehally, J., Wheeler, D.C., Mackay, E.H., et al. 1987. Recurrent acute renal failure with interstitial nephritis due to D-penicillamine. Ren. Fail. 10 (1), 55–57.

Feldmann, M., Pusey, C.D. 2006. Is there a role for TNF-alpha in anti-neutrophil cytoplasmic antibody-associated vasculitis? Lessons from other chronic inflammatory diseases. J. Am. Soc. Nephrol. 17 (5), 1243–1252.

Fernandez, D., Bonilla, E., Mirza, N., et al. 2006. Rapamycin reduces disease activity and normalizes T cell activation-induced calcium fluxing in patients with systemic lupus erythematosus. Arthritis Rheum. 54 (9), 2983–2988.

Ferraro-Peyret, C., Coury, F., Tebib, J.G., et al. 2004. Infliximab therapy in rheumatoid arthritis and ankylosing spondylitis-induced specific antinuclear and antiphospholipid autoantibodies without autoimmune clinical manifestations: a two-year prospective study. Arthritis Res. Ther. 6 (6), R535–R543.

Fornaciari, G., Maccari, S., Borgatti, P.P., et al. 1997. Nephrotic syndrome from 5-ASA for ulcerative colitis? Complicated by carcinoma of the colon and sclerosing cholangitis. J. Clin. Gastroenterol. 24 (1), 37–39.

Gisbert, J.P., Gonzalez-Lama, Y., Mate, J. 2007. 5-Aminosalicylates and renal function in inflammatory bowel disease: a systematic review. Inflamm. Bowel Dis. 13, 629–638.

Griffiths, C.E., Katsambas, A., Dijkmans, B.A., et al. 2006. Update on the use of ciclosporin in immune-mediated dermatoses. Br. J. Dermatol. 155 (Suppl. 2), 1–16.

Hall, C.L. 1989. The natural course of gold and penicillamine nephropathy: a longterm study of 54 patients. Adv. Exp. Med. Biol. 252, 247–256.

Handa, S.P. 1986. Drug-induced acute interstitial nephritis: report of 10 cases. CMAJ 135 (11), 1278–1281.

Harkness, J.A., Blake, D.R. 1982. Penicillamine nephropathy and iron. Lancet 2 (8312), 1368–1369.

Harper, L., Cockwell, P., Howie, A.J., et al. 1997. Focal segmental necrotizing glomerulonephritis in rheumatoid arthritis. QJM 90 (2), 125–132.

Hengge, U.R., Krause, W., Hofmann, H., et al. 2006. Multicentre, phase II trial on the safety and efficacy of topical tacrolimus ointment for the treatment of lichen sclerosus. Br. J. Dermatol. 155 (5), 1021–1028.

Jayne, D.R., Chapel, H., Adu, D., et al. 2000. Intravenous immunoglobulin for ANCA-associated systemic vasculitis with persistent disease activity. QJM 93 (7), 433–439.

Kaneko, Y., Nimmerjahn, F., Ravetch, J.V. 2006. Anti-inflammatory activity of immunoglobulin G resulting from Fc sialylation. Science 313 (5787), 670–673.

Karpinski, J., Jothy, S., Radoux, V., et al. 1997. D-penicillamine-induced crescentic glomerulonephritis and antimyeloperoxidase antibodies in a patient with scleroderma. Case report and review of the literature. Am. J. Nephrol. 17 (6), 528–532.

Kunin, M., Kopolovic, J., Avigdor, A., et al. 2004. Collapsing glomerulopathy induced by long-term treatment with standard-dose pamidronate in a myeloma patient. Nephrol. Dial. Transplant. 19 (3), 723–726.

Lamb, E.J., Tomson, C.R., Roderick, P.J. 2005. Estimating kidney function in adults using formulae. Ann. Clin. Biochem. 42 (Pt 5), 321–345.

Levy, J.B., Pusey, C.D. 2000. Nephrotoxicity of intravenous immunoglobulin. QJM 93 (11), 751–755.

Ludwin, D., Alexopoulou, I., Esdaile, J.M., et al. 1994. Renal biopsy specimens from patients with rheumatoid arthritis and apparently normal renal function after therapy with cyclosporine. Canadian Multicentre Rheumatology Group. Am. J. Kidney Dis. 23 (2), 260–265.

Markowitz, G.S., Appel, G.B., Fine, P.L., et al. 2001. Collapsing focal segmental glomerulosclerosis following treatment with high-dose pamidronate. J. Am. Soc. Nephrol. 12 (6), 1164–1172.

Meys, E., Devogelaer, J.P., Geubel, A., et al. 1992. Fever, hepatitis and acute interstitial nephritis in a patient with rheumatoid arthritis. Concurrent manifestations of azathioprine hypersensitivity. J. Rheumatol. 19 (5), 807–809.

MMWR. 1999. Renal Insufficiency and Failure Associated with Immune Globulin Intravenous Therapy – United States, 1985–1998. MMWR 48, 518–521.

Mor, A., Bingham, C., III Barisoni, L., et al. 2005. Proliferative lupus nephritis and leukocytoclastic vasculitis during treatment with etanercept. J. Rheumatol. 32 (4), 740–743.

Nadiminti, U., Arbiser, J.L. 2005. Rapamycin (sirolimus) as a steroid-sparing agent in dermatomyositis. J. Am. Acad. Dermatol. 52 (2 Suppl. 1), 17–19.

Nanke, Y., Akama, H., Terai, C., et al. 2000. Rapidly progressive glomerulonephritis with D-penicillamine. Am. J. Med. Sci. 320 (6), 398–402.

Nankivell, B.J., Borrows, R.J., Fung, C.L., et al. 2004. Calcineurin inhibitor nephrotoxicity: longitudinal assessment by protocol histology. Transplantation 78 (4), 557–565.

Newman, D.J., Pugia, M.J., Lott, J.A., et al. 2000. Urinary protein and albumin excretion corrected by creatinine and specific gravity. Clin. Chim. Acta 294 (1–2), 139–155.

Orbach, H., Tishler, M., Shoenfeld, Y. 2004. Intravenous immunoglobulin and the kidney—a two-edged sword. Semin. Arthritis Rheum. 34 (3), 593–601.

Parnham, A.P., Dittmer, I., Mathieson, P.W., et al. 1996. Acute allergic reactions associated with azathioprine. Lancet 348 (9026), 542–543.

Pelle, G., Xu, Y., Khoury, N., et al. 2005. Thrombotic microangiopathy in marginal kidneys after sirolimus use. Am. J. Kidney Dis. 46 (6), 1124–1128.

Pelletier, R., Nadasdy, T., Nadasdy, G., et al. 2006. Acute renal failure following kidney transplantation associated with myoglobinuria in patients treated with rapamycin. Transplantation 82 (5), 645–650.

Riley, S.A., Lloyd, D.R., Mani, V. 1992. Tests of renal function in patients with quiescent colitis: effects of drug treatment. Gut 33 (10), 1348–1352.

Rodriguez, F., Krayenbuhl, J.C., Harrison, W.B., et al. 1996. Renal biopsy findings and followup of renal function in rheumatoid arthritis patients treated with cyclosporin A. An update from the International Kidney Biopsy Registry. Arthritis Rheum. 39 (9), 1491–1498.

Roifman, C.M. 1995. Use of intravenous immune globulin in the therapy of children with rheumatological diseases. J. Clin. Immunol. 15 (6 Suppl), 42S–51S.

Roux, C.H., Brocq, O., Albert, C.B.V., et al. 2004. Cutaneous vasculitis and glomerulonephritis in a patient taking the anti-TNF alpha agent etanercept for rheumatoid arthritis. Joint Bone Spine 71 (5), 444–445.

Sakkas, L.I., Chikanza, I.C., Vaughan, R.W., et al. 1993. Gold induced nephropathy in rheumatoid arthritis and HLA class II genes. Ann. Rheum. Dis. 52 (4), 300–301.

Salama, A.D., Pusey, C.D. 2006. Drug insight: rituximab in renal disease and transplantation. Nat. Clin. Pract. Nephrol. 2 (4), 221–230.

Salama, A.D., Sayegh, M.H. 2007. Achieving clinical tolerance. In: B.M. Brenner (Ed.), The Kidney. 8th Edition, Elsevier.

Salvarani, C., Macchioni, P., Olivieri, I., et al. 2001. A comparison of cyclosporine, sulfasalazine, and symptomatic therapy in the treatment of psoriatic arthritis. J. Rheumatol. 28 (10), 2274–2282.

Sati, H.I., Ahya, R., Watson, H.G. 2001. Incidence and associations of acute renal failure complicating high-dose intravenous immunoglobulin therapy. Br. J. Haematol. 113 (2), 556–557.

Schneider-Gold, C., Hartung, H.P., Gold, R. 2006. Mycophenolate mofetil and tacrolimus: new therapeutic options in neuroimmunological diseases. Muscle Nerve 34 (3), 284–291.

Sennesael, J.J., Bosmans, J.L., Bogers, J.P., et al. 2005. Conversion from cyclosporine to sirolimus in stable renal transplant recipients. Transplantation 80 (11), 1578–1585.

Shoenfeld, Y., Katz, U. 2005. IVIg therapy in autoimmunity and related disorders: our experience with a large cohort of patients. Autoimmunity 38 (2), 123–137.

Soares, S.M., Sethi, S. 2006. Impairment of renal function after intravenous immunoglobulin. Nephrol. Dial. Transplant. 21 (3), 816–817.

Stetter, M., Schmidl, M., Krapf, R. 1994. Azathioprine hypersensitivity mimicking Goodpasture's syndrome. Am. J. Kidney Dis. 23 (6), 874–877.

Stokes, M.B., Foster, K., Markowitz, G.S., et al. 2005. Development of glomerulonephritis during anti-TNF-alpha therapy for rheumatoid arthritis. Nephrol. Dial. Transplant. 20 (7), 1400–1406.

Stratton, J.D., Farrington, K. 1998. Relapse of vasculitis, sepsis, or azathioprine allergy? Nephrol. Dial. Transplant. 13 (11), 2927–2928.

Van Staa, T.P., Travis, S., Leufkens, H.G., et al. 2004. 5-Aminosalicylic acids and the risk of renal disease: a large British epidemiologic study. Gastroenterology 126 (7), 1733–1739.

Widemann, B.C., Adamson, P.C. 2006. Understanding and managing methotrexate nephrotoxicity. Oncologist 11 (6), 694–703.

Zandman-Goddard, G., Levy, Y., Shoenfeld, Y. 2005. Intravenous immunoglobulin therapy and systemic lupus erythematosus. Clin. Rev. Allergy Immunol. 29 (3), 219–228.

# PART III:

# The Vasculitides

# CHAPTER 7

# ANCA-Associated Systemic Vasculitides: Mechanisms

Cees G.M. Kallenberg*

*Department of Rheumatology and Clinical Immunology, University Medical Center Groningen, University of Groningen, P.O. Box 30.001, 9700 RB Groningen, The Netherlands*

## 1. Introduction

The ANCA-associated small-vessel vasculitides comprise a group of disorders characterized by necrotizing small-vessel vasculitis, with a paucity of immune deposits, in conjunction with autoantibodies against neutrophil cytoplasmic constituents, in particular proteinase 3 (PR3) and myeloperoxidase (MPO). Glomerulonephritis, with fibrinoid necrosis and crescent formation, is common (Jennette et al., 1994; Jennette and Falk, 1997; Morgan et al., 2006; Bosch et al., 2006). The ANCA-associated systemic vasculitides (ASV) have been defined by the Chapel Hill Consensus Conference (Jennette et al., 1994, Table 1). They include Wegener's granulomatosis (WG), microscopic polyangiitis (MPA), and its renal limited form (idiopathic necrotizing and crescentic glomerulonephritis (iNCGN)), and the Churg–Strauss Syndrome (CSS).

There is increasing evidence that ANCA are involved in the pathogenesis of their associated diseases. This evidence is based not only on clinical correlations between the autoantibodies and these vasculitides, but also on a multitude of in vitro and in vivo experimental data. In this chapter, I will discuss current views on the pathogenesis of ASV.

First, I will review data from clinical studies supporting a role for ANCA in the pathogenesis of ASV. Secondly, in vitro studies will be discussed that relate to mechanisms by which ANCA can induce vasculitis and glomerulonephritis.

Finally, I will discuss in vivo experimental models, both for PR3-ANCA associated vasculitis and for MPO-ANCA associated vasculitis/glomerulonephritis. Based on the data presented, conclusions will be drawn as to the current view on the etiopathogenesis of ASV.

**Table 1**
Classification of the idiopathic vasculitides as proposed by an international study group at the Chapel Hill Consensus Conference on the Nomenclature of Systemic Vasculitis[a]

  I. Large vessel vasculitis
     1. Giant cell (temporal) arteritis
     2. Takayasu arteritis
 II. Medium-sized vessel vasculitis
     1. Polyarteritis nodosa
     2. Kawasaki disease
III. Small-vessel vasculitis
     1. Wegener's granulomatosis
     2. Churg–Strauss syndrome
     3. Microscopic polyangiitis
     4. Henoch Schönlein purpura
     5. Essential cryoglobulinemic vasculitis
     6. Cutaneous leukocytoclastic angiitis

[a] Adapted from Jennette et al. (1994).

---

*Corresponding author.
Tel.: +31-50-3612945; Fax: +31-50-3619308
E-mail address: c.g.m.kallenberg@int.umcg.nl
(C.G.M. Kallenberg).

## 2. ANCA and the idiopathic small-vessel vasculitides: clinical correlates

### 2.1. Sensitivity and specificity of ANCA for the idiopathic pauci-immune small-vessel vaculitides

Autoantibodies directed against neutrophil cytoplasmic constituents were first described by Davies et al. (1982) in a few patients with segmental necrotizing glomerulonephritis. These findings got largely unrecognized until 1985 when Van der Woude et al. described autoantibodies to neutrophil cytoplasm in patients with WG. These autoantibodies, later on designated as cytoplasmic anti-neutrophil cytoplasmic autoantibodies (c-ANCA), were highly sensitive (93%) and specific (97%) for (active) WG (Van der Woude et al., 1985; Cohen Tervaert et al., 1989). c-ANCA produce a cytoplasmic staining pattern with accentuation of the area within the nuclear lobes, by indirect immunofluorescence (IIF) on ethanol-fixed neutrophils. Shortly after their detection, autoantibodies were described that produced a perinuclear staining pattern on this substrate (p-ANCA) (Falk and Jennette, 1988, Fig. 1). These latter autoantibodies, which occurred in patients with pauci-immune crescentic glomerulonephritis, were identified as being directed to MPO (Falk and Jennette, 1988). Shortly thereafter, the target antigen of c-ANCA in WG was identified as proteinase 3 (PR3), a third serine protease from neutrophils besides elastase and cathepsin G (Goldschmeding et al., 1989; Jenne et al., 1990; Niles et al., 1989). Identification of MPO and PR3 as target antigens for ANCA in the vasculitides has allowed the development of antigen-specific assays for standardized qualitative and quantitative assessment of the autoantibodies (Savige et al., 2000). Standardization of assays is, however, still a matter of concern. Further studies showed that PR3-ANCA and MPO-ANCA characterize a group of patients with small-vessel vasculitis in which, in contrast to Henoch–Schönlein purpura and cryoglobulinemia small-vessel vasculitis, immune deposits are generally absent (pauci-immune) (Fig. 2).

The presence of either PR3-ANCA or MPO-ANCA proved, in a meta-analysis (Rao et al., 1995) and a large European study (Hagen et al., 1998), to have a sensitivity of 75–91% for active pauci-immune vasculitis/glomerulonephritis and a specificity as high as 98%. PR3-ANCA positive patients differ from MPO-positive patients in various ways. The former show much more granuloma formation in their lesions, involvement of more organ systems, a faster decline in renal function, and more frequent relapses (Franssen et al., 2000). Thus, PR3-ANCA

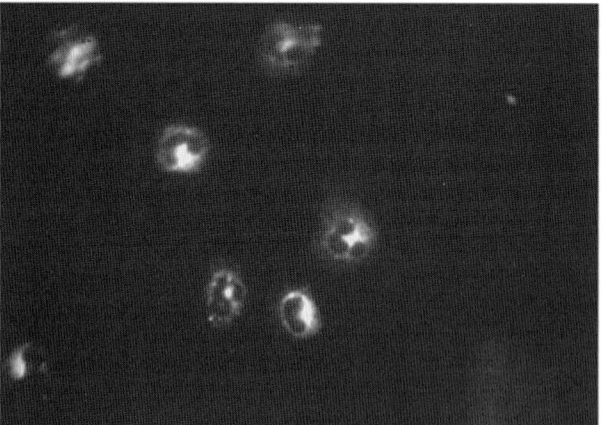 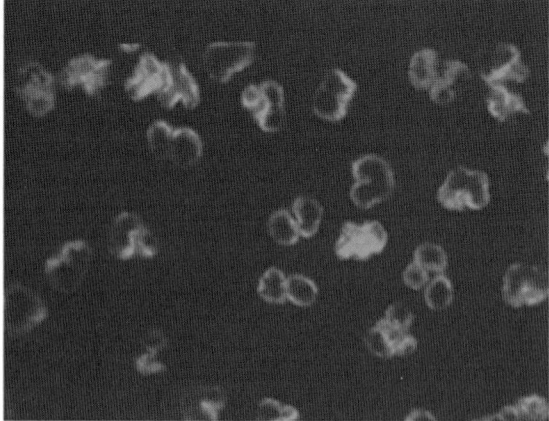

Figure 1. Staining of cytoplasmic components of ethanol-fixed neutrophils by indirect immunofluorescence (IIF) using a serum sample from a patient with active Wegener's granulomatosis (WG) and antibodies to proteinase 3. A characteristic cytoplasmic pattern of fluorescence (c-ANCA) is seen (left). This fluorescence pattern is different from the perinuclear pattern that can be produced by serum samples from patients with anti-MPO antibodies (p-ANCA) (right).

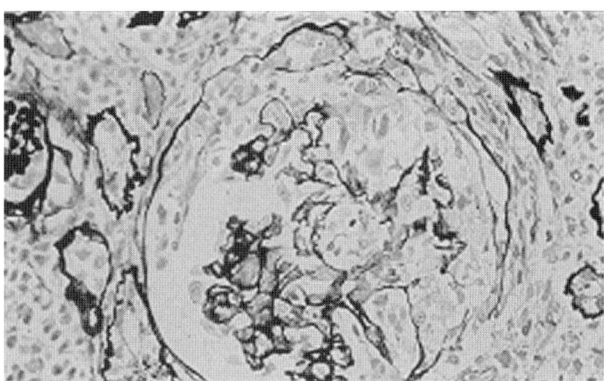
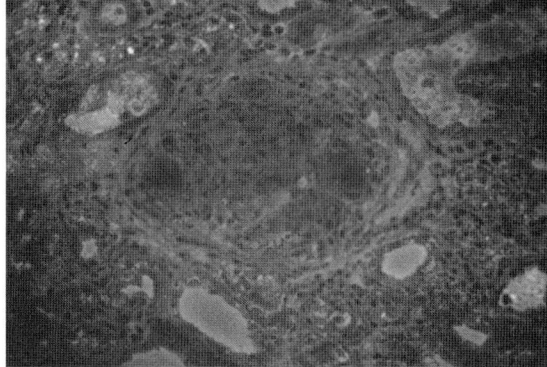

Figure 2. Necrotizing crescentic glomerulonephritis (left, silver staining) with paucity of immune deposits (right, direct immunofluorescence for IgG).

Table 2
Disease associations of PR3-ANCA and MPO-ANCA

| Disease entity | Sensitivity of | |
|---|---|---|
| | PR3-ANCA (%) | MPO-ANCA (%) |
| Wegener's granulomatosus | 70–80 | 10 |
| Microscopic polyangiitis | 30 | 60 |
| Idiopathic crescentic glomerulonephritis | 30 | 64 |
| Churg–Strauss syndrome | <5% | 40 |

Table 3
A hypothetical spectrum of Churg–Strauss Syndrome as based on the presence of anti-neutrophil cytoplasmic autoantibodies (ANCA)

| ANCA-associated subset | ANCA-negative subset |
|---|---|
| Clinical associations | Clinical associations |
|   Necrotizing glomerulonephritis |   Nasal polyposis |
|   Purpura |   Pulmonary infiltrates |
|   Pulmonary hemorrhage |   Cardiomyopathy |
|   Mononeuritis multiplex |   Mono-/polyneuropathy |
| |   Eosinophilic gastritis/enteritis |
| Histopathology | Histopathology |
|   Small-vessel vasculitis |   Tissue infiltration with eosinophils |
| Pathogenesis | Pathogenesis |
|   ANCA-related |   Toxic products from eosinophils |

and MPO-ANCA are markers for different disease expressions. As such, PR3-ANCA is much more frequent in WG, defined as granulomatous inflammation of the respiratory tract and small-vessel necrotizing vasculitis including necrotizing glomerulonephritis, according to the Chapel Hill Consensus Conference (Jennette et al., 1994). MPO-ANCA is predominant in MPA, defined as small-vessel necrotizing vasculitis, in which necrotizing glomerulonephritis and pulmonary capillaritis are common (Jennette et al., 1994, Table 2). As shown in the table, only around 40% of patients with CSS are ANCA-positive, mostly MPO-ANCA. Interestingly, ANCA-positive patients with CSS present with small-vessel vasculitis clinically manifested as mononeuritis multiplex, purpura and glomerulonephritis, whereas the ANCA-negative CSS patients predominantly show tissue infiltration with eosinophils (Sinico et al., 2005; Sable-Fourtassou et al., 2005). This suggests a dichotomy of CSS into two separate disease entities (Table 3, Kallenberg, 2005).

Thus, ANCA directed to PR3 or MPO are very sensitive and highly specific for pauci-immune small-vessel systemic vasculitides. This already suggests a pathogenic role for the autoantibodies. A recent observation has strongly supported a pathogenic role for MPO-ANCA in vivo (Schlieben et al., 2005). It relates to the development, 48 h after delivery, of a pulmonary–renal syndrome in a child born to a woman who got a relapse of MPO-ANCA positive MPA during pregnancy. As the cord blood tested positive for MPO-ANCA, this observation strongly suggested that IgG-class MPO-ANCA alone can induce the symptomatology of MPA.

## 2.2. Do levels of ANCA follow disease activity in ASV?

A second argument, from a clinical point of view, for a pathogenetic role of ANCA could be found in the relation between changes in levels of the autoantibodies and disease activity of the associated disorders. Initial observations (Van der Woude et al., 1985; Cohen Tervaert et al., 1989) already showed that ANCA are more frequently present during active disease than during remission. This has particularly been demonstrated for PR3-ANCA. Nevertheless, conflicting results have been presented for the potential of ANCA titers to predict upcoming relapses (reviewed by Stegeman, 2005; Birck et al., 2006). Discrepancies between studies are largely due to methodological shortcomings of the studies and methodological heterogeneity in the assays performed. In the only large size prospective study (Boomsma et al., 2000) relating titers of (PR3-)ANCA to disease activity in WG, 86 patients were followed for 24 months and sampled at least every 2 months. ANCA were tested by IIF and by ELISA for anti-PR3. A significant rise was defined as a fourfold increase in titer by IIF and a 75% increase by ELISA. Twenty-six out of the 33 relapses, that occurred during the 24 months, were preceded by a rise in anti-PR3 (ELISA), and only 17 by a rise in ANCA as assessed by IIF. Otherwise, 12 out of 38 rises in anti-PR3 by ELISA and 13 out of 30 rises in ANCA by IIF were not followed by a relapse. Thus, changes in levels of ANCA are certainly related to ensuing disease activity (sensitivity 71%, specificity 71%), but the relation is not perfect (Fig. 3).

## 2.3. Induction of ANCA

Presently, we do not know how ANCA are induced. Also, hardly any data are available demonstrating that the development of the autoantibodies

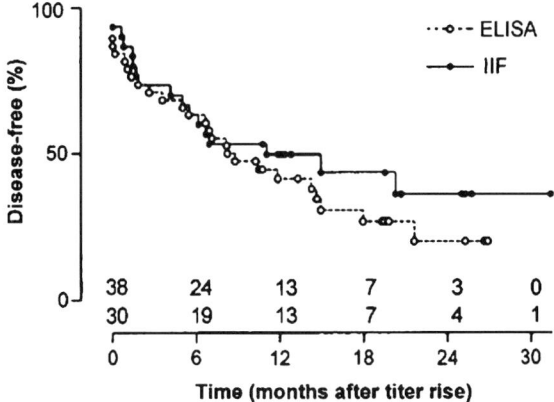

Figure 3. Percentage of patients with WG who did not experience disease relapses in the indicated time period after a rise in antineutrophil cytoplasmic antibodies as measured by either IIF ($n=30$) or antigen-specific enzyme-linked immunosorbent assay (ELISA; $n=38$). The numbers above the horizontal axis indicate the number of patients who were still at risk for a relapse at 6, 12, 18, 24, and 30 months after the rise in antibody levels as detected by ELISA (upper numbers) or IIF (lower numbers). (From Boomsma et al., 2000.)

precedes the clinical expression of the associated diseases. As in many autoimmune diseases, both endogenous and exogenous factors seem to be involved. Various genetic factors, including HLA-genes, have been suggested to be involved (Kallenberg et al., 2002), but no particular (polymorphic) gene has shown a consistent and strong association with the autoantibodies or the ASV. With respect to exogenous factors, various reports have indicated that silica exposure is a risk factor for developing ASV (Cohen Tervaert et al., 1998). In addition, certain drug therapies, particularly propylthiouracil and hydralazine, are associated with the development of MPO-ANCA (Slot et al., 2005). Around 50% of patients who develop MPO-ANCA following propylthiouracil treatment present with vasculitis-like disease, particularly those patients with high-titer and high-affinity MPO-ANCA (Ye et al., 2005). Also, in contrast to drug-induced lupus, ANCA persist in most cases after the drug has been stopped. The mechanisms underlying drug-induced MPO-ANCA production are, however, far from clarified.

With respect to the possible induction of PR3-ANCA, interesting observations have recently been made by Pendergraft et al. (2004). They observed that some patients with PR3-ANCA associated vasculitis also have antibodies to a peptide translated from the middle portion of the antisense DNA strand of PR3 (the protein encoded by the antisense DNA strand was called complementary PR3 (cPR3)). PR3 was shown to bind to cPR3 which led the authors to hypothesize that immunization with cPR3 could induce antibodies that, by idiotypic–antiidiotypic interaction, could, possibly, result in antibodies to PR3. Indeed, mice immunized with cPR3 not only developed antibodies to cPR3 but also to PR3. Thus, an immune response to (peptides of) cPR3 might result in an autoimmune response to PR3. Interestingly, peptides from several micro-organisms, including *Staphylococcus aureus*, show strong homology with peptides of cPR3 (Pendergraft et al., 2004). As carriage of *S. aureus* is strongly associated with persisting of PR3-ANCA and relapsing disease in patients with WG (Stegeman et al., 1994) the bacterium might be involved in the PR3-specific autoimmune response. Further studies have to prove the significance of this concept of cPR3.

As mentioned, nasal carriage of *S. aureus* has been associated with relapsing disease in WG (Stegeman et al., 1994, Fig. 4). The mechanisms underlying this association have not been elucidated but specific (see above) and non-specific, possibly via *S. aureus* derived superantigens, stimulation of the inflammatory autoimmune response has been suggested (Popa et al., 2003).

## 3. ANCA and the small-vessel vasculitides: in vitro evidence for pathogenicity

Falk et al. (1990) were the first to demonstrate that polymorphonuclear granulocytes (PMN) can be activated by ANCA, resulting in their production of reactive oxygen species and release of lysosomal enzymes. In order to be activated by ANCA, PMN must express the major target antigens of ANCA, namely PR3 and MPO, on their membrane.

### 3.1. Membrane expression of PR3 and MPO on neutrophils

In the original study by Falk et al. (1990) it was shown that PMN need to be primed before they can be activated by ANCA. Priming is a process of pre-activation that can be accomplished in vitro with low doses of proinflammatory cytokines, such as tumor necrosis factor-α (TNF-α), interleukin-1 (IL-1), or IL-8, and results in surface expression of the target antigens of ANCA, in particular PR3 and MPO.

Some years ago, it became apparent that, besides being translocated to the cell membrane by proinflammatory stimuli, PR3 can also be constitutively present on the PMN membrane. Non-primed PMN, in vitro, can express PR3 (so-called membrane PR3 or mPR3) either on the total population or on a subset of PMNs (Fig. 5). Individuals can be categorized according to their pattern of mPR3 expression into individuals in whom nearly all PMN express mPR3, individuals with PMN not or hardly expressing mPR3, and individuals in whom two sets of PMN are present, one subset without and one subset with mPR3 expression (Halbwachs-Mecarelli et al., 1995; Witko-Sarsat et al., 1999; Rarok et al., 2002; Schreiber et al., 2003). This pattern of expression, which is specific for PR3 and not seen for MPO and elastase,

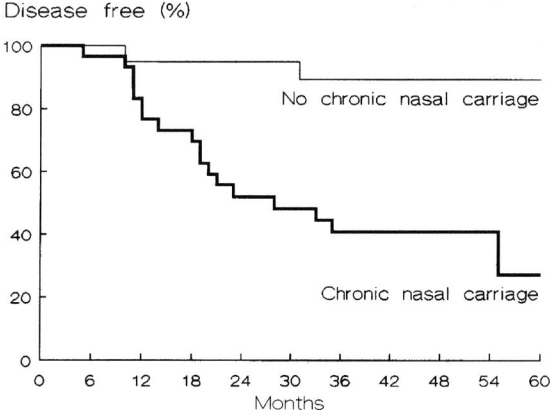

Figure 4. Disease-free interval and carrier status. Disease-free interval of 57 patients with WG grouped according to *Staphylococcus aureus* carrier status. The time of disease free-interval was counted from the beginning of the most recent period of disease activity (either initial diagnosis or relapse; $p<0.001$). (From Stegeman et al., 1994.)

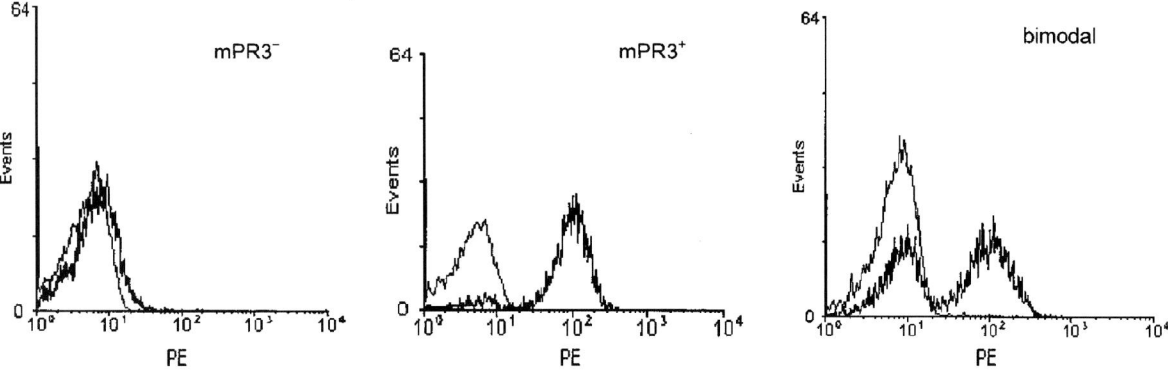

Figure 5. Patterns of PR3 expression on the surface of resting neutrophils as analyzed by flow cytometry. The bold line represents staining with monoclonal anti-PR3 antibody; the thin line indicates non-specific binding of an isotype-matched control. Neutrophils can be negative (left) or positive (middle) for membrane PR3-expression. In some individuals part of the neutrophils are positive and part are negative for membrane PR3-expression. (From van Rossum et al., 2003.)

appears genetically determined (Schreiber et al., 2004).

Interestingly, the frequency of mPR3-expressing PMN and the level of mPR3 expression on non-primed PMN was higher in patients with WG than in controls (Witko-Sarsat et al., 1999; Rarok et al., 2002; Schreiber et al., 2003). Also, increased mPR3 expression in patients with WG was associated with an increased incidence and rate of relapse (Rarok et al., 2002, Fig. 6). How can this genetically determined factor be involved in disease expression of WG? Further studies have shown that mPR3 expressing, non-primed PMN can be activated by ANCA without further priming (Van Rossum et al., 2004), and that mPR3-expressing PMN from patients with ASV show significantly more superoxide generation upon stimulation with ANCA than PMN with low mPR3 expression (Schreiber et al., 2004).

It should be noted that all of the above mentioned studies have been performed in vitro. A recent paper (Abdel-Salam et al., 2004) has suggested that in vivo binding of PR3-ANCA to PMN hardly occurs, due to a very low affinity of PR3-ANCA towards membrane-bound PR3. Using persons with PMN with bimodal expression of mPR3, van Rossum et al. showed, however, that PR3-ANCA in undiluted plasma bound strongly to mPR3 expressing PMN and not to PMN that did not express mPR3 (Van Rossum et al., 2005a, b).

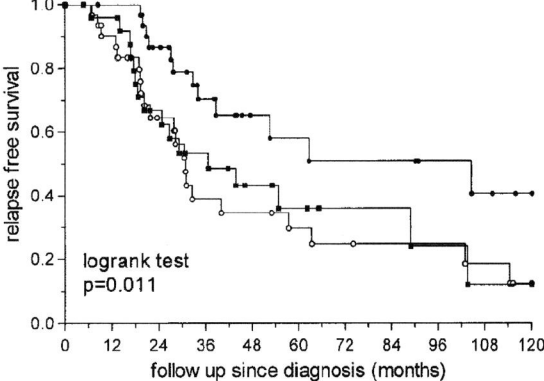

Figure 6. Relapse free survival in WG patients with monomodal low (●, $n=32$), monomodal high (○, $n=31$) and bimodal (■, $n=26$) mPR3 expression. (From Rarok et al., 2002.)

Thus, mPR3 expression seems, also in vivo, a relevant phenomenon.

## 3.2. Pathways involved in ANCA-induced PMN activation

As discussed, ANCA-induced PMN activation requires the expression of PR3 and MPO on the neutrophil membrane. This can be induced by priming with low doses of proinflammatory cytokines which results, at least for PR3, in differential expression of mPR3 (Van Rossum et al., 2005a, b).

Priming is a process that prepares the neutrophil for an appropriate response to a subsequent stimulus and includes, besides expression of the target antigens of ANCA on the neutrophil membrane, a wide range of effects (Rarok et al., 2003, Table 4).

The pathways involved in ANCA-induced PMN activation have not been fully elucidated. Besides specific binding to membrane expressed PR3/MPO, interaction with Fc$\gamma$-receptors seems important. Initial studies have shown that the Fc$\gamma$-RIIA is of major importance as blocking antibodies to this receptor are able to prevent PMN activation by ANCA (Porges et al., 1994; Mulder et al., 1994).

Other studies have shown that the Fc$\gamma$RIIIB is also involved in the initial phase of ANCA-induced PMN activation (Kocher et al., 1998; Ben-Smith et al., 2001). Nevertheless, Kettritz et al. (1997) have suggested that F(ab')$_2$ fragments of ANCA alone, but not Fab fragments, are able to induce some neutrophil activation although Fc$\gamma$-receptor interaction contributes significantly to further activation. The signal transduction routes triggered by ANCA have not been fully elucidated. Fig. 7 depicts the various steps that are probably involved (Rarok et al., 2003). It starts with the priming event which leads to surface

**Table 4**
Effects of priming concentrations of TNF$\alpha$ on the neutrophil

Degranulation of specific granules and secretory vesicles
Up-regulation of PR3 expression on the cell surface
Up-regulation of $\beta_2$ integrins on the cell surface
Clustering of Fc$\gamma$RIIa and $\beta_2$ integrins
Up-regulation of cell surface fMLP receptors
NADPH oxidase complex formation
Shedding of L-selectins from the neutrophil surface

*Source*: From Rarok et al. (2003).

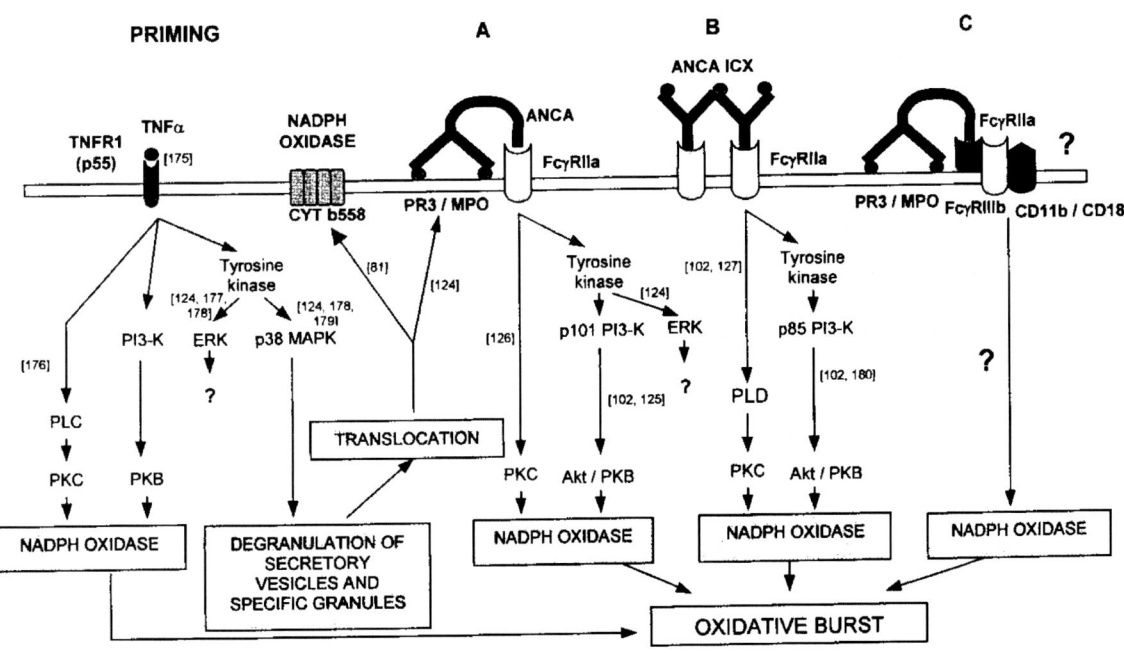

Figure 7. Signal transduction pathways involved in neutrophil activation by ANCA. (A) Activation by monomeric ANCA; (B) activation by ANCA-containing immune complexes; (C) hypothetical mechanism of neutrophil activation by monomeric ANCA, involving "activation clusters." Abbreviations: ANCA, antineutrophil cytoplasm antibodies; CYT b558, cytochrome b$_{558}$; ERK, extracellular signal-regulated kinase; Fc$\gamma$R, Fc$\gamma$ receptor; ICX, immunecomplex; MAPK, mitogen-activated protein kinase; MPO, myeloperoxidase; PI3-K, phosphatidylinositol-3-kinase; PKB, protein kinase B; PKC, protein kinase C; PLD, phospholipase D; PR3, proteinase 3; TNF$\alpha$, tumor necrosis factor-$\alpha$; TNFR1, TNF$\alpha$ receptor-1. Unknown or hypothetical pathways are indicated with a question mark.

expression of the ANCA antigens and NADPH oxidase complex formation. Next, three scenarios are possible. The first one starts with the simultaneous engagement of membrane expressed PR3/MPO by the F(ab')$_2$ binding regions of ANCA and the Fc$\gamma$RIIA by the Fc-part of the autoantibody. The second one starts with complexed PR3-ANCA/PR3 or MPO-ANCA/MPO that interacts with the Fc$\gamma$RIIa on neutrophils. The third pathway uses an activation cluster consisting of Fc$\gamma$RIIA, Fc$\gamma$RIIIB, and the integrins CD11b/CD18. All these pathways finally result in the oxidative burst.

With respect to the interaction between Fc-fragments of ANCA and Fc$\gamma$-receptors on neutrophils, it is relevant to note that subclasses of IgG differentially interact with Fc$\gamma$-receptors. IgG3-subclass interacts most strongly with the second Fc$\gamma$-receptor. Mulder et al. (1995), indeed, showed that IgG3-subclass ANCA were more potent at inducing a neutrophil respiratory burst. Clinically, several reports showed the IgG3-subclass of ANCA to be associated with acute phases of the disease and renal involvement.

## 3.3. ANCA, neutrophils, and endothelial cells

Generally, neutrophils are not activated by monomeric ANCA in the circulation, but they must bind first to the vessel wall and migrate through the endothelial cell layer. In vitro, activation of PMN by PR3- or MPO-ANCA is strongly impaired when PMN adhesion is prevented by stirring or by addition of a blocking anti-CD18 antibody (Reumaux et al., 1995). Otherwise, ANCA can directly induce firm adhesion of rolling PMN as shown in a flow-based adhesion system using a monolayer of activated platelets (Radford et al., 2000). The same authors demonstrated that ANCA are able to induce transmigration of PMN through endothelial cells as studied in a flow system (Radford et al., 2001). Both adhesion and transmigration are $\beta_2$-integrin dependent as they can be blocked by anti-CD11b/CD18 antibodies, and transmigration is reduced by blockade of the chemokine receptor CXCR2 (Calderwood et al., 2005).

Previous studies had already shown that, in vitro, incubation of ANCA, (primed) PMN, and endothelial cells led to endothelial damage (Savage et al., 1992). Furthermore, in vitro incubation of endothelial cells with PR3 induces production of interleukin-8 (IL-8), endothelial cell apoptosis, and endothelial cell detachment and lysis (Berger et al., 1996; Yang et al., 1996; Ballieux et al., 1994). IL-8 production has, indeed, been shown in renal biopsies from patients with ASV (Cockwell et al., 1999) and activated PMN are the major effector cells in glomeruli of these patients (Brouwer et al., 1994).

Taken together, in vitro data strongly support a pathogenic role for PR3-ANCA and MPO-ANCA. In the most likely scenario, neutrophils, once rolling over the endothelial surface, become primed, express PR3/MPO, and interact with ANCA. This interaction leads to firm adhesion (of PMN), transmigration, and also local endothelial damage, all compatible with necrotizing vasculitis and glomerulonephritis. Indeed, numbers of circulating endothelial cells strongly increase during active vasculitis, and can be used as markers for disease activity (Woywodt et al., 2003). Furthermore, these circulating endothelial cells express inflammatory molecules, including neutrophil-activating chemokines, contributing to neutrophil activation and migration (Holmén et al., 2005). These inflammatory endothelial cells suppress the functional capacity of endothelial progenitor cells which are instrumental in repairing damaged blood vessels in vasculitis (Holmén et al., 2005).

## 4. Pathogenicity of ANCA: in vivo experimental evidence

Although the in vitro findings suggest that ANCA are potentially pathogenic, in vivo experimental models are clearly needed to further analyze how these autoantibodies can induce specific lesions in intact animals.

A number of animal models have been developed, mostly with anti-MPO antibodies. As part of a polyclonal autoimmune response anti-MPO were generated in rats exposed to mercuric chloride

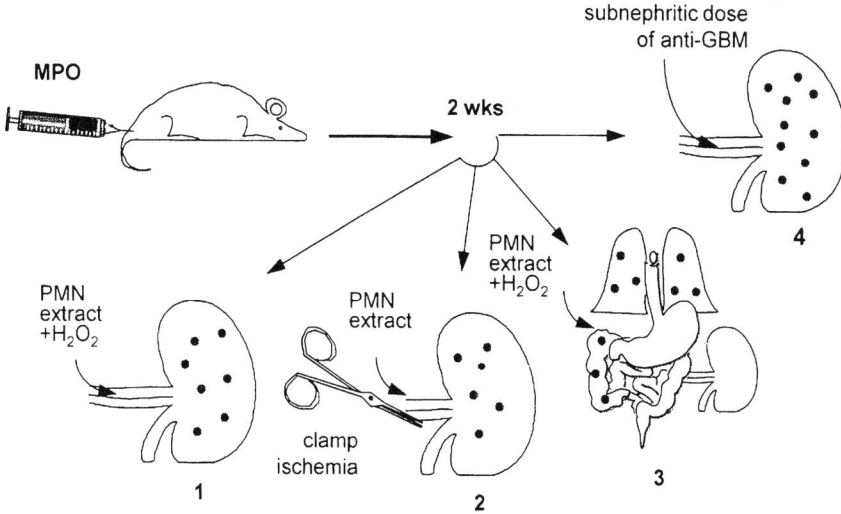

Figure 8. Schematic representation of the animal models for anti-MPO associated vasculitis based on immunization of Brown Norway rats with human MPO. (1) Unilateral renal perfusion of a PMN lysosomal extract and $H_2O_2$ in MPO-immunized rats leads to necrotizing crescentic glomerulonephritis. (2) Unilateral renal perfusion of a PMN lysosomal extract without $H_2O_2$ followed by clamp ischemia in MPO-immunized rats also leads to necrotizing crescentic glomerulonephritis. (3) Systemic injection of a PMN lysosomal extract and $H_2O_2$ in MPO-immunized rats leads to necrotizing vasculitis in the lungs and gut but not in the kidneys. (4) Subnephritogenic anti-GBM disease is aggravated in MPO-immunized rats. (From Heeringa et al., 1998.)

(Mathieson et al., 1992). These rats developed necrotizing leukocytoclastic vasculitis in various organs, particularly the guts, but, due to the polyclonal nature of the autoimmune response, the pathogenic potential of anti-MPO is not clear in this model. A polyclonal response including anti-MPO was associated with the spontaneous development of rapidly progressive crescentic glomerulonephritis and necrotizing vasculitis in an inbred strain of mice, derived from (BXSB × MRL/Mp-lpr/lpr) F1 hybrid mice (Kinjoh et al., 1993). Again, the specific pathogenic role of anti-MPO in this model is not clear.

Immunization of Brown-Norway rats with human MPO in complete Freund's adjuvant resulted in the development of antibodies to human MPO cross-reacting with rat MPO (Brouwer et al., 1993). Lesions did not develop in these rats. However, perfusion of the kidney with products of activated PMN, including proteolytic enzymes, MPO, and its substrate $H_2O_2$, resulted in pauci-immune crescentic glomerulonephritis. In control-immunized rats that were perfused with the same substances, no lesions were apparent (Brouwer et al., 1993). To further prove the phlogistic potential of anti-MPO antibodies, MPO-immunized rats were also injected with a subnephritogenic dose of rabbit anti-glomerular basement membrane (GBM) antibodies. Whereas control immunized rats developed only minor lesions, rats with anti-rat MPO antibodies showed severe renal lesions with fibrinoid necrosis and crescent formation in the glomeruli (Heeringa et al., 1996). A schematic overview of these rat models that show the pathogenic potential of the anti-MPO response, is given in Fig. 8 (Heeringa et al., 1998).

The most convincing evidence for the pathogenic potential of MPO-ANCA comes from a recent animal model using MPO-deficient mice to generate an MPO-directed immune response (Xiao et al., 2002). Immunization of these MPO-deficient mice with mouse MPO led to the development of anti-MPO antibodies. Transfer of spleen cells from these MPO-immunized mice into immunodeficient ($Rag2^{-/-}$) mice led to the development of pauci-immune necrotizing crescentic glomerulonephritis, pulmonary capillaritis, and systemic vasculitis in the recipients (Fig. 9). Transfer of IgG from

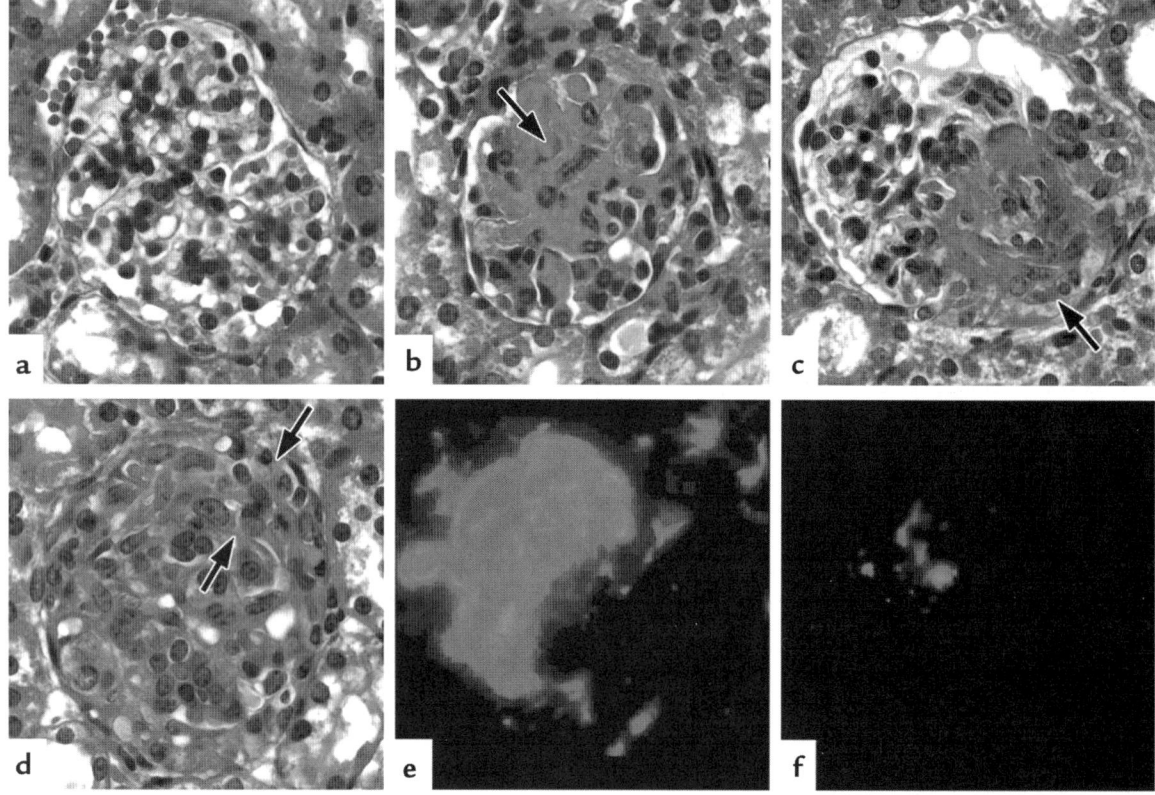

Figure 9. Glomerular lesions in $Rag2^{-/-}$ mice 6 days after receiving anti-MPO IgG. (a) Glomerulus with no lesion. (b) Segmental fibrinoid necrosis (arrow). (c) Segmental fibrinoid necrosis with an adjacent small cellular crescent (arrow). (d) Large circumferential cellular crescent (between arrows) completely surrounding a glomerulus. (e) Immunofluorescence microscopy for fibrin showing prominent staining corresponding to segmental necrosis and crescent formation. (f) Immunofluorescence microscopy for IgG showing a paucity of segmental staining corresponding to an area of segmental necrosis. Masson trichrome staining for light microscopy is shown. (From Xiao et al., 2002.)

MPO-immunized MPO-deficient mice alone into wild type mice resulted in focal necrotizing glomerunephritis in the recipients (Xiao et al., 2002). Pretreatment of the recipients with lipopolysaccharide (LPS) resulted in more diffuse necrotizing and crescentic glomerulonephritis (Huugen et al., 2005). Supposedly, priming of neutrophils and endothelial cells with LPS prepares neutrophils for the activating effect of MPO-ANCA.

This mechanism was further explored by Little et al. (2005). They induced an immune response to autologous MPO in rats by immunization with human MPO (in complete Freund's adjuvant). Rats developed pauci-immune systemic vasculitis. Using intravital microscopy on mesenteric venules (Fig. 10) they showed that MPO-ANCA containing IgG was able to induce firm adhesion and transmigration of leukocytes. Administration of the chemokine CXCL1 led to extensive microvascular hemorrhage. Blockade of TNF by anti-TNFα antibodies resulted in a 43% inhibition of leukocyte transmigration in this model (Little et al., 2006). The essential role of neutrophils in MPO-ANCA associated glomerulonephritis was also demonstrated in the model of Xiao et al. (2002) described before. In this model, mice that were depleted of neutrophils were completely protected from anti-MPO induced glomerulonephritis (Xiao et al., 2005).

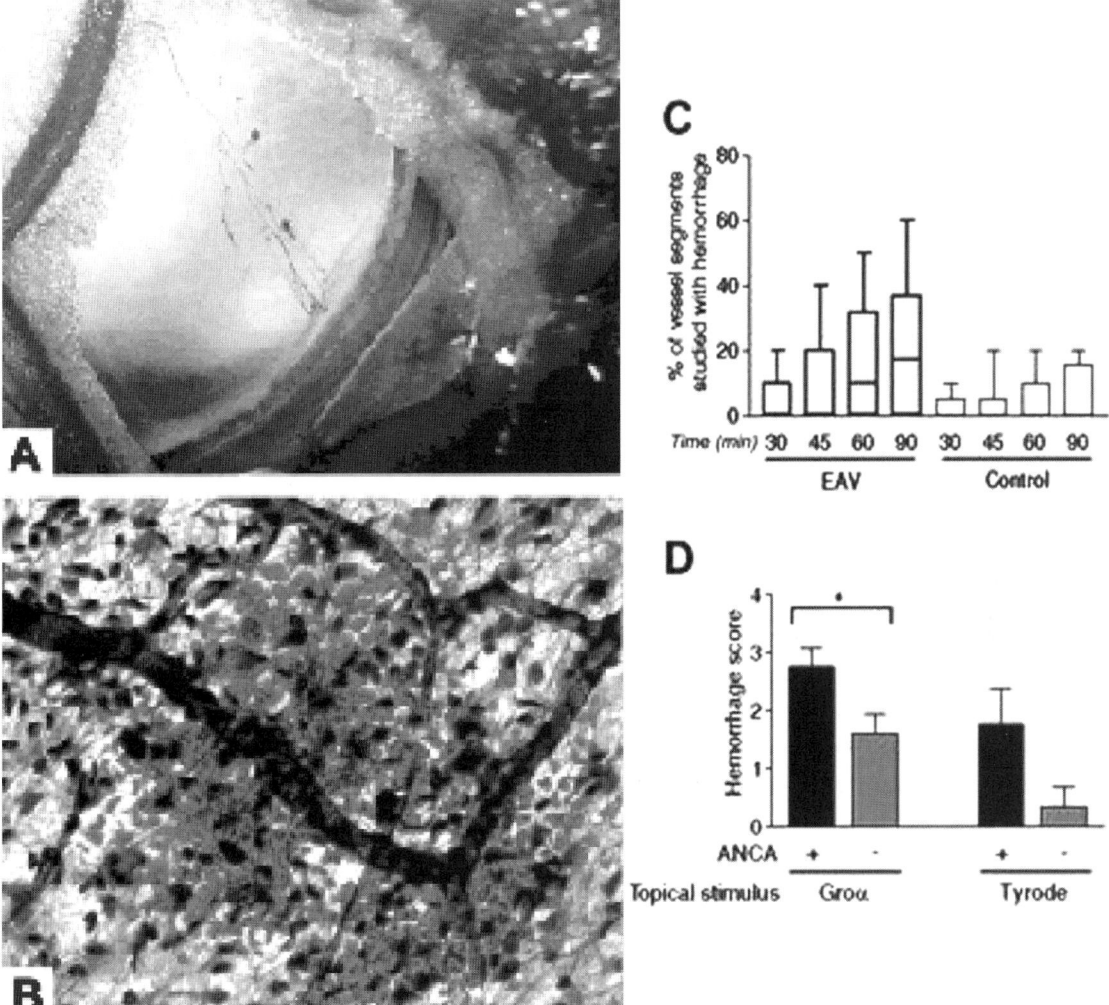

Figure 10. ANCAs induce postcapillary venular hemorrhage. Intravital microscopy was performed on WKY rats 6–7 weeks after immunization with hMPO (EAV rats) or HSA (control rats) (C) or on naive WKY rats with infusion of ANCA-rich or ANCA-negative Ig (D). A representative macroscopic image of petechiae around a mesenteric arcade is shown in panel A (x4; image captured with a Canon IXUS 400; Canon, Tokyo, Japan). The microscopic appearance of this is shown in panel B (H&E stain, UplanApo 20x/0.70 NA). In the active immunization model (C), superfusion with $3 \times 10^{-9}$ M CXCL1 was maintained for 90 min, and hemorrhage was quantified by expressing the number of hemorrhagic venular segments as the percentage of total segments studied at each time point. The data represent the median, interquartile range (box), and range (error bars, $n = 11$ in control group and 13 in EAV group). Of note, although minor degrees of hemorrhage were seen in the control group, the median remained at zero throughout the experiment. In the passive transfer model (D) superfusion fluid was changed in some experiments from Tyrode solution to CXCL1 30 min after Ig infusion, and hemorrhage was quantified after a further 90 min using a global mesenteric visual/analog score ($n = 4$–10 separate rats in each group). Statistically significant differences between groups of rats are shown by asterisks, $*P < .05$. Data in panels C and D are mean ± SEM. (From Little et al., 2005.)

Taken together, the animal models described in this section strongly support the unique role of MPO-ANCA in the development of small-vessel necrotizing vasculitis/glomerulonephritis. The mechanisms involved primarily focus on ANCA-induced neutrophil–endothelial interactions. In contrast to MPO-ANCA associated vasculitis, a satisfying model for PR3-ANCA associated vasculitis with characteristics of human WG is not yet available. Pfister et al. (2004) aimed to develop a model for PR3-ANCA associated vasculitis by immunizing mice deficient for PR3 and elastase with mouse PR3. Mice developed anti-PR3 antibodies that were able to bind to primed mouse neutrophils. Transfer of PR3-ANCA containing IgG from these mice into wild type mice did not, however, induce (systemic) vasculitis. They only observed local increase of inflammation after subcutaneous injection of TNFα in recipients of PR3-ANCA containing IgG compared to control IgG. So, in contrast to MPO-ANCA associated disease, an adequate animal model for PR3-ANCA associated WG is not yet available.

## 5. Pathogenesis of ANCA-associated small-vessel vasculitis: contribution of cell-mediated immunity

The presence of T-cell infiltrates in granulomatous lesions, vasculitic areas, and affected kidneys in WG (Bolton et al., 1987), as well as the possibility of obtaining remission in refractory WG patients by treatment with humanized monoclonal antibodies specific to lymphocyte CD52 and CD4 antigens, or with rabbit anti-thymocyte globulin (Lockwood et al., 1996; Hagen et al., 1995), support the view that T-cells play a major role in the pathogenesis of WG. Indeed, increased serum levels of T-cell activation markers such as soluble interleukin-2 receptor (sIL-2R), soluble CD4, and soluble CD30 have been found in (PR3-)ANCA associated vasculitis with higher levels in patients with active disease (Schmitt et al., 1992; Wang et al., 1997). Upregulation of activation markers, such as CD25 and HLA-DR, on circulating T-cells is present in patients with active disease but also in patients in remission (Popa et al., 1999). These cells were shown to be mainly effector memory cells (Abdulahad et al., 2006). Also in lesional tissue from the respiratory tract in WG, activated memory T-cells have been detected (Balding et al., 2001). Both T-helper-1 and T-helper-2 phenotypes have been described. So, effector memory cells seem operative in (PR3-)ANCA associated vasculitis.

The target antigens of these effector memory cells have not been defined. Previous studies have shown that, in vitro, lymphocytes from patients with either PR3-ANCA or MPO-ANCA proliferate in response to the autoantigens, but only slight differences were noted between patients and controls and no consistent results were obtained (reviewed by Lamprecht, 2005). Also, no particular immunodominant peptides have been detected (Van der Geld et al., 2000).

What in vivo experimental evidence is available to support a role for T-cells in the pathogenesis of ASV? Recent experimental data point to a role of $CD4^+$ effector cells in the pathogenesis of ANCA-associated glomerulonephritis. In an experimental model in mice, Ruth et al. (2006) induced crescentic glomerulonephritis by generating an autoimmune response to mouse-MPO and recruiting neutrophils to glomeruli by injecting anti-GBM antibodies. Depleting $CD4^+$ T-cells in these mice after induction of the MPO-specific autoimmune response but before recruiting neutrophils resulted in a strong attenuation of glomerular crescent formation despite anti-MPO levels being comparable to those in non-depleted mice. So, effector $CD4^+$ T-cells contribute to tissue injury in MPO-ANCA vasculitis/glomerulonephritis. Taken together, clinical, in vitro, and in vivo experimental data strongly suggest that effector T-cells are involved in the pathogenesis of ASV. Their precise targets await further studies.

## 6. Conclusions

Clinical data demonstrate a close association between PR3-ANCA/MPO-ANCA and the pauci-immune small-vessel systemic vasculitides. Also, the dynamics of these autoantibodies correlate with changes in disease expression over time. Although we do not know how the autoantibodies and the diseases are induced, molecular mimicry between peptides complimentary to autoantigens and microbial peptides may play a role. The role of T-cells is less well delineated.

In vitro studies all point to a pathogenic role for PR3-ANCA and MPO-ANCA. The autoantibodies can enhance neutrophil–endothelial interactions and neutrophil activation at the endothelial interface, resulting in endothelial damage. Recent models of MPO-ANCA associated vasulitis/glomerulonephritis have clearly demonstrated the pathogenic role of MPO-ANCA in vivo. These studies have also shown that ANCA-induced neutrophil–endothelial interactions play a dominant role in vivo. These models can explain the pathogenesis of MPO-ANCA associated MPA. Until now, no satisfactory model is available for PR3-ANCA associated WG.

In summary, much progress has been made in the elucidation of the pathogenesis of ANCA-associated vasculitis, but many questions still remain.

## Key points

- ANCA directed against proteinase 3 (PR3) or myeloperoxidase (MPO) are strongly associated with the pauci-immune small-vessel vasculitides; PR3-ANCA are more frequently present in Wegener's granulomatosis (WG) and MPO-ANCA in microscopic polyangiitis.
- Changes in levels of ANCA are related to ensuing disease activity (sensitivity 71%, specificity 71%), but the relation is not perfect.
- In vitro experimental data support a pathogenic role for ANCA: ANCA are able to activate (primed) neutrophils which, in the presence of endothelial cells, leads to damage of the latter cells.
- In vivo experimental data demonstrate that MPO-ANCA are pathogenic by inducing small-vessel vasculitis including the kidney; this is less clear for PR3-ANCA.
- Although cell-mediated immunity is involved as well in the pathogenesis of the associated vasculitides, the precise targets, and underlying mechanisms have only in part been elucidated.

## References

Abdel-Salam, B., Iking-Konert, C., Schneider, M., et al. 2004. Autoantibodies to neutrophil cytoplasmic antigens (ANCA) do not bind to polymorphonuclear neutrophils in blood. Kidney Int. 66, 1009.

Abdulahad, W.H., van der Geld, Y.M., Stegeman, C.A., et al. 2006. Persistent expansion of CD4+ effector memory T cells in Wegener's granulomatosis. Kidney Int. 70, 938.

Balding, C.E., Howie, A.J., Drake-Lee, A.B., et al. 2001. Th2 dominance in nasal mucosa in patients with Wegener's granulomatosis. Clin. Exp. Immunol. 125, 332.

Ballieux, B.E.P.B., Hiemstra, P.S., Klar-Mohamad, N., et al. 1994. Detachment and cytolysis of human endothelial cells by proteinase 3. Eur. J. Immunol. 24, 3211.

Ben-Smith, A., Dove, S.K., Martin, A., et al. 2001. Antineutrophil cytoplasm autoantibodies from patients with systemic vasculitis activate neutrophils through distinct signaling cascades: comparison with conventional Fcgamma receptor ligation. Blood 98, 1448.

Berger, S.P., Seelen, M.A., Hiemstra, P.S., et al. 1996. Proteinase 3, the major autoantigen of Wegener's granulomatosis, enhances IL-8 production by endothelial cells in vitro. J. Am. Soc. Nephrol. 7, 694.

Birck, R., Schmitt, W.H., Kaelsch, I.A., et al. 2006. Serial ANCA determinations for monitoring disease activity in patients with ANCA-associated vasculitis: systematic review. Am. J. Kidney Dis. 47, 15.

Bolton, W.K., Innes, D.J., Jr., Sturgill, B.C., et al. 1987. T-cells and macrophages in rapidly progressive glomerulonephritis: clinicopathologic correlations. Kidney Int. 32, 869.

Boomsma, M.M., Stegeman, C.A., van der Leij, M.J., et al. 2000. Prediction of relapses in Wegener's granulomatosis by measurement of antineutrophil cytoplasmic antibody levels: a prospective study. Arthritis Rheum. 43, 2025.

Bosch, X., Guilabert, A., Font, J. 2006. Antineutrophil cytoplasmic antibodies. Lancet 368, 404.

Brouwer, E., Huitema, M.G., Klok, P.A., et al. 1993. Anti-myeloperoxidase associated proliferative glomerulonephritis: an animal model. J. Exp. Med. 177, 905.

Brouwer, E., Huitema, M.G., Mulder, A.H.L., et al. 1994. Neutrophil activation in vitro and in vivo in Wegener's granulomatosis. Kidney Int. 45, 1120.

Calderwood, J.W., Williams, J.M., Morgan, M.D., et al. 2005. ANCA induces $\beta_2$ integrin and CXC chemokine-dependent neutrophil–endothelial cell interactions that mimic those of highly cytokine-activated endothelium. J. Leuc. Biol. 77, 33.

Cockwell, P., Brooks, C.J., Adu, D., et al. 1999. Interleukin-8: a pathogenetic role in antineutrophil cytoplasmic autoantibody-associated glomerulonephritis. Kidney Int. 55, 852.

Cohen Tervaert, J.W., Stegeman, C.A., Kallenberg, C.G.M. 1998. Silicon exposure and vasculitis. Curr. Opin. Rheumatol. 10, 12.

Cohen Tervaert, J.W., van der Woude, F.J., Fauci, A.S., et al. 1989. Association between active Wegener's granulomatosis and anticytoplasmic antibodies. Arch. Int. Med. 149, 2461.

Davies, D.J., Moran, J.E., Niall, J.F., et al. 1982. Segmental necrotizing glomerulonephritis with antineutrophil antibody: possible arbovirus aetiology. Br. Med. J. 285, 606.

Falk, R.J., Jennette, J.C. 1988. Anti-neutrophil cytoplasmic autoantibodies with specificity for myeloperoxidase in patients with systemic vasculitis and idiopathic necrotizing and crescentic glomerulonephritis. N. Engl. J. Med. 318, 1651.

Falk, R.J., Terrell, R.S., Charles, L.A., et al. 1990. Antineutrophil cytoplasmic autoantibodies induce neutrophils to degranulate and produce oxygen radicals in vitro. Proc. Natl. Acad. Sci. USA 87, 4115.

Franssen, C.F., Stegeman, C.A., Kallenberg, C.G.M., et al. 2000. Antiproteinase 3- and antimyeloperoxidase-associated vasculitis. Kidney Int. 57, 2195.

Goldschmeding, R., van der Schoot, C.E., ten Bokkel Huinink, D., et al. 1989. Wegener's Granulomatosis autoantibodies identify a novel DFP-binding protein in the lysosomes of normal human neutrophils. J. Clin. Invest. 84, 1577.

Halbwachs-Mecarelli, L., Bessou, G., Lesavre, P., et al. 1995. Bimodal distribution of proteinase 3 (PR3) surface expression reflects a constitutive heterogeneity in the polymorphonuclear neutrophil pool. FEBS Lett. 374, 29.

Hagen, E.C., Daha, M.R., Hermans, J., et al. 1998. Diagnostic value of standardized assays for anti-neutrophil cytoplasmic antibodies in idiopathic systemic vasculitis. EC/BCR project for ANCA assay standardization. Kidney Int. 53, 743.

Hagen, E.C., de Keizer, R.J., Andrassy, K., et al. 1995. Compassionate treatment of Wegener's granulomatosis with rabbit anti-thymocyte globulin. Clin. Nephrol. 43, 351.

Heeringa, P., Brouwer, E., Cohen Tervaert, J.W., et al. 1998. Animal models of anti-neutrophil cytoplasmic antibody associated vasculitis. Kidney Int. 53, 253.

Heeringa, P., Brouwer, E., Klok, P.A., et al. 1996. Autoantibodies to myeloperoxidase aggravate mild antiglomerular-basement-membrane-mediated glomerular injury in the rat. Am. J. Pathol. 149, 1695.

Holmén, C., Elsheikh, E., Stenvinkel, P., et al. 2005. Circulating inflammatory endothelial cells contribute to endothelial progenitor cell dysfunction in patients with vasculitis and kidney involvement. J. Am. Soc. Nephrol. 16, 3110.

Huugen, D., Xiao, H., van Esch, A., et al. 2005. Aggravation of anti-myeloperoxidase antibody-induced glomerulonephritis by bacterial lipopolysaccharide: role of tumor necrosis factor-alpha. Am. J. Pathol. 167, 47.

Jenne, D.E., Tschopp, J., Lüdemann, J., et al. 1990. Wegener's autoantigen decoded. Nature 346, 520.

Jennette, J.C., Falk, R.J. 1997. Small vessel vasculitis. N. Engl. J. Med. 137, 1512.

Jennette, J.C., Falk, R.J., Andrassy, K., et al. 1994. Nomenclature of systemic vasculitides. Proposal of an international consensus conference. Arthritis Rheum. 37, 187.

Kallenberg, C.G.M. 2005. Churg–Strauss Syndrome: just one disease entity? Arthritis Rheum. 52, 2589.

Kallenberg, C.G.M., Rarok, A.A., Stegeman, C.A. 2002. Genetics of ANCA-associated vasculitides. Cleve. Clin. J. Med. 69(Suppl. 2), SII61.

Kettritz, R., Jennette, J.C., Falk, R.J. 1997. Crosslinking of ANCA-antigens stimulates superoxide release by human neutrophils. J. Am. Soc. Nephrol. 8, 386.

Kinjoh, K., Kyogoku, M., Good, R.A. 1993. Genetic selection for crescent formation yields mouse strain with rapidly progressive glomerulonephritis and small vessel vasculitis. Proc. Natl. Acad. Sci. USA 90, 3413.

Kocher, M., Edberg, J.C., Fleit, H.B., et al. 1998. Antineutrophil cytoplasmic antibodies preferentially engage Fc gammaRIIIb on human neutrophils. J. Immunol. 161, 6909.

Lamprecht, P. 2005. Off balance: T-cells in antineutrophil cytoplasmic antibody-associated vasculitides. Clin. Exp. Immunol. 141, 201–210.

Little, M.A., Bhangal, G., Smyth, C.L., et al. 2006. Therapeutic effect of anti-TNF-α antibodies in an experimental model of anti-neutrophil cytoplasm antibody-associated systemic vasculitis. J. Am. Soc. Nephrol. 17, 160.

Little, M.A., Smyth, C.L., Yadav, R., et al. 2005. Antineutrophil cytoplasm antibodies directed against myeloperoxidase augment leukocyte–microvascular interaction in vivo. Blood 106, 2050.

Lockwood, C.M., Thiru, S., Stewart, S., et al. 1996. Treatment of refractory Wegener's granulomatosis with humanized monoclonal antibodies. Q. J. M. 89, 903.

Mathieson, P.W., Thiru, S., Oliveira, D.B. 1992. Mercuric chloride-treated brown Norway rats develop widespread tissue injury including necrotizing vasculitis. Lab. Invest. 67, 121.

Morgan, M.D., Harper, L., Williams, J., et al. 2006. Antineutrophil cytoplasm-associated glomerulonephritis. J. Am. Soc. Nephrol. 17, 1224.

Mulder, A.H.L., Heeringa, P., Brouwer, E., et al. 1994. Activation of granulocytes by anti-neutrophil cytoplasmic antibodies (ANCA): a Fc RII-dependent process. Clin. Exp. Immunol. 98, 270.

Mulder, A.H.L., Stegeman, C.A., Kallenberg, C.G.M. 1995. Activation of granulocytes by anti-neutrophil cytoplasmic antibodies (ANCA) in Wegener's granulomatosis: a predominant role for the IgG3 subclass of ANCA. Clin. Exp. Immunol. 101, 227.

Niles, J.L., McCluskey, R.T., Ahmad, M.F., et al. 1989. Wegener's granulomatosis autoantigen is a novel neutrophil serine proteinase. Blood 74, 1888.

Pendergraft, W.F., III, Preston, G.A., Shah, R.R., et al. 2004. Autoimmunity is triggered by cPR-3 (105–201), a protein complementary to human autoantigen proteinase-3. Nat. Med. 10, 72.

Pfister, H., Ollert, M., Frohlich, L.F., et al. 2004. Antineutrophil cytoplasmic autoantibodies against the murine homologue of proteinase 3 (Wegener autoantigen) are pathogenic in vivo. Blood 104, 1411.

Popa, E.R., Stegeman, C.A., Bos, N.A., et al. 1999. Differential B- and T-cell activation in Wegener's granulomatosis. J. Allergy Clin. Immunol. 103, 885.

Popa, E.R., Stegeman, C.A., Bos, N.A., et al. 2003. Staphylococcal superantigens and T cell expansions in Wegener's granulomatosis. Clin. Exp. Immunol. 132, 496.

Porges, A.J., Redecha, P.B., Kimberly, W.T. 1994. Antineutrophil cytoplasmic antibodies engage and activate human neutrophils via Fc gamma RIIa. J. Immunol. 153, 1271.

Radford, D.J., Luu, N.T., Hewins, P., et al. 2001. Antineutrophil cytoplasmic antibodies stabilize adhesion and promote migration of flowing neutrophils on endothelial cells. Arthritis Rheum. 44, 2851.

Radford, D.J., Savage, C.O.S., Nash, G.B. 2000. Treatment of rolling neutrophils with antineutrophil cytoplasmic antibodies causes conversion to firm integrin-mediated adhesion. Arthritis Rheum. 43, 1337.

Rao, J.K., Weinberger, M., Oddone, E.Z., et al. 1995. The role of antineutrophil cytoplasmic antibody testing in the diagnosis of Wegener granulomatosis. Ann. Intern. Med. 123, 925.

Rarok, A.A., Stegeman, C.A., Limburg, P.C., et al. 2002. Neutrophil membrane expression of proteinase 3 (PR3) is related to relapse in PR3-ANCA-associated vasculitis. J. Am. Soc. Nephrol. 13, 2232.

Rarok, A.A., Limburg, P.C., Kallenberg, C.G. 2003. Neutrophil-activating potential of antineutrophil cytoplasm autoantibodies. J. Leukoc. Biol. 74, 3.

Reumaux, D., Vossebeld, P.J., Roos, D., et al. 1995. Effect of tumor necrosis factor-induced integrin activation on Fc gamma receptor II-mediated signal transduction: relevance for activation of neutrophils by anti-proteinase 3 or anti-myeloperoxidase antibodies. Blood 86, 3189.

Ruth, A.J., Kitching, A.R., Kwan, R.Y.Q., et al. 2006. Antineutrophil cytoplasmic antibodies and effector $CD4^+$ cells play nonredundant roles in anti-myeloperoxidase crescentic glomerulonephritis. J. Am. Soc. Nephrol. 17, 1940.

Sable-Fourtassou, R., Cohen, P., Mahr, A., et al. 2005. Antineutrophil cytoplasmic antibodies and the Churg–Strauss syndrome. Ann. Intern. Med. 143, 632.

Savage, C.O., Pottinger, B.E., Gaskin, G., et al. 1992. Autoantibodies developing to myeloperoxidase and proteinase 3 in systemic vasculitis stimulate neutrophil cytotoxicity toward cultured endothelial cells. Am. J. Pathol. 141, 335.

Savige, J., Davies, D., Falk, R.J., et al. 2000. Antineutrophil cytoplasmic antibodies and associated diseases: a review of the clinical and laboratory features. Kidney Int. 57, 846.

Schlieben, D.J., Korbet, S.M., Kimura, R.E., et al. 2005. Pulmonary–renal syndrome in a newborn with placental transmission of ANCAs. Am. J. Kidney Dis. 45, 758.

Schmitt, W.H., Heesen, C., Csernok, E., et al. 1992. Elevated serum levels of soluble interleukin-2 receptor in patients with Wegener's granulomatosis. Association with disease activity. Arthritis Rheum. 35, 1088.

Schreiber, A., Busjahn, A., Luft, F.C., et al. 2003. Membrane expression of proteinase 3 is genetically determined. J. Am. Soc. Nephrol. 14, 68.

Schreiber, A., Luft, F.C., Kettritz, R. 2004. Membrane proteinase 3 expression and ANCA-induced neutrophil activation. Kidney Int. 65, 2172.

Sinico, R.A., Di Toma, L., Maggiore, U., et al. 2005. Prevalence and clinical significance of antineutrophil cytoplasmic antibodies in Churg–Strauss syndrome. Arthritis Rheum. 52, 2926.

Slot, M.C., Links, T.P., Stegeman, C.A., et al. 2005. Occurrence of antineutrophil cytoplasmic antibodies and associated vasculitis in patients with hyperthyroidism treated with antithyroid drugs. Arthritis Rheum. 53, 108.

Stegeman, C.A. 2005. Predictive value of antineutrophil cytoplasmic antibodies in small-vessel vasculitis: is the glass half full or half empty? J. Rheumatol. 32, 2075.

Stegeman, C.A., Cohen Tervaert, J.W., Sluiter, W.J., et al. 1994. Association of nasal carriage of *Staphylococcus aureus* and higher relapse in Wegener's granulomatosis. Ann. Intern. Med. 120, 12.

van der Geld, Y.M., Huitema, M.G., Franssen, C.F., et al. 2000. In vitro T lymphocyte responses to proteinase 3 (PR3) and linear peptides of PR3 in patients with Wegener's granulomatosis (WG). Clin. Exp. Immunol. 122, 504.

van Rossum, A.P., van der Geld, Y.M., Limburg, P.C., et al. 2005a. Human anti-neutrophil cytoplasm autoantibodies to proteinase 3 (PR3-ANCA) bind to neutrophils. Kidney Int. 68, 537.

van Rossum, A.P., Limburg, P.C., Kallenberg, C.G.M. 2003. Membrane proteinase 3 expression on resting neutrophils as a pathogenic factor in PR3-ANCA-associated vasculitis. Clin. Exp. Rheumatol. 21(6 (Suppl 32)), S64.

van Rossum, A.P., Limburg, P.C., Kallenberg, C.G.M. 2005b. Activation, apoptosis and clearance of neutrophils in Wegener's granulomatosis. Ann. N.Y. Acad. Sci. 1051, 1.

van Rossum, A.P., Rarok, A.A., Huitema, M.G., et al. 2004. Constitutive membrane expression of proteinase 3 (PR3) and neutrophil activation by anti-PR3 antibodies. J. Leukoc. Biol. 76, 1162.

van der Woude, F.J., Rasmussen, N., Lobatto, S., et al. 1985. Autoantibodies to neutrophils and monocytes: a new tool for diagnosis and a marker of disease activity in Wegener's granulomatosis. Lancet ii, 425.

Wang, G., Hansen, H., Tatsis, E., et al. 1997. High plasma levels of the soluble form of CD30 activation molecule reflect disease activity in patients with Wegener's granulomatosis. Am. J. Med. 102, 517.

Witko-Sarsat, V., Lesavre, P., Lopez, S., et al. 1999. A large subset of neutrophils expressing membrane proteinase 3 is a risk factor for vasculitis and rheumatoid arthritis. J. Am. Soc. Nephrol. 10, 1224.

Woywodt, A., Streiber, F., de Groot, K., et al. 2003. Circulating endothelial cells as markers for ANCA-associated small-vessel vasculitis. Lancet 361, 206.

Xiao, H., Heeringa, P., Hu, P., et al. 2002. Antineutrophil cytoplasmic autoantibodies specific for myeloperoxidase cause glomerulonephritis and vasculitis in mice. J. Clin. Invest. 110, 955.

Xiao, H., Heeringa, P., Liu, Z., et al. 2005. The role of neutrophils in the induction of glomerulonephritis by anti-myeloperoxidase antibodies. Am. J. Pathol. 167, 39.

Yang, J.J., Kettritz, R., Falk, R.J., et al. 1996. Apoptosis of endothelial cells induced by the neutrophil serine proteases proteinase 3 and elastase. Am. J. Pathol. 149, 1617.

Ye, H., Gao, Y., Guo, X.H., et al. 2005. Titre and affinity of propylthiouracil-induced anti-myeloperoxidase antibodies are closely associated with the development of clinical vasculitis. Clin. Exp. Immunol. 142, 116.

CHAPTER 8

# ANCA-Associated Vasculitis: Clinical Features and Treatment

David Jayne*

*Renal Medicine, Renal Unit, Department of Medicine, Addenbrooke's Hospital, Cambridge CB2 2QQ, UK*

## 1. Introduction

Primary systemic vasculitis comprises a group of disorders of unknown cause united by the common histopathological finding of blood vessel inflammation, necrosis, and thrombosis (Jennette et al., 1994). The most frequent subgroup of primary systemic vasculitis is that associated with circulating autoantibodies to neutrophil cytoplasmic antigens (ANCA), with involvement of microscopic blood vessels without immune deposits in the vessel walls, "pauci-immune micro-vasculitis" (Lane et al., 2005a, b). ANCA-associated vasculitis (AASV) includes the syndromes of Wegener's granulomatosis and microscopic polyangiitis (Hellmich et al., 2007). A minority of patients with Churg–Strauss angiitis are also ANCA positive, and a "forme-fruste" of microscopic polyangiitis, renal-limited vasculitis, is also recognized (Sable-Fourtassou et al., 2005).

Renal involvement in AASV occurs in 70% cases and is of particular clinical importance because it is the most common cause of the clinical syndrome of rapidly progressive glomerulonephritis, accounting for 4% of the cases of end-stage renal disease, but this process is reversible if diagnosed early and treated appropriately. The typical renal lesion of vasculitis is a glomerular capillaritis leading to a segmental, necrotizing glomerulonephritis with epithelioid crescent formation (Hauer et al., 2002a, b). Less frequently, this lesion occurs with arteritis of extra-glomerular vessels in the kidney (Hauer et al., 2002a, b). It has become increasingly clear that renal vasculitis is more common with age and this disease is probably the most common primary cause of renal failure in the elderly (Rychlik et al., 2004).

Major current issues in the management of vasculitis are diagnostic delay, the toxicity of treatment and its contribution to morbidity and mortality, and the propensity of AASV to relapse. The multi-system nature of this chronic, relapsing disease, the risks of vital organ failure, death, and treatment toxicity place unique demands on healthcare systems. Collaborative research networks have harmonized and optimized the therapy of vasculitis and newer therapies are providing hope for improved outcomes in the future 2005 (Jayne and Rasmussen, 1997).

### 1.1. Classification of vasculitis

Vasculitis occurs as a primary disease or secondary to drug reactions, infections, or malignancy. It may also occur as a component of another auto-inflammatory disease such as rheumatoid arthritis, systemic lupus erythematosus (SLE), or Behcet's disease. This situation is complicated because apparent primary systemic vasculitic disorders, especially microscopic polyangiitis associated with ANCA, may be triggered by causes of secondary vasculitis. This has been described for both infective endocarditis and rheumatoid arthritis.

---

*Corresponding author.
Tel.: +44-1223-586796; Fax: +44-1223-586506
E-mail address: dj106@cam.ac.uk

© 2008 Elsevier B.V. All rights reserved.
DOI: 10.1016/S1571-5078(07)07008-0

Reports of secondary renal vasculitis frequently involve the elderly, but this has not been systematically studied (Ulm et al., 2006).

The terminology of the primary vasculitic disorders has been defined by consensus statements and they have been classified according to the predominant vessel size involved and the presence or absence of ANCA (Watts et al., 2007; Jennette et al., 1994). Renal vasculitis is a common feature of the small-vessel vasculitides, whether or not ANCA is present. When it occurs in Churg–Strauss angiitis the features are similar to those in microscopic polyangiitis; in polyarteritis nodosa, a glomerulonephritis would reassign the diagnosis to microscopic polyangiitis (Sinico et al., 2006). Both giant cell arteritis and Takayasu's arteritis involve the aorta and its major branches; large vessel arteritis in the elderly is ascribed to giant cell arteritis, but when renal involvement has occurred there has usually been evidence of a concurrent small-vessel vasculitis (Muller et al., 2004).

For patients presenting with the syndrome of rapidly progressive glomerulonephritis, deteriorating renal function, and a crescentic glomerulonephritis on biopsy, classification depends on the nature of the glomerular immune deposits and the presence of circulating antibodies (Table 1) (Zauner et al., 2002). Linear immune fluorescence and anti-glomerular basement membrane antibodies are characteristic of anti-GBM disease; speckled deposits of immunoglobulin and complement imply an immune complex process such as SLE or Henoch–Schönlein purpura, while a pauci-immune appearance is associated with circulating ANCA and a diagnosis of vasculitis. Some 10% of pauci-immune crescentic nephritis patients are ANCA negative, and this group has previously been called, "idiopathic rapidly progressive or crescentic glomerulonephritis" (Eisenberger et al., 2005).

## 1.2. Epidemiology of vasculitis

The incidence of primary systemic vasculitis is approximately 40/million/year, with the ANCA-associated group comprising 15–20/million/year (Watts and Scott, 2004). An apparent increasing incidence has been explained by improved detection, especially in the elderly, and where long-term epidemiology studies have been performed, no increase in incidence has been seen. Prevalence rates of ANCA vasculitis range from 90 to 400/million (Lane et al., 2005a, b). Both Wegener's granulomatosis and microscopic polyangiitis have an increased incidence with age, being very rare in children. Where the association with age in Wegener's granulomatosis is similar for those aged 50–60 and in older age groups, the incidence of microscopic polyangiitis continues to rise and is highest in the oldest age groups (Fig. 1). Renal involvement is more common in microscopic polyangiitis, at over 90%, and in Wegener's granulomatosis the proportion with renal involvement increases with age (Krafcik et al., 1996). As a consequence of the increased incidence with age the proportion of kidney biopsies displaying a crescentic nephritis rises from 5% in those under 60 years to over 11% in those over 60 years of age (Rychlik et al., 2004). This association implies an aetiological contribution of an aging immune system, and the possible involvement of environmental factors. Silica exposure

**Table 1**
The classification of rapidly progressive glomerulonephritis according to renal immune fluorescence findings and circulating serological abnormalities

|  | Renal immunofluorescence | Compatible serology | Diagnosis |
| --- | --- | --- | --- |
| Type I | Linear | Anti-GBM antibodies | Anti-GBM disease |
| Type II | Granular | ANA, anti-dsDNA antibodies | Systemic lupus erythematosus |
|  |  | Cryoglobulins | Cryoglobulinaemia |
|  |  | Low complement levels | Henoch–Schönlein purpura |
| Type III | "Pauci-immune" (absent or scanty deposits) | ANCA | Vasculitis |

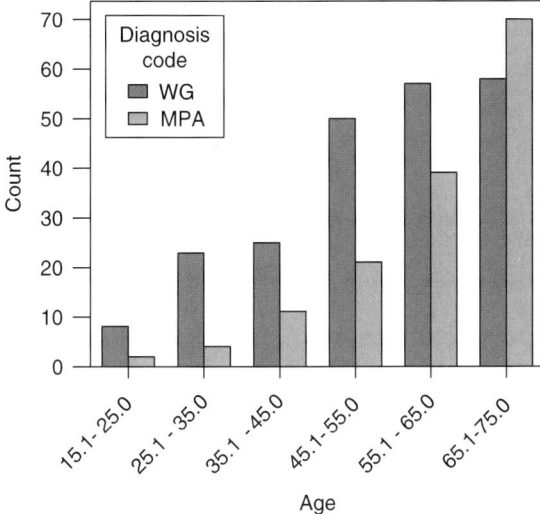

Figure 1. Frequency of Wegener's granulomatosis and microscopic polyangiitis according to the patients' age at diagnosis. Number of patients for each decade enrolled into three clinical trials. (Data from the European Vasculitis Study Group (EUVAS)—Jayne and Rasmussen, 1997.)

increases the incidence of microscopic polyangiitis and an association with farming, especially with animals, has also been demonstrated. The relative frequencies of Wegener's granulomatosis and microscopic polyangiitis are influenced by latitude, with Wegener's granulomatosis being more frequent in colder climates in both the North and South hemisphere (Watts and Scott, 2004). In addition, there are ethnic differences, with Wegener's granulomatosis being less common in eastern Asian and black populations (Mahr et al., 2006). The lack of a major immunogenetic contribution and the late age of onset differentiates ANCA-associated autoimmunity from other autoantibody-associated autoimmune diseases.

## 1.3. ANCA testing

ANCA were reported in association with rapidly progressive glomerulonephritis in 1982, and subsequently associated with Wegener's granulomatosis in 1985 and microscopic polyangiitis in 1987 (Davies et al., 1982; Feehally et al., 1987; van der Woude et al., 1985). Several patters of binding were recognized, a cytoplasmic or C-ANCA pattern, a peri-nuclear or P-ANCA pattern, and an atypical pattern, X-ANCA (Savige et al., 1999). Between 1988 and 1990, the target antigens for C-ANCA and P-ANCA were characterized as an elastinolytic serine protease, proteinase 3 (PR3-ANCA), and myeloperoxidase (MPO-ANCA), respectively (Falk and Jennette, 1988; Ludemann et al., 1990). Solid phase assays for PR3-ANCA and MPO-ANCA are now combined with indirect immunofluorescence and positivity in both assay systems carries a sensitivity for AASV of approximately 80% and specificity of 70–95% depending on the clinical context (Hagen et al., 1998). PR3-ANCA measured by "capture" ELISA have an increased specificity and the antibody binding level at diagnosis carries prognostic significance (Csernok et al., 2004; Westman et al., 1998a, b).

## 1.4. ANCA and pathogenesis

AASV predominantly affects small blood vessels, with glomerular and alveolar capillaritis accounting for renal and pulmonary vasculitis, the most common manifestations in the elderly. The pathogenetic role of ANCA remains controversial because this pathology can occur without circulating ANCA, immune deposits are rarely present, and ANCA can persist without disease activity. Experimental studies have demonstrated unequivocally that ANCA can induce neutrophil activation, cytokine release, and mediate endothelial cytotoxicity (Hewins and Savage, 2003). Both spontaneous and induced animal models have confirmed the pathogenicity of ANCA (Little et al., 2006; Xiao et al., 2002). MPO-ANCA is more common in the elderly than PR3 ANCA (Wang et al., 2004). MPO-ANCA is also found in vasculitis associated with environmental exposure, or occurring secondary to chronic infections. This points to a greater role of environmental stimuli for vasculitis occurring in the elderly. In contrast, genetic factors may be less important in the elderly, as the association of polymorphisms of alpha 1 anti-trypsin and Fc gamma R III with vasculitis are only found with PR3-ANCA positive patients. Dysregulated antigen presentation occurs in Wegener's granulomatosis and persistent circulating T-cell and B-cell activation are typically present (Abdulahad et al., 2006). Bacterial antigens have been proposed to play a role in Wegener's granulomatosis, possibly through molecular mimicry, but the lack of an immunogenetic association implies that environmental drives are likely to be numerous and varied between patients (Popa et al., 2007). The inflammatory infiltrate at vasculitic foci is neutrophil rich and interventions which deplete neutrophils, including experimental chemokine blockade or the drugs cyclophosphamide and deoxyspergualin are effective therapies (Birck et al., 2003). Autoantibodies to endothelial antigens are found in over 50% of vasculitis patients, but their targets have not been defined and contribution to pathogenesis is unclear (Frampton et al., 1990). Wegener's granulomatosis is characterized by poorly formed granulomata, in a peri-vascular distribution with frequent giant cells.

## 1.5. Drives and trigger factors

Identification of reversible elements that contribute to vasculitis is part of the primary evaluation at presentation. In Wegener's granulomatosis intercurrent bacterial infection of damaged upper respiratory tract mucosa is frequent and appropriate antibiotic treatment will aid disease control (Stegeman et al., 1994). Whether *Staphylococcus aureus* has a role in aetiology is controversial, but its presence is associated with increased risk of disease relapse and prolonged sulfamethoxazole/trimethoprim reduces relapse rates in Wegener's granulomatosis (Boomsma et al., 2000; Popa et al., 2007). The respiratory tract in Wegener's granulomatosis becomes damaged and prone to recurrent infection, which in turn exacerbates vasculitic activity. Aggressive attention to the diagnosis and treatment of respiratory tract infection is an important factor in achieving vasculitic control. Chronic virus infection, especially with hepatitis B and C viruses can cause polyarteritis and are better treated with anti-viral therapy then immunosuppression. Penicillamine, hydralazine, propyl thiouracil, and minocycline have been implicated as causes of drug-induced AASV, and remission has followed their withdrawal without the need for other interventions. Malignancy, bacterial abscesses, and tuberculosis are rare causes of polyarteritis syndromes.

## 2. Clinical features

Wegener described a triad of upper respiratory tract (ear, nose, and throat), lung, and renal disease (Wegener, 1936). Symptomatic disease of the upper respiratory tract is almost universal in Wegner's granulomatosis, but any organ may be involved. Microscopic polyangiitis typically involves the kidney with other sites less frequently affected, but may spare the kidney, in these circumstances ANCA may be negative. The frequency of organ involvement in incident patients with AASV is shown in Table 2.

## 2.1. Disease assessment

Attempts have been made to subgroup patients with vasculitis according to the extent and severity

Table 2
The frequency of organ involvement at presentation in Wegener's granulomatosis and microscopic polyangiitis

|  | Wegener's granulomatosis $N=224$ | Microscopic polyangiitis $N=161$ | |
| --- | --- | --- | --- |
| Constitutional | 97 | 92 | |
| Skin | 26 | 20 | |
| Eye | 44 | 15 | $P<0.001$ |
| Ear, nose and throat | 77 | 21 | $P<0.001$ |
| Chest | 56 | 48 | |
| Heart | 5 | 7 | |
| Kidney | 69 | 96 | $P<0.001$ |
| Nervous system | 24 | 13 | $P=0.01$ |
| BVAS | 18 | 16 | $P=0.03$ |

*Note*: BVAS = Birmingham vasculitis activity score. Pooled data from the European Vasculitis Study group (De Groot et al., 2005; Jayne et al., 2003, 2007).

of disease and several systems have been developed. They include the "five factor score" which identified factors predictive of a poor prognosis and comprised proteinuria, impaired renal function, cardiac or gastro-intestinal vasculitis and central nervous system vasculitis; the disease extent index, a numerical score of the number of systems involved; and a multi-item list of clinical features weighted for their importance, designed for clinical trials, the Birmingham Vasculitis Activity Score (BVAS) (Cohen et al., 2007; Guillevin et al., 2003; Luqmani et al., 1994). The European Vasculitis study group (EUVAS) has sub-classified ANCA vasculitis at presentation into three groups: "early systemic", "generalized" and "severe", according to the presence and severity of renal disease (Table 3 (www.vasculitis.org)) (Jayne and Rasmussen, 1997). In three concurrent studies, the average age of each group rose with the severity of the vasculitis.

## 2.2. Prodrome

Prior to diagnosis most patients give a history of several months of constitutional and focal symptoms. Constitutional symptoms include fatigue, malaise, polymyalgia, polyarthralgia, weight loss, fevers, and night sweats. Focal symptoms include headaches, deafness, eye pain, cough, flitting arthritis, purpuric rash, and numbness. The non-specific nature of these symptoms contributes to the diagnostic delay in vasculitis.

## 2.3. The kidney

The absence of specific symptoms of renal disease results in diagnostic delay, and patients with renal limited vasculitis present with more advanced renal failure than those with extra-renal disease. During the prodromal phase urinary abnormalities will be present and should be sought in all patients with unexplained illness. Without early detection patients present with symptoms and signs of uraemia, the average delay from onset of symptoms is 6–9 months. Glomerular haematuria and proteinuria is always present in renal vasculitis, but may be confused with prostatic disease or urinary tract infection. Atypical presentations including "failure to thrive" and unexpected, asymptomatic renal impairment may be more common in the elderly.

Renal histology is essential in the absence of ANCA positivity in order to make a secure diagnosis. There is a debate as to the diagnostic value of renal biopsy when the ANCA is positive and clinical presentation is typical. However, false

Table 3
Subgrouping of patients with AASV at diagnosis according to disease severity and treatment response

| Subgroup | Organ involvement | Constitutional symptoms | ANCA status | EUVAS trial | Age at entry |
| --- | --- | --- | --- | --- | --- |
| Localized | One site, typically the upper respiratory tract in Wegener's granulomatosis | No | +/− | | |
| Early systemic | Any, except renal or imminent vital organ failure | Yes | +/− | NORAM | 55 |
| Generalized (or renal) | Imminent vital organ failure or renal with creatinine <500 μmol/l | Yes | + | CYCAZAREM | 60 |
| Severe | Vital organ failure, typically renal with creatinine >500 μmol/l | Yes | + | MEPEX | 66 |
| Refractory | Progressive disease despite conventional therapy | Yes | +/− | SOLUTION | |

*Note*: Randomized controlled trials performed by the European Vasculitis Study Group and average age at entry of each subgroup (Jayne and Rasmussen, 1997).

positive ANCAs have been reported in myeloma, atheroembolic disease, and chronic infections, so the absence of biopsy confirmation increases the risk of an incorrect diagnosis (Esnault et al., 1990). In practice, the start of treatment need not be delayed for a biopsy result.

The typical renal biopsy features in AASV are a pauci-immune necrotizing glomerulonephritis with crescent formation. The proportion of affected glomeruli in a biopsy are predictive of outcome as is the severity of tubulo-interstitial fibrosis (Falk et al., 2000; Hauer et al., 2002a, b). In Wegener's granulomatosis acute tubular changes are more frequent, scarring is less apparent, and the prognosis is better. There has been debate as to whether treatment should be guided by histological features, and the suggestion that those with advanced, chronic changes should receive less aggressive treatment in view of a poorer prognosis. This has not been examined in an interventional study and the relatively poor correlation between histological changes and renal outcome for individual patients argues against adjusting treatment according to the biopsy severity (de Lind van Wijngaarden et al., 2006).

Renal vasculitis is more common in the elderly with AASV, and is more severe, with a lower glomerular filtration rate at diagnosis (Fig. 2). Some 5% of AASV cases with renal vasculitis have co-existent anti-glomerular basement membrane antibodies in the circulation and linear IgG deposits on the glomerular basement membrane (Jayne et al., 1990). Such patients have a more aggressive renal presentation and are more likely to have pulmonary capillaritis. Although described as pauci-immune, one third of AASV patients have detectable glomerular immune deposits which may have prognostic significance (Neumann et al., 2003) (Fig. 3).

## 2.4. The respiratory tract

Over 50% of patients with AASV will have respiratory tract involvement with three principle patterns of disease (Lane et al., 2005a, b). An alveolar capillaritis, analogous to the glomerular

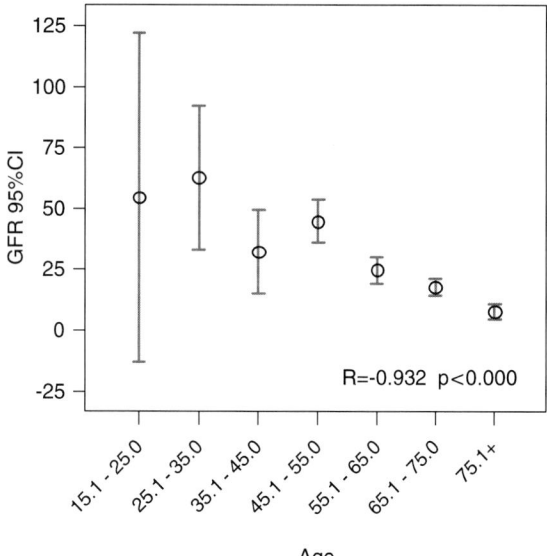

**Figure 2.** Glomerular filtration rate (mean) at diagnosis according to the patients' age. (Data from the EUVAS—Jayne and Rasmussen, 1997.)

capillaritis seen in the kidney, presents with haemoptysis, cough, dyspnoea, and radiological infiltrates. This presentation occurs both in Wegener's granulomatosis and microscopic polyangiitis, usually in conjunction with renal vasculitis when it is termed "pulmonary–renal syndrome" (Gallagher et al., 2002; Specks, 2001). This presentation can be severe with respiratory failure due to massive lung hemorrhage, in which case it will be accompanied by a fall in hemoglobin, and an increase in carbon monoxide transfer factor (Ewan et al., 1976). Bronchoscopy usually reveals fresh bleeding and broncho-alveolar lavage, increasingly blood stained fluid. Transbronchial biopsy may reveal vasculitis but haemosiderin laden macrophages are typically present.

The second pattern of disease is endobronchial inflammation and stenosis found exclusively in Wegener's granulomatosis (Gottschlich et al., 2006). For unknown reasons, these manifestations often develop some time after the diagnosis and the most common site is the sub-glottis, causing sub-glottic stenosis. The tracheo-bronchial inflammation causes a cough, sputum production, and haemoptysis and the stenosis presents as exertional

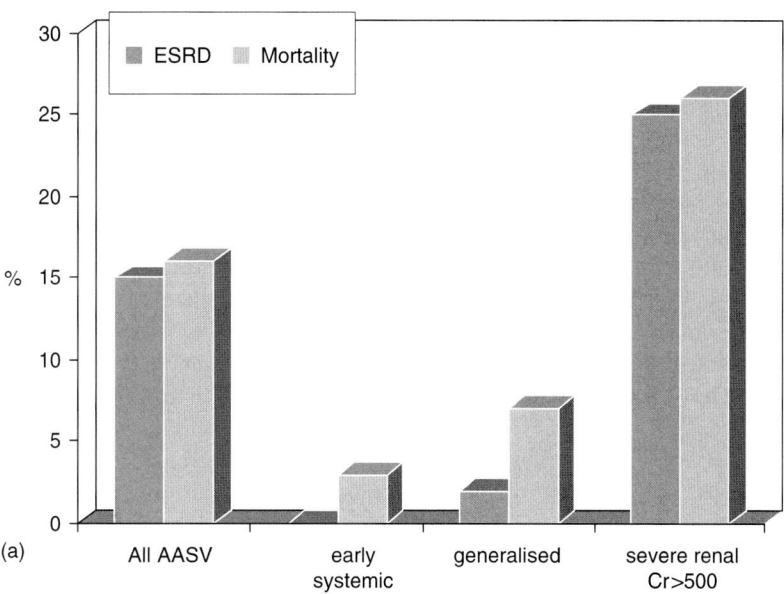

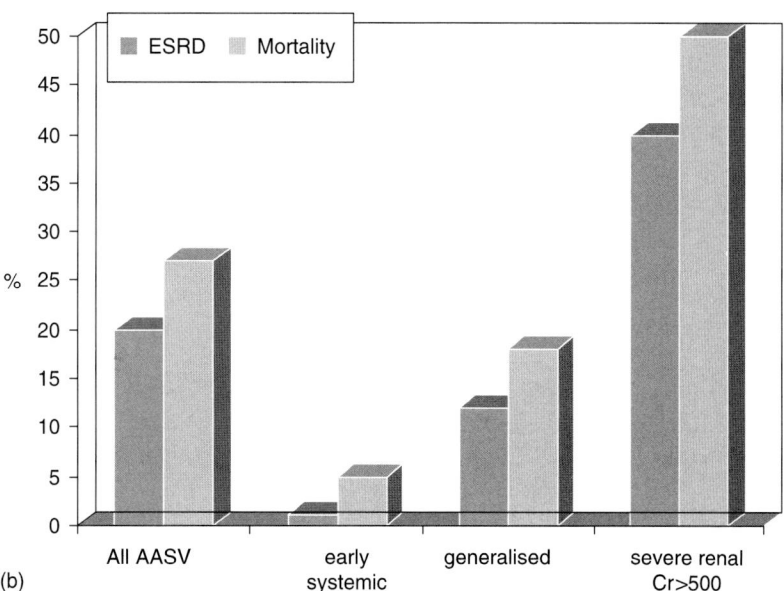

**Figure 3.** Mortality and end-stage renal disease rates at 1 and 5 years of ANCA-associated systemic vasculitis according to disease severity at entry (Jayne, 2003).

dyspnoea. This may be missed in a patient who is otherwise well, or attributed to asthma or intercurrent infection. Lung function testing with a "flow volume loop" is useful in monitoring but can be surprisingly normal. There is no improvement with bronchodilators, stenoses can be seen on plain X-ray or spiral CT scanning, but again direct visualization by bronchoscopy is the key to diagnosis and also provides an opportunity for microbiological evaluation.

The third manifestation is pulmonary cavitation seen in Wegener's granulomatosis. This first appears as nodules on X-ray which increase in size and then cavitate. They are usually multi-focal and in both lung fields. CT scanning is very much more sensitive in their detection than plain X-ray. When large and chronic they distort the local anatomy and heal with visible scarring. They may be complicated by local haemorrhage and secondary bacterial or fungal infection.

A recently described, additional manifestation is pulmonary fibrosis (Homma et al., 2004). It is unclear whether this is caused by vasculitis, is a response to lung haemorrhage, or is an associated pathology. It is most commonly found in microscopic polyangiitis associated with MPO-ANCA and is usually present at the time of diagnosis. Its course is often progressive despite remission of vasculitis.

## 2.5. Other organs

Involvement of the nose in Wegener's granulomatosis causes obstruction by necrotic inflammation tissue and excess mucus production (Gottschlich et al., 2006). There is pain and epistaxis with sinus mucosal thickening which progresses to sinus obliteration. Eustachian tube dysfunction leads to middle ear disease, secondary infection, and deafness. Damage to the ciliary epithelium of the nose impairs physiological nasal hygiene, causing crusting and epistaxis even when the vasculitis is controlled. Vasculitic destruction of the nasal cartilage induces nasal pain and collapse of the bridge of the nose. Inner ear involvement causing deafness may occur infrequently.

Episcleritis is a common finding in active systemic vasculitis and even when not clinically apparent, abnormalities of retinal blood flow are seen on angiography. Frank scleritis and scleral necrosis caused by vasculitis can disrupt the integrity of the eyeball, but the most common cause of visual loss is retinal vein thrombosis in the absence of obvious retinitis. Rarely the optic nerve or chiasm is involved, causing a rapid onset of uniocular or binocular blindness. Deposition of inflammatory tissue behind the eye, "retro-orbital granulomata", leads to propotosis and may also threaten sight, as is seen in Wegener's granulomatosis.

Peripheral neuropathy occurs in 20% and this may be more common with nerve conduction studies (Cattaneo et al., 2007). Cerebral vasculitis is very rare, although thrombotic stroke is more common. Meningeal involvement in Wegener's granulomatosis causes severe headache and cranial nerve lesions and is clearly seen on gadolinium-enhanced MR scanning, while pituitary vasculitis is rare and results in pituitary failure. Gastro-intestinal involvement with pain, haemorrhage, and perforation is secondary to a micro-vasculitis of the gut wall and is most frequent in the terminal ileum. Culture negative endocarditis and valvular destruction are rare and must be differentiated from infective endocarditis causing a secondary vasculitis (Iqbal et al., 2005; Roberts et al., 2006). It is unclear whether myocarditis or small-vessel coronary arteritis is a manifestation of AASV.

## 2.6. Investigations and diagnosis

The diagnosis depends on the triad of clinical features, serology, and histology. ANCA positivity, confirmed by a positive proteinase 3 ANCA or myeloperoxidase ANCA, has a high predictive value for the diagnosis of vasculitis in the absence of another chronic inflammatory process (Hagen et al., 1998). A negative ANCA does not exclude the diagnosis of vasculitis, immune-complex-associated diseases including SLE should be considered, as they may be missed in the elderly. Further investigations aim to determine the severity and extent of organ dysfunction, confirm a vasculitic diagnosis, and exclude secondary causes and mimics of vasculitis. Ninety percent of patients with AASV are ANCA positive at diagnosis, both by indirect immunofluorescence and PR3-ANCA or MPO-ANCA by ELISA. Those with localized disease, no renal involvement, or those who have been previously treated are more likely to be ANCA negative. False positive ANCA testing occurs and is more frequent in pulmonary or gastro-intestinal presentations caused by chronic inflammatory lung disease or inflammatory bowel disease. There is a specificity of over 95% for ANCA positivity for renal vasculitis when evidence for nephritis exists (Choi et al., 2001). Important causes of secondary vasculitis have been outlined above, but infections with tuberculosis and endocarditis may cause particular difficulty. Mimics of vasculitic syndromes include athero-embolic disease, anti-phospholipid syndrome, and multiple myeloma as well as other chronic infections.

## 3. Treatment

### 3.1. Background

The goals of therapy in the primary systemic vasculitides are to control the overt manifestations of disease activity thereby preventing vital organ damage and restoring the patient to their pre-morbid state of health. Because treatment is not curative, and vasculitis has a tendency to relapse on drug reduction or withdrawal, treatment has to be prolonged (Boomsma et al., 2000; Booth et al., 2003). Without therapy, mortality at 12 months exceeds 80%; the introduction of corticosteroids heralded the modern therapeutic era, but even high dose are often ineffective (Walton, 1958). Their combination with the immune suppressives, azathioprine, methotrexate and particularly cyclophosphamide, a decade later, allowed more reliable disease control or remission (Fauci et al., 1971; Leib et al., 1979).

There is considerable variability in severity, treatment responsiveness, and relapse risk between vasculitis patients that complicates the design of therapeutic regimens. The use of long-term daily oral cyclophosphamide for at least 1 year after attaining disease control, popularized by studies from the National Institutes of Health in the USA, was associated with a high risk of bladder tumors and lymphoproliferative disease (Hoffman et al., 1992). An alternative approach to therapy has used cyclophosphamide and high-dose steroids for a shorter period of time to gain remission and alternative immunosuppressives and lower steroid doses to maintain remission (Jayne et al., 2003).

A recent consensus statement by EUVAS and the European League against rheumatism (EULAR), has defined disease states in vasculitis and disease assessment methodology (Hellmich et al., 2007). Remission is the absence of overt signs of disease activity sustained over a period of time with moderate or low steroid dosing. Remission does not imply the withdrawal of therapy. As therapy is suppressive and disease relapse may follow treatment reduction, this definition is not robust. Furthermore, it is often difficult to judge the level of disease activity, for example, in renal vasculitis or in Wegener's granulomatosis affecting the nasopharynx. This definition does not take into account irreversible scars of disease, the presence of adverse effects of therapy, or the patient's functional status. Partial remission indicates a stabilization and reduction in intensity without resolution of all disease activity.

Consensus guidelines for the management of vasculitis are now emerging based on the increasing body of evidence produced by clinical trials performed over the last 20 years.

### 3.2. Approaches to remission induction

In the absence of curative therapies current regimens aim to suppress manifestations of disease activity, with the combination of corticosteroids and cyclophosphamide being accepted as the, "standard of care". A sequential approach with switching to azathioprine or methotrexate after remission has been achieved, between 3 and 6 months from diagnosis, obtains similar results at 1 to 2 years, when compared to continued cyclophosphamide and considerably reduces cyclophosphamide exposure

(Jayne et al., 2003). However subsequent relapse rates, particularly after the withdrawal of therapy, are higher with sequential designs, which indicate that there is a balance between the improved long-term disease control with higher cyclophosphamide exposure and the higher toxicity, and probably higher mortality, of such regimens (Sanders et al., 2006).

Alternative agents, including plasma exchange, intravenous immunoglobulin, and tumor necrosis alpha (TNFα) blockade have been added to the "standard of care", or used as an alternative in induction regimens to improve efficacy or reduce toxicity. Preliminary studies have attempted curative strategies by employing lymphocyte depletion or immunoablation with stem-cell transplantation (Daikeler et al., 2007; Lockwood et al., 2003). These strategies aim to destroy autoreactive T-cells and predict that immune reconstitution will restore tolerance to the previously pathogenic autoantigens. More recently, selective B-cell depletion has shown considerable promise for remission induction and maintenance, and has highlighted the pathogenic role B-cells play in vasculitis (Smith et al., 2006).

## 3.3. Remission and relapse

Current remission induction regimens lead to a partial or full remission in 80–90% of patients within 6 months, but persisting low-disease activity states are recognized, especially in Wegener's granulomatosis, quality of life remains depressed during remission, and prolonged therapy is required to avoid relapse (Hellmich et al., 2007). By 5 years, 50% of patients will have experienced at least one relapse (Booth et al., 2003). Risk factors for relapse include a diagnosis of Wegener's granulomatosis, involvement of the ear nose and throat, lack of kidney involvement, persistent ANCA positivity, reduction or withdrawal of therapy, and colonization with *S. aureus* (Boomsma et al., 2000). The consequences of relapse are varied with minor relapse implying moderate intensification of therapy with little risk of late sequelae, and major relapse carrying a high risk of contributing to permanent damage and incapacity. Thus management during the remission phase aims to balance the risks of relapse with those of continued therapy and is improved by careful monitoring and early detection or prediction of relapse. The cumulative exposure to cyclophosphamide in a frequently relapsing patient will raise the malignancy risk and makes bone marrow suppression, causing drug intolerance, more likely (Westman et al., 1998a, b).

## 3.4. Therapeutic agents: steroids and immune suppressives

### 3.4.1. Corticosteroids

The wide range of anti-inflammatory actions of corticosteroids are useful for the early control of disease activity in vasculitis but as sole therapy they are ineffective at remission induction in generalized Wegener's granulomatosis or polyarteritis nodosa. They have been recommended for localized and cutaneous disease, but this has not been studied in detail. In combination with cyclophosphamide, oral prednisolone is typically commenced at 1 mg/kg/day, with varying rates of taper and time to withdrawal (Jayne and Rasmussen, 1997).

A potential benefit of "pulsed" intravenous methyl prednisolone has been demonstrated in renal vasculitis, and its use may allow lower oral corticosteroid dosing and more rapid disease control (Bolton and Sturgill, 1989). A major concern is the contribution of corticosteroids to the risk of severe infection, bone disease, and long-term disability (Hoffman et al., 1992).

Current evidence suggests that the infective risk of vasculitis remission induction regimens involving cyclophosphamide, is directly related to the prednisolone dose, and an important aim of future therapeutic strategies is to reduce corticosteroid exposure.

### 3.4.2. Methotrexate

Approaches to avoid cyclophosphamide in "early systemic" vasculitis have used methotrexate and other immunosuppressives (de Groot et al., 1996;

Langford et al., 2000; Sneller et al., 1995). A consensus regimen with oral methotrexate, 22.5–25 mg/week, demonstrated an equivalent response rate at 6 months to a cyclophosphamide-based protocol (89% methotrexate vs. 95% cyclophosphamide) (De Groot et al., 2005). On subgroup analysis, those patients with more extensive disease at diagnosis, typically of the lower respiratory tract, took longer to enter remission if they were from the methotrexate group. High relapse rates have been reported despite continued methotrexate, and if immune suppressives are withdrawn relapse rates in methotrexate treated patients are higher than in those who had received cyclophosphamide (Reinhold-Keller et al., 2002). Experience from other diseases suggests methotrexate will be safer than cyclophosphamide, however, infective adverse events remain frequent although cytopaenias, especially neutropaenia are rare. Gastric intolerance can prevent this being achieved, while higher doses of 30–40 mg/week have been used outside clinical trials. Intestinal side effects can be reduced by parenteral administration, but it is unclear whether this route is more efficacious. Folic acid is recommended to prevent hematological toxicity, again it is not known whether this influences efficacy. The possibility of methotrexate pneumonitis complicates the treatment of pulmonary vasculitis and hepatotoxicty is more common than with cyclophosphamide (Sneller et al., 1995).

### 3.4.3. Cyclophosphamide

The toxicity of long-term oral cyclophosphamide use in vasculitis, especially bladder and lymphoproliferative malignancies, has had a major influence on current regimens (Hoffman et al., 1992; Talar-Williams et al., 1996). Two routes of administration are used, daily oral tablets typically at 2 mg/kg/day or intermittent intravenous boluses. Because the malignancy risk of cyclophosphamide is dependent on the cumulative dose, and is clearly raised after 1 year of daily oral dosing, discontinuation once remission has been achieved is attractive (Westman et al., 1998a, b). Remission rates of 80% at 3 months and 93% at 6 months have been obtained with daily oral cyclophosphamide in AASV (Jayne et al., 2003). There are potential advantages of intravenous bolus therapy when compared to a daily oral regimen: protection of the urinary bladder, less than 50% of the cumulative exposure, and less risk of severe neutropaenia. Several, small trials have compared these regimens, and a pooled analysis concluded that there was no difference in the hard end-points of renal failure or death, subsequent relapse was higher with bolus therapy and infective risk was higher with daily oral use (de Groot et al., 2001). The use of an alternative immune suppressive to maintain remission may avoid the problems over relapse, but concerns over the relative efficacy of these two routes for remission induction remain. The EUVAS group has designed a consensus intravenous bolus regimen that has identical remission and relapse rates to daily oral regimens, but with lower rates of leucopaenia and infection (de Groot and Jayne, 2005). The frequency of severe infections associated with neutropaenia is the major early complication of cyclophosphamide and most frequent cause of early death (Booth et al., 2003). This event is associated with older age and renal failure. The elimination of cyclophosphamide is delayed in renal impairment and it has now become clear that cyclophosphamide dosing should be reduced for both age and renal impairment (Haubitz et al., 2002).

Earlier, uncontrolled studies of intravenous cyclophosphamide in relapsing Wegener's granulomatosis did not suggest superior efficacy when compared to daily oral use in this setting, and one small study found that vasculitis persisting despite intravenous bolus therapy responded to daily oral cyclophosphamide (de Groot et al., 2001). For polyarteritis nodosa with a poor prognosis, a recent trial has compared 6 to 12 monthly pulses of cyclophosphamide and found the remission rate to be higher and relapse rate lower for the 12-month regimen (Guillevin et al., 2003).

### 3.4.4. Other immunosuppressives

Azathioprine and mycophenolate mofetil (MMF) are anti-proliferative drugs which inhibit purine metabolism. Azathioprine has been shown to be effective for remission maintenance in vasculitis, after remission induction with cyclophosphamide (Jayne et al., 2003). Historical studies have pointed to the efficacy of azathioprine as a remission-inducing drug, but this has not been studied in detail (Leib et al., 1979). It seems plausible that azathioprine and MMF will be of similar, or possibly greater, efficacy than methotrexate for remission induction of early systemic vasculitis. Azathioprine and methotrexate are of equal efficacy for remission maintenance after cyclophosphamide induction. Studies of MMF have been small or retrospective and have involved patients with refractory disease. Results have been varied, with a majority experiencing an improvement in disease control, at least in the short-term (Joy et al., 2005; Koukoulaki and Jayne, 2006; Stassen et al., 2007). Ongoing studies are evaluating MMF both for induction and maintenance therapy. Less data supports the use of the calcineurin inhibitors ciclosporin and tacrolimus or sirolimus. There have been occasional reports of remission in refractory Wegener's granulomatosis following etoposide (D'Cruz et al., 1992; Morton et al., 2000).

Deoxyspergualin is a novel immune suppressive with anti-proliferative and anti-immune effects that has led to remission in experimental vasculitis, and in patients with relapsing and refractory AASV (Schmitt et al., 2005). Its mechanism of action is uncertain, with pleomorphic effects on monocytes and lymphocytes. Daily deoxyspergualin dosing results in neutropaenia, which is rapidly reversible on drug withdrawal. Regimens have used up to six, monthly, cycles of 2 to 3 weeks daily dosing followed by a washout period. Remission rates in refractory disease are high but disease relapse following withdrawal occurs in over one third within 6 months despite maintenance azathioprine (Schmitt et al., 2005).

A randomized comparison of leflunomide to methotrexate for remission maintenance after induction with cyclophosphamide was stopped early due to an excess of major relapses in the methotrexate group (Metzler et al., 2007). At this stage, leflunomide was associated with more toxic events and there was no clear conclusion as to which was the superior drug. Further studies with leflunomide are warranted, and it is now a further option as a second-line remission sustaining agent.

## 3.5. Therapeutic agents: plasma exchange, immunoglobulin, and therapeutic antibodies

### 3.5.1. Plasma exchange

Following demonstration of the ability of plasma exchange to remove pathogenic autoantibodies in anti-glomerular basement membrane disease, it was used in other forms of rapidly progressive glomerulonephritis (Lockwood et al., 1976). Small studies with conflicting results failed to make a convincing case for routine use of this expensive therapy (Cole et al., 1992; Frasca et al., 2003; Guillevin et al., 1991; Korbet et al., 2007; Nakamura et al., 2004; Pusey et al., 1991; Szpirt, 1996; Zauner et al., 2002). A recent EUVAS trial found an increased rate of renal recovery after seven, 4 L plasma exchanges, of 80% in surviving patients for those presenting in renal failure, creatinine over 500 μmol/L (Jayne et al., 2007). In this study, plasma exchange was compared to the addition of 3000 mg of pulsed methyl prednisolone to daily oral cyclophosphamide and oral prednisolone. Since the pathogenetic potential of ANCA has been confirmed, a logical rationale for plasma exchange now exists, however the optimal duration of plasma exchange and the role of ANCA monitoring during this therapy is not known (Tesar et al., 1998; Xiao et al., 2002).

Diffuse alveolar haemorrhage is the most common life-threatening vasculitis manifestation. In common with renal vasculitis, it is closely related to ANCA positivity and a role for plasma exchange has also been suggested (Nguyen et al., 2005). Removal of coagulation factors has the potential to exacerbate lung haemorrhage, so this indication remains controversial. Whether plasma exchange has a role in milder renal vasculitis or other vasculitic manifestations is unknown.

### 3.5.2. Intravenous immunoglobulin (IVIg)

When used as an additional therapy to steroids and an immune suppressive in relapsing or refractory vasculitis, IVIg is superior to placebo in controlling vasculitic activity and reducing C-reactive protein levels (Jayne et al., 2000). The responses to IVIg are variable and usually of short duration and its expense and the nephrotoxicity of some preparations complicate its use (Levy and Pusey, 2000). No clear indication has emerged, but in situations where the risks of immune suppressives are of particular concern, such as, ongoing infections, or the severely ill patient in the intensive care unit, IVIg may be a useful addition to a remission induction protocol. One small study has found IVIg alone to be beneficial in new patients and an ongoing study uses IVIg alone for the initial control of renal vasculitis (Ito-Ihara et al., 2006).

### 3.5.3. Tumor necrosis factor (TNF) blockade

There are strong theoretical and experimental reasons for exploring TNFα blockade in AASV (Feldmann and Pusey, 2006). Several anecdotal reports and one uncontrolled study have found the addition of anti-TNFα agents, Infliximab (Centocor, USA) or Etanercept (Wyeth, USA), to aid remission induction (Booth et al., 2002) (Wegener' Etanercept Research Group, 2005). The WGET study compared the addition of etanercept or placebo to "standard" induction and maintenance regimens for Wegener's granulomatosis over a 2-year period and found no benefit of etanercept (2005) (Wegener's Etanercept Research Group, 2005). An infliximab study in renal vasculitis suggested that remission induction was quicker and steroid use lower, than in conventionally treated patients (Booth et al., 2004). This study also showed that prolonged use of Infliximab revealed escape of disease control and an increased incidence of severe bacterial and fungal infections. Thus, there may be a role for TNFα blockade in remission induction and as a steroid-sparing agent, subjects not examined in the WGET study. It is also possible that infliximab is more effective in vasculitis than etanercept, analogous to the results in inflammatory bowel disease.

### 3.5.4. Lymphocyte depletion

The pathogenic role of T-cells has been supported by remissions seen after anti-thymocyte globulin (ATG) and the anti-CD52 monoclonal antibody, Alemtuzumab (Roche, UK) (Schmitt et al., 2004; Walsh et al., in press). ATG was associated with frequent severe adverse events and a mean time to relapse of 9 months (Schmitt et al., 2004). The development of an anti-globulin response precludes re-treatment. This is not a problem with Alemtuzumab, and in a series of anecdotal studies prolonged treatment free remissions were obtained in 71 patients with relapsing AASV (Walsh et al., in press). The high level of immune suppression after Alemtuzumab was associated with opportunistic infections and increased mortality in the elderly or those with renal failure. Surviving patients did well with prolonged treatment free remissions and little indication of any delayed toxicity.

B-cell depletion with the anti-CD20 monoclonal antibody, Rituximab (Roche, UK) is a licensed therapy for rheumatoid arthritis and is under detailed investigation for SLE and vasculitis. It appears safe and three prospective studies have reported high remission rates in refractory disease (Table 4) (Keogh et al., 2006; Smith et al., 2006; Stasi et al., 2006). Rituximab induces a variable period of peripheral B-cell depletion, typically 6–9 months, accompanied by falls in ANCA levels. Relapses have occurred after an average of 13 months, but repeat treatment is also effective (Smith et al., 2006). Rising ANCA levels appear predictive of relapse in this setting, but there is not a close association with the return of B-cells (Keogh et al., 2006). Current protocols have varied in their rituximab dosing regimen, and in the use of concurrent or continued immunosuppression. Potential problems with rituximab include the development of anti-chimeric antibodies and hypogammaglobulinaemia with repeated administration.

## 3.6. Disease monitoring and the adverse effects of therapy

Regular assessment of vasculitic activity and treatment toxicity are required to optimize disease control and minimize treatment-related effects. Sequential measurement of the inflammatory markers C-reactive protein and erythrocyte sedimentation rate provide information on vasculitic activity, in the absence of infection, but carry little

**Table 4**
Prospective clinical trials of rituximab in ANCA-associated vasculitis

| Study | Number of patients (number of nephritis) | Dose of RTX | Concomitant treatments | Remission | B-cell depletion | ANCA serology | Relapse (months) |
|---|---|---|---|---|---|---|---|
| Aries et al. (2006) | 8 (2) | 375 mg/m$^2$ every 4 weeks × 4 | CYC, MMF, MTX, GC | 2/8 CR, 1/8 PR | 8/8 | 0/8 became negative | NR |
| Eriksson (2005) | 9 (7) | 500 mg weekly × 4 | MMF, AZA, CYC, GC | 8/9 CR, 1/9 PR | 9/9 | 0/7 became negative | 2 (12, 13) |
| Keogh et al. (2005) | 11 (4) | 375 mg/m$^2$ weekly × 4 | PLEX, GC | 10/11 CR 1/11 PR | 11/11 | 8/11 became negative | 2 (7, 12) |
| Keogh et al. (2005) | 10 (7) | 375 mg/m$^2$ weekly × 4 | GC | 10/10 CR | 10/10 | 6/10 became negative | 1 (9) |
| Omdal et al. (2005) | 3 (3) | 375 mg/m$^2$ weekly × 4 | NR | 3/3 CR | 3/3 | 0/3 became negative | 3/3 (8, 13, 15) |
| Smith et al. (2006) | 11 (6) | 375 mg/m$^2$ weekly × 4 | MMF, GC | 9/11 CR, 1/11 PR | 11/11 | 6/10 became negative | 6/10 (median 16.5) |
| Stasi et al. (2006) | 10 (6) | 375 mg/m$^2$ weekly × 4 | GC | 9/10 CR, 1/10 PR | 10/10 | 8/10 became negative | 3/10 (12, 16, 24) |
| Henes et al. (2007) | 6 | 375 mg/m$^2$ weekly × 4 | Leflunomide, GC | 5/6 CR, 1/6 PR | 6/6 | 4/4 became negative | 3/6 (3, 3, 18) |
| Brihaye et al. (2007) | 8 | 375 mg/m$^2$ weekly × 4 | MTX/AZA, GC | 3/8 CR, 3/8 PR 2/8 NR | 8/8 | 4/6 became negative | 1/8 (12) |

prognostic value (Jayne et al., 1995). Pro-calcitonin is elevated in bacterial infection, but is not raised in active vasculitis and provides superior discrimination to C-reactive protein. ANCA levels fall with therapy and persisting ANCA positivity after induction therapy is strongly linked with an increased risk of later relapse (Sanders et al., 2006). The extent to which rising ANCA levels predict relapse is controversial and is influenced by patient variability, concurrent therapy, and the nature of the ANCA assay (Jayne et al., 1995). The optimal duration of immunosuppressive and steroid therapy has not been determined. Current guidelines recommend 2–4 years of therapy, although for a minority of patients, earlier drug withdrawal may be justified and for patients with a history or relapse, indefinite therapy may be required.

The toxicity of current protocols contributes to mortality and chronic disability (Exley et al., 1997). The frequency of adverse effects is related to age and renal function and infection is the major problem affecting remission induction protocols (Jayne, 2003). Cyclophosphamide-induced neutropaenia is directly associated with infective mortality and should be avoided by careful monitoring and dose adjustment (Booth et al., 2003). In the presence of cyclophosphamide, the infective risk associated with the steroid dose is reduced by more rapid steroid tapering. Prophylaxis against *Pneumocystis jiruvecii* pneumonia, fungal infections, steroid-induced peptic ulceration, and osteoporosis has become routine (Jayne and Rasmussen, 1997).

## 3.7. The outcome of AASV

Age and renal function at diagnosis are strongly predictive of mortality and risk of end-stage renal disease (Fig. 2) (Booth et al., 2003; Jayne, 2003). This reflects the need for prompt diagnosis and for improved therapies in the elderly with renal disease, in whom early mortality is particularly high. When reviewing all cases of AASV, patient survival at 1 and 5 years is 84 and 64% respectively, of whom 15 and 23% will have developed end-stage renal disease by 1 and 5 years. This implies a standardized mortality ratio of between 2.5 and 4 when compared to an age-adjusted control population, and the mortality with ESRD is higher than for other causes of renal failure (Booth et al., 2003). The long-term consequences of disease-related damage, disability, loss of quality of life, and economic implications have not been accurately quantified.

## 4. Summary

The concept of AASV has proved attractive and clinically useful in defining the most frequent subgroup of primary systemic vasculitis. The availability of ANCA testing has facilitated earlier diagnosis and has been of prognostic value. Although AASV has heterogeneous presentations, there are important similarities in the response to treatment and long-term outcomes. The development of collaborative research networks has permitted more randomized controlled trials, the agreement of consensus protocols and treatment guidelines. Results of the randomized trials have now described a standard approach to the therapy of AASV, with the combination of steroids and cyclophosphamide to gain remission, and switching to an alternative immunosuppressive for remission maintenance. Intravenous pulse is safer than daily oral cyclophosphamide and may be equally effective. These regimens achieve remission in over 90% of naïve patients, but can be less effective or less well tolerated in the treatment of relapsing disease. Patients without imminent vital organ dysfunction respond to alternative immunosuppressives, and the most experience has been with methotrexate. Adverse event rates are high and dictate careful monitoring to minimize the infective risk, early steroid tapering, and a search for safer agents. Future trials will aim to reduce adverse event rates, improve quality of life, and obtain more sustained remissions.

The addition of plasma exchange has been demonstrated to be of value in severe renal vasculitis, and the additions of intravenous immunoglobulin and TNFα blockade are under further evaluation. T-cell depletion with therapeutic antibodies has been effective in preliminary studies and merits further attention, and B-cell depletion is offering exciting prospects of safe, long-term disease control. The late consequences of vasculitis are being more carefully explored by registry studies, but economic evaluation of vasculitis, necessary for cost-effectiveness analyses has not been performed. The prospects for vasculitis patients are improving but progress is slow due to a low public profile and little direct pharmaceutical investment.

---

**Key points**

- The kidney is the most important target of injury in ANCA-associated vasculitis.
- Renal outcome is influenced by age and serum creatinine at diagnosis.
- Diagnostic delay is an important factor in poor outcomes.
- Current therapies are toxic and only partially effective.
- There is a particular problem with the toxicity for current therapies in the elderly who present with more severe renal disease.
- Mycophenolate mofetil, leflunomide and rituximab are alternative therapies for remission maintenance or relapsing disease.

---

## References

Abdulahad, W.H., van der Geld, Y.M., Stegeman, C.A., et al. 2006. Persistent expansion of CD4+ effector memory T cells in Wegener's granulomatosis. Kidney Int. 70, 938–947.

Aries, P.M., Lamprecht, P., Gross, W.L. 2006. Rituximab in refractory Wegener's granulomatosis: favorable or not? Am. J. Respir. Crit. Care Med. 173, 815–816.

Birck, R., Warnatz, K., Lorenz, H.M., et al. 2003. 15-Deoxyspergualin in patients with refractory ANCA-associated systemic vasculitis: a six-month open-label trial to evaluate safety and efficacy. J. Am. Soc. Nephrol. 14, 440–447.

Bolton, W.K., Sturgill, B.C. 1989. Methylprednisolone therapy for acute crescentic rapidly progressive glomerulonephritis. Am. J. Nephrol. 9, 368–375.

Boomsma, M.M., Stegeman, C.A., van der Leij, M.J., et al. 2000. Prediction of relapses in Wegener's granulomatosis by measurement of antineutrophil cytoplasmic antibody levels: a prospective study. Arthritis Rheum. 43, 2025–2033.

Booth, A., Harper, L., Hammad, T., et al. 2004. Prospective study of TNFalpha blockade with infliximab in antineutrophil cytoplasmic antibody-associated systemic vasculitis. J. Am. Soc. Nephrol. 15, 717–721.

Booth, A.D., Almond, M.K., Burns, A., et al. 2003. Outcome of ANCA-associated renal vasculitis: a 5-year retrospective study. Am. J. Kidney Dis. 41, 776–784.

Booth, A.D., Jefferson, H.J., Ayliffe, W., et al. 2002. Safety and efficacy of TNFalpha blockade in relapsing vasculitis. Ann. Rheum. Dis. 61, 559.

Brihaye, B., Aouba, A., Pagnoux, C., et al. 2007. Adjunction of rituximab to steroids and immunosuppressants for refractory/relapsing Wegener's granulomatosis: a study on 8 patients. Clin. Exp. Rheumatol. 25, S23–S27.

Cattaneo, L., Chierici, E., Pavone, L., et al. 2007. Peripheral neuropathy in Wegener's granulomatosis, Churg–Strauss syndrome and microscopic polyangiitis. J. Neurol. Neurosurg. Psychiatry 13, 13.

Choi, H.K., Liu, S., Merkel, P.A., et al. 2001. Diagnostic performance of antineutrophil cytoplasmic antibody tests for idiopathic vasculitides: metaanalysis with a focus on antimyeloperoxidase antibodies. J. Rheumatol. 28, 1584–1590.

Cohen, P., Pagnoux, C., Mahr, A., et al. 2007. Churg–Strauss syndrome with poor-prognosis factors: a prospective multicenter trial comparing glucocorticoids and six or twelve cyclophosphamide pulses in forty-eight patients. Arthritis Rheum. 57, 686–693.

Cole, E., Cattran, D., Magil, A., et al. 1992. A prospective randomized trial of plasma exchange as additive therapy in idiopathic crescentic glomerulonephritis. The Canadian Apheresis Study Group. Am. J. Kidney Dis. 20, 261–269.

Csernok, E., Holle, J., Hellmich, B., et al. 2004. Evaluation of capture ELISA for detection of antineutrophil cytoplasmic antibodies directed against proteinase 3 in Wegener's granulomatosis: first results from a multicentre study. Rheumatology (Oxford) 43, 174–180.

Daikeler, T., Kotter, I., Bocelli Tyndall, C., et al. 2007. Haematopoietic stem cell transplantation for vasculitis including Behcet's disease and polychondritis: a retrospective analysis of patients recorded in the European Bone Marrow Transplantation and European League Against Rheumatism databases and a review of the literature. Ann. Rheum. Dis. 66, 202–207.

Davies, D.J., Moran, J.E., Niall, J.F., et al. 1982. Segmental necrotising glomerulonephritis with antineutrophil antibody: possible arbovirus aetiology? Br. Med. J. (Clin. Res. Ed.) 285, 606.

D'Cruz, D., Payne, H., Timothy, A., et al. 1992. Response of cyclophosphamide-resistant Wegener's granulomatosis to etoposide. Lancet 340, 425–426.

de Groot, K., Adu, D., Savage, C.O. 2001. The value of pulse cyclophosphamide in ANCA-associated vasculitis: meta-analysis and critical review. Nephrol. Dial. Transplant. 16, 2018–2027.

de Groot, K., Jayne, D. 2005. What is new in the therapy of ANCA-associated vasculitides? Take home messages from the 12th workshop on ANCA and systemic vasculitides. Clin. Nephrol. 64, 480–484.

De Groot, K., Rasmussen, N., Bacon, P.A., et al. 2005. Randomized trial of cyclophosphamide versus methotrexate for induction of remission in early systemic antineutrophil cytoplasmic antibody-associated vasculitis. Arthritis Rheum. 52, 2461–2469.

de Groot, K., Reinhold-Keller, E., Tatsis, E., et al. 1996. Therapy for the maintenance of remission in sixty-five patients with generalized Wegener's granulomatosis. Methotrexate versus trimethoprim/sulfamethoxazole. Arthritis Rheum. 39, 2052–2061.

de Lind van Wijngaarden, R.A., Hauer, H.A., Wolterbeek, R., et al. 2006. Clinical and histologic determinants of renal outcome in ANCA-associated vasculitis: a prospective analysis of 100 patients with severe renal involvement. J. Am. Soc. Nephrol. 17, 2264–2274.

Eisenberger, U., Fakhouri, F., Vanhille, P., et al. 2005. ANCA-negative pauci-immune renal vasculitis: histology and outcome. Nephrol. Dial. Transplant. 20, 1392–1399.

Eriksson, P. 2005. Nine patients with anti-neutrophil cytoplasmic antibody-positive vasculitis successfully treated with rituximab. J. Intern. Med. 257, 540–548.

Esnault, V.L., Jayne, D.R., Keogan, M.T., et al. 1990. Anti-neutrophil cytoplasm antibodies in patients with monoclonal gammopathies. J. Clin. Lab. Immunol. 32, 153–159.

Ewan, P.W., Jones, H.A., Rhodes, C.G., et al. 1976. Detection of intrapulmonary hemorrhage with carbon monoxide uptake. Application in goodpasture's syndrome. N. Engl. J. Med. 295, 1391–1396.

Exley, A.R., Carruthers, D.M., Luqmani, R.A., et al. 1997. Damage occurs early in systemic vasculitis and is an index of outcome. Q. J. Med. 90, 391–399.

Falk, R.J., Jennette, J.C. 1988. Anti-neutrophil cytoplasmic autoantibodies with specificity for myeloperoxidase in patients with systemic vasculitis and idiopathic necrotizing and crescentic glomerulonephritis. N. Engl. J. Med. 318, 1651–1657.

Falk, R.J., Nachman, P.H., Hogan, S.L., et al. 2000. ANCA glomerulonephritis and vasculitis: a Chapel Hill perspective. Semin. Nephrol. 20, 233–243.

Fauci, A.S., Wolff, S.M., Johnson, J.S. 1971. Effect of cyclophosphamide upon the immune response in Wegener's granulomatosis. N. Engl. J. Med. 285, 1493–1496.

Feehally, J., Wheeler, D.C., Walls, J., et al. 1987. A case of microscopic polyarteritis associated with antineutrophil cytoplasmic antibodies. Clin. Nephrol. 27, 214–215.

Feldmann, M., Pusey, C.D. 2006. Is there a role for TNF-alpha in anti-neutrophil cytoplasmic antibody-associated vasculitis? Lessons from other chronic inflammatory diseases. J. Am. Soc. Nephrol. 17, 1243–1252.

Frampton, G., Jayne, D.R., Perry, G.J., et al. 1990. Autoantibodies to endothelial cells and neutrophil cytoplasmic antigens in systemic vasculitis. Clin. Exp. Immunol. 82, 227–232.

Frasca, G.M., Soverini, M.L., Falaschini, A., et al. 2003. Plasma exchange treatment improves prognosis of antineutrophil cytoplasmic antibody-associated crescentic glomerulonephritis: a case-control study in 26 patients from a single center. Ther. Apher. Dial. 7, 540–546.

Gallagher, H., Kwan, J.T., Jayne, D.R. 2002. Pulmonary renal syndrome: a 4-year, single-center experience. Am. J. Kidney Dis. 39, 42–47.

Gottschlich, S., Ambrosch, P., Kramkowski, D., et al. 2006. Head and neck manifestations of Wegener's granulomatosis. Rhinology 44, 227–233.

Guillevin, L., Cohen, P., Mahr, A., et al. 2003. Treatment of polyarteritis nodosa and microscopic polyangiitis with poor prognosis factors: a prospective trial comparing glucocorticoids and six or twelve cyclophosphamide pulses in sixty-five patients. Arthritis Rheum. 49, 93–100.

Guillevin, L., Jarrousse, B., Lok, C., et al. 1991. Longterm followup after treatment of polyarteritis nodosa and Churg–Strauss angiitis with comparison of steroids, plasma exchange and cyclophosphamide to steroids and plasma exchange. A prospective randomized trial of 71 patients. The cooperative study group for polyarteritis Nodosa. J. Rheumatol. 18, 567–574.

Hagen, E.C., Daha, M.R., Hermans, J., et al. 1998. Diagnostic value of standardized assays for anti-neutrophil cytoplasmic antibodies in idiopathic systemic vasculitis. EC/BCR Project for ANCA Assay Standardization. Kidney Int. 53, 743–753.

Haubitz, M., Bohnenstengel, F., Brunkhorst, R., et al. 2002. Cyclophosphamide pharmacokinetics and dose requirements in patients with renal insufficiency. Kidney Int. 61, 1495–1501.

Hauer, H.A., Bajema, I.M., Van Houwelingen, H.C., et al. 2002a. Determinants of outcome in ANCA-associated glomerulonephritis: a prospective clinico-histopathological analysis of 96 patients. Kidney Int. 62, 1732–1742.

Hauer, H.A., Bajema, I.M., van Houwelingen, H.C., et al. 2002b. Renal histology in ANCA-associated vasculitis: differences between diagnostic and serologic subgroups. Kidney Int. 61, 80–89.

Hellmich, B., Flossmann, O., Gross, W.L., et al. 2007. EULAR recommendations for conducting clinical studies and/or clinical trials in systemic vasculitis: focus on anti-neutrophil cytoplasm antibody-associated vasculitis. Ann. Rheum. Dis. 66, 605–617.

Henes, J.C., Fritz, J., Koch, S., et al. 2007. Rituximab for treatment-resistant extensive Wegener's granulomatosis-additive effects of a maintenance treatment with leflunomide. Clin. Rheumatol. 15, 15.

Hewins, P., Savage, C.O. 2003. ANCA and neutrophil biology. Kidney Blood Press. Res. 26, 221–225.

Hoffman, G.S., Kerr, G.S., Leavitt, R.Y., et al. 1992. Wegener granulomatosis: an analysis of 158 patients. Ann. Intern. Med. 116, 488–498.

Homma, S., Matsushita, H., Nakata, K. 2004. Pulmonary fibrosis in myeloperoxidase antineutrophil cytoplasmic antibody-associated vasculitides. Respirology 9, 190–196.

Iqbal, M.B., Fisher, N.G., Fox, K.M. 2005. Vasculitis masquerading as aortic valve endocarditis. Heart 91, e37.

Ito-Ihara, T., Ono, T., Nogaki, F., et al. 2006. Clinical efficacy of intravenous immunoglobulin for patients with MPO-ANCA-associated rapidly progressive glomerulonephritis. Nephron. Clin. Pract. 102, c35–c42.

Jayne, D. 2003. Current attitudes to the therapy of vasculitis. Kidney Blood Press. Res. 26, 231–239.

Jayne, D., Rasmussen, N., Andrassy, K., et al. 2003. A randomized trial of maintenance therapy for vasculitis associated with antineutrophil cytoplasmic autoantibodies. N. Engl. J. Med. 349, 36–44.

Jayne, D.R., Chapel, H., Adu, D., et al. 2000. Intravenous immunoglobulin for ANCA-associated systemic vasculitis with persistent disease activity. Q. J. Med. 93, 433–439.

Jayne, D.R., Gaskin, G., Pusey, C.D., et al. 1995. ANCA and predicting relapse in systemic vasculitis. Q. J. Med. 88, 127–133.

Jayne, D.R., Gaskin, G., Rasmussen, N., et al. 2007. Randomized trial of plasma exchange or high-dosage methylprednisolone as adjunctive therapy for severe renal vasculitis. J. Am. Soc. Nephrol. 20, 20.

Jayne, D.R., Marshall, P.D., Jones, S.J., et al. 1990. Autoantibodies to GBM and neutrophil cytoplasm in rapidly progressive glomerulonephritis. Kidney Int. 37, 965–970.

Jayne, D.R., Rasmussen, N. 1997. Treatment of antineutrophil cytoplasm autoantibody-associated systemic vasculitis: initiatives of the European Community Systemic Vasculitis Clinical Trials Study Group. Mayo Clin. Proc. 72, 737–747.

Jennette, J.C., Falk, R.J., Andrassy, K., et al. 1994. Proposal of an international consensus conference. Nomenclature of systemic vasculitides. Arthritis Rheum. 37, 187–192.

Joy, M.S., Hogan, S.L., Jennette, J.C., et al. 2005. A pilot study using mycophenolate mofetil in relapsing or resistant ANCA small vessel vasculitis. Nephrol. Dial. Transplant. 20, 2725–2732.

Keogh, K.A., Wylam, M.E., Stone, J.H., et al. 2005. Induction of remission by B lymphocyte depletion in eleven patients with refractory antineutrophil cytoplasmic antibody-associated vasculitis. Arthritis Rheum. 52, 262–268.

Keogh, K.A., Ytterberg, S.R., Fervenza, F.C., et al. 2006. Rituximab for refractory Wegener's granulomatosis: report of a prospective, open-label pilot trial. Am. J. Respir. Crit. Care Med. 173, 180–187.

Korbet, S.M., Schwartz, M.M., Evans, J., et al. 2007. Severe lupus nephritis: racial differences in presentation and outcome. J. Am. Soc. Nephrol. 18, 244–254.

Koukoulaki, M., Jayne, D.R. 2006. Mycophenolate mofetil in anti-neutrophil cytoplasm antibodies-associated systemic vasculitis. Nephron. Clin. Pract. 102, c100–c107.

Krafcik, S.S., Covin, R.B., Lynch, J.P. 3rd, et al. 1996. Wegener's granulomatosis in the elderly. Chest 109, 430–437.

Lane, S.E., Watts, R., Scott, D.G. 2005. Epidemiology of systemic vasculitis. Curr. Rheumatol. Rep. 7, 270–275.

Lane, S.E., Watts, R.A., Shepstone, L., et al. 2005. Primary systemic vasculitis: clinical features and mortality. Q. J. Med. 98, 97–111.

Langford, C.A., Talar-Williams, C., Sneller, M.C. 2000. Use of methotrexate and glucocorticoids in the treatment of Wegener's granulomatosis. Long-term renal outcome in patients with glomerulonephritis. Arthritis Rheum. 43, 1836–1840.

Leib, E.S., Restivo, C., Paulus, H.E. 1979. Immunosuppressive and corticosteroid therapy of polyarteritis nodosa. Am. J. Med. 67, 941–947.

Levy, J.B., Pusey, C.D. 2000. Nephrotoxicity of intravenous immunoglobulin. Q. J. Med. 93, 751–755.

Little, M.A., Bhangal, G., Smyth, C.L., et al. 2006. Therapeutic effect of anti-TNF-alpha antibodies in an experimental model of anti-neutrophil cytoplasm antibody-associated systemic vasculitis. J. Am. Soc. Nephrol. 17, 160–169.

Lockwood, C.M., Hale, G., Waldman, H., et al. 2003. Remission induction in Behcet's disease following lymphocyte depletion by the anti-CD52 antibody CAMPATH 1-H. Rheumatology (Oxford) 42, 1539–1544.

Lockwood, C.M., Rees, A.J., Pearson, T.A., et al. 1976. Immunosuppression and plasma-exchange in the treatment of Goodpasture's syndrome. Lancet 1, 711–715.

Ludemann, J., Utecht, B., Gross, W.L. 1990. Anti-neutrophil cytoplasm antibodies in Wegener's granulomatosis recognize an elastinolytic enzyme. J. Exp. Med. 171, 357–362.

Luqmani, R.A., Bacon, P.A., Moots, R.J., et al. 1994. Birmingham Vasculitis Activity Score (BVAS) in systemic necrotizing vasculitis. Q. J. Med. 87, 671–678.

Mahr, A.D., Neogi, T., Merkel, P.A. 2006. Epidemiology of Wegener's granulomatosis: lessons from descriptive studies and analyses of genetic and environmental risk determinants. Clin. Exp. Rheumatol. 24, S82–S91.

Metzler, C., Miehle, N., Manger, K., et al. 2007. Elevated relapse rate under oral methotrexate versus leflunomide for maintenance of remission in Wegener's granulomatosis. Rheumatology (Oxford) 46, 1087–1091.

Morton, S.J., Lanyon, P.C., Powell, R.J. 2000. Etoposide in Wegener's granulomatosis. Rheumatology (Oxford) 39, 810–811.

Muller, E., Schneider, W., Kettritz, U., et al. 2004. Temporal arteritis with pauci-immune glomerulonephritis: a systemic disease. Clin. Nephrol. 62, 384–386.

Nakamura, T., Matsuda, T., Kawagoe, Y., et al. 2004. Plasmapheresis with immunosuppressive therapy vs immunosuppressive therapy alone for rapidly progressive anti-neutrophil cytoplasmic autoantibody-associated glomerulonephritis. Nephrol. Dial. Transplant. 19, 1935–1937.

Neumann, I., Regele, H., Kain, R., et al. 2003. Glomerular immune deposits are associated with increased proteinuria in patients with ANCA-associated crescentic nephritis. Nephrol. Dial. Transplant. 18, 524–531.

Nguyen, T., Martin, M.K., Indrikovs, A.J. 2005. Plasmapheresis for diffuse alveolar hemorrhage in a patient with Wegener's granulomatosis: case report and review of the literature. J. Clin. Apher. 20, 230–234.

Omdal, R., Wildhagen, K., Hansen, T., et al. 2005. Anti-CD20 therapy of treatment-resistant Wegener's granulomatosis: favourable but temporary response. Scand. J. Rheumatol. 34, 229–232.

Popa, E.R., Stegeman, C.A., Abdulahad, W.H., et al. 2007. Staphylococcal toxic-shock-syndrome-toxin-1 as a risk factor for disease relapse in Wegener's granulomatosis. Rheumatology (Oxford) 46, 1029–1033.

Pusey, C.D., Rees, A.J., Evans, D.J., et al. 1991. Plasma exchange in focal necrotizing glomerulonephritis without anti-GBM antibodies. Kidney Int. 40, 757–763.

Reinhold-Keller, E., Fink, C.O., Herlyn, K., et al. 2002. High rate of renal relapse in 71 patients with Wegener's granulomatosis under maintenance of remission with low-dose methotrexate. Arthritis Rheum. 47, 326–332.

Roberts, W.C., Ko, J.M., Moore, T.R., et al. 2006. Causes of pure aortic regurgitation in patients having isolated aortic valve replacement at a single US tertiary hospital (1993 to 2005). Circulation 114, 422–429.

Rychlik, I., Jancova, E., Tesar, V., et al. 2004. The Czech registry of renal biopsies. Occurrence of renal diseases in the years 1994–2000. Nephrol. Dial. Transplant. 19, 3040–3049.

Sable-Fourtassou, R., Cohen, P., Mahr, A., et al. 2005. Antineutrophil cytoplasmic antibodies and the Churg–Strauss syndrome. Ann. Intern. Med. 143, 632–638.

Sanders, J.S., Huitma, M.G., Kallenberg, C.G., et al. 2006. Prediction of relapses in PR3-ANCA-associated vasculitis by assessing responses of ANCA titres to treatment. Rheumatology (Oxford) 45, 724–729.

Savige, J., Gillis, D., Benson, E., et al. 1999. International consensus statement on testing and reporting of Antineutrophil Cytoplasmic Antibodies (ANCA). Am. J. Clin. Pathol. 111, 507–513.

Schmitt, W.H., Birck, R., Heinzel, P.A., et al. 2005. Prolonged treatment of refractory Wegener's granulomatosis with 15-deoxyspergualin: an open study in seven patients. Nephrol. Dial. Transplant. 20, 1083–1092.

Schmitt, W.H., Hagen, E.C., Neumann, I., et al. 2004. Treatment of refractory Wegener's granulomatosis with antithymocyte globulin (ATG): an open study in 15 patients. Kidney Int. 65, 1440–1448.

Sinico, R.A., Di Toma, L., Maggiore, U., et al. 2006. Renal involvement in Churg–Strauss syndrome. Am. J. Kidney Dis. 47, 770–779.

Smith, K.G., Jones, R.B., Burns, S.M., et al. 2006. Long-term comparison of rituximab treatment for refractory systemic lupus erythematosus and vasculitis: remission, relapse, and re-treatment. Arthritis Rheum. 54, 2970–2982.

Sneller, M.C., Hoffman, G.S., Talar-Williams, C., et al. 1995. An analysis of forty-two Wegener's granulomatosis patients treated with methotrexate and prednisone. Arthritis Rheum. 38, 608–613.

Specks, U. 2001. Diffuse alveolar hemorrhage syndromes. Curr. Opin. Rheumatol. 13, 12–17.

Stasi, R., Stipa, E., Poeta, G.D., et al. 2006. Long-term observation of patients with anti-neutrophil cytoplasmic antibody-associated vasculitis treated with rituximab. Rheumatology 21, 21.

Stassen, P.M., Cohen Tervaert, J.W., Stegeman, C.A. 2007. Induction of remission in active anti-neutrophil cytoplasmic antibody-associated vasculitis with mycophenolate mofetil in patients who cannot be treated with cyclophosphamide. Ann. Rheum. Dis. 66, 798–802.

Stegeman, C.A., Tervaert, J.W., Sluiter, W.J., et al. 1994. Association of chronic nasal carriage of *Staphylococcus aureus* and higher relapse rates in Wegener granulomatosis. Ann. Intern. Med. 120, 12–17.

Szpirt, W.R.N. 1996. Plasma exchange and cyclosporin A in Wegener's granulomatosis. Int. J. Artif. Organs 10, 501–505.

Talar-Williams, C., Hijazi, Y.M., Walther, M.M., et al. 1996. Cyclophosphamide-induced cystitis and bladder cancer in patients with Wegener granulomatosis. Ann. Intern. Med. 124, 477–484.

Tesar, V., Jelinkova, E., Masek, Z., et al. 1998. Influence of plasma exchange on serum levels of cytokines and adhesion molecules in ANCA-positive renal vasculitis. Blood Purif. 16, 72–80.

The Wegener's Etanercept Trail (WGET) Research Group, 2005. Etanercept plus standard therapy for Wegener's granulomatosis. N. Engl. J. Med. 352, 351–361.

Ulm, S., Hummel, M., Emig, M., et al. 2006. Leukocytoclastic vasculitis and acute renal failure after influenza vaccination in an elderly patient with myelodysplastic syndrome. Onkologie 29, 470–472.

van der Woude, F.J., Rasmussen, N., Lobatto, S., et al. 1985. Autoantibodies against neutrophils and monocytes: tool for diagnosis and marker of disease activity in Wegener's granulomatosis. Lancet 1, 425–429.

Walsh, M., Chaudhry, A., Jayne, D. (in press). Long-term follow-up of patients with refractory ANCA-associated vasculitis treated with Alemtuzumab (CAMPATH 1-H). Ann. Rheum. Dis.

Walton, E.W. 1958. Giant-cell granuloma of the respiratory tract (Wegener's granulomatosis). Br. Med. J. 2, 265–270.

Wang, Y., Zhao, M.H., Yu, J., et al. 2004. The clinical and pathological characteristics of Chinese elderly patients with anti-neutrophil cytoplasmic autoantibodies associated small vessel vasculitis. Exp. Gerontol. 39, 1401–1405.

Watts, R., Lane, S., Hanslik, T., et al. 2007. Development and validation of a consensus methodology for the classification of the ANCA-associated vasculitides and polyarteritis nodosa for epidemiological studies. Ann. Rheum. Dis. 66, 222–227.

Watts, R.A., Scott, D.G. 2004. Epidemiology of the vasculitides. Semin. Respir. Crit. Care Med. 25, 455–464.

Wegener, F. 1936. Uber generaliste, septische efaberkrankungen. Dtsch. Pathol. Ges. 29, 202–210.

Westman, K.W., Bygren, P.G., Olsson, H., et al. 1998. Relapse rate, renal survival, and cancer morbidity in patients with Wegener's granulomatosis or microscopic polyangiitis with renal involvement. J. Am. Soc. Nephrol. 9, 842–852.

Westman, K.W., Selga, D., Bygren, P., et al. 1998. Clinical evaluation of a capture ELISA for detection of proteinase-3 antineutrophil cytoplasmic antibody. Kidney Int. 53, 1230–1236.

Xiao, H., Heeringa, P., Hu, P., et al. 2002. Antineutrophil cytoplasmic autoantibodies specific for myeloperoxidase cause glomerulonephritis and vasculitis in mice. J. Clin. Invest. 110, 955–963.

Zauner, I., Bach, D., Braun, N., et al. 2002. Predictive value of initial histology and effect of plasmapheresis on long-term prognosis of rapidly progressive glomerulonephritis. Am. J. Kidney Dis. 39, 28–35.

# CHAPTER 9

## Large and Medium Vessel Vasculitis: Mechanisms

Elisabeth Nordborg*, Claes Nordborg

*Department of Pathology, Sahlgrenska University Hospital, SE-413 45 Göteborg, Sweden*

## 1. Introduction

Takayasu's arteritis and giant cell arteritis (GCA) are chronic granulomatous vasculitides of unknown origin, targeting large- and middle-sized arteries (Björnsson, 2002). Takayasu's arteritis is mainly diagnosed in Southeast Asian female patients, during their second or third decade (Johnston et al., 2002), whereas GCA typically is a disease of elderly women of Nordic heritage (Nordborg and Nordborg, 2003). Characteristically, Takayasu's arteritis targets the aorta and its major branches, including the aortic valve. GCA, on the other hand, shows a strong preference for the cranial branches of the aorta, particularly the branches of the external and internal carotid arteries (Björnsson, 2002). Aortitis is seen in both entities although it is more common in Takayasu's arteritis (Gravinis, 2000). The typical macroscopic findings in Takayasu's arteritis are stenotic lesions caused by intimal proliferation and fibrotic contraction of the media and adventitia. Thrombosis, dissecting hemorrhage, diffuse dilatation, and vessel wall rupture occur almost exclusively in Takayasu's arteritis (Johnston et al., 2002); in GCA, dissecting hemorrhage and the formation of saccular aneurysms are restricted to the aorta. In full-blown GCA, the intima is markedly thickened, which causes severe luminal stenosis. However, thrombotic occlusion is exceptional.

There is a significant histological overlap between Takayasu's arteritis and GCA (Björnsson, 2002). Inflammatory cells invade all layers of the vessel wall in both Takayasu's arteritis and GCA, and as a rule the infiltrates are alternating with uninflamed skip lesions. The inflammatory cells are recruited via adventitial microvessels, and they invade the denser media tissue, resulting in structural disruption. Giant cells are seen in both Takayasu's arteritis and in GCA. However, despite its name, the identification of giant cells is not a prerequisite for the diagnosis in GCA; temporal artery specimens contain giant cells in about two-thirds of the cases at the very most.

## 2. Takayasu's arteritis: pathogenesis

The cause of Takayasu's arteritis remains unclear. The inflammatory infiltrate is composed of dendritic cells (DCs), macrophages, various subsets of T-cells ($\alpha\beta$, $\gamma\delta$, cytotoxic T-cells), and natural killer cells which enter the vessel wall via the vasa vasorum (Miyata, 2005; Seko, 2002). It has been proposed that DCs, activated by an as yet unidentified stimulus, recruit T-cells to the vessel wall. Interferon gamma (IFN-$\gamma$) produced by Th1 cells is indispensable for the formation of granulomas. In Takayasu's arteritis T-cells may have additional effector functions. The release of perforin, a protein that is able to directly

---

*Corresponding author.
Tel.: +46-31-342-10-00; Fax: +46-31-417283
E-mail address: nordborg@swipnet.se

damage cells by polymerizing to their surface, by natural killer cells, γδ T-cells and cytotoxic T-cells, may contribute to the vessel wall damage (Seko et al., 1994). Furthermore, vessel wall injury is caused by the release of matrix metalloproteinases (MMPs), reactive oxygen intermediates, and nitrosative stress (Miyata, 2005; Seko, 2002). The local production of growth factors such as vascular endothelial growth factor (VEGF) and platelet-derived growth factor (PDGF) contribute to intimal hyperplasia with prominent occlusive and stenotic lesions as a result.

## 3. Giant cell arteritis: pathogenesis

Despite differences in clinical manifestations, many pathogenetic principles are similar in Takayasu's arteritis and GCA, and similar rules apply in diagnostic and therapeutic approaches. The pathogenetic pathways have, however, been more thoroughly investigated in GCA, much due to the accessibility of the temporal artery. The following section therefore, will focus on GCA.

### 3.1. The immunopathogenesis

It is generally accepted that the vascular inflammation in GCA is driven by the orchestrated activity of DCs, T-lymphocytes, and activated macrophages. B-cells are rare and granulocytes are not a feature of GCA. The vasa vasorum of the adventitia, the capillary network supplying the vessel wall, have been regarded as the portal of entry for the inflammatory cells into the vessel wall (Nordborg and Nordborg, 1998; Weyand and Goronzy, 2003).

Activation of the T-cells occurs in the adventitia, where selected CD4+ T-cells undergo clonal expansion, suggesting antigen-driven responses (Weyand et. al., 1994; Weyand and Goronzy, 1995). However, no specific antigen has so far been detected. These T-cells, located in the tunica adventitia release IFN-γ, a critical cytokine which regulates the differentiation and function of tissue-infiltrating macrophages (Wagner et al., 1996; Weyand and Goronzy, 2003). Macrophages residing in different layers of the arterial wall are committed to distinct and non-overlapping functional pathways. Macrophages of the adventitia produce the proinflammatory cytokines interleukin (IL)-1β and IL-6, equipped to support T-cell activation, whereas those of the media synthesize MMPs and angiogenic and growth factors. Release of reactive oxygen intermediates and secretion of nitric oxide synthase are events related to macrophages of the intima which further contribute to tissue damage in GCA (Rittner et al., 1999). Resident cells of the arterial wall respond to the immune insult mediated by tissue-infiltrating cells by the migration and proliferation of myofibroblasts, which leads to severe intimal hyperplasia. In the aorta, the inflammatory infiltrate causes focal destruction of the media and the loss of elastic lamellae. This focal loss of elasticity and contractile power is held to be the cause of aneurysmal dilatation, dissection and hemorrhage in the aortic wall (Fig. 1) (Petursdottir et al., 1996). Secondary scarring of the inflammatory lesions in the aorta consists of collagen and disorganized smooth-muscle fibers (Petursdottir et al., 1996).

Two different types of multinucleated giant cells are encountered in the vascular lesions in GCA. The foreign-body giant cells are exclusively found in granulomas, associated with calcified parts of the lamina elastica interna (LEI), whereas the Langhans giant cells may be found in all layers of the wall, with a clear preponderance for the media–intima border. The mechanisms behind the formation of the two types of giant cell are not completely understood, and the stimuli controlling their activity remain to be elucidated.

### 3.2. Dendritic cells

The inflammatory activity of the vascular lesion is driven by adaptive immune responses. A crucial question is which mechanisms are involved in the initial T-cell activation and which cells are the

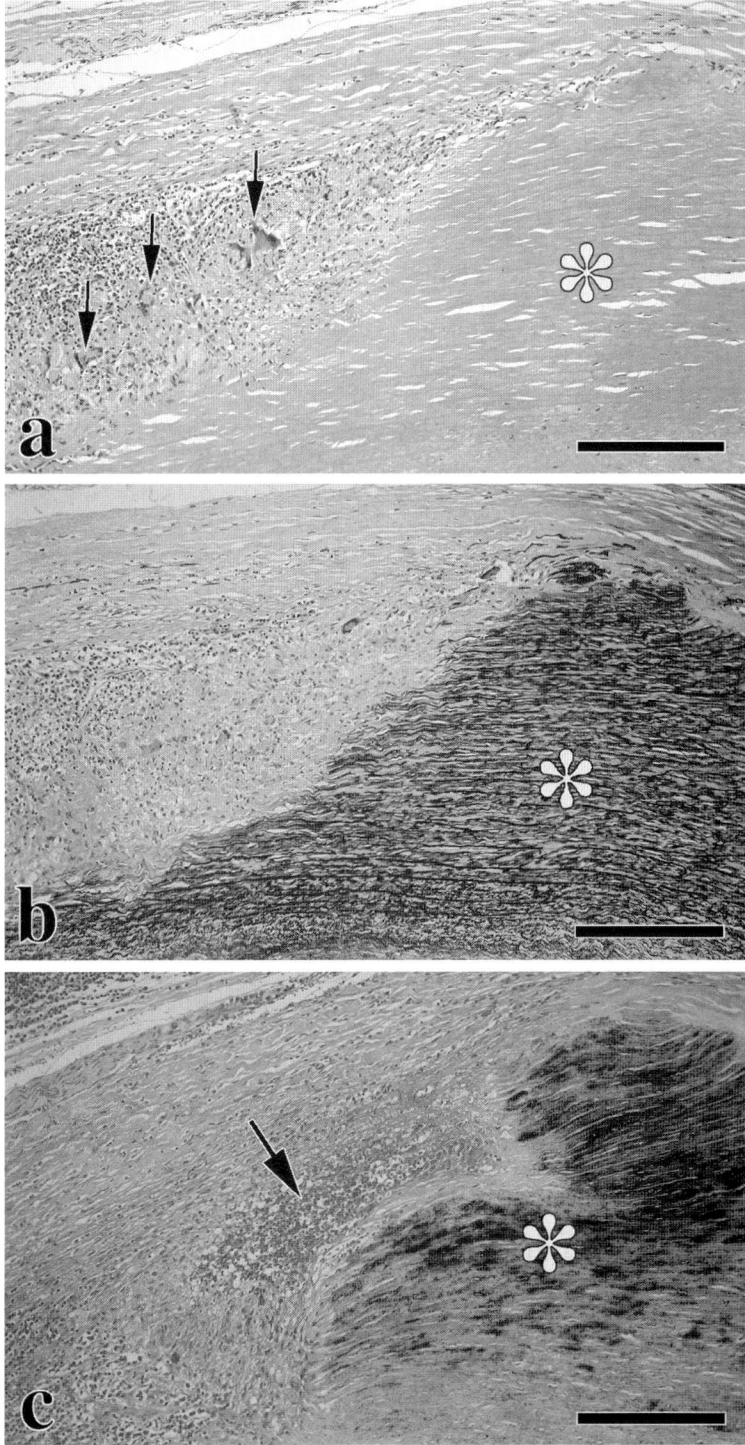

**Figure 1.** Giant cell aortitis. (a) Inflammation with multinucleated giant cells (arrows) adjacent to atrophic part of the media, in which no smooth-muscle cell nuclei are seen (asterisk). (Hematoxylin and Eosin; bar: 370 μm.) (b) Same area. Note the preserved, dark elastic lamellae in the atrophic part (asterisk), and the loss of elastic lamellae in the inflamed tissue. (Elastin; bar: 370 μm.) (c) Same area. Note the dark calcification in the atrophic part of the media (asterisk) and recent bleeding (arrow) in the inflamed tissue. (van Kossa; bar: 370 μm.)

antigen-presenting cells. During recent years it has become evident that the DCs, are critical to the activation of T-cells. These cells belong to a heterogeneous family of leukocytes with the ability to integrate innate information and convey it to lymphocytes (Reis e Sousa, 2004). The early innate signaling by DCs seems to be a prerequisite for the activation of both T- and B-cells. Consequently, the innate immunological pathway evidently *precedes* and seems to be critical for the activation of adaptive immune responses (Janeway, 1989). However, the communication between innate and adaptive immune mechanisms are intricate and complex and recent contributions show that also adaptive signals in some instances are capable of inducing DC activation (Manickasingham and Reis e Sousa, 2000; Mailliard et al., 2002).

The function of DCs in health and disease has been elucidated. In the arterial wall of medium-sized vessels there is normally a resident population of DCs in the adventitia of healthy individuals. These cells are strictly located in the adventitia, close to the outer border of the media. Characteristically, they lack CD83, indicating that they are in a resting state (Zhou and Tedder, 1995). Immature DCs play a role in the maintenance of T-cell unresponsiveness, called immunoprivilege, which is extremely important in the prevention of inappropriate autoimmunity (Huang and Mac Pherson, 2001; Randolph, 2000; Steinman and Nussenzweig, 2002). The function of the immature adventitial DCs is thought to contribute to immunosurveillance. However, it is unknown which types of antigen they sample, and which precise signals determine their maturation.

The functional capabilities of DCs change fundamentally as they transform from a resting to an active state. On encountering antigen in tissues their phagocytic properties are down-regulated and they switch to an antigen-presenting cell type (Sallusto and Lanzavecchia, 2000; Inaba et al., 2000). They modify their profile of chemokine receptors and migrate toward secondary lymphoid tissues via lymphatics (Steinman and Nussenzweig, 2002; Guermonprez et al., 2002) to initiate priming of naïve T-cells.

## 3.3. Dendritic cells in GCA

Studies by Weyand et al. (2005) have contributed to our knowledge of the function of DCs in medium-sized arteries, particularly the temporal artery. In full-blown GCA, the DCs are greatly increased in number and they populate not only the adventitia but also the media. Moreover, in GCA the DCs are no longer immature since they have acquired the activation marker CD83 and produce the chemokines CCL19 and CCL21. Furthermore, the DCs also express CCR7, resulting in their entrapment within the vasculitic lesion (Ma-Krupa et al., 2002) thereby, continuously taking an active part in driving the vasculitic process. In patients with PMR, the subclinical form of GCA, the DCs are also activated and capable of triggering T-cells, despite the lack of an inflammatory infiltrate in the vessel wall (Ma-Krupa et al., 2002). Such activation indicates that adventitial DCs may also be of importance in the early disease phase in GCA.

Experimental studies by Weyand et al. (Ma-Krupa et al., 2004), using human GCA artery-severe combined immunodeficiency (SCID) mouse chimeras, showed that the depletion of CD83+ DCs essentially abrogated the vasculitic lesions in the arterial wall, which may indicate that the DCs are not only the critical antigen-presenting cells but may also be a prerequisite for the sustained disease process. These results demonstrate the crucial role of DCs in the pathogenesis of GCA. A change in the functional status of the adventitial DCs is an early event in the disease process. Activation of adventitial DCs initiates and maintains T-cell responses in the artery and breaks self-tolerance in GCA (Ma-Krupa et al., 2004).

Which factors might break the resting state of adventitial DCs? Infectious agents, toxins, drugs, and autoantigens in arteries would qualify. An underlying infection as a trigger of GCA has repeatedly been suggested (Elling et al., 1996, 2000; Duhaut et al., 1999; Nordborg et al., 1998; Mitchell and Font, 2001; Helweg-Larsen et al., 2002; Regan et al., 2002). However, so far no material of infectious origin has been detected in the vessel wall. Experimental data (Ma-Krupa et al., 2004) revealed that immature adventitial DCs in healthy arteries were activated and highly responsive to systemic injection of lipopolysaccharide (LPS) with ensuing DC activation, T-cell recruitment and T-cell stimulation in the arterial wall. These observations show that blood-borne stimuli are sufficient triggers to initiate wall inflammation in temporal arteries. Vasculogenic antigens might derive from a systemic infectious event far from the blood vessel. Any episode of bacterial infection leading to release of LPS is able to stimulate adventitial DCs and thereby initiate the disease process. Microbial components and inflammatory cytokines have long been known to profoundly affect DC phenotype and function. However, the pathways involved in infection sensing by DCs still remain elusive.

A triggering antigen might also originate from the vessel wall itself. Although, the DCs have been shown to be the principal antigen-presenting cells once clinical symptoms are evident in GCA, the mechanisms preceding the overt disease state are not known. There might be other cells responsible for antigen presentation in the pre-clinical phase of GCA (Theofilopoulos et al., 2005). Furthermore, DCs are known to become activated in response to alterations in the internal milieu or in response to different self-molecules (Gallucci et al., 1999; Liu et al., 2001).

Although considerable progress has been made during the last decade in the understanding of pathogenetic mechanisms in GCA, the majority of studies have been performed on temporal arteries with full-blown inflammation. Consequently, the pathogenetic processes before the outbreak of the inflammatory reaction or during its early stages are less well understood. In the future, hopefully, new technologies will help to clarify the early immunopathogenesis of GCA in greater detail.

## 3.4. The morphology of GCA

A number of morphological investigations have provided new information regarding the pathogenesis of GCA. The use of plastic embedding and semi-thin serial sectioning of temporal arteries have been informative when it comes to the role of elastin-associated calcification. Semi-thin plastic sections give a more detailed image than paraffin sections, and small calcifications are better preserved and not displaced when sectioned in this hard medium.

## 3.5. Light microscopy: two phases of inflammation

Morphologically, two different types of inflammatory reactions are found in the temporal arteries from patients fulfilling the ACR criteria for GCA (Nordborg et al., 1991, 2000). One is a *foreign-body giant-cell reaction*, directed at small calcifications of the internal elastic membrane (IEM) (Figs. 2 and 3). These are not to be confused with the Mönckeberg-type of calcifications, which are localized entirely in the media (Mönckeberg, 1902). The foreign-body type of inflammation is focal, affecting only part of the arterial circumference (Fig. 4). Light-microscopically, large, polygonal cells, which accumulate around IEM calcifications, fuse to form foreign-body giant cells (Figs. 2 and 5). The foreign-body giant cells enclose and disintegrate the calcifications (Figs. 2, 3, and 5). In some biopsies, this type of foreign-body reaction is found in calcified, atrophic arterial segments, devoid of other inflammatory cells. However, more often small, lymphocyte-like cells are seen in pockets on the surface of the giant cells, and varying numbers of mononuclear cells surround them (Figs. 2 and 5) (Nordborg et al., 1991, 2000). The fact that IEM calcifications, and the foreign-body giant cell reaction against them, are strictly focal might explain the focality of the inflammatory process in GCA and might be the underlying cause of the occurrence of skip lesions.

In the other, more common *diffuse type of inflammation*, the different layers of the arterial wall are invaded by mononuclear inflammatory cells in the whole circumference of the vessel. In this phase, the Langhans type of giant cell may be

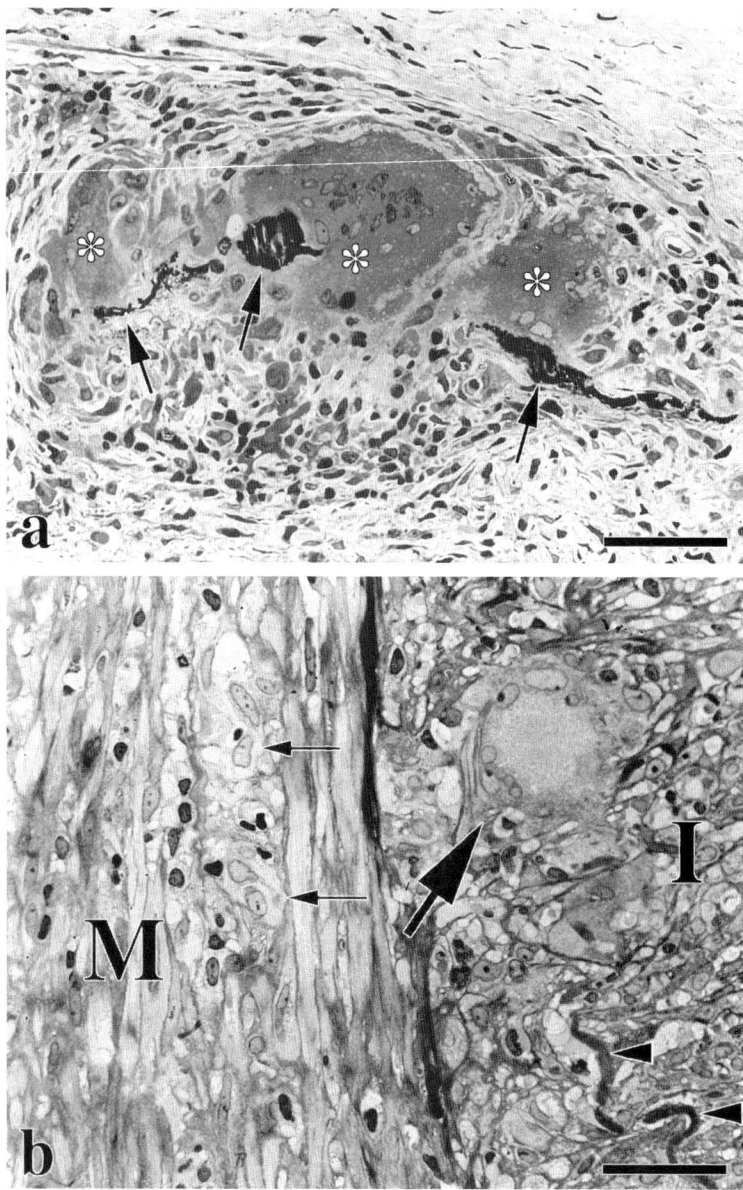

**Figure 2.** Inflammatory phases in GCA. (a) Focal, foreign-body giant-cell reaction. Granulomatous accumulation of large polygonal cells and foreign-body giant cells (asterisks) around black, calcified parts of the internal elastic membrane (IEM, arrows). The larger calcification is enclosed in a giant cell. The giant cell nuclei are randomly distributed. Note surrounding small, lymphocyte-like cells. (Semi-thin plastic section. Richardson; bar: 80 μm.) (b) Diffuse inflammation. Langhans giant cell (arrow) at the border between media (M) and intima (I). The giant cell nuclei are peripherally distributed. There are numerous large, pale macrophages (small arrows) in the media and intima. There are no enclosed fragments of the IEM in the giant cell cytoplasm, and there is no calcification. Arrowheads: IEM. (Semi-thin plastic section. Richardson; bar: 63 μm.)

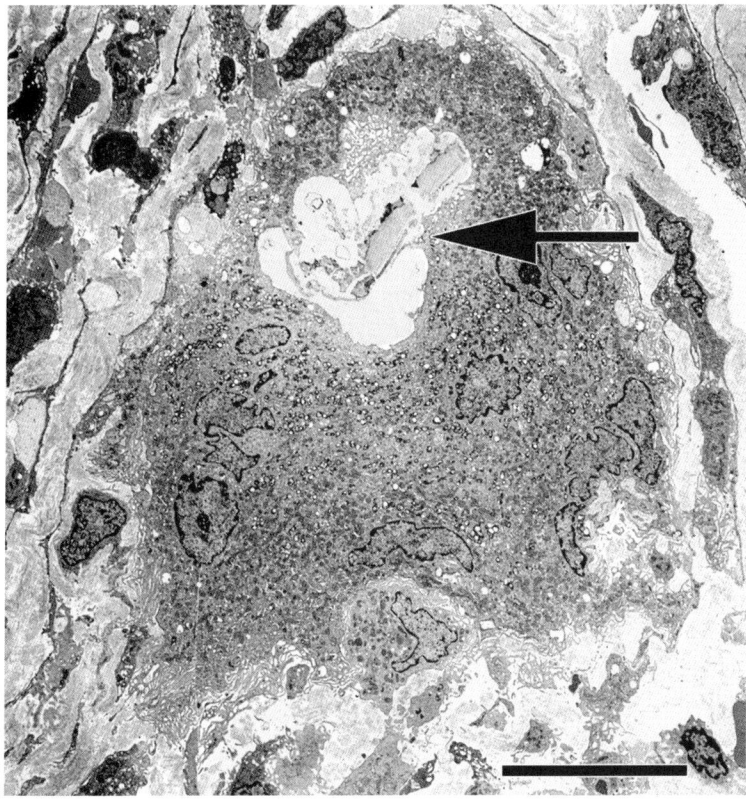

**Figure 3.** Electron micrograph of foreign-body giant cell in GCA. Foreign-body giant cell with a vacuole (arrow) containing a fragment of the IEM with dark, calcified surface. (Bar: 11 μm.)

seen, mainly at the media–intima border. This type of giant cell is neither associated with nor attacks calcified parts of the IEM (Fig. 2). A mixture of the two phases is seen in some biopsies (Nordborg et al., 1991, 2000).

The two types of inflammation may be found not only in temporal arteries from patients with a clinical diagnosis of temporal arteritis (TA), but also in patients with polymyalgia rheumatica (PMR). Both the foreign-body giant-cell reaction to calcified IEM, and the diffuse type of inflammation are seen. However, the inflammation is generally more restricted and less common in PMR than in TA, and it is *always* found in atrophic, calcified segments of the artery, which further indicates that IEM calcification plays a pathogenetic role in GCA/PMR. Inflammation was found in 40.7% of the PMR biopsies, when temporal arteries were sectioned serially with a 50 μm interval. In clinical practice, the interval between investigated sections is generally 2 mm or more; the small lesions in PMR may therefore easily be missed (Nordborg and Nordborg, 1995).

There is reason to believe that the focal foreign-body giant-cell reaction is an early phase of the inflammatory process in GCA. First, the circumference of the arteries displaying the full-blown diffuse inflammatory reaction is approximately 70% greater than that of the arteries displaying the focal foreign-body type of reaction (Nordborg et al., 1991). GCA causes arterial dilatation which is positively related to the degree of inflammation (Nordborg and Petursdottir, 2000). Therefore, the dilated, diffusely inflamed arteries should

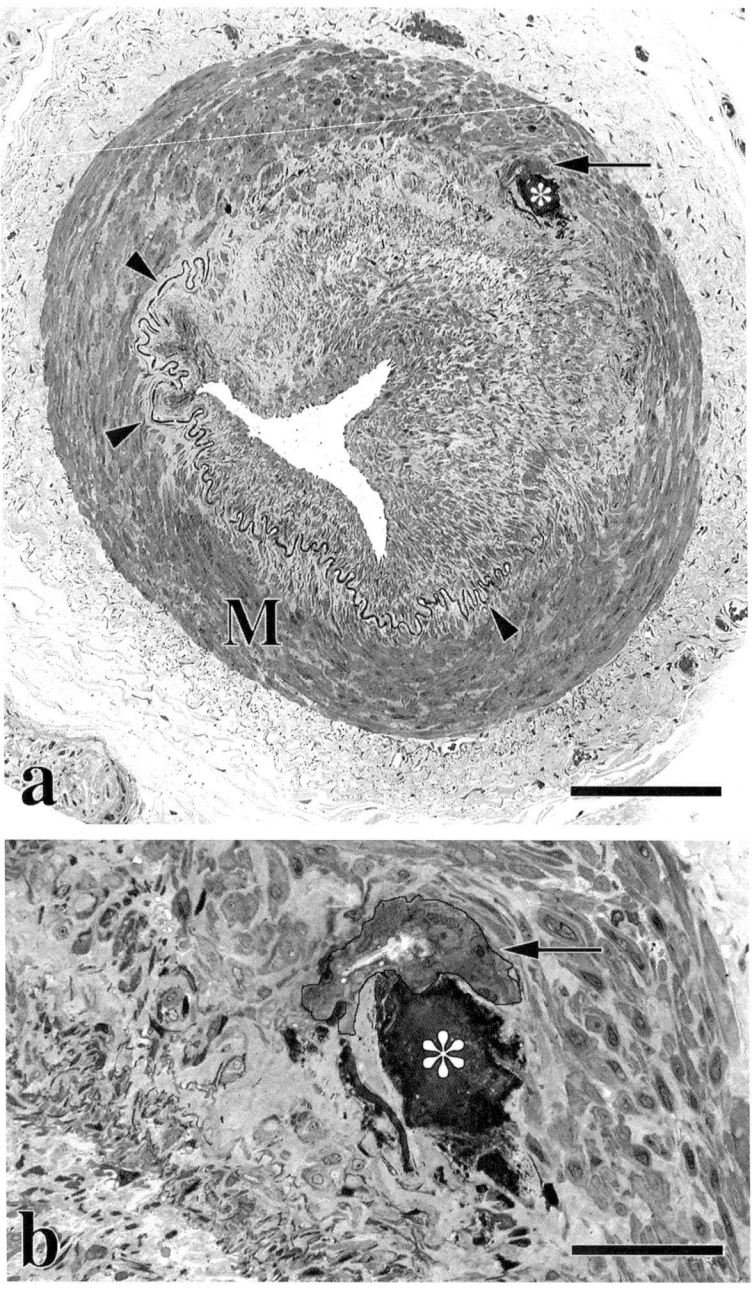

**Figure 4.** Early formation of foreign-body giant cell in GCA. (a) Early foreign-body giant cell (arrow) adjacent to a small focal calcification (asterisk) at the media–intima border. Note asymmetric thickening of the intima, and, in the contralateral half of the circumference, preserved IEM (arrowheads) and media (M). (Semi-thin plastic section. Richardson; bar: 430 μm.) (b) Detail of (a). Note the calcification (asterisk), and delineated giant cell (arrow). (Semi-thin plastic section. Richardson; bar: 108 μm.)

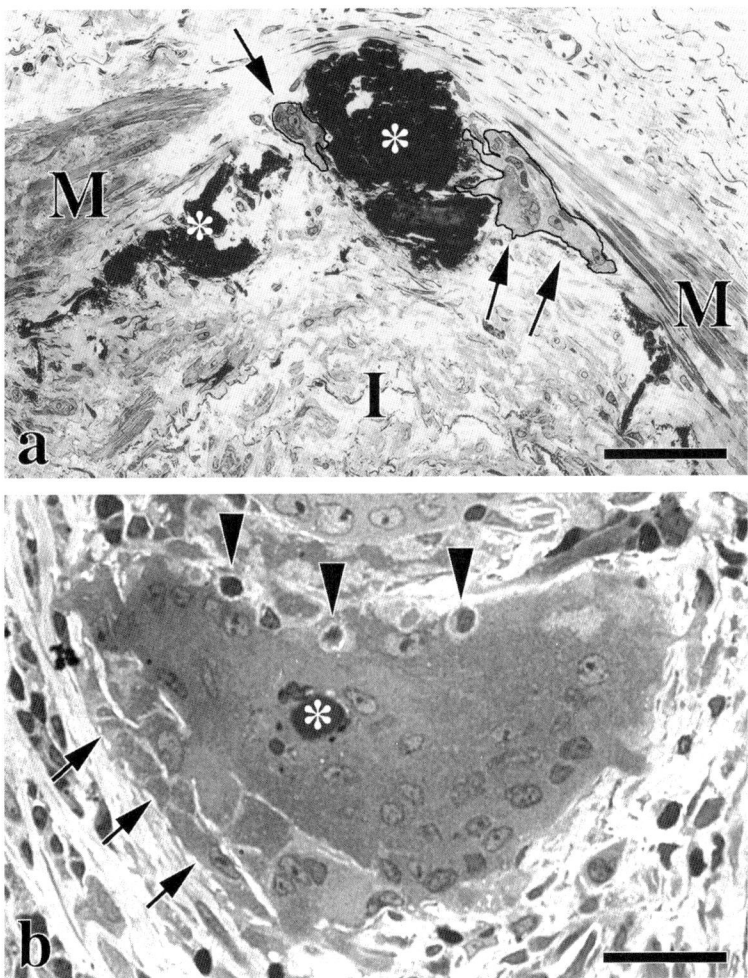

**Figure 5.** Foreign-body giant cells in GCA. (a) Early foreign-body giant cells (arrows, delineated) around black, calcified parts of the IEM (asterisks). Note the proximity between giant cells and media smooth-muscle cells. M: media. I: Intima. (Semi-thin plastic section. Richardson; bar: 60 μm.) (b) Foreign-body giant cell with numerous randomly distributed nuclei. Note large polygonal cells (arrows), which appear partly to be fused with the giant cell, and mononuclear, lymphocyte-like cells in pockets on its surface (arrowheads). Asterisk: enclosed calcified fragment. (Semi-thin plastic section. Richardson; bar: 26 μm.)

represent a later, more pronounced stage of the disease than the focally inflamed arteries. Second, the inflammatory process in GCA eventually leads to the destruction of the arterial wall and, generally, to a total loss of the IEM (Lie et al., 1970). However, in the focal foreign-body inflammatory phase, uninvolved parts of the circumference display well-preserved portions of media and IEM (Fig. 4).

### 3.6. The calcification of elastic membranes

An investigation of negative temporal artery biopsies from patients, aged 51 or more, who proved to have other clinical diagnoses than GCA or PMR revealed that focal calcifications of the IEM appear in the general population, growing more common with age, and being 2.62 times more common in women than in men

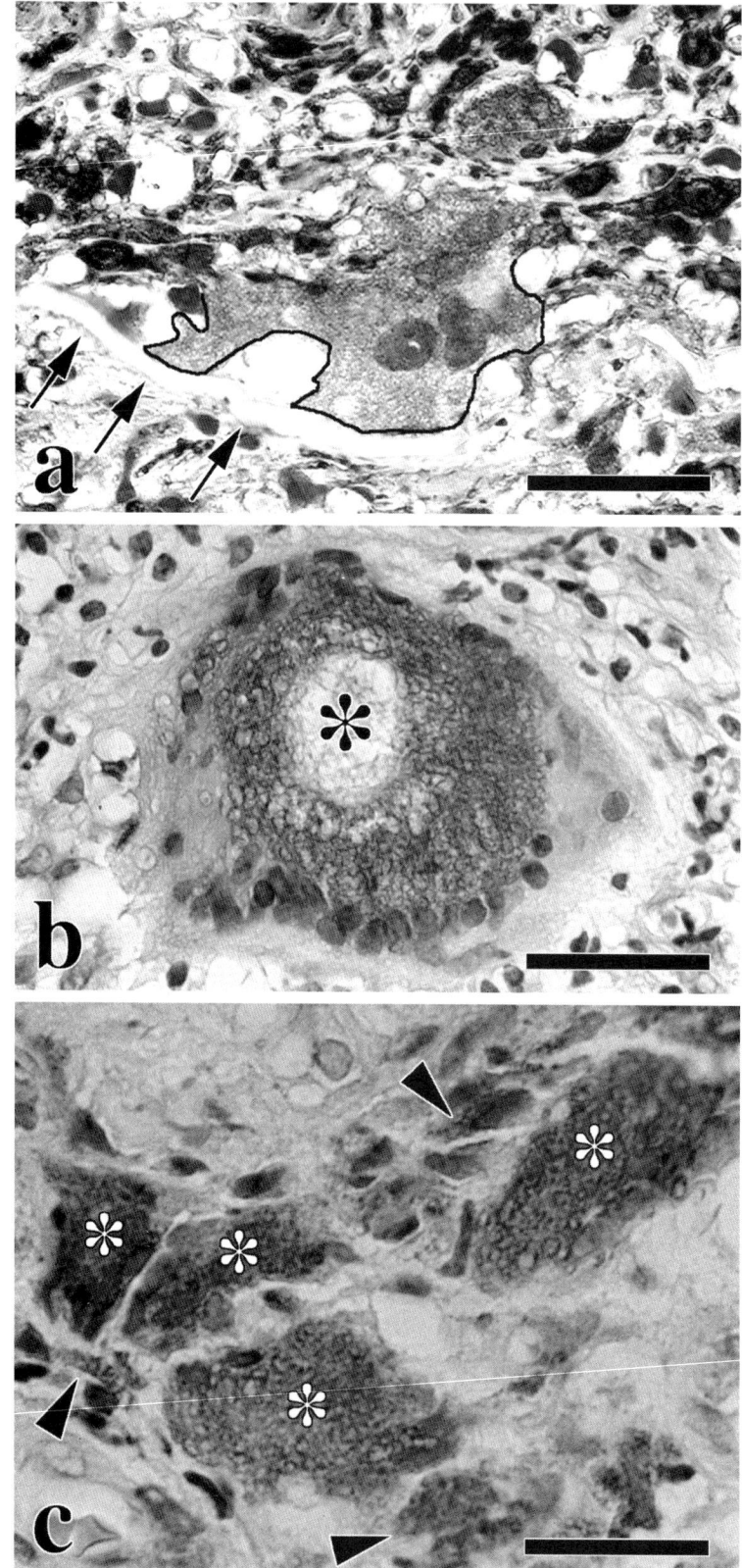

(Nordborg et al., 2001). Thus, the age and sex distribution of IEM calcifications in the general population proved to be similar to the age and sex distribution of GCA. The presence of calcifications was not related to diabetes mellitus or hypertension. Neither did they correlate significantly with atherosclerosis in other arteries (Nordborg et al., 2001).

GCA affects arteries with elastic membranes, that is medium size, muscular arteries with an IEM, and larger arteries with multiple elastic lamellae in their media such as the aorta. In the temporal arteries, the foreign-body giant-cell reaction is exclusively directed at IEM calcifications (Figs. 2–5), and the focal IEM calcifications are significantly greater in GCA and PMR than in controls (Nordborg et al., 1991). Analogous to the inflammatory process in the temporal artery, the inflammation in the aorta is directed at atrophic, calcified parts of the media (Fig. 1) (Petursdottir et al., 1996).

Thus, histopathological and epidemiological observations indicate that focal, elastin-associated calcification might be a pre-requisite for GCA, which many older people carry. A key question regarding the early pathogenesis of GCA would then be why only some of those individuals react against their calcifications, and why only some of the calcifications in an artery are attacked by foreign-body giant cells.

## 3.7. The histogenesis of giant cells

In *light microscopy of semi-thin plastic sections*, foreign-body giant cells have an irregular shape with randomly distributed nuclei. They are found in association with IEM calcifications, which they often enclose, and fragments of calcified elastic membranes are often found in large vacuoles in the giant cell cytoplasm (Figs. 2–5). They appear to be formed by the fusion of large, polygonal cells, which are closely associated with and similar to vascular smooth-muscle cells (Figs. 2 and 5). In contrast, the Langhans type of giant cell is not associated with IEM calcifications, and may be seen in all layers of the vessel wall, although most commonly at the media–intima border. This type of giant cell generally has peripherally distributed nuclei and a pale cytoplasm devoid of elastin-containing vacuoles (Fig. 2) (Nordborg et al., 1991, 1997).

*Immunocytochemically*, the Langhans type of giant cell and its surrounding inflammatory cells display a strong and uniform cytoplasmic immunoreactivity for the macrophage marker CD68, whereas the expression of this marker is uneven, and generally central in the foreign-body giant cells (Fig. 6). Immunostaining for alpha smooth-muscle actin shows a poor delineation between the vascular smooth-muscle cells and the foreign-body giant cells (Fig. 6), whereas this delineation is sharp when it comes to the Langhans type of giant cell (Nordborg et al., 1991, 1997). Both types of giant cell express HLA-DR (unpublished data).

*Ultrastructurally*, the foreign-body giant cells are surrounded by large polygonal cells with which they apparently fuse; innumerable thin intertwining processes are found between the cell surfaces (Nordborg et al., 1997). These surrounding cells are devoid of lysosomes suggesting they are unlikely to be monocytes or macrophages. Moreover, in the foreign-body giant cells, lysosomes tend to concentrate in the central part of the cytoplasm, not peripherally as might be expected if macrophages were added by fusion. The cells that fuse with the foreign-body giant cells do not show obvious ultrastructural smooth-muscle features, although they express smooth-muscle actin

**Figure 6.** Giant cell immunocytochemistry in GCA. (a) Brown expression of α smooth-muscle actin in vascular smooth-muscle cells and in a foreign-body giant cell (partly delineated). Note the diffuse border between the giant cell and adjacent cells, which show strong expression of α smooth-muscle actin. Arrows: IEM. (Anti-α-smooth-muscle actin and hematoxylin; bar: 30 μm.) (b) Foreign-body giant cell, showing central vacuole (asterisk), and brown CD68-expression. The periphery of the giant cell is largely immunonegative, and there is very sparse CD68 expression in its surrounding. (Anti-CD68 and hematoxylin; bar: 25 μm.) (c) Langhans giant cells (asterisks). Note the complete cytoplasmic CD68 expression in the giant cells, and numerous surrounding CD68-expressing macrophages (arrowheads). (Anti-CD68 and hematoxylin; bar: 25 μm.)

immunocytochemically. However, large, polygonal cells which form clusters close to IEM calcifications show, to a varying degree, ultrastructural features of smooth-muscle cells such as micropinocytotic vesicles, a fibrillary cytoplasm, and cytoplasmic densities. In contrast to the foreign-body giant cells, the lysosomes are numerous and evenly distributed in the Langhans giant cells and in the cells surrounding them (Nordborg et al., 1991, 1997).

## 3.8. Inflammation and vessel wall morphometry

The inflammatory reaction in GCA causes not only substantial arterial dilatation but also a marked thickening of the intima as reported in the first histopathological description of the disease by Horton et al. (1932). The intimal thickening is induced by the release of IFN-$\gamma$ and of factors such as PDGF and VEGF, produced by macrophages, giant cells, and smooth-muscle cells (Kaiser et al., 1998). The positive relationship between the degree of inflammation and intimal thickening has been morphometrically assessed (Nordborg and Petursdottir, 2000). Ischemic damage in GCA, such as retinal infarction and stroke, are caused by intimal thickening and luminal stenosis in the corresponding cranial arteries. Occlusive thrombosis is not a complication in GCA.

## 3.9. Neovascularization

Inflammation is also a major determinant of neovascularization in GCA. A significant positive relationship was observed between the degree of inflammation and the degree of vascularization in the media and in the outer and inner layers of the intima. Some of the new microvessels are formed by the budding of the adventitial vasa vasorum (angiogenesis). In some biopsies, the microvessels formed a prominent plexus in the intima without apparent connection with microvessels in the adventitia/media, and there were no signs of endothelial budding from the arterial lumen.

This observation might indicate an additional influence on neovascularization, the nature of which remains to be investigated (Nordborg et al., 2006). Ischemic complications are less common in GCA patients with prominent neovascularization of the temporal artery and with pronounced tissue and serum angiogenic activity (Cid et al., 2002; Hernandez-Rodriguez et al., 2003). The extent to which this beneficial effect is related to the formation of new vessels in the arterial wall and in peripheral vascular beds respectively remains to be investigated.

## 3.10. Concluding remarks

The earliest phase of the inflammatory process in GCA has been morphologically described in detail. However, whereas there is much new information about the full-blown inflammation, little is known about the immunology of the early inflammatory events and the actual initiation of the inflammatory process. Our observations indicate that vascular smooth-muscle cells change their phenotype and fuse to form foreign-body giant cells. The foreign-body giant cells that attack IEM calcifications during the early phase show a strong HLA-DR expression. The lymphocytes which surround the giant cells and which are found in pockets on their surface, express interleukin-2 receptor, indicating that antigen is presented by the foreign-body giant cells (unpublished data). Experimental data have shown that vascular smooth-muscle cells may change phenotype, and that they may have an antigen presenting capacity with an ensuing T-cell activation in atherosclerosis (Stemme et al., 1990; Suttles et al., 1995; Andreeva et al., 1997; Hansson, 2001). How the activity of foreign-body giant cells is linked to the presumably later development of Langhan's giant cells in GCA is not known. Further studies are required to increase the understanding of the immunological roles not only of the mononuclear inflammatory cells but also of foreign-body giant cells, vascular smooth-muscle cells, DCs, and calcification in this initial phase of GCA.

## Key points

**The pathogenesis of Takayasu's arteritis and GCA**

### Takayasu's arteritis
- Inflammatory infiltrate composed of DCs, macrophages and various subsets of perforin-producing T-cells ($\alpha\beta$, $\gamma\delta$, cytotoxic T-cells) and natural killer cells.
- Inflammatory cells enter the vessel wall via the vasa vasorum.
- DCs are proposed to recruit and activate T-cells.

### Giant cell arteritis
- Inflammatory infiltrate dominated by T-lymphocytes and activated macrophages, which produce pro-inflammatory cytokines and tissue-damaging factors.
- Inflammatory cells enter the vessel wall via the vasa vasorum.
- DCs play a crucial role in the pathogenesis of GCA. Activated adventitial DCs initiate and maintain T-cell responses in the artery and breaks self-tolerance in GCA.
- The pathways involved in the activation of DCs still remain elusive.
- Morphologically, the initial inflammatory event in GCA is a foreign-body giant-cell reaction against small calcifications of the IEM, followed by a diffuse invasion of mononuclear cells.
- In the aorta, the inflammation is directed at atrophic, calcified parts of the media.
- In the general population, the age and sex distribution of small IEM calcifications is the same as the age and sex distribution of GCA.
- A key question is why only some individuals react against their calcifications and why only some of the calcifications in an artery are attacked by foreign-body giant cells.

## References

Andreeva, E.R., Pugach, I.M., Orekhov, A.N. 1997. Subendothelial smooth muscle cells of human aorta express macrophage antigen in situ in vitro. Atherosclerosis 135, 19.

Björnsson, J. 2002. Histopathology of primary vasculitic disorders. In: G.S. Hoffman, C.M. Weyand (Eds.), Inflammatory diseases of blood vessels. Marcel Dekker, Inc., New York, pp. 255–265.

Cid, M.C., Hernandez-Rodriguez, J., Esteban, M.J., Cebrian, M., Ghy, Y.S., Font, C., Urbano-Marquez, A., Grau, J.M., Kleinman, H.K. 2002. Tissue and serum angiogenetic activity is associated with low prevalence of ischemic complications in patients with giant cell arteritis. Circulation 106, 1664.

Duhaut, P., Bosshard, S., Calvet, A., Pinede, L., Demolombe-Rague, S., Dumontet, C., Loire, R., Seydoux, D., Ninet, J., Pasquier, J., Aymard, M. 1999. Giant cell arteritis and polymyalgia rheumatica, and viral hypothesis: a multicenter, prospective case-control study. J. Rheumatol. 26, 361.

Elling, P., Olsson, A.T., Elling, H. 1996. Synchronous variations of the incidence of temporal arteritis and polymyalgia rheumatica in different regions of Denmark: association with epidemics of *Mycoplasma pneumoniae* infection. J. Rheumatol. 23, 112.

Elling, P., Olsson, A.T., Elling, H. 2000. Human *Parvovirus* and giant cell arteritis: a selective arteritic impact? Clin. Exp. Rheumatol. 18 (Suppl. 20), s12.

Gallucci, S., Lolkema, M., Matzinger, P. 1999. Natural adjuvants: endogenous activators of dendritic cells. Nat. Med. 5, 1249.

Gravinis, M.B. 2000. Giant cell arteritis and Takayasu aortitis: morphologic, pathogenetic and etiologic factors. Int. J. Cardiol. 75 (Suppl. 1), S21.

Guermonprez, P., Valladeau, J., Zitvogel, L., Thery, C., Amigorena, S. 2002. Antigen presentation and T cell stimulation by dendritic cells. Annu. Rev. Immunol. 20, 621.

Hansson, G.K. 2001. Immune mechanisms in atherosclerosis. Arterioscler. Thromb. Vasc. Biol. 21, 1896.

Helweg-Larsen, J., Tarp, N., Obel, N., Baslung, B. 2002. No evidence of parvovirus B19, *Chlamydia pneumoniae*, or human herpes virus infection in temporal artery biopsies in patients with giant cell arteritis. Rheumatology 41, 445.

Hernandez-Rodriguez, J., Segarra, M., Vilardell, C., Sanchez, M., Garcia-Martinez, A., Esteban, M.J., Urbano-Marquez, A., Grau, J.M., Colomer, D., Kleinman, H.K., Cid, M.C. 2003. Elevated production of interleukin-6 is associated with a lower incidence of disease-related ischemic events in patients with giant cell arteritis. Angiogenetic activity of interleukin-6 as a potential protective mechanism. Circulation 107, 2428.

Horton, B.T., Magath, T.B., Brown, G.E. 1932. An undescribed form of arteritis of the temporal vessel. Proc. Mayo. Clin. 7, 700.

Huang, F.P., Mac Pherson, G.G. 2001. Continuing education of the immune system-dendritic cells, immune regulation and tolerance. Curr. Mol. Med. 1, 457.

Inaba, K.S., Turley, S., Iyoda, T., Yamaide, F., Shimoyama, S., Reis e Sousa, C., German, R.N., Mellman, I., Steinman, R.M. 2000. The formation of immunogenic major histocompatibility complex class II-peptide ligands in lysosomal compartments of dendritic cells is regulated by inflammatory stimuli. J. Exp. Med. 191, 927.

Janeway, C.A., Jr. 1989. Approaching the asymptote? Evolution and revolution in immunology. Cold. Spring. Harb. Symp. Quant. Biol. 54, 1.

Johnston, S.I., Lock, R.J., Gompels, M.M. 2002. Takayasu arteritis: a review. J. Clin. Pathol. 55, 481.

Kaiser, M., Weyand, C.M., Björnsson, J., Goronzy, J.J. 1998. Platelet-derived growth factor, intimal hyperplasia, and ischemic complications in giant cell arteritis. Arthritis Rheum. 41, 623.

Lie, J.T., Brown, A.L., Carter, E.T. 1970. Spectrum of aging changes in temporal arteries. Its significance, in interpretation of biopsy of temporal artery. Arch. Path. 90, 278.

Liu, Y.J., Kanzler, H., Soumelis, V., Gilliet, M. 2001. Dendritic cell lineage, plasticity and cross-regulation. Nat. Immunol. 2, 585.

Mailliard, R.B., Egawa, S., Cai, Q., Kalinska, A., Bykovskaya, S.N., Lotze, M.T., Kapsenberg, M.L., Storkus, W.J. 2002. Complementary dendritic cell-activating function of CD8+ and CD4+ T cells: helper role of CD8+ T cells in the development of T helper type-1 responses. J. Exp. Med. 195, 473.

Ma-Krupa, W.M., Dewan, M., Jeon, M.S., Kurtin, P.J., Young, B.R., Goronzy, J.J., Weyand, C.M. 2002. Trapping of misdirected dendritic cells in the granulomatous lesions of giant cell arteritis. Am. J. Pathol. 161, 1815.

Ma-Krupa, W.M., Jeon, M.S., Spoerl, S., Tedder, T., Goronzy, J.J., Weyand, C.M. 2004. Activation of arterial wall dendritic cells and breakdown of self-tolerance in giant cell arteritis. J. Exp. Med. 199, 173.

Manickasingham, S., Reis e Sousa, C. 2000. Microbial and T cell-derived stimuli regulate antigen presentation by dendritic cells in vivo. J. Immunol. 165, 5027.

Mitchell, B.M., Font, R.J. 2001. Detection of *Varicella zoster* virus DNA in some patients with giant cell arteritis. Invest. Ophthalmol. Vis. Sci. 42, 2572.

Miyata, T. 2005. Takayasu's arteritis. In: H. Kallimo (Ed.), Pathology & Genetics: Cerebrovascular Diseases. Allen Press, Inc., Lawrence, KS.

Mönckeberg, J.G. 1902. Über die reine Mediaverkalkung der Extremitätenarterien und ihr Verhalten zur Arteriosklerose. Virchows Arch. Pathol. Anat. 171, 141.

Nordborg, C., Larsson, K., Nordborg, E. 2006. A stereological study of neovascularisation in temporal arteritis. J. Rheumatol. 33, 2020.

Nordborg, C., Nordborg, E., Petursdottir, V. 2000. Giant cell arteritis. Epidemiology, etiology and pathogenesis. APMIS 108, 713.

Nordborg, C., Nordborg, E., Petursdottir, V., Fyhr, I.-M. 2001. Calcification of the internal elastic membrane in temporal arteries: Its relation to age and gender. Clin. Exp. Rheumatol. 19, 565.

Nordborg, C., Nordborg, E., Petursdottir, V., La Guardia, J., Mahalingam, R., Wellish, M., Gilden, D.H. 1998. Search for *Varicella zoster* virus in giant cell arteritis. Ann. Neurol. 44, 413.

Nordborg, C., Petursdottir, V. 2000. Vessel wall morphometry in giant cell arteritis. Arthritis Care Res. 13, 286.

Nordborg, E., Bengtsson, B.-Å., Nordborg, C. 1991. Temporal artery morphology and morphometry in giant cell arteritis. APMIS 99, 1013.

Nordborg, E., Bengtsson, B.Å., Petursdottir, V., Nordborg, C. 1997. Morphological aspects of giant cells in giant cell arteritis: An electron-microscopic and immunocytochemical study. Clin. Exp. Rheumatol. 15, 129.

Nordborg, E., Nordborg, C. 1995. The influence of sectional interval on the reliability of temporal artery biopsies in polymyalgia rheumatica. Clin. Rheumatol. 14, 330.

Nordborg, E., Nordborg, C. 1998. The inflammatory reaction in giant cell arteritis: An immunohistochemical investigation. Clin. Exp. Rheumatol. 16, 165.

Nordborg, E., Nordborg, C. 2003. Giant cell arteritis: epidemiological clues to its pathogenesis and an update of its treatment. Rheumatology 42, 413.

Petursdottir, V., Nordborg, E., Nordborg, C. 1996. Atrophy of the aortic media in giant cell arteritis. APMIS 104, 191.

Randolph, G.I. 2000. Dendritic cell migration to lymph nodes; cytokines, chemokines and lipid mediators. Semin. Immunol. 13, 267.

Regan, M.J., Wood, B.J., Hsieh, Y.H., Theodore, M.L., Quinn, T.C., Hellmann, D.C., Green, W.R., Gaydos, C.A., Stone, J.H. 2002. Temporal arteritis and *Chlamydia pneumoniae*: failure to detect the organism by polymerase chain reaction in ninety cases and ninety controls. Arthritis Rheum. 46, 1056.

Reis e Sousa, C. 2004. Activation of dendritic cells: translating innate into adaptive immunity. Curr. Opin. Immunol. 16, 21.

Rittner, H.L., Kaiser, M., Brack, L.I., Szweda, J.J., Goronzy, J.J., Weyand, C.M. 1999. Tissue-destructive macrophages in giant cell arteritis. Circ. Res. 84, 1050.

Sallusto, F., Lanzavecchia, A. 2000. Understanding dendritic cell and T-lymphocyte traffic through the analysis of chemokine receptor expression. Immunol. Rev. 177, 134.

Seko, Y. 2002. Takayasu's arteritis: pathogenesis. In: G.S. Hoffman, C.M. Weyand (Eds.), Inflammatory Diseases of Blood Vessels. Marcel Dekker, Inc., New York, p. 455.

Seko, Y., Minota, S., Kawasaki, A., Shinkai, Y., Maeda, K., Yagita, H., Okumora, K., Sato, O., Takagi, A., Tada, Y., Yazaki, Y. 1994. Perforin-secreting killer cell infiltration and expression of a 65-kDa heat-shock protein in aortic tissue of patients with Takayasu's arteritis. J. Clin. Invest. 93, 750.

Steinman, R.M., Nussenzweig, M.C. 2002. Avoiding horror autotoxicus: the importance of dendritic cells in peripheral T cell tolerance. Proc. Natl. Acad. Sci. USA 99, 351.

Stemme, S., Fager, G., Hansson, G.K. 1990. MHC class II antigen expression in human vascular smooth muscle cells is induced by interferon-gamma and modulated by tumour necrosis factor and lymphotoxin. Immunology 60, 243.

Suttles, J., Miller, R.W., Moyer, C.F. 1995. T-cell vascular smooth muscle interactions: antigen-specific activation and cell cycle blockade of T helper clones by cloned vascular smooth muscle cells. Exp. Cell. Res. 218, 331.

Theofilopoulos, A.N., Baccala, R., Beutler, B., Kono, D.H. 2005. Type I interferons (alpha/beta) in immunity and autoimmunity. Annu. Rev. Immunol. 23, 307.

Wagner, A.D., Björnsson, J., Bartley, G.B., Goronzy, J.J., Weyand, C.M. 1996. Interferon-gamma-producing T cells in giant cell vasculitis represent a minority of tissue-infiltrating cells and are located distant from the site of pathology. Am. J. Pathol. 148, 1925.

Weyand, C.M., Goronzy, J.J. 1995. Giant cell arteritis as an antigen-driven disease. Rheum. Dis. Clin. North. Am. 21, 1027.

Weyand, C.M., Goronzy, J.J. 2003. Medium- and large-vessel vasculitis, mechanisms of disease-review article. N. Engl. J. Med. 349, 160.

Weyand, C.M., Ma-Krupa, W., Pryshchep, O., Gröschel, S., Bernardino, R., Goronzy, J.J. 2005. Vascular dendritic cells in giant cell arteritis. Ann. N.Y. Acad. Sci. 1062, 195.

Weyand, C.M., Schonberger, J., Oppitz, U., Hunder, N.N., Hicock, K.C., Goronzy, J.J. 1994. Distinct vascular lesions in giant cell arteritis share identical T-cell clonotypes. J. Exp. Med. 179, 951.

Zhou, L.J., Tedder, T.F. 1995. Human blood dendritic cells selectively express CD83, a member of the immunoglobulin superfamily. J. Immunol. 154, 3821.

# CHAPTER 10

# Large and Medium Vessel Vasculitis: Clinical Features and Treatment

Eamonn S. Molloy*, Gary S. Hoffman

*Center for Vasculitis Care and Research, Department of Rheumatic and Immunologic Diseases/Desk A50, Cleveland Clinic Foundation, 9500 Euclid Avenue, Cleveland, OH 44195, USA*

## 1. Introduction

The systemic vasculitides are a heterogeneous group of disorders characterized by inflammation of blood vessels. They are typically classified according to the predominant vessel size involved, the nature of the inflammatory lesion and the organ systems that are most frequently affected (Hunder et al., 1990a; Jennette et al., 1994). Giant cell arteritis (GCA) and Takayasu's arteritis (TAK) are the most classical examples of inflammatory diseases of large vessels. However, large vessel vasculitis can also be a component of diseases that also affect other caliber vessels such as Behçet's syndrome, sarcoidosis, Cogan's syndrome (CS), and Kawasaki's disease (KD). In addition, other disorders may mimic large vessel vasculitis and should be considered in the differential diagnosis of patients presenting with features suggestive of large vessel vasculitis and renal disease (see Table 1). Polyarteritis nodosa (PAN) is strictly a medium vessel disease. Most renal disease complicating vasculitis is due to glomerulonephritis, which may be a component of Henoch–Schonlein purpura, Wegener's granulomatosis, microscopic polyangiitis, Churg–Strauss syndrome (CSS), viral-associated vasculitis, and idiopathic cryoglobulinemia. These entities are discussed in Chapters 7, 8, 12, and 13. This chapter will instead focus on large and medium-sized vessel diseases that may lead to renal disease because of regional or global renal ischemia. Very rarely these entities may also involve glomerular capillaries (i.e., cause glomerulonephritis).

Table 1
Differential diagnosis of large vessel vasculitis

| Differential diagnosis of large vessel vasculitis |
| --- |
| Diseases characterized by large vessel vasculitis |
|   Takayasu's arteritis |
|   Giant cell arteritis |
| Diseases that may cause large vessel vasculitis[a] |
|   Cogan's syndrome |
|   Behçet's disease |
|   Kawasaki's disease |
|   Sarcoidosis |
|   Chronic idiopathic periaortitis/inflammatory abdominal aortic aneurysm |
|   Other inflammatory disorders (e.g., rheumatoid arthritis, systemic lupus erythematosus, seronegative spondyloarthropathies, relapsing polychondritis) |
| Diseases that may mimic large vessel vasculitis |
|   Atherosclerosis[b] |
|   Infectious causes (e.g., syphilis, tuberculosis, mycotic aneurysm)[b] |
|   Heritable disorders (e.g., Ehler–Danlos syndrome type IV, Marfan's syndrome) |
|   Fibromuscular dysplasia |
|   Iatrogenic (e.g., post-radiation therapy) |

[a] These diseases may also affect medium-sized and small vessels.

[b] Inflammation is present in each of these, but is secondary to known causes (e.g., infectious agents, lipid deposition and oxidation).

*Corresponding author.
Tel.: +216-445-6996; Fax: +216-445-7569
E-mail address: molloye@ccf.org

## 2. Takayasu's arteritis

### 2.1. Clinical features

TAK is an idiopathic systemic inflammatory disease characterized by vasculitis affecting the aorta and its primary branches. TAK predominantly affects women of reproductive age, with mean age at diagnosis in the third decade in most series (Ishikawa, 1988; Kerr et al., 1994; Nakao et al., 1967; Subramanyan et al., 1989; Vanoli et al., 2005; Zheng et al., 1990). However, its occurrence has been recognized in older patients, males and in all races (Hoffman, 1996). The subclavian and carotid arteries are the most frequently affected branch vessels, although any part(s) of the aorta and its major branches may be involved. Affected vessels most frequently (75%) develop luminal narrowing and occlusion due to myointimal proliferation and secondary atherosclerosis. Aneurysms constitute approximately 25% of lesions. They are most common in the thoracic aorta, especially in its ascending and arch regions.

Typical clinical features of TAK are listed in Table 2. There is considerable variability in the presenting symptoms in TAK patients. About half of all patients may have constitutional symptoms. Limb claudication, neurologic, cardiac, or gastrointestinal symptoms may develop due to vessel stenosis or occlusion. However, the absence of such symptoms does not preclude the existence of significant abnormalities of the arteries in question, as sub-clinical changes may not yet have produced significant ischemia or may vary with the degree of usage of the affected limb and the development of collateral vessels over time.

Physical examination of patients suspected of having TAK must include a thorough examination of the vascular system that assesses symmetry of pulses and blood pressure in all four extremities and auscultation of all major arteries for bruits. Vessels may also be tender (e.g., carotidynia). If there is large vessel stenosis of major vessels, blood pressure measurements in that limb may not accurately reflect aortic pressures and central hypertension may be unrecognized and untreated as a result. In some cases, where the circulation to all four extremities is attenuated, the only reliable blood pressure measurements will be readings taken in the aorta during catheter-based angiography.

Careful cardiac auscultation should be performed to detect aortic regurgitation, which commonly occurs due to dilatation of the aortic root. Other cardiac manifestations include arrhythmias, cardiomyopathy, congestive heart failure, coronary artery stenoses, angina, myocardial infarction, and sudden death. Involvement of carotid and vertebral arteries can result in transient ischemic attacks, blindness, or stroke. However, symptoms of cerebrovascular insufficiency can be non-specific and easily overlooked (e.g., dizziness, vertigo, lightheadedness, near-syncope). Visual symptoms may occur due to decreased perfusion of the retinal artery and/or anterior ischemic optic neuropathy resulting from occlusion of the internal carotid or common carotid artery. However, more common causes of visual impairment in TAK are hypertensive retinopathy, glaucoma, and cataract formation

Table 2
Clinical features of Takayasu's arteritis

| Abnormality | Frequency (%) |
|---|---|
| Dizziness/lightheadedness | 18–50 |
| Syncope | 13–25 |
| Transient ischemic attack/stroke | 5–17 |
| Visual disturbances | 8–20 |
| Headache | 18–57 |
| Carotidynia | 10–35 |
| Vascular bruits | 23–96 |
| Pulse deficit | 22–96 |
| Blood pressure asymmetry | 13–65 |
| Claudication | 29–40 |
| Congestive cardiac failure | 5–12 |
| Hypertension | 17–72 |
| Aortic valve regurgitation | 8–24 |
| Chest pain | 13–25 |
| Dyspnea | 11–72 |
| Palpitations | 19–43 |
| Myalgias | 5–25 |
| Arthralgias | 5–53 |
| Weight loss | 4–22 |
| Malaise | 29–60 |
| Fever | 8–44 |
| Erythema nodosum | 0–16 |

*Source*: Hall et al. (1985), Ishikawa (1978), Jain et al. (1996), Kerr et al. (1994), Lupi-Herrera et al. (1977), Maksimowicz-McKinnon et al. (2007), Shelhamer et al. (1985), Vanoli et al. (2005).

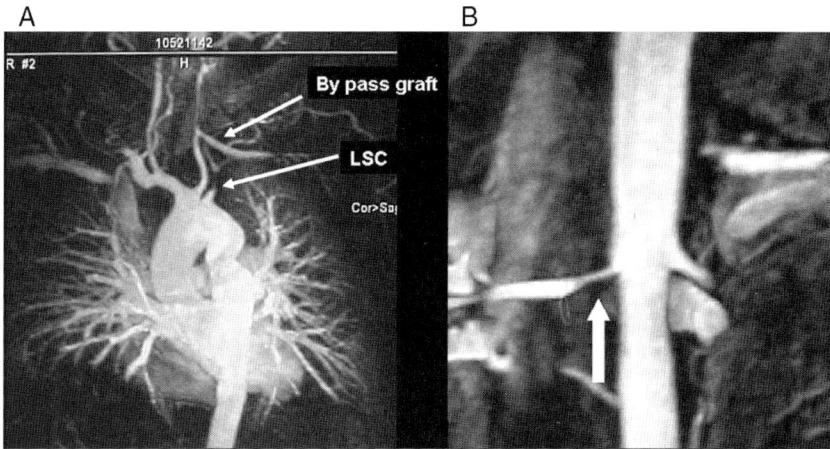

Figure 1. (A) Magnetic resonance angiogram (MRA) in a patient with Takayasu's arteritis (TAK). Failed bypass from the left subclavian artery (LSC) to left carotid. LSC occlusion followed the bypass, resulting in retrograde flow through the bypass graft. SC stenosis is the most common lesion in TAK. This illustrates why bypass to the arch vessels should originate from the ascending aorta. (B) MRA in a patient with TAK demonstrating right renal artery stenosis.

(due at least in part to corticosteroid therapy). Pulmonary involvement in TAK is increasingly being recognized and most commonly is manifested as stenoses of larger branches of the pulmonary arteries and pulmonary hypertension.

## 2.2. Diagnosis

The observed variability in systemic and vascular symptoms from large series is probably in part due to retrospective collection of data and lack of standardized data collection. There may be regional/ethnic variations in disease expression; for example, in India, there is an increased frequency of disease in men, and abnormalities of the abdominal aorta and renal arteries are more common than among American and Japanese patients (Jain et al., 1996). Delays in diagnosis of TAK no doubt are due to the rarity of disease and absence of systematic approaches to evaluation of ischemic symptoms in children and young adults. TAK may eventually be diagnosed following the serendipitous finding of a diminished pulse or blood pressure or a bruit on routine physical examination. Diagnosis of TAK is based on the demonstration of typical vascular lesions on angiography in a patient with a compatible clinical presentation. Competing diagnoses (see Table 1) must also be ruled out.

Acute phase reactants may be normal in patients with active disease and cannot either confirm or refute the diagnosis of TAK. While catheter-directed angiography is the gold standard for vessel imaging in TAK patients, it is increasingly being supplanted by non-invasive modalities, particularly magnetic resonance angiography (MRA, Tso et al., 2002) and computed tomography angiography (Figs. 1 and 2). Positron emission tomography (PET) scanning (Gotway et al., 2005; Moreno et al., 2005) provides implied data about vascular inflammation, but the performance characteristics of this technique in TAK are still being defined.

## 2.3. Definition of disease relapse

The definition of disease activity and relapse is critical to the evaluation of the therapeutic response in TAK patients. It has previously been demonstrated that in just under half of TAK patients in whom medical therapy was maximized prior to surgery, as assessed by absence of symptoms and normalization of acute phase reactants, persistent inflammation was found on pathologic examination of surgical specimens (Kerr et al., 1994; Lagneau et al., 1987). Therefore, while clinical symptoms and acute phase markers can have utility in determining level of disease activity in some

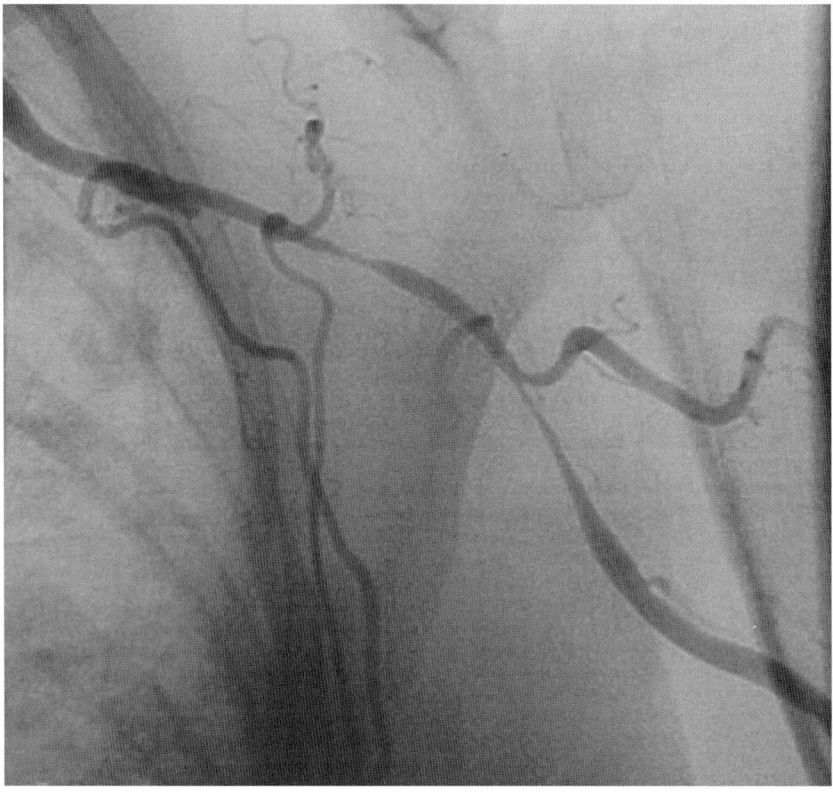

**Figure 2.** Catheter-directed angiogram of a patient with giant cell arteritis demonstrating stenoses of the left subclavian and left axillary artery. (Reproduced with permission from Mandell and Hoffman (2005).)

patients, they cannot be relied on for all patients. Clearly, pathologic specimens cannot be routinely obtained for the assessment of disease activity unless there is a specific indication for surgery. Invasive angiography has long been the diagnostic gold standard investigation for TAK, but is impractical for repeated monitoring because of the associated risks, including hemorrhage, arterial injury, infection, and contrast nephropathy as well as the risks associated with ionizing radiation. There is an unmet need for anatomic high resolution, non-invasive vascular imaging techniques that reliably detect vascular inflammation for the routine assessment of disease activity in TAK.

Magnetic resonance imaging (MRI) is increasingly being used to monitor disease activity in TAK patients (Tso et al., 2002). MRI can detect anatomic abnormalities such as luminal stenosis, aneurysm formation, vessel wall thickening, and collateral vessel formation. MRI can also detect signal changes or brightness in the vessel wall, which may be attributable to neovascularization of vasa vasora, edema, and/or inflammation. Efforts are ongoing to determine the sensitivity and specificity of brightness on MRI for inflammation.

Vessel stenoses or aneurysms are not generally considered reversible lesions, sub-total vessel narrowing may be worsened by development of secondary atherosclerosis and aneurysm size can increase as a result of mechanical factors. Consequently, the persistence or worsening of a previously identified vessel lesion on follow-up vascular imaging cannot be construed as evidence of ongoing or increased disease activity. Instead, the interim development of a new lesion in a previously unaffected location should be regarded

## 2.4. Renal involvement

The most common renal manifestation of TAK is renal artery stenosis (RAS). RAS is an important cause of secondary hypertension. In TAK, RAS may be caused by vasculitis and/or secondary atherosclerosis. RAS has been reported in up to 80% of TAK patients, and may be unilateral or bilateral (Castellote et al., 1995; Hall et al., 1985; Jain et al., 1996; Kerr et al., 1994). RAS may result in hypertension and chronic renal failure due to ischemic renal disease. Stenosis of the suprarenal aorta may mimic the presentation of bilateral RAS. Such patients may or may not have evidence of bilateral lower limb ischemia. The diagnosis of TAK should be considered in all young patients with increased blood pressure, visceral ischemic symptoms, and especially in those diagnosed with RAS. The presence of RAS in TAK patients is a particular concern during pregnancy, given the frequent occurrence of pregnancy-induced hypertension with attendant complications (Chugh et al., 1992; Sharma et al., 2000b). Renal imaging may be abnormal in up to two-thirds, with common findings including significantly reduced renal size and non-functioning kidney (Chugh et al., 1992). Asymmetrical renal size noted on abdominal imaging is suggestive of unilateral RAS. Doppler ultrasonography is thought by some to be useful for the diagnosis and monitoring of RAS. Although RAS can be demonstrated by MRA, it is most accurately assessed by invasive angiography.

A number of other renal manifestations have been reported in TAK; however, given the rarity of these cases, it is unclear whether they are pathogenetically linked with TAK. These include involvement of medium-sized intrarenal arteries resulting in proteinuria and chronic renal failure (Munir et al., 2000). AA amyloidosis has also been reported, frequently leading to the nephrotic syndrome (Ates et al., 1996; Dash et al., 1984; Espinosa et al., 1994; Graham et al., 1985; Jain et al., 1992; Makino et al., 1994; Rath et al., 1996; Sousa et al., 1993; van der Meulen et al., 1989; Wada et al., 1999). Glomerular disease has rarely been reported in TAK patients; reported presentation includes nephritis, proteinuria, or the nephrotic syndrome. The reported patterns of injury have included focal segmental glomerulosclerosis (Tiryaki et al., 2007; Zilleruelo et al., 1978), IgA nephropathy (Cavatorta et al., 1995; Kanahara et al., 1999), and mesangio-proliferative (Greene et al., 1986b; Kuroda et al., 2004; Lai et al., 1986; Takagi et al., 1984; Yoshimura et al., 1985), membranoproliferative (Koumi et al., 1990; Yoshikawa et al., 1988) and crescentic glomerulonephritis (Arita et al., 1998; Hellmann et al., 1987; Logar et al., 1994).

## 2.5. Treatment

There are no controlled comparative trials to guide the treatment of TAK. The available data regarding the medical and surgical treatment of TAK were recently reviewed (Liang and Hoffman, 2005). For most patients with active disease and lesions that are not organ threatening, initial treatment is with glucocorticoid monotherapy, typically prednisone 1 mg/kg/day. If remission is not achieved or relapse occurs on steroid tapering, cytotoxic therapy is indicated. Methotrexate is at least partially effective in this setting (Hoffman et al., 1994). Cyclophosphamide, because of its greater toxicity, is reserved for severe manifestations and/or refractory disease (Shelhamer et al., 1985). Azathioprine may be efficacious (Valsakumar et al., 2003). Mycophenolate mofetil was found to be of benefit in one small case series (Daina et al., 1999), but was not found useful by others (Hoffman et al., 2004). The experience with anti-tumor necrosis factor therapy has been encouraging to date (Hoffman et al., 2004). In addition, because of the association of TAK with accelerated atherosclerosis, all patients should be treated with low-dose aspirin unless contraindicated, with aggressive management of other vascular risk factors such as hyperlipidemia and hypertension.

Indications for surgery in TAK patients include severe symptomatic vessel stenoses or occlusion (e.g., cerebrovascular disease), aneurysm enlargement or rupture, and advanced or critical coronary artery disease or valvular heart disease. A number of authors have reported surgical outcomes in TAK patients (Kerr et al., 1994; Lagneau et al., 1987; Liang et al., 2004; Miyata et al., 2003; Pajari et al., 1986; Weaver et al., 1990). Results appear to be better with use of autologous rather than synthetic grafts. In general, the use of percutaneous transluminal angioplasty is not favored because of high rates of restenosis (Fava et al., 1993; Kerr et al., 1994; Liang et al., 2004; Weaver et al., 1990), although good results have been reported in some series (Sharma et al., 2000a; Tyagi et al., 1993, 1998).

RAS in TAK has been successfully treated with percutaneous transluminal angioplasty (Sharma et al., 1998; Tyagi et al., 1993), although long-term success rates may be sub-optimal (Fava et al., 1993; Liang et al., 2004). Overall, long-term outcomes appear to be more favorable with bypass procedures (Kerr et al., 1994; Lagneau and Michel, 1985; Liang et al., 2004; Maksimowicz-McKinnon et al., 2007; Teoh, 1999; Weaver et al., 2004). Renal transplantation has previously been successfully performed in a TAK patient with ischemic nephropathy (Basri and Shaheen, 2003).

## 3. Giant cell arteritis

### 3.1. Clinical features

GCA is a large vessel systemic vasculitis that affects patients over age 50 years, with a mean age at onset in most series being about 74 years. GCA has a predilection for involvement of the extra-cranial branches of the carotid arteries, but can involve intracranial branches of the carotid artery and any part of the aorta and its major branches. The typical clinical features of GCA gathered from the largest published series are listed in Table 3. Complications include blindness (up to 30%), stroke ($\sim$5%) as well as development of thoracic and abdominal aortic aneurysms (15–20%).

Laboratory abnormalities are non-specific, including elevation of acute phase reactants. However, in approximately 10% of cases, acute phase reactants may be normal. Therefore, laboratory testing cannot be relied on to either "rule-in" or "rule-out" GCA in patients in whom it is suspected on clinical grounds. The diagnosis of GCA may be confirmed by temporal artery biopsy. Granulomatous GCA is seen in approximately 50% of biopsies, with the remainder typically showing mononuclear cell-predominant infiltrates without giant cells (Lie, 1990). There is a false negative rate of at least 10–15% for temporal artery biopsy (Klein et al., 1976). It is not essential to perform this procedure in patients in whom the pre-biopsy probability of GCA is sufficiently high.

**Table 3**
Clinical features of giant cell arteritis

| Abnormality | Frequency (%) |
| --- | --- |
| Headache (new, localized) | 60–90 |
| Scalp tenderness | 44–67 |
| Fever | 10–48 |
| Visual signs/symptoms | 23–40 |
| Permanent visual loss | 8–30 |
| Polymyalgia rheumatica | 36–53 |
| Claudication | |
|    Extremity | 2–8 |
|    Jaw | 18–67 |
|    Tongue and/or on deglutition | 3–7 |
| Dysphagia | 5 |
| Vertigo | 7–12 |
| Tenderness of temporal artery | 55–69 |
| Absent temporal artery pulse | 40–51 |
| Thoracoabdominal aneurysms | 15–20 |
| Stroke | 2–7 |

*Source*: Caselli et al. (1988), Gonzalez-Gay et al. (2005), Greene et al. (1986a), Hamilton et al. (1971), Hunder et al. (1990b), Huston et al. (1978), Klein et al. (1975), Nesher et al. (2004).

### 3.2. Renal involvement

Renal manifestations are not typically considered a feature of GCA. In general, impairment of renal function in a patient with GCA is unlikely to be due to GCA. Therefore, a rising serum creatinine or the presence of heavy proteinuria in a GCA patient should prompt consideration of a renal co-morbidity. Although benign microscopic hematuria in the absence of biopsy proof of GN has been reported in GCA (Manna et al., 1997; Vanderschueren et al., 2002), its significance is uncertain. This elderly population has a high incidence of atrophy of genitourinary mucosa and of renal genitourinary co-morbidities that may contribute to this finding. Rare renal manifestations of GCA include RAS, although this appears to be far less frequent than in TAK. In a necropsy study of 16 GCA patients, 4 of the 26 renal arteries examined had evidence of arteritic involvement (Ostberg, 1972). There are few reports of overt RAS in GCA (Justo-Muradas et al., 2000; Lin and Hsueh, 1995). The nephrotic syndrome has also been reported in GCA in the setting of focal segmental glomerulonephritis (Pascual et al., 1994), membranous glomerulonephritis (Truong et al., 1985), and amyloidosis (Escriba et al., 2000; Monteagudo et al., 1997; Moraga et al., 2001; Strasser et al., 2000). There have been reports of necrotizing glomerulonephritis, with and without crescent formation, and necrotizing renal arteritis occurring in the setting of biopsy-proven temporal artery inflammation (Canton et al., 1992; Elling and Kristensen, 1980; Govil et al., 1998; Lenz et al., 1998; Montoliu et al., 1997; Muller et al., 2004; O'Neill et al., 1976; Pascual et al., 1994). However, given the rarity of these reports, it may be that these were cases of systemic small or medium vessel vasculitis (e.g., Wegener's granulomatosis or microscopic polyangiitis) with temporal artery involvement (Genereau et al., 1999). Patients with such a presentation should be treated aggressively with steroids and other immunosuppressants to maximize recovery of renal function.

## 3.3. Treatment

Corticosteroid therapy remains the cornerstone of pharmacologic therapy of GCA. If there are any symptoms suggestive of impending cranial ischemic complications, intravenous steroids should be administered immediately. If cranial ischemic complications have already developed, a narrow "window" of 24–48 h exists, within which improvement may be seen after starting high-dose corticosteroid therapy. Oral steroids should be commenced in all other patients where there is a strong clinical suspicion of GCA. Steroid therapy should not be delayed pending the performance of a temporal artery biopsy, as positive biopsy findings can be expected for at least 2 weeks beyond the commencement of steroid therapy. GCA generally responds well to steroid therapy, although many patients will remain steroid-dependent. Several randomized controlled trials have examined the utility of potential steroid-sparing agents such as methotrexate (Hoffman et al., 2002; Jover et al., 2001; Spiera et al., 2001), azathioprine (de Silva and Hazleman, 1986), and infliximab (Hoffman et al., 2007). However, to date, no convincing data has been reported to support the use of any of these agents in the treatment of GCA. Current strategies to minimize corticosteroid toxicity include use of appropriate measures to prevent reduction of bone mineral density and gastrointestinal toxicity in at-risk patients.

Recent data support the use of low-dose aspirin for the prevention of cranial ischemic events in GCA patients (Lee et al., 2006; Nesher et al., 2004). In a retrospective study of 175 GCA patients, Nesher et al. found a significant reduction in the incidence of ocular and cerebral ischemic events at the time of diagnosis in patients taking aspirin, compared to those who were not taking aspirin (8 vs. 40%, respectively). Among the 166 patients treated with glucocorticoids that were followed up for at least 3 months, cranial ischemic complications developed in only 3% of the aspirin-treated patients, compared with 13% of the patients treated with prednisone only. These differences were present despite the increased prevalence of risk factors for cerebrovascular disease in the aspirin treated group (39 vs. 20%). This work was corroborated by the observations of Lee et al. (2006). There was no significant increase in adverse events noted in the aspirin treated patients in either study. Therefore, all GCA patients should be treated with low-dose aspirin unless there is a specific contra-indication.

## 4. Cogan's syndrome

### 4.1. Clinical features

CS is a rare inflammatory disorder that predominantly affects young adults (St Clair and McCallum, 1999). Onset of disease frequently occurs in the aftermath of an upper respiratory tract infection. It is characterized by the presence of ocular inflammation (classically interstitial keratitis) and audio-vestibular dysfunction. While these two cardinal disease features are thought to be a consequence of non-vasculitic inflammation, they are accompanied by a systemic vasculitis in up to 15% of cases. Although this is typically a large vessel vasculitis resembling TAK, small-to-medium vessel involvement has also been described.

## 4.2. Renal involvement

Renal manifestations are unusual in CS and generally result directly from vasculitis. RAS is the most frequently reported renal manifestation of CS (Allen et al., 1990; Cochrane and Tatoulis, 1991; Gaubitz et al., 2001; Grasland et al., 2004; Vella et al., 1997; Vollertsen et al., 1986). When small vessel vasculitis predominates, a picture resembling pauci-immune glomerulonephritis or diffuse proliferative glomerulonephritis may be seen (Udayaraj et al., 2004). Other reported renal manifestations of CS include fatal renal artery rupture (Thomas, 1992), membranoproliferative glomerulonephritis leading to end-stage renal disease (Grasland et al., 2004), and renal amyloidosis in a patient with long-standing CS (Grasland et al., 2004).

## 4.3. Treatment

There are no controlled trials to guide treatment of CS. Eye disease, depending on severity, may be managed with topical or systemic corticosteroids (Chynn and Jakobiec, 1996). Systemic therapy is required for audiovestibular and systemic manifestations and severe eye disease. Prompt treatment with corticosteroids may ameliorate hearing loss in addition to other clinical features (Vollertsen et al., 1986). Although additional immunosuppressive therapies such as cyclophosphamide, methotrexate, azathioprine, and cyclosporine have been frequently employed, there is insufficient evidence to evaluate their efficacy. Cochlear implants may improve quality of life in patients with permanent hearing loss.

# 5. Sarcoid vasculitis

## 5.1. Clinical features

Sarcoidosis is a multi-system disorder, the histologic hallmark of which is non-caseating granulomatous inflammation. Less often, patients may develop necrotizing granulomatous lesions. While pulmonary involvement is most frequent, any tissue in the body may be affected. Large and medium vessel vasculitis has rarely been reported in association with sarcoidosis (Barbour and Roberts, 1987; Bottcher, 1959; Deneberg, 1965; Faye-Petersen et al., 1991; Fernandes et al., 2000; Fink and Cimaz, 1997; Gedalia et al., 1996; Korkmaz et al., 1999; Maeda et al., 1983; Marcussen and Lund, 1989; Rose et al., 1990; Shintaku et al., 1989; Weiler et al., 2000). Small vessel vasculitis can also occur (Fernandes et al., 2000). Large vessel involvement may mimic TAK, although large vessel aneurysms occur more frequently in sarcoid vasculitis (Fernandes et al., 2000). Large vessel vasculitis in sarcoidosis appears to have a predilection for African-American and Asian individuals (Fernandes et al., 2000). Reported complications of large vessel vasculitis in sarcoidosis include myocardial infarction, cerebrovascular accident, aortic dissection, and limb and mesenteric ischemia and peripheral gangrene.

While there are no pathognomonic clinical features to differentiate sarcoid vasculitis from other forms of large vessel vasculitis, the diagnosis can generally be made on the basis of associated clinical findings, such as hilar adenopathy, erythema nodosum, arthritis/periarthritis, and uveitis. Although granulomatous inflammation of blood vessels is also a feature of TAK and GCA, demonstration of well-formed non-caseating granulomata on histologic examination of extravascular tissue may be helpful in distinguishing sarcoid vasculitis from these other forms of large vessel vasculitis.

## 5.2. Renal involvement

Renal disease in sarcoidosis may be due to nephrocalcinosis, granulomatous inflammation, interstitial nephritis, glomerulonephritis, and ischemia from RAS (Gobel et al., 2001; Muther et al., 1981). In patients with sarcoidosis and large vessel vasculitis, renal artery involvement is common, with both RAS and aneurysm formation reported (Fernandes et al., 2000; Gross et al., 1986; Murai et al., 1986; Rotenstein et al., 1982; Umemoto et al., 1997). Renal manifestations in sarcoidosis are also discussed in Chapter 22.

## 5.3. Treatment

Corticosteroid and cytotoxic therapies appear to be of benefit in sarcoid vasculitis, but relapses are common (Fernandes et al., 2000). Surgical intervention may be required in selected cases. In general, the approach to treatment of large vessel vasculitis associated with sarcoidosis is similar to that outlined above for TAK.

## 6. Behçet's disease

### 6.1. Clinical features

Behçet's disease (BD) is a multi-system disorder initially described as a triad of recurrent ulceration of the oral and genital mucosa and relapsing uveitis. Involvement of the skin, joints, and the gastrointestinal, genitourinary, and nervous systems are also well described. Vasculitis is thought to be responsible for the features of BD, which may affect arteries and/or veins of all sizes. While small vessel involvement predominates, large vessel vasculitis is seen in up to one-third of BD patients (Calamia et al., 2005; Cooper et al., 1994; Gurler et al., 1997; Hamza, 1987; Shahram et al., 2003a). Patients with involvement of large vessels in one area are more likely to have similar involvement in other parts of the circulation. Aneurysm formation in BD occurs more often in the abdominal aorta, lower extremity vessels, and pulmonary arteries, but any vessel may be affected (Ceyran et al., 2003; Hamza, 1987; Lakhanpal et al., 1985). Arterial obstruction may be due to either thrombosis or stenosis. Thrombotic and inflammatory occlusion of large veins may include the venae cavae. While large vessel vasculitis in BD can mimic TAK (Matsumoto et al., 1991), there appears to be a greater incidence of aneurysms in BD. In contrast to TAK, large vessel vasculitis in BD patients has a strong predilection for young male patients. The presence of venous thromboses or migratory superficial thrombophlebitis in a patient with large vessel vasculitis should also prompt consideration of BD rather than TAK. However, because BD typically includes many characteristic features such as mucosal ulcers, a variety of skin lesions, and inflammatory ocular disease, distinguishing BD from TAK is usually not difficult.

### 6.2. Renal involvement

Despite the wide spectrum of disease manifestations of BD, clinically apparent renal involvement is relatively rare (Gurler et al., 1997; Shahram et al., 2003a). Shahram et al. (2003b) reported that proteinuria and/or hematuria were found in 475 of 4386 BD patients (10.8%). These abnormalities were transient in most cases. Renal biopsy was performed in 14 patients, showing glomerulonephritis in 12 cases and amyloidosis in 2. Interpretation of urinalysis in BD patients is complicated by the frequent occurrence of genitourinary lesions (e.g., genital ulcers, epididymitis). Akpolat et al. (2002) analyzed 159 patients with BD and renal disease in the literature.. They found 69 cases of AA amyloid, 51 of glomerulonephritis, 35 of renal vascular disease, and 4 cases of interstitial nephritis. The "renal vascular disease" group included 12 cases of renal artery aneurysm, 12 cases of RAS or occlusion, 7 cases of renal vein thrombosis, and 4 cases of biopsy-proven (non-glomerular) small vessel vasculitis. Large vessel vasculitis was found to be more common in patients with amyloidosis than in BD patients without amyloidosis. This is consistent with the hypothesis that BD patients with large vessel vasculitis more frequently have a systemic inflammatory response, as indicated by constitutional symptoms and abnormalities of acute phase reactants, than patients without large vessel involvement (Calamia et al., 2005). Large vessel involvement in BD patients may result in RAS and/or supra-renal aortic stenosis, thereby leading to renovascular hypertension. Renal involvement in BD is discussed further in Chapter 22.

## 6.3. Treatment

The approach to treatment of large vessel vasculitis in BD is similar to that described above for TAK. Surgical intervention is frequently complicated by a "pathergic" response leading to recurrent disease, graft occlusion, and/or anastomotic aneurysms (Ceyran et al., 2003; Saba et al., 2003). This emphasizes the particular importance of controlling inflammation pre-operatively in BD patients. Endovascular repair techniques have been used in an attempt to limit the morbidity and mortality associated with surgical procedures. A number of reports attest to the potential efficacy and safety of these techniques in BD patients (Bautista-Hernandez et al., 2004; Kizilkilic et al., 2003; Nitecki et al., 2004; Robenshtok and Krause, 2004; Silistreli et al., 2004); however, more information is required regarding the long-term outcomes before such approaches can be routinely recommended for vascular lesions in BD.

## 7. Polyarteritis nodosa

### 7.1. Clinical features

PAN is a systemic necrotizing arteritis of medium-sized and small muscular arteries. PAN may be indolent and mild, or severe and rapidly progressive. The Chapel Hill International Consensus Conference (CHCC) emphasized that (classic) PAN does not involve the glomerular capillaries, or small vessels in any organ system, a criterion that serves to distinguish PAN from microscopic polyangiitis (MPA) (Jennette et al., 1994). Typical clinical features in PAN include constitutional symptoms such as weight loss and fever. Organ systems frequently involved are the skin, peripheral nerves, kidneys, gut, genitourinary system, and joints (Fig. 3). Other findings include muscle, ocular, and central nervous system involvement. As most large series of patients with "polyarteritis" combine PAN with MPA, CSS, and/or viral-associated vasculitis, it is difficult to accurately predict the frequency of the clinical features listed above in PAN. The absence of pulmonary capillary involvement and consequent pulmonary hemorrhage is useful in distinguishing PAN from the small vessel vasculitides such as Wegener's granulomatosis (WG), MPA, or CSS. Another distinguishing feature is the fact that patients with classic PAN rarely (<10%) suffer relapses (Guillevin et al., 1996), in contrast to patients with WG or MPA (Jayne et al., 2003). By definition, PAN is idiopathic (Jennette et al., 1994). However, an identical disease phenotype can complicate infection with either the hepatitis B or C viruses, which has important implications for therapy. Diagnosis of PAN is based on the typical constellation of clinical features along with angiographic findings consistent with medium-sized vessel vasculitis and/or necrotizing vasculitis of muscular arteries on biopsy (Fig. 3). Typical angiographic features include multiple microaneurysms and irregular constrictions and/or occlusion of smaller arteries (Fig. 3). There are no diagnostic laboratory tests for PAN. A positive anti-neutrophil cytoplasmic antibody test, particularly with specificity for proteinase 3 or myeloperoxidase, points strongly away from a diagnosis of PAN and toward WG or MPA.

### 7.2. Renal involvement

The frequency of kidney involvement in PAN is difficult to ascertain because many previous reports considered PAN and MPA together (Cohen et al., 1980; Fortin et al., 1995; Guillevin et al., 1992; Leib et al., 1979; Scott et al., 1982). Two more recent studies have considered these as separate entities (el-Reshaid et al., 1997; Kirkland et al., 1997). A Kuwaiti study described the renal manifestations in 16 patients with classic PAN (el-Reshaid et al., 1997). Eleven patients had chronic renal insufficiency with variable severity of proteinuria, two patients had rapidly progressive renal failure with evidence on renal biopsy of necrotizing arteritis (but not glomerulonephritis), two patients had nephrotic syndrome, and one patient had asymptomatic urinary abnormalities.

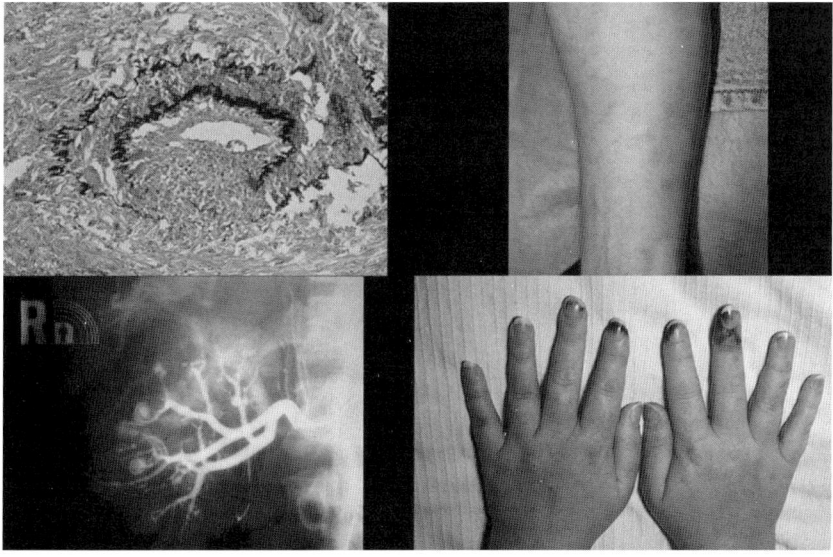

**Figure 3.** A patient with polyarteritis nodosa with (painful) erythematous nodular skin lesions (top right), peripheral gangrene due to severe digital artery involvement (bottom right), renal angiogram with multiple aneurysms and occlusive lesions (bottom left) and histologic evidence of necrotizing arteritis of a muscular artery with destruction of the internal elastic lamina and intimal thickening and stenosis (top left). (Reproduced with permission from Mandell and Hoffman (2005).)

Renal function stabilized or improved in all patients with immunosuppressive therapy and no patients required maintenance dialysis; there were no deaths in this group during a median follow-up of 16 months. A smaller study found that two/five patients with classic PAN had either proteinuria or azotemia (Kirkland et al., 1997). A more recent study of ten patients with classic PAN included seven patients with renal involvement (Selga et al., 2006). Of these, all seven had proteinuria, non-glomerular hematuria, and/or renal microaneurysms on angiography. Five patients had hypertension (three with malignant hypertension), but only two had azotemia. Renal biopsy was not performed in these patients because of the typical findings of classic PAN on angiography and the absence of dysmorphic red blood cells and red blood cell casts on urine microscopy (Selga et al., 2006). However, it is unlikely that all the patients described in these studies had classic PAN, as opposed to MPA, given the significant proteinuria reported in some of these cases, which is more suggestive of glomerulonephritis than glomerular ischemia. Furthermore, the ability of the finding of microaneurysms at renal/mesenteric angiography to discriminate between classic PAN and MPA has not been rigorously studied.

Hypertension is a common finding in PAN and is thought to relate to renal ischemia due to luminal narrowing of affected vessels, with consequent activation of the renin–angiotensin–aldosterone system (Stockigt et al., 1979). Renal microaneurysms may rupture giving rise to perinephric, subcapsular, or intrarenal hematomas or renal infarctions (Hekali et al., 1985; Peterson et al., 1970; Schlesinger et al., 1989). Renal infarctions may be clinically silent and renal insufficiency may ensue over the course of months to years (Lhote and Guillevin, 1995). Other reported renal manifestations include spontaneous bilateral renal rupture (Romijn et al., 1989), papillary necrosis due to calyceal artery involvement (Heaton and Bourke, 1976), bilateral renal artery dissection (Hekali et al., 1984), and ureteral stenosis due to peri-ureteric vasculitis and fibrosis (Azar et al., 1989; Glanz and Grunebaum, 1976).

While renal biopsy may reveal evidence of involvement of medium-sized arteries (without glomerulonephritis), sampling error is common. The presence of renal microaneurysms increases the potential for hemorrhagic complications. Therefore, closed renal biopsy is not recommended to confirm the diagnosis of PAN. If abdominal angiography failed to support the diagnosis and there was no other site amenable to biopsy, an open renal biopsy might be considered because of the ability to control bleeding complications from aneurysms. However, this situation rarely arises.

## 7.3. Treatment

The main determinants of treatment of patients with a presentation suggestive of PAN are the presence of chronic viral infection, rate of disease progression, and the distribution of involved organs (Guillevin, 1999). In patients with PAN-like vasculitis associated with HBV or HCV infection, antiviral therapy, and judicious use of glucocorticoids may be effective in controlling the disease.

Milder forms of PAN may be treated with glucocorticoids alone, typically at doses of 1 mg/kg/day. However, in the presence of critical organ- or life-threatening disease, intravenous glucocorticoids, and cytotoxic therapy should be initiated. Surgical intervention may be required for gastrointestinal complications such as bowel perforation or hemorrhage.

## 8. Kawasaki's disease

### 8.1. Clinical features

KD, also known as mucocutaneous lymph node syndrome, is a form of medium vessel (and less often large vessel) vasculitis that preferentially affects children under the age of 5 years (Kawasaki, 2002). Most frequently KD is a self-limited condition. Clinical features of KD are listed in Table 4. However, more severe complications such as cardiac involvement, gastrointestinal involvement, and peripheral gangrene can develop in a proportion of patients, leading to significant morbidity and mortality. Cardiac disease occurs in 20–25% of untreated patients and is the principal determinant

Table 4
Clinical features of Kawasaki's disease

| Abnormality |
| --- |
| Diagnostic criteria for KD |
|   Otherwise unexplained Fever ≥5 days |
|   Plus at least four of the following: |
|   Rash |
|   Cervical lymphadenopathy |
|   Extremity changes: swelling/erythema/desquamation |
|   Bilateral conjunctival injection |
|   Mucus membrane changes: injection or fissuring of lips, injected pharynx or 'strawberry' tongue |
| "Incomplete" KD |
|   Fever plus at least two of the other clinical criteria listed above |
| Other features |
|   Cardiac involvement (20–25%) |
|   Articular involvement (polyarticular/pauciarticular) 33% |
|   Anterior uveitis |
|   Aseptic meningitis |
|   Gastrointestinal involvement (e.g., gallbladder hydrops, small bowel obstruction, ileus, hepatitis, pancreatitis) |
|   Peripheral gangrene (rare) |

*Source*: Burns and Glode (2004), Burns et al. (1986), Kawasaki (1979).

of prognosis. Echocardiographic abnormalities of coronary arteries may be appreciable as early as day 7 after onset of the illness. Pericarditis, myocarditis, and endocarditis can also occur. Mortality in the acute phase of KD has been estimated at 2%. The main cause of death is myocardial infarction, typically resulting from thrombotic occlusion of a coronary aneurysm. Aneurysms in other arteries such as the aorta, axillary, iliac, and renal arteries have also been reported, typically occurring in patients that also have coronary artery aneurysms (Foster et al., 2000; Fuyama et al., 1996; Odagiri et al., 1989; Sasaguri and Kato, 1982). Recent reports also suggest that there may be a link with accelerated atherosclerosis in adulthood (Cheung et al., 2004a, b, 2007; Ikemoto et al., 2005).

### 8.2. Renal involvement

Renal manifestations are rare in KD. Microscopic examination of urine commonly demonstrates sterile pyuria of urethral origin (Kawasaki, 2002). Other less frequently reported findings include proteinuria (typically mild), nephrotic syndrome, acute interstitial nephritis, and acute renal failure (Rhodes et al., 1998; Bonany et al., 2002; Ferriero and Wolfsdorf, 1981; Hicks and Melish, 1986; Joh et al., 1997; Mac Ardle et al., 1983; Nardi et al., 1985; Salcedo et al., 1988; Veiga et al., 1992). The last of these can occur in response to a variety of insults including hemolytic–uremic syndrome and immune-complex deposition, but is most commonly due to acute interstitial nephritis. Reported abnormalities on renal ultrasound include increased cortical echogenicity, renal hypertrophy, and enhanced corticomedullary differentiation (Nardi et al., 1985). Renovascular hypertension may develop as a result of renal artery or abdominal aortic involvement (Foster et al., 2000; Fuyama et al., 1996; Odagiri et al., 1989).

## 8.3. Treatment

Prompt diagnosis and treatment of KD can ameliorate the associated cardiac morbidity and mortality. However, despite the standard therapy of high-dose intravenous immunoglobulin (IVIG, in a single dose of 2 g/kg) and aspirin (50–100 mg/kg/day), coronary artery aneurysms still occur in 5% of affected children (Dajani et al., 1994). Use of corticosteroids in the initial stages of KD is controversial. A meta-analysis of eight studies that examined the efficacy of corticosteroids in prevention of coronary aneurysms in KD patients concluded that there was a reduction in the incidence of aneurysms (OR: 0.57, 95%, CI: 0.37–0.80) (Wooditch and Aronoff, 2005). However, because of concerns regarding methodologic flaws in these studies, a multi-center randomized controlled trial is being performed, the results of which should clarify the role of corticosteroids in the initial treatment of KD.

There is no evidence-based data to guide the treatment of patients refractory to the therapy outlined above. Re-treatment with a second infusion of IVIG and continued use of aspirin has been recommended (Kawasaki, 2002). The use of oral or pulse intravenous corticosteroids, cyclosporine, cyclophosphamide, and infliximab has also been reported to be efficacious in small numbers of patients with refractory KD. While continued low-dose aspirin therapy (3–5 mg/kg/day) seems prudent for patients with coronary aneurysms, a role for anti-coagulation has not been clearly established (Levy et al., 2005). Coronary artery bypass surgery and cardiac transplantation are occasionally required.

Acute renal failure in KD requires standard supportive care and if necessary, dialysis may be required (Joh et al., 1997; Mac Ardle et al., 1983). No specific recommendation can be made with regard to the use of immunosuppressive therapy in this setting. However, for some patients treated with standard therapy alone, long-term outcome was good with recovery of renal function (Bonany et al., 2002; Mac Ardle et al., 1983; Veiga et al., 1992). There are no reports of renal transplantation in KD patients. Surgical bypass (following failed percutaneous angioplasty) resulted in normalization of blood pressure in a patient with renovascular hypertension due to ostial stenosis of the renal artery (Foster et al., 2000).

## 9. Conclusions

Vasculitides that are categorized as large and medium vessel diseases generally do not cause glomerulonephritis. Classification systems for vasculitis lean heavily on separation of entities based on vessel size and clinical and histologic features. While helpful, this is also an oversimplification. Evidence for this criticism is found among patients in whom large vessel disease can occasionally be associated with small vessel vasculitis (e.g., TAK and glomerulonephritis or cutaneous vasculitis). Recommendations for treatment have been derived in some cases from multi-center randomized controlled trials (GCA, KD) but in many instances (TAK, CS, sarcoid vasculitis), treatment has been empirically derived. The most important development in vasculitis research in the past 20 years has been the emergence of large multi-center consortia that will allow these rare diseases to be studied in a more rigorous manner in the future.

## Key points

- The most common mechanism of renal disease in large and medium vessel vasculitides is regional or global renal ischemia; they are rarely associated with glomerulonephritis.
- Careful clinical assessment and judicious interpretation of laboratory and imaging data is essential in the diagnosis and management of patients with vasculitis.
- Non-invasive imaging modalities such as MRI are increasingly used in place of conventional catheter-directed angiography in the assessment of large vessel vasculitis; however, such non-invasive techniques have insufficient resolution to be relied on for the assessment of medium-sized vessels.
- Although in some cases (GCA, KD), recommendations for therapy are based on multi-center randomized controlled trials, for other forms of large and medium vessel vasculitis, treatment guidelines are largely derived from case series and observational studies. The recent establishment of multi-center collaborative groups will facilitate more rigorous study of these rare diseases in the future.

# References

Akpolat, T., Akkoyunlu, M., Akpolat, I., et al. 2002. Renal Behcet's disease: a cumulative analysis. Semin. Arthritis Rheum. 31, 317–337.

Allen, N.B., Cox, C.C., Cobo, M., et al. 1990. Use of immunosuppressive agents in the treatment of severe ocular and vascular manifestations of Cogan's syndrome. Am. J. Med. 88, 296–301.

Arita, M., Iwane, M., Nakamura, Y., et al. 1998. Anticoagulants in Takayasu's arteritis associated with crescentic glomerulonephritis and nephrotic syndrome: a case report. Angiology 49, 75–78.

Ates, K., Erturk, S., Diker, E., et al. 1996. Renal amyloidosis complicating Takayasu's arteritis: a case report. Nephron. 73, 111–112.

Azar, N., Guillevin, L., Huong Du, L.T., et al. 1989. Symptomatic urogenital manifestations of polyarteritis nodosa and Churg-Strauss angiitis: analysis of 8 of 165 patients. J. Urol. 142, 136–138.

Barbour, D.J., Roberts, W.C. 1987. Aneurysm of the pulmonary trunk unassociated with intracardiac or great vessel left-to-right shunting. Am. J. Cardiol. 59, 192–194.

Basri, N.A., Shaheen, F.A. 2003. Renal transplantation for Takayasu's Arteritis: a case report. Transplant. Proc. 35, 2617–2618.

Bautista-Hernandez, V., Gutierrez, F., Capel, A., et al. 2004. Endovascular repair of concomitant celiac trunk and abdominal aortic aneurysms in a patient with Behcet's disease. J. Endovasc. Ther. 11, 222–225.

Bonany, P.J., Bilkis, M.D., Gallo, G., et al. 2002. Acute renal failure in typical Kawasaki disease. Pediatr. Nephrol. 17, 329–331.

Bottcher, E. 1959. Disseminated sarcoidosis with a marked granulomatous arteritis. Arch. Pathol. 68, 419–423.

Burns, J.C., Glode, M.P. 2004. Kawasaki syndrome. Lancet 364, 533–544.

Burns, J.C., Wiggins, J.W., Jr. Toews, W.H., et al. 1986. Clinical spectrum of Kawasaki disease in infants younger than 6 months of age. J. Pediatr. 109, 759–763.

Calamia, K.T., Schirmer, M., Melikoglu, M. 2005. Major vessel involvement in Behcet disease. Curr. Opin. Rheumatol. 17, 1–8.

Canton, C.G., Bernis, C., Paraiso, V., et al. 1992. Renal failure in temporal arteritis. Am. J. Nephrol. 12, 380–383.

Caselli, R.J., Hunder, G.G., Whisnant, J.P. 1988. Neurologic disease in biopsy-proven giant cell (temporal) arteritis. Neurology 38, 352–359.

Castellote, E., Romero, R., Bonet, J., et al. 1995. Takayasu's arteritis as a cause of renovascular hypertension in a non-Asian population. J. Hum. Hypertens. 9, 841–845.

Cavatorta, F., Campisi, S., Trabassi, E., et al. 1995. IgA nephropathy associated with Takayasu's arteritis: report of a case and review of the literature. Am. J. Nephrol. 15, 165–167.

Ceyran, H., Akcali, Y., Kahraman, C. 2003. Surgical treatment of vasculo-Behcet's disease. A review of patients with concomitant multiple aneurysms and venous lesions. Vasa. 32, 149–153.

Cheung, Y.F., Wong, S.J., Ho, M.H. 2007. Relationship between carotid intima-media thickness and arterial stiffness in children after Kawasaki disease. Arch. Dis. Child 92, 43–47.

Cheung, Y.F., Ho, M.H., Tam, S.C., et al. 2004a. Increased high sensitivity C reactive protein concentrations and increased arterial stiffness in children with a history of Kawasaki disease. Heart 90, 1281–1285.

Cheung, Y.F., Yung, T.C., Tam, S.C., et al. 2004b. Novel and traditional cardiovascular risk factors in children after Kawasaki disease: implications for premature atherosclerosis. J. Am. Coll. Cardiol. 43, 120–124.

Chugh, K.S., Jain, S., Sakhuja, V., et al. 1992. Renovascular hypertension due to Takayasu's arteritis among Indian patients. Q. J. Med. 85, 833–843.

Chynn, E.W., Jakobiec, F.A. 1996. Cogan's syndrome: ophthalmic, audiovestibular, and systemic manifestations and therapy. Int. Ophthalmol. Clin. 36, 61–72.

Cochrane, A.D., Tatoulis, J. 1991. Cogan's syndrome with aortitis, aortic regurgitation, and aortic arch vessel stenoses. Ann. Thorac. Surg. 52, 1166–1167.

Cohen, R.D., Conn, D.L., Ilstrup, D.M. 1980. Clinical features, prognosis, and response to treatment in polyarteritis. Mayo Clin. Proc. 55, 146–155.

Cooper, A.M., Naughton, M.N., Williams, B.D. 1994. Chronic arterial occlusion associated with Behcet's disease. Br. J. Rheumatol. 33, 170–172.

Daina, E., Schieppati, A., Remuzzi, G. 1999. Mycophenolate mofetil for the treatment of Takayasu arteritis: report of three cases. Ann. Intern. Med. 130, 422–426.

Dajani, A.S., Taubert, K.A., Takahashi, M., et al. 1994. Guidelines for long-term management of patients with Kawasaki disease. Report from the Committee on Rheumatic Fever, Endocarditis, and Kawasaki Disease, Council on Cardiovascular Disease in the Young, American Heart Association. Circulation 89, 916–922.

Dash, S.C., Sharma, R.K., Malhotra, K.K., et al. 1984. Renal amyloidosis and non-specific aorto-arteritis—a hitherto undescribed association. Postgrad. Med. J. 60, 626–628.

Deneberg, M. 1965. Sarcoidosis of the myocardium and aorta: a case report. Am. J. Clin. Pathol. 43, 445–449.

De Silva, M., Hazleman, B.L. 1986. Azathioprine in giant cell arteritis/polymyalgia rheumatica: a double-blind study. Ann. Rheum. Dis. 45, 136–138.

Elling, H., Kristensen, I.B. 1980. Fatal renal failure in polymyalgia rheumatica caused by disseminated giant cell arteritis. Scand. J. Rheumatol. 9, 206–208.

el-Reshaid, K., Kapoor, M.M., el-Reshaid, W., et al. 1997. The spectrum of renal disease associated with microscopic polyangiitis and classic polyarteritis nodosa in Kuwait. Nephrol. Dial. Transplant. 12, 1874–1882.

Escriba, A., Morales, E., Albizua, E., et al. 2000. Secondary (AA-type) amyloidosis in patients with polymyalgia rheumatica. Am. J. Kidney Dis. 35, 137–140.

Espinosa, M., Rodriguez, M., Martin-Malo, A., et al. 1994. A case of Takayasu's arteritis, nephrotic syndrome, and systemic amyloidosis. Nephrol. Dial. Transplant. 9, 1486–1488.

Fava, M.P., Foradori, G.B., Garcia, C.B., et al. 1993. Percutaneous transluminal angioplasty in patients with Takayasu arteritis: five-year experience. J. Vasc. Interv. Radiol. 4, 649–652.

Faye-Petersen, O., Frankel, S.R., Schulman, P.E., et al. 1991. Giant cell vasculitis with extravascular granulomas in an adolescent. Pediatr. Pathol. 11, 281–295.

Fernandes, S.R., Singsen, B.H., Hoffman, G.S. 2000. Sarcoidosis and systemic vasculitis. Semin. Arthritis Rheum. 30, 33–46.

Ferriero, D.M., Wolfsdorf, J.I. 1981. Hemolytic uremic syndrome associated with Kawasaki disease. Pediatrics 68, 405–406.

Fink, C.W., Cimaz, R. 1997. Early onset sarcoidosis: not a benign disease. J. Rheumatol. 24, 174–177.

Fortin, P.R., Larson, M.G., Watters, A.K., et al. 1995. Prognostic factors in systemic necrotizing vasculitis of the polyarteritis nodosa group—a review of 45 cases. J. Rheumatol. 22, 78–84.

Foster, B.J., Bernard, C., Drummond, K.N. 2000. Kawasaki disease complicated by renal artery stenosis. Arch. Dis. Child. 83, 253–255.

Fuyama, Y., Hamada, R., Uehara, R., et al. 1996. Long-term follow up of abdominal aortic aneurysm complicating Kawasaki disease: comparison of the effectiveness of different imaging methods. Acta Paediatr. Jpn. 38, 252–255.

Gaubitz, M., Lubben, B., Seidel, M., et al. 2001. Cogan's syndrome: organ-specific autoimmune disease or systemic vasculitis? A report of two cases and review of the literature. Clin. Exp. Rheumatol. 19, 463–469.

Gedalia, A., Shetty, A.K., Ward, K., et al. 1996. Abdominal aortic aneurysm associated with childhood sarcoidosis. J. Rheumatol. 23, 757–759.

Genereau, T., Lortholary, O., Pottier, M.A., et al. 1999. Temporal artery biopsy: a diagnostic tool for systemic necrotizing vasculitis. French Vasculitis Study Group. Arthritis Rheum. 42, 2674–2681.

Glanz, I., Grunebaum, M. 1976. Ureteral changes in polyarteritis nodosa as seen during excretory urography. J. Urol. 116, 731–733.

Gobel, U., Kettritz, R., Schneider, W., et al. 2001. The protean face of renal sarcoidosis. J. Am. Soc. Nephrol. 12, 616–623.

Gonzalez-Gay, M.A., Barros, S., Lopez-Diaz, M.J., et al. 2005. Giant cell arteritis: disease patterns of clinical presentation in a series of 240 patients. Medicine (Baltimore) 84, 269–276.

Gotway, M.B., Araoz, P.A., Macedo, T.A., et al. 2005. Imaging findings in Takayasu's arteritis. Am. J. Roentgenol. 184, 1945–1950.

Govil, Y.K., Sabanathan, K., Scott, D. 1998. Giant cell arteritis presenting as renal vasculitis. Postgrad. Med. J. 74, 170–171.

Graham, A.N., Delahunt, B., Renouf, J.J., et al. 1985. Takayasu's disease associated with generalised amyloidosis. Aust. NZ J. Med. 15, 343–345.

Grasland, A., Pouchot, J., Hachulla, E., et al. 2004. Typical and atypical Cogan's syndrome: 32 cases and review of the literature. Rheumatology (Oxford) 43, 1007–1015.

Greene, G.M., Lain, D., Sherwin, R.M., et al. 1986a. Giant cell arteritis of the legs. Clinical isolation of severe disease with gangrene and amputations. Am. J. Med. 81, 727–733.

Greene, N.B., Baughman, R.P., Kim, C.K. 1986b. Takayasu's arteritis associated with interstitial lung disease and glomerulonephritis. Chest 89, 605–606.

Gross, K.R., Malleson, P.N., Culham, G., et al. 1986. Vasculopathy with renal artery stenosis in a child with sarcoidosis. J. Pediatr. 108, 724–726.

Guillevin, L. 1999. Treatment of classic polyarteritis nodosa in 1999. Nephrol. Dial. Transplant. 14, 2077–2079.

Guillevin, L., Lhote, F., Gayraud, M., et al. 1996. Prognostic factors in polyarteritis nodosa and Churg-Strauss syndrome. A prospective study in 342 patients. Medicine (Baltimore) 75, 17–28.

Guillevin, L., Lhote, F., Jarrousse, B., et al. 1992. Treatment of polyarteritis nodosa and Churg-Strauss syndrome. A meta-analysis of 3 prospective controlled trials including 182 patients over 12 years. Ann. Med. Interne (Paris) 143, 405–416.

Gurler, A., Boyvat, A., Tursen, U. 1997. Clinical manifestations of Behcet's disease: an analysis of 2147 patients. Yonsei Med. J. 38, 423–427.

Hall, S., Barr, W., Lie, J.T., et al. 1985. Takayasu arteritis. A study of 32 North American patients. Medicine (Baltimore) 64, 89–99.

Hamilton, C.R., Jr. Shelley, W.M., Tumulty, P.A. 1971. Giant cell arteritis: including temporal arteritis and polymyalgia rheumatica. Medicine (Baltimore) 50, 1–27.

Hamza, M. 1987. Large artery involvement in Behcet's disease. J. Rheumatol. 14, 554–559.

Heaton, J.M., Bourke, E. 1976. Papillary necrosis associated with calyceal arteritis. Nephron. 16, 57–63.

Hekali, P., Kivisaari, L., Standerskjold-Nordenstam, C.G., et al. 1985. Renal complications of polyarteritis nodosa: CT findings. J. Comput. Assist. Tomogr. 9, 333–338.

Hekali, P.E., Pajari, R.I., Kivisaari, M.L., et al. 1984. Bilateral renal artery dissections: unusual complication of polyarteritis nodosa. Eur. J. Radiol. 4, 6–8.

Hellmann, D.B., Hardy, K., Lindenfeld, S., et al. 1987. Takayasu's arteritis associated with crescentic glomerulonephritis. Arthritis Rheum. 30, 451–454.

Hicks, R.V., Melish, M.E. 1986. Kawasaki syndrome. Pediatr. Clin. North Am. 33, 1151–1175.

Hoffman, G.S. 1996. Takayasu arteritis: lessons from the American National Institutes of Health experience. Int. J. Cardiol. 54 (Suppl), S99–S102.

Hoffman, G.S., Cid, M.C., Hellmann, D.B., et al. 2002. A multicenter, randomized, double-blind, placebo-controlled trial of adjuvant methotrexate treatment for giant cell arteritis. Arthritis Rheum. 46, 1309–1318.

Hoffman, G.S., Cid, M.C., Rendt-Zagar, K.E., et al. 2007. Infliximab for Maintenance of Glucocorticosteroid-Induced Remission of Giant Cell Arteritis: A Randomized Trial. Ann. Intern. Med. 146, 621–630.

Hoffman, G.S., Leavitt, R.Y., Kerr, G.S., et al. 1994. Treatment of glucocorticoid-resistant or relapsing Takayasu arteritis with methotrexate. Arthritis Rheum. 37, 578–582.

Hoffman, G.S., Merkel, P.A., Brasington, R.D., et al. 2004. Anti-tumor necrosis factor therapy in patients with difficult to treat Takayasu arteritis. Arthritis Rheum. 50, 2296–2304.

Hunder, G.G., Arend, W.P., Bloch, D.A., et al. 1990a. The American College of Rheumatology 1990 criteria for the classification of vasculitis. Introduction. Arthritis Rheum. 33, 1065–1067.

Hunder, G.G., Bloch, D.A., Michel, B.A., et al. 1990b. The American College of Rheumatology 1990 criteria for the classification of giant cell arteritis. Arthritis Rheum. 33, 1122–1128.

Huston, K.A., Hunder, G.G., Lie, J.T., et al. 1978. Temporal arteritis: a 25-year epidemiologic, clinical, and pathologic study. Ann. Intern. Med. 88, 162–167.

Ikemoto, Y., Ogino, H., Teraguchi, M., et al. 2005. Evaluation of preclinical atherosclerosis by flow-mediated dilatation of the brachial artery and carotid artery analysis in patients with a history of Kawasaki disease. Pediatr. Cardiol. 26, 782–786.

Ishikawa, K. 1978. Natural history and classification of occlusive thromboaortopathy (Takayasu's disease). Circulation 57, 27–35.

Ishikawa, K. 1988. Diagnostic approach and proposed criteria for the clinical diagnosis of Takayasu's arteriopathy. J. Am. Coll. Cardiol. 12, 964–972.

Jain, S., Kumari, S., Ganguly, N.K., et al. 1996. Current status of Takayasu arteritis in India. Int. J. Cardiol. 54 (Suppl), S111–S116.

Jain, S., Taraphdar, A., Joshi, K., et al. 1992. Renal amyloidosis complicating Takayasu's arteritis: a rare association. Nephrol. Dial. Transplant. 7, 1133–1135.

Jayne, D., Rasmussen, N., Andrassy, K., et al. 2003. A randomized trial of maintenance therapy for vasculitis associated with antineutrophil cytoplasmic autoantibodies. N. Engl. J. Med. 349, 36–44.

Jennette, J.C., Falk, R.J., Andrassy, K., et al. 1994. Nomenclature of systemic vasculitides. Proposal of an international consensus conference. Arthritis Rheum. 37, 187–192.

Joh, K., Kanetsuna, Y., Ishikawa, Y., et al. 1997. Diffuse mesangial sclerosis associated with Kawasaki disease: an analysis of alpha chains (alpha 1-alpha 6) of human type IV collagen in the renal basement membrane. Virchows Arch. 430, 489–494.

Jover, J.A., Hernandez-Garcia, C., Morado, I.C., et al. 2001. Combined treatment of giant-cell arteritis with methotrexate and prednisone. a randomized, double-blind, placebo-controlled trial. Ann. Intern. Med. 134, 106–114.

Justo-Muradas, I., Perez-Suarez, M., Saracibar, E., et al. 2000. Hypokalemic metabolic alkalosis secondary to giant cell arteritis. Nephron. 86, 524–525.

Kanahara, K., Yorioka, N., Ogata, S., et al. 1999. A case of aortitis syndrome and IgA nephropathy: possible role of human leukocyte antigens in both diseases. Hiroshima J. Med. Sci. 48, 25–29.

Kawasaki, T. 1979. Clinical signs and symptoms of mucocutaneous lymph node syndrome (Kawasaki disease). Jpn. J. Med. Sci. Biol. 32, 237–238.

Kawasaki, T. 2002. Kawasaki's disease. In: G.V. Ball, S.L. Bridges (Eds.), Vasculitis 1. Oxford University Press, New York, pp. 329–339.

Kerr, G.S., Hallahan, C.W., Giordano, J., et al. 1994. Takayasu arteritis. Ann. Intern. Med. 120, 919–929.

Kirkland, G.S., Savige, J., Wilson, D., et al. 1997. Classical polyarteritis nodosa and microscopic polyarteritis with medium vessel involvement—a comparison of the clinical and laboratory features. Clin. Nephrol. 47, 176–180.

Kizilkilic, O., Albayram, S., Adaletli, I., et al. 2003. Endovascular treatment of Behcet's disease-associated intracranial aneurysms: report of two cases and review of the literature. Neuroradiology 45, 328–334.

Klein, R.G., Campbell, R.J., Hunder, G.G., et al. 1976. Skip lesions in temporal arteritis. Mayo Clin. Proc. 51, 504–510.

Klein, R.G., Hunder, G.G., Stanson, A.W., et al. 1975. Large artery involvement in giant cell (temporal) arteritis. Ann. Intern. Med. 83, 806–812.

Korkmaz, C., Efe, B., Tel, N., et al. 1999. Sarcoidosis with palpable nodular myositis, periostitis and large-vessel vasculitis stimulating Takayasu's arteritis. Rheumatology (Oxford) 38, 287–288.

Koumi, S., Endo, T., Okumura, H., et al. 1990. A case of Takayasu's arteritis associated with membranoproliferative glomerulonephritis and nephrotic syndrome. Nephron. 54, 344–346.

Kuroda, T., Ohbayashi, H., Murakami, S., et al. 2004. A case of Takayasu arteritis complicated with glomerulonephropathy mimicking membranoproliferative glomerulonephritis. Clin. Rheumatol. 23, 536–540.

Lagneau, P., Michel, J.B. 1985. Surgical management and results of renal artery revascularization. Int. Angiol. 4, 329–333.

Lagneau, P., Michel, J.B., Vuong, P.N. 1987. Surgical treatment of Takayasu's disease. Ann. Surg. 205, 157–166.

Lai, K.N., Chan, K.W., Ho, C.P. 1986. Glomerulonephritis associated with Takayasu's arteritis: report of three cases and review of literature. Am. J. Kidney Dis. 7, 197–204.

Lakhanpal, S., Tani, K., Lie, J.T., et al. 1985. Pathologic features of Behcet's syndrome: a review of Japanese autopsy registry data. Hum. Pathol. 16, 790–795.

Lee, M.S., Smith, S.P., Goler, A., et al. 2006. Anti-platelet and anti-coagulant therapy in patients with giant cell arteritis. Arthritis Rheum. 54, 3306–3309.

Leib, E.S., Restivo, C., Paulus, H.E. 1979. Immunosuppressive and corticosteroid therapy of polyarteritis nodosa. Am. J. Med. 67, 941–947.

Lenz, T., Schmidt, R., Scherberich, J.E., et al. 1998. Renal failure in giant cell vasculitis. Am. J. Kidney Dis. 31, 1044–1047.

Levy, D.M., Silverman, E.D., Massicotte, M.P., et al. 2005. Longterm outcomes in patients with giant aneurysms secondary to Kawasaki disease. J. Rheumatol. 32, 928–934.

Lhote, F., Guillevin, L. 1995. Polyarteritis nodosa, microscopic polyangiitis, and Churg-Strauss syndrome. Clinical aspects and treatment. Rheum. Dis. Clin. North Am. 21, 911–947.

Liang, P., Hoffman, G.S. 2005. Advances in the medical and surgical treatment of Takayasu arteritis. Curr. Opin. Rheumatol. 17, 16–24.

Liang, P., Tan-Ong, M., Hoffman, G.S. 2004. Takayasu's arteritis: vascular interventions and outcomes. J. Rheumatol. 31, 102–106.

Lie, J.T. 1990. Illustrated histopathologic classification criteria for selected vasculitis syndromes. American College of Rheumatology Subcommittee on Classification of Vasculitis. Arthritis Rheum. 33, 1074–1087.

Lin, J.L., Hsueh, S. 1995. Giant cell arteritis induced renal artery aneurysm. Clin. Nephrol. 43, 66–68.

Logar, D., Rozman, B., Vizjak, A., et al. 1994. Arteritis of both carotid arteries in a patient with focal, crescentic glomerulonephritis and anti-neutrophil cytoplasmic autoantibodies. Br. J. Rheumatol. 33, 167–169.

Lupi-Herrera, E., Sanchez-Torres, G., Marcushamer, J., et al. 1977. Takayasu's arteritis. Clinical study of 107 cases. Am. Heart J. 93, 94–103.

Mac Ardle, B.M., Chambers, T.L., Weller, S.D., et al. 1983. Acute renal failure in Kawasaki disease. J. R. Soc. Med. 76, 615–616.

Maeda, S., Murao, S., Sugiyama, T., et al. 1983. Generalized sarcoidosis with "sarcoid aortitis". Acta Pathol. Jpn. 33, 183–188.

Makino, H., Nagake, Y., Murakami, K., et al. 1994. Remission of nephrotic syndrome in a patient with renal amyloidosis associated with Takayasu's arteritis after treatment with dimethylsulphoxide. Ann. Rheum. Dis. 53, 842–843.

Maksimowicz-McKinnon, K., Clark, T.M., Hoffman, G.S. 2007. Takayasu's arteritis: limitations of therapy and guarded prognosis in an American cohort. Arthritis Rheum. 56, 1000–1009.

Mandell, B.F., Hoffman, G.S. 2005. Rheumatic diseases and the cardiovascular system. In: D.P. Zipes, P. Libby, R.O. Bonow (Eds.), Braunwald's Heart Disease: a textbook of cardiovascular medicine. 7th ed., Braunwald E. Elsevier Saunders, Philadelphia, PA., p. 2104.

Manna, R., Cristiano, G., Todaro, L., et al. 1997. Microscopic haematuria: a diagnostic aid in giant-cell arteritis? Lancet. 350, 1226.

Marcussen, N., Lund, C. 1989. Combined sarcoidosis and disseminated visceral giant cell vasculitis. Pathol. Res. Pract. 184, 325–330.

Matsumoto, T., Uekusa, T., Fukuda, Y. 1991. Vasculo-Behcet's disease: a pathologic study of eight cases. Hum. Pathol. 22, 45–51.

Miyata, T., Sato, O., Koyama, H., et al. 2003. Long-term survival after surgical treatment of patients with Takayasu's arteritis. Circulation 108, 1474–1480.

Monteagudo, M., Vidal, G., Andreu, J., et al. 1997. Giant cell (temporal) arteritis and secondary renal amyloidosis: report of 2 cases. J. Rheumatol. 24, 605–607.

Montoliu, J., Amoedo, M.L., Panades, M.J., et al. 1997. Lessons to be learned from patients with vasculitis. Nephrol. Dial. Transplant. 12, 2781–2786.

Moraga, I., Sicilia, J.J., Blanco, J., et al. 2001. Giant cell arteritis and renal amyloidosis: report of a case. Clin. Nephrol. 56, 402–406.

Moreno, D., Yuste, J.R., Rodriguez, M., et al. 2005. Positron emission tomography use in the diagnosis and follow up of Takayasu's arteritis. Ann. Rheum. Dis. 64, 1091–1093.

Muller, E., Schneider, W., Kettritz, U., et al. 2004. Temporal arteritis with pauci-immune glomerulonephritis: a systemic disease. Clin. Nephrol. 62, 384–386.

Munir, I., Uflacker, R., Milutinovic, J. 2000. Takayasu's arteritis associated with intrarenal vessel involvement. Am. J. Kidney Dis. 35, 950–953.

Murai, T., Imai, M., Inui, M., et al. 1986. Generalized granulomatous arteritis with aortic dissection. Zentralbl. Allg. Pathol. 132, 41–47.

Muther, R.S., McCarron, D.A., Bennett, W.M. 1981. Renal manifestations of sarcoidosis. Arch. Intern. Med. 141, 643–645.

Nakao, K., Ikeda, M., Kimata, S., et al. 1967. Takayasu's arteritis. Clinical report of eighty-four cases and immunological studies of seven cases. Circulation 35, 1141–1155.

Nardi, P.M., Haller, J.O., Friedman, A.P., et al. 1985. Renal manifestations of Kawasaki's disease. Pediatr. Radiol. 15, 116–118.

Nesher, G., Berkun, Y., Mates, M., et al. 2004. Low-dose aspirin and prevention of cranial ischemic complications in giant cell arteritis. Arthritis Rheum. 50, 1332–1337.

Nitecki, S.S., Ofer, A., Karram, T., et al. 2004. Abdominal aortic aneurysm in Behcet's disease: new treatment options for an old and challenging problem. Isr. Med. Assoc. J. 6, 152–155.

Odagiri, S., Yoshida, Y., Kawahara, H., et al. 1989. Abdominal aortic aneurysm in a 3-year-old child: a case report and review of the Japanese-language literature. Surgery 106, 481–485.

O'Neill, W.M., Jr. Hammar, S.P., Bloomer, A. 1976. Giant cell arteritis with visceral angiitis. Arch. Intern. Med. 136, 1157–1160.

Ostberg, G. 1972. Morphological changes in the large arteries in polymyalgia arteritica. Acta Med. Scand. (Suppl. 533), 135–159.

Pajari, R., Hekali, P., Harjola, P.T. 1986. Treatment of Takayasu's arteritis: an analysis of 29 operated patients. Thorac. Cardiovasc. Surg. 34, 176–181.

Pascual, J., Quereda, C., Liano, F., et al. 1994. End-stage renal disease after necrotising glomerulonephritis in an elderly patient with temporal arteritis. Nephron. 66, 236–237.

Peterson, C., Jr. Willerson, J.T., Doppman, J.L., et al. 1970. Polyarteritis nodosa with bilateral renal artery aneurysms and perirenal haematomas: angiographic and nephrotomographic features. Br. J. Radiol. 43, 62–66.

Rath, B., Gupta, S., Tyagi, S., et al. 1996. Pulseless disease with renal amyloidosis. Pediatr. Nephrol. 10, 129–130.

Rhodes, J., King, M.E., Aretz, H.T. 1998. Case records of the Massachusetts General Hospital. Weekly clinicopathological exercises. Case 36-1998. An 11-year-old girl with fever, hypotension, and azotemia. N. Engl. J. Med. 339, 1619–1626.

Robenshtok, E., Krause, I. 2004. Arterial involvement in Behcet's disease—the search for new treatment strategies. Isr. Med. Assoc. J. 6, 162–163.

Romijn, J.A., Blaauwgeers, J.L., van Lieshout, J.J., et al. 1989. Bilateral kidney rupture with severe retroperitoneal bleeding in polyarteritis nodosa. Neth. J. Med. 35, 260–266.

Rose, C.D., Eichenfield, A.H., Goldsmith, D.P., et al. 1990. Early onset sarcoidosis with aortitis—"juvenile systemic granulomatosis?" J. Rheumatol. 17, 102–106.

Rotenstein, D., Gibbas, D.L., Majmudar, B., et al. 1982. Familial granulomatous arteritis with polyarthritis of juvenile onset. N. Engl. J. Med. 306, 86–90.

Saba, D., Saricaoglu, H., Bayram, A.S., et al. 2003. Arterial lesions in Behcet's disease. Vasa. 32, 75–81.

Salcedo, J.R., Greenberg, L., Kapur, S. 1988. Renal histology of mucocutaneous lymph node syndrome (Kawasaki disease). Clin. Nephrol. 29, 47–51.

Sasaguri, Y., Kato, H. 1982. Regression of aneurysms in Kawasaki disease: a pathological study. J. Pediatr. 100, 225–231.

Schlesinger, M., Oren, S., Fano, M., et al. 1989. Perirenal and renal subcapsular haematoma as presenting symptoms of polyarteritis nodosa. Postgrad. Med. J. 65, 681–683.

Scott, D.G., Bacon, P.A., Elliott, P.J., et al. 1982. Systemic vasculitis in a district general hospital 1972–1980: clinical and laboratory features, classification and prognosis of 80 cases. Q. J. Med. 51, 292–311.

Selga, D., Mohammad, A., Sturfelt, G., Segelmark, M. 2006. Polyarteritis nodosa when applying the Chapel Hill nomenclature–descriptive study on ten patients. Rheumatology 45, 1276–1281.

Shahram, F., Assadi, K., Davatchi, F., et al. 2003a. Chronology of clinical manifestations in Behcet's disease. Analysis of 4024 cases. Adv. Exp. Med. Biol. 528, 85–89.

Shahram, F., Davatchi, F., Nadji, A., et al. 2003b. Urine abnormalities in Behcet's disease. Study of 4704 cases. Adv. Exp. Med. Biol. 528, 477–478.

Sharma, B.K., Jain, S., Bali, H.K., et al. 2000a. A follow-up study of balloon angioplasty and de-novo stenting in Takayasu arteritis. Int. J. Cardiol. 75 (Suppl. 1), S147–S152.

Sharma, B.K., Jain, S., Vasishta, K. 2000b. Outcome of pregnancy in Takayasu arteritis. Int. J. Cardiol. 75 (Suppl. 1), S159–S162.

Sharma, S., Gupta, H., Saxena, A., et al. 1998. Results of renal angioplasty in nonspecific aortoarteritis (Takayasu disease). J. Vasc. Interv. Radiol. 9, 429–435.

Shelhamer, J.H., Volkman, D.J., Parrillo, J.E., et al. 1985. Takayasu's arteritis and its therapy. Ann. Intern. Med. 103, 121–126.

Shintaku, M., Mase, K., Ohtsuki, H., et al. 1989. Generalized sarcoidlike granulomas with systemic angiitis, crescentic glomerulonephritis, and pulmonary hemorrhage. Report of an autopsy case. Arch. Pathol. Lab. Med. 113, 1295–1298.

Silistreli, E., Karabay, O., Erdal, C., et al. 2004. Behcet's disease: treatment of popliteal pseudoaneurysm by an endovascular stent graft implantation. Ann. Vasc. Surg. 18, 118–120.

Sousa, A.E., Lucas, M., Tavora, I., et al. 1993. Takayasu's disease presenting as a nephrotic syndrome due to amyloidosis. Postgrad. Med. J. 69, 488–489.

Spiera, R.F., Mitnick, H.J., Kupersmith, M., et al. 2001. A prospective, double-blind, randomized, placebo controlled trial of methotrexate in the treatment of giant cell arteritis (GCA). Clin. Exp. Rheumatol. 19, 495–501.

St Clair, E.W., McCallum, R.M. 1999. Cogan's syndrome. Curr. Opin. Rheumatol. 11, 47–52.

Stockigt, J.R., Topliss, D.J., Hewett, M.J. 1979. High-renin hypertension in necrotizing vasculitis. N. Engl. J. Med. 300, 1218.

Strasser, F., Hailemariam, S., Weinreich, T., et al. 2000. Giant cell arteritis "causing" AA-amyloidosis with rapid renal failure. Schweiz. Med. Wochenschr. 130, 1606–1609.

Subramanyan, R., Joy, J., Balakrishnan, K.G. 1989. Natural history of aortoarteritis (Takayasu's disease). Circulation 80, 429–437.

Takagi, M., Ikeda, T., Kimura, K., et al. 1984. Renal histological studies in patients with Takayasu's arteritis. Report of 3 cases. Nephron. 36, 68–73.

Teoh, M.K. 1999. Takayasu's arteritis with renovascular hypertension: results of surgical treatment. Cardiovasc. Surg. 7, 626–632.

Thomas, H.G. 1992. Case report: clinical and radiological features of Cogan's syndrome—non-syphilitic interstitial keratitis, audiovestibular symptoms and systemic manifestations. Clin. Radiol. 45, 418–421.

Tiryaki, O., Buyukhatipoglu, H., Onat, A.M., Kervancioglu, S., Cologlu, S., Usalan, C. 2007. Takayasu arteritis: association with focal segmental glomerulosclerosis. Clin. Rheumatol. 26, 609–611.

Truong, L., Kopelman, R.G., Williams, G.S., et al. 1985. Temporal arteritis and renal disease. Case report and review of the literature. Am. J. Med. 78, 171–175.

Tso, E., Flamm, S.D., White, R.D., et al. 2002. Takayasu arteritis: utility and limitations of magnetic resonance imaging in diagnosis and treatment. Arthritis Rheum. 46, 1634–1642.

Tyagi, S., Singh, B., Kaul, U.A., et al. 1993. Balloon angioplasty for renovascular hypertension in Takayasu's arteritis. Am. Heart J. 125, 1386–1393.

Tyagi, S., Verma, P.K., Gambhir, D.S., et al. 1998. Early and long-term results of subclavian angioplasty in aortoarteritis (Takayasu disease): comparison with atherosclerosis. Cardiovasc. Intervent. Radiol. 21, 219–224.

Udayaraj, U.P., Hand, M.F., Shilliday, I.R., et al. 2004. Renal involvement in Cogan's syndrome. Nephrol. Dial. Transplant. 19, 2420–2421.

Umemoto, M., Take, H., Yamaguchi, H., et al. 1997. Juvenile systemic granulomatosis manifesting as premature aging syndrome and renal failure. J. Rheumatol. 24, 393–395.

Valsakumar, A.K., Valappil, U.C., Jorapur, V., et al. 2003. Role of immunosuppressive therapy on clinical, immunological, and angiographic outcome in active Takayasu's arteritis. J. Rheumatol. 30, 1793–1798.

van der Meulen, J., Gupta, R.K., Peregrin, J.H., et al. 1989. Takayasu's arteritis and nephrotic syndrome in a patient with crossed renal ectopia. Neth. J. Med. 34, 142–147.

Vanderschueren, S., Depoot, I., Knockaert, D.C., et al. 2002. Microscopic haematuria in giant cell arteritis. Clin. Rheumatol. 21, 373–377.

Vanoli, M., Daina, E., Salvarani, C., et al. 2005. Takayasu's arteritis: a study of 104 Italian patients. Arthritis Rheum. 53, 100–107.

Veiga, P.A., Pieroni, D., Baier, W., et al. 1992. Association of Kawasaki disease and interstitial nephritis. Pediatr. Nephrol. 6, 421–423.

Vella, J.P., O'Callaghan, J., Hickey, D., et al. 1997. Renal artery stenosis complicating Cogan's syndrome. Clin. Nephrol. 47, 407–408.

Vollertsen, R.S., McDonald, T.J., Younge, B.R., et al. 1986. Cogan's syndrome: 18 cases and a review of the literature. Mayo Clin. Proc. 61, 344–361.

Wada, Y., Nishida, H., Kohno, K., et al. 1999. AA amyloidosis in Takayasu's arteritis—long-term survival on maintenance haemodialysis. Nephrol. Dial. Transplant. 14, 2478–2481.

Weaver, F.A., Kumar, S.R., Yellin, A.E., et al. 2004. Renal revascularization in Takayasu arteritis-induced renal artery stenosis. J. Vasc. Surg. 39, 749–757.

Weaver, F.A., Yellin, A.E., Campen, D.H., et al. 1990. Surgical procedures in the management of Takayasu's arteritis. J. Vasc. Surg. 12, 429–437. discussion 438–439.

Weiler, V., Redtenbacher, S., Bancher, C., et al. 2000. Concurrence of sarcoidosis and aortitis: case report and review of the literature. Ann. Rheum. Dis. 59, 850–853.

Wooditch, A.C., Aronoff, S.C. 2005. Effect of initial corticosteroid therapy on coronary artery aneurysm formation in Kawasaki disease: a meta-analysis of 862 children. Pediatrics 116, 989–995.

Yoshikawa, Y., Truong, L.D., Mattioli, C.A., et al. 1988. Membranoproliferative glomerulonephritis in Takayasu's arteritis. Am. J. Nephrol. 8, 240–244.

Yoshimura, M., Kida, H., Saito, Y., et al. 1985. Peculiar glomerular lesions in Takayasu's arteritis. Clin. Nephrol. 24, 120–127.

Zheng, D.Y., Liu, L.S., Fan, D.J. 1990. Clinical studies in 500 patients with aortoarteritis. Chin. Med. J. (England) 103, 536–540.

Zilleruelo, G.E., Ferrer, P., Garcia, O.L., et al. 1978. Takayasu's arteritis associated with glomerulonephritis. A case report. Am. J. Dis. Child. 132, 1009–1013.

# CHAPTER 11

# Anti-GBM Disease: Mechanisms, Clinical Features, and Treatment

Lorna Henderson, Neil Turner*

*Renal and Autoimmunity Group, Centre for Inflammation, University of Edinburgh, Hugh Robson Building, George Square, Edinburgh EH8 9XD, Scotland, UK*

## 1. Introduction

Anti-glomerular basement membrane (anti-GBM) disease is the best-defined renal organ-specific autoimmune disease. The disease is strongly associated with autoantibody formation to a specific target found in the glomerular and alveolar basement membranes and is characterized by a rapidly progressive glomerulonephritis (RPGN) which is often associated with pulmonary hemorrhage, though either may occur alone.

In 1919 Ernest Goodpasture first described the clinical syndrome of pulmonary hemorrhage associated with glomerulonephritis as a result of an autopsy on an 18-year-old man during the 1918 influenza pandemic (Goodpasture, 1919). Little more was heard of this syndrome until 1958, when Stanton and Tange described a group of nine patients with similar findings and gave Goodpasture's name to the condition (Stanton and Tange, 1958).

There are multiple causes of the association between glomerulonephritis and pulmonary hemorrhage. The term Goodpasture's disease is reserved for individuals who have disease in association with antibodies to the glomerular basement membrane (GBM), either bound directly to the target organ or in the circulation. In early series, mortality was very high and irreversible renal failure a common outcome. The introduction of cyclophosphamide and plasma exchange however transformed therapy, and this became the first unequivocally effective therapy for inflammatory renal disease (Lockwood et al., 1976).

## 2. Epidemiology

Goodpasture's syndrome is uncommon, with an incidence of up to 1 case per million population per annum in the UK, based on the identification of anti-GBM antibodies by immunoassay and in biopsy specimens. It has been reported to account for up to 5% of cases of glomerulonephritis (Wilson and Dixon, 1973; New Zealand Glomerulonephritis Study Group, 1989), but 10–20% of crescentic glomerulonephritis (Couser, 1988; Andrassy et al., 1991). The disease is more common in White and certain other racial groups including the indigenous population of New Zealand (Teague et al., 1978). It seems to be rare in South Asian and Black races, but cases have been reported in Japan and China.

The distribution by gender is approximately equal, with a slight preponderance of males to females. The age at presentation can vary from first to ninth decade. There is however a bimodal distribution, with a greater number of individuals presenting around 30 years and a second peak at around 60 (Savage et al., 1986). The youngest case presented at 11-months-old and several patients in their 9th decade have been described, although presentations at such extremes are very rare. This age and gender distribution is somewhat dissimilar

---

*Corresponding author.
Tel.: 0131-242-9167; Fax: +44 131 242 1233
E-mail address: neil.turner@ed.ac.uk

© 2008 Elsevier B.V. All rights reserved.
DOI: 10.1016/S1571-5078(07)07011-0

to that of other organ-specific autoimmune disorders. Pulmonary hemorrhage appears more common in the young, and in males, and lone glomerulonephritis is more common in older patients and in women. While the disease can present at any time, its incidence appears to increase in the spring and early summer.

Clustering of cases has been described in three reports (Simpson et al., 1982; Perez et al., 1974; Williams et al., 1988). Within our own unit in Edinburgh, two cases presented within a few months of each other in unrelated individuals who were in fact next door neighbors. Such reports lend support to the hypothesis that exposure to an infective or other exogenous agent is involved in the pathogenesis (see later). To date however, no such pathogen has been identified. One of the greatest difficulties in analyzing potential exogenous agents is the likelihood that any infective agent may exacerbate tissue injury caused by existing disease, leading to its clinical presentation without necessarily causing it.

Disease associations may give some clues to aetiology. Several are disorders in which there may be increased production or destruction of the target antigen in GBM (Table 1). Associations with other autoimmune disorders are uncommon. The occurrence of anti-GBM disease in up to 5% of patients with Alport's syndrome after renal transplantation is an informative special circumstance which is discussed further below.

A strong class II MHC association has been described, with over 80% of patients carrying HLA-DR15. A negative association exists with DR7 and possibly DR1. Class II MHC associations are found to varying degrees in almost all autoimmune diseases and this is discussed further below.

## 3. Clinical features

Typically patients present with fulminant disease of short duration although minor symptoms, usually of pulmonary disease, may have been present for weeks and occasionally much longer. A sudden crescendo of disease intensity is common and it is often only when this occurs that the disease is diagnosed. In such patients, the time window in which treatment can be instigated to salvage renal function and even life, is short (Glassock, 1999; Turner and Rees, 1998).

Affected individuals may also present with a benign history of malaise, headaches, fever, myalgia, arthralgia, and weight loss, although these are generally mild. This is in contrast to most cases of vasculitis presenting with pulmonary renal syndrome, in which clinical features are more severe. Anemia (usually microcytic and hypochromic) is common and frequently symptomatic, and is most likely a reflection of sub-clinical pulmonary hemorrhage.

### 3.1. Pulmonary disease

Patients may present with pulmonary or renal disease alone. Pulmonary hemorrhage used to be reported in two-thirds of patients, but recent series suggest the prevalence has fallen to 50% or less. Typically, pulmonary hemorrhage presents as haemoptysis that may be episodic. However pulmonary hemorrhage can occur without haemoptysis, which is often a poor guide to the quantity of pulmonary bleeding. Lung hemorrhage

Table 1
Diseases recurrently associated with Goodpasture's disease

| Disease | Number of reports (approximately) |
| --- | --- |
| ANCA-associated vasculitis (mostly with anti-myeloperoxidase ANCA) | Hundreds |
| Membranous nephropathy | <20 |
| Diabetes mellitus | 10 |
| Lithotripsy to intrarenal stones | 3 |
| (Alport's syndrome following renal transplantation) | (Tens) |

*Note*: Alport's syndrome following transplantation is bracketed as it is predominantly an alloimmune rather than an autoimmune example of anti-GBM disease.

can cause haemoptysis relatively early, leading patients to seek medical attention when signs of renal involvement may be minimal, resulting in paradoxical observation that pulmonary hemorrhage may be associated with a better renal outcome.

In contrast with renal injury, pulmonary hemorrhage does not correlate well with circulating levels of antibody (Wilson and Dixon, 1981; Simpson et al., 1982). Although Goodpasture antigen is present on both alveolar and GBM, there is a lack of direct contact between antibody and alveolar basement membrane, either because intrinsic properties of the basement membrane prevent access to the autoantigen, or because the unfenestrated (or thinly fenestrated) endothelium that lines alveolar capillaries provides a greater barrier than the fenestrated endothelium in glomeruli (Lerner et al., 1967; Mcphaul and Dixon, 1970).

It is postulated that a second insult is required before circulating antibodies are allowed access (Jennings et al., 1981; Downie et al., 1982; Yamamoto and Wilson, 1987). Cigarette smoking or exposure to other inhaled toxins have been associated with pulmonary hemorrhage in Goodpasture's disease, and anecdotally a prompt recurrence of disease has been noted on the resumption of smoking in patients in whom the disease was seemingly under control. Pulmonary edema and infection have also been shown to provoke lung hemorrhage in Goodpasture's disease (Briggs et al., 1979; Rees et al., 1979; Bailey et al., 1981; Simpson et al., 1982). Pulmonary hemorrhage does however have a tendency to remit and relapse spontaneously (Schindler et al., 1998; Schmidt et al., 1999), which often complicates interpretation of associated exposure and response to therapy.

Although physical examination can be normal, the more severely affected are tachypnoeic and/or cyanosed. Fresh blood can be expectorated and dry inspiratory crackles, most prominently over the lower lung fields, can be heard on auscultation, occasionally accompanied by areas of bronchial breathing. Most episodes of hemorrhage are associated with radiological changes, usually affecting central lung fields, with peripheral and upper-lobe sparing. Abnormalities are often symmetrical and rarely confined by fissures, which should raise the suspicion of consolidation, either alone or superimposed on hemorrhage. Shadowing caused by bleeding often starts to resolve within 48 h, but may last longer. Changes are usually gone within 2 weeks. Diagnosis of hemorrhage can be supported by a sudden unexplained drop in hemoglobin, as well as by characteristic radiological changes. Bleeding into the lung causes an acute increase in the transfer factor corrected for lung volume and hemoglobin ($K_{CO}$), and this is the most specific test for lung hemorrhage, although not all patients may be well enough for this investigation in the acute setting.

## 3.2. Renal disease

Patients may present with renal disease alone, although some develop clinical or sub-clinical pulmonary hemorrhage later. As the symptoms of minor renal disease are non-specific, it is common for presentation of isolated renal disease to occur at an advanced and often irreversible stage. Renal disease is much less likely to have a relapsing and remitting course, although renal involvement can occasionally remit spontaneously if mild. If significant renal damage has occurred, spontaneous remission is extremely unlikely and deterioration often rapid.

Abnormalities of urinary sediment, usually in the form of microscopic haematuria, are the earliest signs of renal damage. At this stage, serum urea and creatinine are often normal and urine abnormalities may remit and relapse without specific treatment. At a more advanced stage, urine contains many dysmorphic red cells and red cell casts. Patients can present with subacute renal disease, leading to nephrotic syndrome together with haematuria and variable renal impairment, although mild or rapidly progressive renal disease is much more common. Loin pain can occur if nephritis is severe and macroscopic haematuria is common. Hypertension is uncommon and oliguria suggests that renal damage is already at an advanced stage and the prognosis is poor.

The kidneys are typically of normal size or, in acute disease, may be enlarged. No other characteristic morphological findings are seen on renal imaging. Even where the diagnosis appears obvious, renal biopsy (Figs. 1 and 2) should be performed for prognostic reasons and to aid decisions about therapy.

Anti-GBM antibodies fixed to other basement membranes have been reported rarely. The eye is an exception, where retinal detachment has been described in at least four cases (Jampol et al., 1975; Boucher et al., 1987; Sharma, 1998) associated with antibody fixation to Bruch's membrane and the basement membrane of choroidal vessels (Jampol et al., 1975). Fixation of antibody to the choroid plexus (which also has a fenestrated endothelium) may also be quite common, although whether this has any clinical relevance, such as causing the convulsions seen in some patients, remains unclear.

## 4. Diagnosis

Diagnosis is based on the demonstration of anti-GBM antibodies, either in the circulation or fixed to basement membrane of affected organs on biopsy.

### 4.1. Antibodies

The most sensitive technique for antibody detection is direct immunohistological examination of the renal biopsy, provided the sample is adequate and the glomeruli are not too severely damaged.

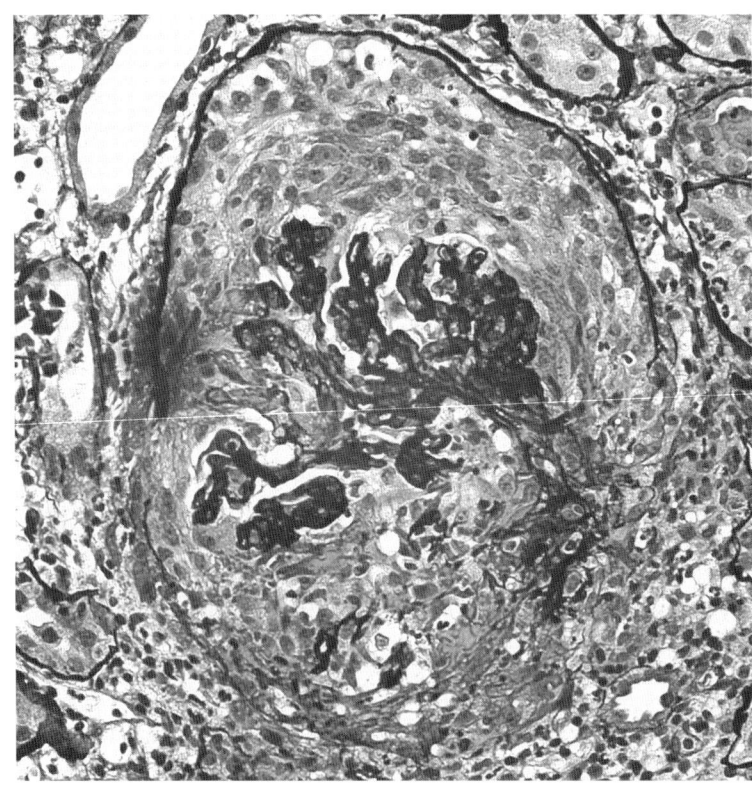

**Figure 1.** Crescentic nephritis in anti-GBM disease. A highly cellular crescent with fibrin deposition from GBM fractures, and fibrin thrombi can also be seen in some capillaries at 9 O'Clock. The lower segment of the glomerular tuft has been almost completely destroyed, and Bowman's capsule also contains many breaks over its lower circumference. (Courtesy of Dr. Chris Bellamy.)

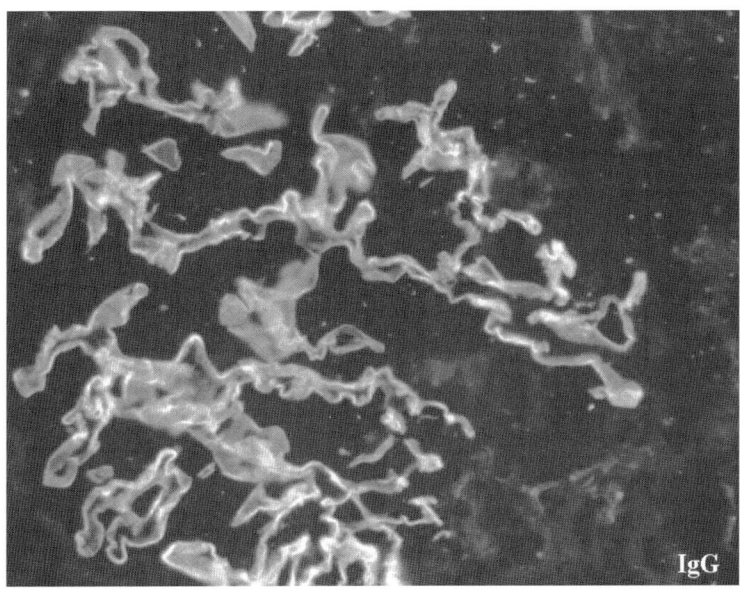

**Figure 2.** Linear deposition of IgG shown by direct immunofluorescence in a patient with crescentic nephritis caused by anti-GBM disease. (Courtesy of Dr. Chris Bellamy.)

Although linear fixation of IgG to the GBM is described in several circumstances, linear fixation in the setting of a crescentic nephritis is specific to anti-GBM disease, or to systemic vasculitis associated with anti-GBM disease (Turner and Rees, 1998). Direct immunohistochemistry of the lung biopsy is less reliable, as antibody fixation is often patchy. Indirect immunohistochemistry using patients' sera and sections of normal kidney is relatively insensitive.

Immunoassays for circulating antibodies are often used, and while helpful, may have varying reliability (Litwin et al., 1996). They can give false positive or negative results, depending on antigen preparation and samples used to calibrate the assay. For this reason, if there is any doubt, Western blotting should be performed at a reference center. Circulating antibody is usually IgG1 and IgG4 (Segelmark et al., 1990). There have been occasional reports in which IgA alone was detected. As systemic vasculitis can present in a similar fashion and indeed even overlap with anti-GBM disease, anti-neutrophil cytoplasm antibodies (ANCA) should always be measured along with anti-GBM antibodies.

## 4.2. Renal biopsy

The earliest changes on biopsy are of segmental mesangial cell expansion and hypercellularity. Changes then typically progress to a focal and segmental glomerular necrosis, with destruction of the GBM and cellular proliferation leading to crescent formation (Fig. 1). Crescents are generally at the same stage of evolution, unlike the picture in systemic vasculitis. Vasculitis on biopsy suggests the simultaneous presence of ANCA-related disease. As lesions progress, an interstitial nephritis with subsequent fibrosis and tubular atrophy develops.

Linear binding of antibody to GBM is found in all patients regardless of disease severity (Fig. 2). Antibody may also be detected on the basement membrane of the distal convoluted tubule and the collecting duct. IgG is virtually always detected, but other immunoglobulins are found in addition in around 30% of cases. Linear C3 is seen in 60–70%. On rare occasions, IgA or IgM alone are reported. IgA antibody in the circulation and on the GBM, in association with lung hemorrhage and RPGN, has been documented.

On electron microscopy, the GBM usually demonstrates widespread irregular broadening, and breaks in the GBM are common. Endothelial and epithelial cells are swollen and there may be effacement of the foot processes. At a later stage, subepithelial deposits have also been described.

## 4.3. Pulmonary biopsy

Linear fixation of immunoglobulin can be detected at autopsy in patients with pulmonary hemorrhage. However, binding is patchy and hence bronchial biopsy is unreliable for diagnostic use in anti-GBM disease.

## 5. Mechanisms

### 5.1. Aetiology

The clinical outline presented above provides clues that are helpful in approaching the pathogenesis of the disease. It illustrates that:

1. Breaking of tolerance is rare.
2. Association with other autoimmune diseases is rare.
3. Increased turnover or destruction of basement membrane may be implicated in disease initiation.
4. Antibody formation is consistent and likely to be a central part of the pathogenesis of the disease.
5. HLA genes are a strong predisposing factor in disease susceptibility

The clinical syndrome of autoimmune disease caused by activation of T-cells, B-cells, or both, in the absence of infection, is the consequence of the failure of safety mechanisms established under the heading of tolerance. For years the presentation of autoimmunity was thought to be based on the clonal deletion of autoreactive cells, leaving a repertoire of T- and B-cells capable of recognizing solely foreign antigen. Current understanding has shifted and acknowledges that a degree of autoreactivity is likely to be physiological (Dighiero and Rose, 1999), and indeed crucial to normal immune function.

Autoantigen has been demonstrated to help form the repertoire of mature lymphocytes, and continuous exposure to low-level antigen is necessary to allow the survival of naïve T- and B-cells in the periphery. In theory, as there is no fundamental difference in the structure between self and foreign antigen, lymphocytes may have evolved not to distinguish self from foreign antigen, but to respond to antigen in certain microenviroments such as in the presence of inflammatory cytokines (Silverstein and Rose, 2000).

The challenge then is to understand how this physiological process becomes pathological. More is known about Goodpasture's disease than any other autoimmune renal disorder. Some information comes from animal studies, but in this disease there are also invaluable clinical studies and results from laboratory investigation of the human antigen, antibodies, and lymphocytes.

### 5.2. Antigen

Basement membranes are specialized and complex structures, usually found at the boundary between cells and connective tissue stroma. The membranes themselves can influence the fate of cells, the polarization of subcellular constituents, and the location of cell receptors and transporters. The majority of the components of the basement membrane are ubiquitous to all basement membranes, while others have a more restricted distribution, probably related to more specific functions within the respective basement membrane (Miner, 1999). Within the kidney, the GBM is a key component of the ultrafiltration barrier. It is assembled through interweaving of collagen IV with laminins, nidogen, and sulphated proteoglycans.

Collagen IV (Fig. 3) was first isolated by Kefalides from GBM in 1966. It belongs to a family of collagenous proteins with at least 25 members. The genes *COL4A1* to *COL4A6* encoding the six chains of collagen IV, $\alpha 1(IV)$–$\alpha 6(IV)$, which form three sets of triple helical molecules

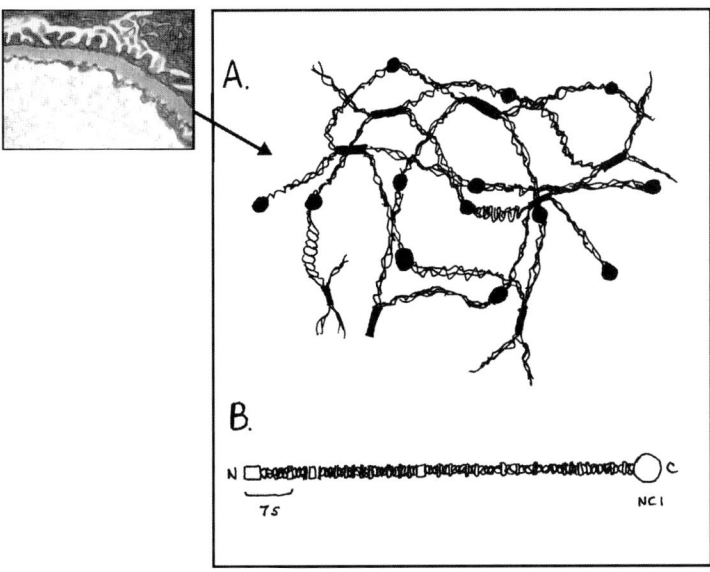

**Figure 3.** Type IV collagen is the major protein of basement membranes. Its triple helical protomers have multiple non-collagenous interruptions that make the fibers non-linear, with kinks and tertiary coils and the head-to-head and tail-to-tail interactions form an open meshwork. The Goodpasture antigen lies in the C-terminal, non-collagenous domain.

(protomers), α1α1α2, α3α4α5, and α5α5α6, selectively expressed in different membranes at different stages of embryonic development. These protomers create fishnet-like collagenous networks by covalent associations, as dimers head-to-head and tetramers tail-to-tail. The α1α1α2 network is present in almost all basement membranes, while the other networks have a much more tissue-specific distribution, with that of α3α4α5 being particularly limited. It is found especially in basement membranes, formed by fusion of epithelial and endothelial cell basement membranes or those involved in gas or fluid exchange or transfer. These networks occur in the GBM and some tubular basement membranes in the kidneys and in the lungs testis, cochlea, and eye (Cashman et al., 1988). Glomerular epithelial cells seem to be responsible for the synthesis of α3α4α5 collagens in the formation of GBM.

Hudson and co-workers recognized that most of the circulating antibodies in patients with anti-GBM disease were directed against a non-collagenous (NC1) domain of a new type IV collagen chain that they termed α3 (Wieslander et al., 1984; Saus et al., 1988). This was confirmed by cDNA cloning, which showed that the 230 amino acid carboxy terminal domain α3(IV)NC1 was the consistent target of autoantibodies in all patients with anti-GBM disease (Turner et al., 1992).

## 5.3. Antibodies and B-cell epitopes

In detailed studies with recombinant proteins some patients show additional, usually minor reactivity to other NC1 domains, but while reactivity with α3(IV)NC1 is consistent and restricted, much of the reactivity of any one patient can be blocked by other patients' sera or even by single monoclonal antibodies (Hellmark et al., 1994). Antibodies may make up 1–5% of circulating IgG in patients with active disease (unpublished observations). Within α3(IV)NC1 there is a dominant, consistent epitope termed $E_A$ at residues 17–31, towards the N-terminal end of the NC1 domain close to the triple helical region, and a subdominant epitope $E_B$ in the second hemidomain at 127–141 (Ryan et al., 1998; Netzer et al., 1999; Hellmark et al., 1999; Borza et al., 2000; David et al., 2001). The epitope is highly conformational, rendering early studies using synthetic peptides or bacterially

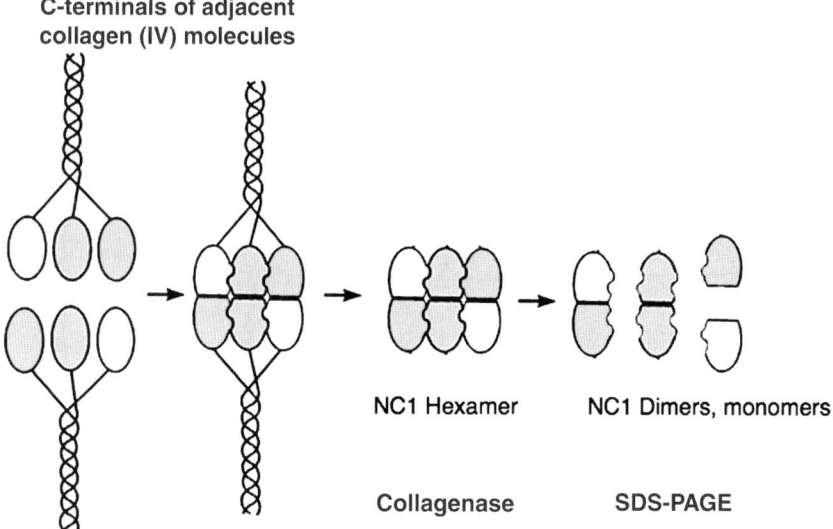

**Figure 4.** The NC1 domains of adjacent α3α4α5 protomers are tightly associated as hexamers. Digestion with enzymes that break down collagens releases hexamers intact and this process is presumably part of normal basement membrane turnover and of destructive proteolysis during inflammation. Dissociation of NC1 hexamers (e.g. for SDS–PAGE chromatography or by low pH) releases dimers and monomers of the constituent alpha chain NC1 domains and exposes further antibody-binding epitopes. Persisting dimers are composed of monomers covalently linked by disulfide and other covalent linkages.

produced antigen unreliable. There is a degree of concealment or crypticity of the B-cell epitope in the fully folded NC1 domain, which can be purified from GBM as a hexamer containing the NC1 domains of two adjacent α3α4α5 protomers (Borza et al., 2000; Wieslander et al., 1985) (Fig. 4). However, in vivo circulating antibodies bind to the normal GBM of experimental animals, including primates, and to the apparently normal GBM of humans. Detailed studies suggest that subtle differences in the covalent bonding between monomers of adjacent fibrils may influence the accessibility of the epitope, with many more sites becoming available when the molecule is dissociated (Borza et al., 2005).

## 5.4. Regulatory and effector T-cell epitopes and their generation

Tolerance to self antigens is maintained by regulatory T-cells, as well as by deletion of cells with a high affinity for presented peptides of self antigens. The α3 chain of type IV collagen has been demonstrated to be "promiscuously" expressed in the thymus, in common with many other known autoantigens (Salama et al., 2001; Wong et al., 2001). Expression of the α5 chain is more widespread, and it seems likely that tolerance to it would be more secure. Although the percentage of T-cells capable of recognizing the alpha chain deleted in the thymus is not clear, it is known that a small percentage do survive into the periphery. Peripheral blood T lymphocytes in both healthy individuals and patients with disease are capable of proliferating to α3(IV)NC1 when incubated in its presence in vitro (Derry et al., 1995; Salama et al., 2001). T-cells that proliferate in healthy individuals are much less abundant than in those with active disease or those in the recovery stage of disease (Salama et al., 2001). Cairns et al. demonstrated that the T-cells of patients recognized a different set of epitopes on α3(IV)NC1 than those derived from healthy controls. The relative proportions of anergic and regulatory cells is not yet known (Cairns et al., 2003).

Extensive work in our laboratory has used biochemical techniques to identify peptides that appear bound to HLA-DR15 on the surface of B cells that have processed recombinant Goodpasture antigen. This avoids the confounding effects of tolerance when using conventional lymphocyte responsiveness assays to define peptides presented. Three nested sets of peptides were identified, each centered on core sequences of nine-amino-acid long MHC-binding motifs. The peptides have intermediate affinity for the presenting HLA-DR15 molecules, confirming that antigen processing pathways exert a strong influence on the peptides presented (Phelps et al., 1996, 1998). Importantly, these are different from the peptides recognized by patients with active anti-GBM disease (Cairns et al., 2003). Recent observations suggest that the disease-associated peptides are not the specific subjects of immune tolerance, because in normal antigen processing they are destroyed very early in an obligatory first "unlocking" step in proteolysis by Cathepsin D/E (Zou et al., 2007). This dependence on a specific unlocking step has been described for other globular proteins including another potential autoantigen, myelin basic protein (Manoury et al., 2002), but with dependence on a different proteolytic enzyme, asparginyl endopeptidase (AEP). Using a specific and consistent unlocking step might be immunologically important, as it will help antigen presenting cells generate a predictable rather than random set of peptides in early antigen processing, allowing a subset of all possible peptides to be the subject of immune responses. The implications of these findings are that anti-GBM disease initiation will require an altered antigen processing mechanism or pathway.

## 5.5. Initiation of the autoimmune response

In experimental animals, initiating an autoimmune response requires several actions, and these are highly informative when considering how autoimmune diseases may be intitiated in man:

- Choose a susceptible strain—where genetic susceptibility has been mapped, multiple loci are usually involved, for example in the Wistar–Kyoto rat which is particularly susceptible to crescentic nephritis and vasculitis (Reynolds et al., 2002). It is clear that this is also true in human autoimmune diseases (Chapter 1). The only well-established genetic association in Goodpasture's disease so far is HLA linkage. There are reports of discordance in monozygotic twins, and this is generally true for autoimmune diseases, showing that at least a second, if not third, hit is required on a background of genetic susceptibility. Reports of clusters of cases mentioned above provide strong circumstantial evidence for an exogenous factor—but no factor has been identified in any of these clusters.
- Immunize with a *slightly modified* antigen—to induce an immune response that can cross-react with a self protein. The most common strategy is to use antigen prepared from another species so that there are some sequence differences, but post-translational, chemical, or structural alterations may also suffice. B lymphocytes may be important in generating this type of cross-reactivity. It is frequently hypothesized, though rarely proven, that molecular mimicry by microorganisms is an important initiating element in autoimmune diseases (reviewed by Wucherpfennig, 2001). Looking for linear sequence similarities is probably an oversimplification, as T-cells see shapes not sequences, and T-cell clones may be stimulated by peptides of quite different sequence (Wucherpfennig and Stromiger, 1995). Antigen modifications may also follow chemical or other modifications, including somatic mutations of self proteins.
- Use an adjuvant—without an adjuvant, immune responses in animals are frequently absent or benign. The stimulation of toll-like receptors, and possibly other pathways, can critically influence the outcome of the interaction between an antigen presenting cell and interacting lymphocytes, switching from the default response of tolerance to one of active immunity—the "danger hypothesis" (Gallucci and Matzinger, 2001). If the mimicry hypothesis is favored, the same microorganism may

also provide the adjuvant stimulus. However, there is no demonstrable consistent relationship between specific infections and most autoimmune diseases.

The associations of Goodpasture's disease with small-vessel vasculitis, lithotripsy, and to a lesser extent membranous nephropathy and possibly diabetes, support the idea that a quantitative or qualitative change in antigen presentation may be important. Lithotripsy is known to cause renal trauma; as the kidney moves with respiration it is almost impossible to prevent some exposure to shock waves and potential tissue damage when fragmenting intrarenal stones (Evan et al., 1991; Jaeger et al., 1995). In diabetes and membranous nephropathy, the thickened and abnormal GBM contains an increased amount of Goodpasture antigen. As discussed above, there is good reason to suspect that a change in antigen presentation occurs in disease initiation, permitting generation of disease-associated peptides, which are abnormally presented, and to which there is no (or less) tolerance.

## 6. Mechanisms of injury

Though the pendulum has swung forward and back, it is clear that both cell-mediated and antibody-dependent mechanisms are integral to the damage seen in anti-GBM disease.

### 6.1. Injury caused by antibodies

In 1967, Lerner, Glassock, and Dixon demonstrated that anti-GBM antibodies were nephrotoxic. Nephritic kidneys from patients with anti-GBM disease were acid-eluted in order to obtain purified antibody. The antibody was injected into unilaterally nephrectomized squirrel monkeys, which subsequently developed fulminant glomerulonephritis and renal failure. In humans, pathogenicity of circulating anti-GBM antibodies was suggested by the close association of circulating antibodies and disease, as well as by the titre of antibody and severity and subsequent resolution of disease (Simpson et al., 1982; Savage et al., 1986; Herody et al., 1993).

In genetically engineered mice that produce human IgG antibodies, immunization with α3(IV) NC1 domains results in the production of human anti-GBM antibodies and a proliferative glomerulonephritis (Meyers et al., 2002). It should be noted, that in this model, the changes produced by antibodies alone were not of a crescentic nephritis. In the WKY rat, transfer of antibodies has been demonstrated to transfer disease (discussed further below).

Human anti-GBM antibodies, usually of the IgG-complement-fixing class or rarely IgA, are of particularly high affinity and remain attached to the GBM for prolonged periods (Rutgers et al., 2000). Anti-GBM antibody binding to GBM activates complement, leading to cell injury and inflammation. The cleavage of C3 generates C3 fragments and ultimately the membrane attack complex (C5b-9), which inserts into cell membranes where it may lyse cells or activate them to secrete cytokines. Subsequent recruitment of cellular effectors is critical to further damage.

### 6.2. Injury caused by T lymphocytes

The evidence to suggest that cell-mediated immunity has an important role to play in aggressive glomerulonephritis has been summarized by Bolton (Bolton, 2002). Lymphocytes are seen in biopsies, and the IgG subclass distribution of autoantibodies IgG1 and IgG4 suggest a T-cell-dependent process. The strong association of disease with HLA Class II alleles, in vitro evidence of cell mediated immunity and the observation that effective treatments also act on cell-mediated immunity provide additional support.

In animal models of injury caused by anti-GBM disease, CD4+ and CD8+ T-cells, and intrinsic renal epithelium, induce the migration of macrophages and neutrophils into the kidney (Tipping et al., 1997; Wu et al., 2002; Timoshanko et al., 2001). IL-12 and IFN-γ mediate crescent formation (Timoshanko et al., 2001, 2002). The initial inflammatory reaction in the glomerulus produces proteinuria and the attendant downstream consequences for tubular epithelium, namely the development of interstitial nephritis and the subsequent fibrosis (Abbate et al., 1998).

Studies of murine models show the importance of inducing a Th1 response if pathology is to develop, and suggests T-cells may be important, not only in providing help for autoantibody production, but also for driving glomerular inflammation (Huang et al., 1997). In particular, disease could be passively transferred with anti-α3(IV)NC1 antibody from nephritogenic strains to syngeneic recipients, but not to TCR-deficient mice, suggesting crescentic nephritis requires cell-mediated immunity. (Tipping and Holdsworth, 2006).

In the last few years, a rat model of experimental allergic glomerulonephritis (EAG) has allowed greater understanding of the potential role of T-cells in immunopathogenesis. The Wistar Kyoto (WKY) rat model of EAG, originally described by Sado (Sado et al., 1998), demonstrates that EAG can be generated in animals without antibody production, that disease can be transferred by T-cells alone, and can be induced by peptide immunization where antibody binding to the GBM is undetectable (Robertson et al., 2005). Interestingly, diseases can be transferred by antibodies in the WKY rat, (Chen et al., 2003; Sado et al., 1992) perhaps through altered antigen presentation leading to generation of new aggressive T-cells in the recipient animal.

The T-cell epitope responsible for EAG in WKY rats is in the amino-terminal third of α3(IV)NC1, where the human antibody epitope is to be found (Bolton et al., 2005a, b), but this is distinct from the T-cell epitopes identified in patients (Cairns et al., 2003). Remarkably, immunization with a minimal peptide can induce disease in which antibodies are formed as a secondary phenomenon, or without antibody generation at all. The length of the peptide influences the formation of anti-GBM antibody and the presence of certain amino acid residues at position 19 appears to be critical for disease induction (Bolton et al., 2005a, b). The potential for immunotherapy directed at T-cells is highlighted by the success of tolerogenic intervention with oral α3(IV)NC1 administration in attenuating nephritis and the associated Th1 response in disease susceptible rats (Reynolds et al., 2005).

## 6.3. Factors modulating injury

Intercurrent infection has long been known to increase the intensity of the inflammatory response and end organ damage (Rees et al., 1978). These clinical observations are supported by experimental evidence (e.g. Karkar and Rees, 1997).

# 7. Genetic influences

## 7.1. HLA

Epidemiological studies have demonstrated that genetic factors are crucial determinants of susceptibility to autoimmune disease. The majority of autoimmune diseases are multigenic. In isolation, these polymorphisms or mutations are usually subclinical. Only when present with other susceptibility genes do they contribute to autoimmunity, and even then, some kind of "second hit" is required to initiate the disease process.

In common with other human autoimmune diseases, Goodpasture's has been associated with inheritance of specific class II HLA alleles (Phelps et al., 2000). HLA class II molecules consist of an alpha and beta chain, with the greatest variability in the beta chain. They are encoded at the DR, DP, and DQ loci on chromosome 6. DR specificities are determined exclusively by differences in the $\beta$ chain encoded by the DRB1 locus. DR2 requires DRB1*15 or DRB1*16 at the B1 locus, the former of which accounts for >80% of the DR specificity in the northern European caucasoids most commonly affected by this disease. Meta-analysis has confirmed that anti-GBM disease is strongly associated with DRB1*1501, and has clarified weaker associations with alleles DRB1*04 and DRB1*03. Weaker negative associations are also seen with DRB1*07 and DRB1*01.

Susceptibility to Goodpasture's disease is shown to be influenced by a combination of DRB1 alleles inherited on maternal and paternal chromosomes. Gene dosage does not affect susceptibility, as it is similarly increased in homozygous or heterozygous individuals for DRB1*1501. The effect also includes neutralization of the susceptibility enhancing effect of DRB1*1501 by co-inherited DRB1*07. Thus, DRB1 and 7 confer dominant protection against anti-GBM disease. This strongly suggests an interaction, most likely occurring between the class II molecules they encode. The obvious assumption is that there might be competition for the disease-causing peptide. However, the explanation could also lie in the opposite interpretation, that a tolerance-inducing peptide is particularly well presented by the protective alleles and poorly presented by DR15.

*7.2. Other genetic factors*

In animal models, variation in gene copy number has drawn increasing attention in recent years as a source of individual differences in genome sequence and has thus been proposed as a driving force for genomic evolution and phenotypic variation (Ohno et al., 1968; Glazier et al., 2002; Eichler and Patel, 2002).

Aitman et al. demonstrated that copy number variations of the orthologous rat and human *Fcgr3* genes is a determinant of susceptibility to immune-mediated glomerulonephritis. Loss of the rat specific *Fcgr3* paralogue, *Fcgr3*-related sequence was a determinant of macrophage overactivity and GN in Wistar–Kyoto rats. An orthologue of rat *Fcgr3* was associated with GN in the human disease systemic lupus erythematosus, proving the importance of genomic plasticity in the evolution of genetically susceptible phenotypes including susceptibility to human disease. It remains to be seen whether a similar polymorphism can occur in anti-GBM disease (Aitman et al., 2006), but it is notable that patients with Goodpasture's disease only very rarely have other autoimmune diseases, as might be expected if they had a significant widespread alteration of regulatory signaling. However, this area will be the subject of intense scrutiny in the near future.

## 8. Treatment

Early data suggested that without treatment the prognosis of Goodpasture's disease was poor, especially in the presence of established renal impairment. Indeed, most patients died of pulmonary hemorrhage or renal failure. Before the 1970s, treatment regimes varied from corticosteroids and azathioprine to bilateral nephrectomy as a last resort therapy for intractable pulmonary hemorrhage (Turner and Rees, 1998). Furthermore, success rates were variable, conflicting, and hard to interpret, particularly as pulmonary hemorrhage has a tendency to spontaneously remit and relapse. Wilson and Dixon's retrospective analysis of survivors suggested that treatment with corticosteroids was more likely to be associated with preservation of renal function than development of end stage renal failure (Wilson and Dixon, 1973). Anecdotal reports suggested the addition of more powerful immunosuppressive agents may confer greater benefits (Couser, 1974).

As evidence emerged for a direct pathogenic role for circulating antibodies in disease, a potentially highly toxic combination treatment was devised and tested on patients, based on the rationale of removing circulating pathogenic antibodies as rapidly as possible, whilst simultaneously inhibiting their synthesis. This combination strategy was introduced in the mid 1970s (Lockwood et al., 1976) and consisted of three elements: intensive plasma exchange to remove antibodies, cytotoxic therapy with cyclophosphamide to prevent their synthesis, and corticosteroids as an adjunctive anti-inflammatory agent. Initial results were extremely encouraging. Patients, who would otherwise have had a poor prognosis, showed termination of hemorrhage within days, and recovery or preservation of renal function. Extension of these initial studies resulted in similarly impressive results being reported. (Briggs et al., 1979; Simpson et al., 1982; Walker et al., 1985).

Plasma exchange combined with cyclophosphamide and corticosteroids remains the mainstay of treatment for Goodpasture's disease and most centers use similar protocols. Although the original regime introduced by Lockwood included azathioprine as well as cyclophosphamide, the latter is now usually used alone with equal effect and greater safety. The intensity of treatment has varied, with some using less cyclophosphamide and/or less plasma exchange, with potentially less impressive outcomes, although fair comparison of series from different centers and countries is difficult.

In the only controlled trial carried out in 1985, Johnson et al. randomized nine patients to receive oral prednisolone and cyclophosphamide, six of whom failed to recover renal function and eight to receive additional low-intensity plasma exchange, two of whom failed to recover renal function. The interpretation of this study was complicated by the fact that the latter group had less severe disease at the time of presentation. Both plasma exchange and cyclophosphamide regimes used were less intensive than current recommendations, and only 69% of patients with creatinine <6.8 mg/dl recovered.

Plasma exchange regimes have differed substantially over the years. However, if antibody removal is indeed the therapeutic mode of action one may expect the more intensive regimes to be of greater benefit. Although there is little doubt that improved patient survival in recent series is attributable to better supportive care, and to a greater experience with immunosuppressive therapy, it is apparent that renal survival remains poor. In addition, in recent years the limits of effectiveness of this therapy and its potential hazards have been delineated, with infection being the most common cause of morbidity, often in relation to neutropenia.

Early treatment is often difficult for a disease that evolves rapidly and is only diagnosed once organ damage is established. There is a clear relationship between severity of renal disease at presentation and outcome. Those who are dialysis requiring, oliguric, or have serum creatinine >500–600 μmol/l (6–7 mg/dl), 100% crescents or advanced renal fibrosis have a low probability of regaining useful renal function, and for this reason a prompt reduction rather than intensification in therapy is advocated, unless there is concomitant pulmonary hemorrhage, as the risks of therapy far outweigh the slight possibility of renal recovery. However ameliorating factors (such as very acute disease, acute tubular necrosis) should also be taken into account.

This is in direct contrast with RPGN caused by systemic vasculitides (microscopic polyarteritis or Wegners), where in oliguric renal failure or in biopsies with 100% crescents, function may still be salvaged by treatments similar to those used in Goodpasture's Disease (Hind et al., 1983; Bolton and Sturgill, 1989). If ANCA (most commonly against neutrophil granule enzyme MPO) is found as well as anti-GBM antibody, the renal prognosis may be better, although this conclusion in some series is not echoed by others.

## 8.1. Other therapies

Early accounts suggested azathioprine alone provided inadequate immunosuppression to modify disease. Cyclosporin (Querin et al., 1992) appears to be effective in preventing relapse post-transplantation, but there are conflicting reports (Pepys et al., 1982). Mycophenolate mofetil may be a better agent with reports of its success in a patient intolerant of cyclophosphamide (García-Cantón et al., 2000).

Although prednisolone is still a key element of therapy, the use of pulsed methyl prednisolone is controversial. Pulsed IV methyl prednisolone has been used widely in RPGN of other types. In anti-GBM disease it has been used in place of plasma exchange. A non-randomized study of pulsed methyl prednisolone without concurrent immunosuppression in crescentic nephritis included 17 Goodpasture's patients (Bolton and Sturgill, 1989). Of four non-oliguric patients treated, only two retained renal function. Williams reported failures of pulsed corticosteroids in controlling pulmonary hemorrhage (Williams et al., 1988), and Johnson felt it may treat pulmonary hemorrhage while having no effect on renal disease (Johnson et al., 1985). The major concern of high-dose corticosteroid therapy is the increased risk of secondary and opportunistic infections. In animal models, infection may precipitate or exacerbate pulmonary hemorrhage and aggravate renal injury. For this reason the safety and efficiency of high-dose steroids is not established as an alternative to plasma exchange.

Plasma exchange allows the removal of circulating antibodies. However, proving its efficacy is difficult as when used without other reagents its effect on antibody titres is transient as a result of rapid re-synthesis of autoantibodies. For this reason, there is no indication for the use of plasma exchange alone (Proskey et al., 1970; Guillen et al., 1995). Immunoadsorption against staphylococcal protein A to adsorb circulating IgG (Bygren et al., 1985; Laczika et al., 2000), lowers antibody titres more rapidly than plasma exchange and preliminary evidence shows that is may be beneficial even in those who are dialysis-dependent. It has a number of therapeutic advantages (complement and clotting factors not depleted, expensive and potentially harmful replacement colloid solutions avoided). However, the evidence is limited to isolated case reports in which protein A or sepharose-coupled anti-human IgG was used to selectively remove IgG, and no real comparison was made. Immunoadsorption is also a complicated and time-consuming technique and not widely available.

The best approach is to use intensive plasma exchange (and/or immunoadsorption with protein A) in all patients with renal impairment felt to be salvageable and in all with continuing/recurrent pulmonary hemorrhage. It should be maintained until antibody titres have reached background values, and restarted in the setting of rising creatinine or recurrent pulmonary haemorrhage in association with elevated antibody titre.

## 9. Future treatments

Work in rodent models in recent years has revealed a number of novel and potentially useful therapies in the treatment of Goodpasture's disease. We highlight a few here.

### 9.1. Blocking CD80/CD28 T-cell co-stimulatory pathway

The increasing evidence for T-cell involvement in disease has led to the targeting of the T-cell effector arm of the immune system. Using a rodent model of anti-GBM disease, one study investigated the ability of the fusion protein CTLA4-Ig to block CD80/CD28 T-cell co-stimulatory pathway. This approach completely prevented the development of crescentic nephritis (Reynolds et al., 2000). However, it should be noted that these treatments are often given from disease onset, and it is not clear how closely these models mimic human disease and immune responses.

### 9.2. Inhibition of TGF-$\beta$

A recent study using the WKY rat model of anti-GBM nephritis investigated the effects of a natural regulator of haemopoesis, $N$-acetyl-seryl-aspartyl-lysyl-proline (Ac-SDKP), known to inhibit TGF-$\beta$ action in mesangial cells; an action thought to be pivotal in the development and progression of GN. The administration of Ac-SDKP significantly ameliorated the progression of renal dysfunction and fibrosis even in those with established nephritis, suggesting a potentially novel and useful therapy in the treatment of progressive renal disease (Omata et al., 2006).

### 9.3. Antigen-specific treatment strategies

Work by Reynolds et al. in the WKY rat model of EAG demonstrated for the first time that mucosal tolerance could be induced by nasal administration of recombinant rat alpha3(IV)NC1, which prevented crescentic glomerulonephritis (Reynolds et al., 2005).

### 9.4. Regulatory T-cells

Wolf et al. transferred CD4+ CD25+ T-cells (Tregs) into mice that were previously immunized with rabbit IgG and subsequently received an injection of anti-GBM rabbit serum. They demonstrated significant attenuation in the development of proteinuria, when compared to animals that received an injection of CD4+ CD25− T-cells. Injection of Tregs also attenuated glomerular damage and reduced CD4+ and CD8+ T-cells as well as macrophage infiltration. However, immune complex formation was not prevented by Tregs (Wolf et al., 2005).

## 10. Transplantation in Goodpasture's disease and Alport's syndrome

There is a generally accepted policy of not transplanting patients with Goodpasture's disease in the face of continuing presence of detectable autoantibodies, or for several months after their disappearance. Hence, there have been no recent reports of post-transplant recurrence while taking immunosuppression. Moreover, recurrence of Goodpasture's disease is rare. There is a classic report of recurrent disease in a transplant from an identical twin, and this was controlled by the introduction of chemotherapy (Almkuist et al., 1981).

In many patients with Alport's syndrome, particularly when it is of early onset, Goodpasture antigen is immunohistochemically reduced or absent from GBM (McCoy et al., 1982). The most common explanation is a deletion or mutation of the *COL4A5* gene on the X chromosome encoding the α5 chain of type IV collagen, α5(IV), but autosomal Alport's syndrome may be caused by mutations in *COL4A3* or *COL4A4*. This destabilizes the α3α4α5 type IV collagen trimer which makes up the majority of normal GBM, and Alport GBM therefore never changes from the fetal pattern, containing the generic α1α1α2 trimer. Disease-causing mutations lead to inability to form stable α3α4α5 type IV collagen fibrils, and some lead to complete lack of exposure of the immune system to any of the sequence of the normal chain. Transplantation of a normal kidney in these patients may then trigger development of an anti-GBM immune response to "new" antigen in the donor kidney. Linear IgG fixation to the GBM occurs quite commonly, but only a small proportion of patients develop crescentic nephritis, and lung haemorrhage generally does not occur. The disease tends to be more aggressive in a subsequent transplant, so that second and subsequent grafts are usually lost in days to weeks to crescentic nephritis. Although this is predominantly an alloimmune response rather than true autoimmune disease, observations in this group of patients have been informative about disease processes (Browne et al., 2004):

- Disease is more likely in patients with an underlying gene deletion rather than a point mutation.
- Antibodies are directed predominantly toward the NC1 domain of the molecule that is mutated or deleted, i.e. the one to which tolerance has not been established before transplantation, most commonly α5(IV)NC1 (Brainwood et al., 1998).
- The disease caused by anti-α5(IV)NC1 is essentially the same as anti-α3(IV)NC1 disease, so the "special" thing about α3(IV)NC1 in spontaneous anti-GBM disease is the fact that tolerance to it can be more easily broken, not that attack on it can uniquely cause disease. This has also been shown in the WKY rat model of EAG (Sado et al., 1998).
- Even in these circumstances of alloimmunity, disease is not consistent; additional genetic cofactors and/or a "second hit" are required. This applies even to families with gene deletions.
- Lymphocytolytic therapies (anti-lymphocyte globulin, alemtuzumab) may modify the appearance of the disease, but they do not cure or prevent it.
- Therapies aimed at lowering antibody titres alone are also ineffective, although delayed therapy and the aggressive nature of the disease lowers the certainty of this conclusion.

**Key points**

- Anti-GBM disease is associated with autoantibody formation to a specific basement membrane autoantigen but cell mediated mechanisms are central.
- Clinical manifestations are usually of a RPGN, often with pulmonary haemorrhage.
- Genetic influences are important with a strong association of the disease with HLA DR15.
- The disease is typically "single shot" and its initiation may be triggered by altered antigen presentation.

# References

Abbate, A., Zoja, C., Corna, D., Capitanio, M., Bertani, T., Remuzzi, G. 1998. In progressive nephropathies, overload of tubular cells with filtered proteins translates glomerular permeability dysfunction into cellular signals of interstitial inflammation. J. Am. Soc. Nephrol. 9 (7), 1213.

Aitman, T.J., Dong, R., Vyse, T.J., Norsworthy, P.J., Johnson, M.D., Smith, J., Mangion, J., Roberton-Lowe, C., Marshall, A.J., Petretto, E., Hodges, M.D., Bhangal, G., Patel, S.G., Sheehan-Rooney, K., Duda, M., Cook, P.R., Evans, D.J., Domin, J., Flint, J., Boyle, J.J., Pusey, C.D., Cook, H.T. 2006. Copy number polymorphism in Fcgr3 predisposes to glomerulonephritis in rats and humans. Nature 16;439 (7078), 851–855. Fascinating mapping exercise of susceptibilty to the disease in the WKY rat model; with one of the genes involved identified. Not necessarily the same in man.

Almkuist, R.D., Buckalew, V.M., Jr. Hirszel, P., Maher, J.F., James, P.M., Wilson, C.B. 1981. Recurrence of anti-GBM antibody mediated glomerulonephritis in an isograft. Clin. Immunol. Immunopathol. 18, 54.

Andrassy, K., Kuster, S., Waldherr, R., Ritz, E. 1991. Rapidly progressive nephritis: analysis of prevalence and clinical course. Nephron. 59, 206.

Bailey, R.R., Simpson, I.J., Lynn, K.L., Neale, T.J., Doak, P.B., McGiven, A.R. 1981. Goodpasture's syndrome with normal renal function. Clin. Nephrol. 15, 211.

Bolton, W.K. 2002. What sensitized cells just might be doing in glomerulonephritis. J. Clin. Invest. 109 (6), 713.

Bolton, W.K., Sturgill, B.C. 1989. Methylprednisolone therapy for acute crescentic rapidly progressive glomerulonephritis. Am. J. Nephrol. 9, 368.

Bolton, W.K., Chen, L., Hellmark, T., Fox, J., Wieslander, J. 2005a. Molecular mapping of the Goodpasture's epitope for glomerulonephritisTrans. Am. Clin. Climatol. Assoc. 116, 229, discussion 237.

Bolton, W.K., Chen, L., Hellmark, T., Wieslander, J., Fox, J.W. 2005b. Epitope spreading and autoimmune glomerulonephritis in rats induced by a T cell epitope of Goodpasture's antigen. J. Am. Soc. Nephrol. 16 (9), 2657.

Borza, D.B., Bondar, O., Colon, S., Todd, P., Sado, Y., Neilson, E.G., Hudson, B.G. 2005. Goodpasture autoantibodies unmask cryptic epitopes by selectively dissociating autoantigen complexes lacking structural reinforcement: novel mechanisms for immune privilege and autoimmune pathogenesis. J. Biol. Chem. 280 (29), 27147.

Borza, D.B., Netzer, K.O., Leinonen, A., Todd, P., Cervera, J., Saus, J., Hudson, B.G. 2000. The goodpasture autoantigen. Identification of multiple cryptic epitopes on the NC1 domain of the alpha3(IV) collagen chain. J. Biol. Chem. 275 (8), 6030.

Boucher, A., Droz, D., Adafer, E., Noel, L.H. 1987. Relationship between the integrity of Bowman's capsule and the composition of cellular crescents in human crescentic glomerulonephritis. Lab. Invest. 56, 526.

Brainwood, D., Kashtan, C., Gubler, M.C., Turner, A.N. 1998. Targets of alloantibodies in Alport anti-glomerular basement membrane disease after renal transplantation. Kidney Int. 53 (3), 762.

Briggs, W.A., Johnson, J.P., Teichman, S., Yeager, H.C., Wilson, C.B. 1979. Anti-GBM antibody mediated glomerulonephritis and Goodpasture's syndrome. Medicine (Baltimore) 58, 348.

Browne, G., Brown, P.A., Tomson, C.R., Fleming, S., Allen, A., Herriot, R., Pusey, C.D., Rees, A.J., Turner, A.N. 2004. Retransplantation in Alport post-translation anti-GBM disease. Kidney Int. 65 (2), 675.

Bygren, P., Freiburghaus, C., Lindholm, T., Simonsen, O., Thysell, H., Wieslander, J. 1985. Goodpasture's syndrome treated with staphylococcal protein A immunoadsorption. Lancet ii, 1295.

Cairns, L.S., Phelps, R.G., Bowie, L., Hall, A.M., Saweirs, W.W., Rees, A.J., Barker, R.N. 2003. The fine specificity and cytokine profile of T-helper cells responsive to the alpha3 chain of type IV collagen in Goodpasture's disease. J. Am. Soc. Nephrol. 14 (11), 2801. The only study to map patient's lymphocyte responses precisely.

Cashman, S.J., Pusey, C.D., Evans, D.J. 1988. Extraglomerular distribution of immunoreactive Goodpasture antigen. J. Pathol. 155 (1), 61.

Chen, L., Hellmark, T., Wieslander, J., Bolton, W.K. 2003. Immunodominant epitopes of alpha3(IV)NC1 induce autoimmune glomerulonephritis in rats. Kidney Int. 64 (6), 2108.

Couser, W.G. 1974. Goodpasture's syndrome: a response to nitrogen mustard. Am. J. Med. Sci. 268, 175.

Couser, W.G. 1988. Rapidly progressive glomerulonephritis: classification, pathogenetic mechanisms, and therapy. Am. J. Kidney Dis. 11, 449.

David, M., Borza, D.B., Leinonen, A., Belmont, J.M., Hudson, B.G. 2001. Hydrophobic amino acid residues are critical for the immunodominant epitope of the Goodpasture autoantigen. A molecular basis for the cryptic nature of the epitope. J. Biol. Chem. 276 (9), 6370.

Derry, C.J., Ross, C.N., Lombardi, G., Mason, P.D., Rees, A.J., Lechler, R.I., Pusey, C.D. 1995. Analysis of T cell responses to the autoantigen in Goodpasture's disease. Clin. Exp. Immunol. 100, 262.

Dighiero, G., Rose, N.R. 1999. Critical self-epitopes are key to the understanding of self-tolerance and autoimmunity. Immunol. Today 20 (9), 423.

Downie, G.H., Roholt, O.A., Jennings, L., Brentjens, J.R., Andres, G.A. 1982. Experimental anti-alveolar basement membrane antibody-mediated pneumonitis. II. Role of endothelial damage and repair, induction of autologous phase, and kinetics of antibody deposition in Lewis rats. J. Immunol. 129, 2647.

Eichler, E.E., Patel, N.H. 2002. Finding genes that underlie complex traits. Science 20; 298 (5602), 2345.

Evan, A.P., Willis, L.R., Connors, B., Reed, G., McAteer, J.A., Lingeman, J.E. 1991. Shock wave lithotripsy-induced renal injury. Am. J. Kidney Dis. 17, 445.

Gallucci, S., Matzinger, P. 2001. Danger signals: SOS to the immune system. Curr. Opin. Immunol. 13, 114.

García Cantón, C., Toledo, A., Palomar, R., Fernandez, F., Lopez, J., Moreno, A., Esparza, N., Suria, S., Rossique, P., Diaz, J.M., Checa, D. 2000. Goodpasture's syndrome treated with mycophenolate mofetil. Nephrol. Dial. Transplant. 15, 920.

Goodpasture, E.W. 1919. The significance of certain pulmonary lesions in relation to the etiology of influenza. Am. J. Med. Sci. 158, 863.

Glassock, R.J. 1999. Anti-GBM disease. In: B.M. Brenner (Ed.), Benner and Rector's The Kidney, WB Saunders, Philadelphia.

Glazier, A.M., Nadeau, J.H., Aitman, T.J. 2002. Finding genes that underlie complex traits. Science 298 (5602), 2345.

Guillen, E.L., Ruiz, A.M., Fernandez, M.A., Losa, A.M. 1995. Goodpasture syndrome: re-exacerbations associated with intercurrent infections. Rev. Clin. Esp. 195, 761.

Hellmark, T., Johansson, C., Wieslander, J. 1994. Characterization of anti-GBM antibodies involved in Goodpasture's syndrome. Kidney Int. 46, 823.

Hellmark, T.H., Burkhardt, H., Wieslander, J. 1999. Goodpasture disease. Characterization of a single conformational epitope as the target of pathogenic autoantibodies. J. Biol. Chem. 274, 25862.

Herody, M., Bobrie, G., Gourain, C., Grunfeld, J.P., Noel, L.H. 1993. Anti-GBM disease: predictive value of clinical, histological and serological data. Clin. Nephrol. 40, 249.

Hind, C.R., Paraskevakou, H., Lockwood, C.M., Evans, D.J., Peters, D.K., Rees, A.J. 1983. Prognosis after immunosuppression of patients with crescentic nephritis requiring dialysis. Lancet i, 263.

Huang, X.R., Tipping, P.G., Shou, L., Holdsworth, S.R. 1997. Th1 responsiveness to nephritogenic antigens determines susceptibility to crescentic glomerulonephritis in mice. Kidney Int. 51 (1), 94.

Jaeger, P., Redha, F., Marquardt, K., Uhlschmid, G., Hauri, D. 1995. Morphological and functional changes in canine kidneys following extracorporeal shock-wave treatment. Urol. Int. 54, 48.

Jampol, L.M., Lahov, M., Albert, D.M., Craft, J. 1975. Ocular clinical findings and basement membrane changes in Goodpasture's syndrome. Am. J. Ophthalmol. 79, 452.

Jennings, L., Roholt, O.A., Pressman, D., Blau, M., Andres, G.A., Brentjens, J.R. 1981. Experimental anti-alveolar basement membrane antibody-mediated pneumonitis. I. The role of increased permeability of the alveolar capillary wall induced by oxygen. J. Immunol. 127, 129.

Johnson, J.P., Moore, J., Jr. Austin, H.A., Balow, J.E., Antonovych, T.T., Wilson, C.B. 1985. Therapy of antiglomerular basement membrane antibody disease: analysis of prognostic significance of clinical, pathologic and treatment factors. Medicine (Baltimore) 64 (4), 219.

Karkar, A.M., Rees, A.J. 1997. Influence of endotoxin contamination on anti-GBM antibody induce glomerular injury in rats. Kidney Int. 52 (6), 1579.

Kefalides, N.A. 1966. A collagen of unusual composition and a glycoprotein isolated from canine glomerular basement membrane. Biochem. Biophys. Res. Commun. 22 (1), 26.

Laczika, K., Knapp, S., Derfler, K., Soleiman, A., Horl, W.H., Druml, W. 2000. Immunoadsorption in Goodpasture's syndrome. Am. J. Kidney Dis. 36, 392.

Lerner, R.A., Glassock, R.J., Dixon, F.J. 1967. The role of antiglomerular basement membrane antibody in the pathogenesis of human glomerulonephritisJ. Exp. Med. 126, 989–1004. The original evidence that anti-GBM antibodies can mediate tissue injury in anti-GBM disease. Doesn't show that they act alone though.

Litwin, C.M., Mouritsen, C.L., Wilfahrt, P.A., Schroder, M.C., Hill, H.R. 1996. Anti-GBM disease: role of enzyme-linked immunosorbent assays in diagnosis. Biochem. Mol. Med. 59 (1), 52.

Lockwood, C.M., Rees, A.J., Pearson, T.A., Evans, D.J., Peters, D.K., Wilson, C.B. 1976. Immunosuppression and plasma-exchange in the treatment of Goodpasture's syndrome. Lancet i, 711.

Manoury, B., Mazzeo, D., Fugger, L., Viner, N., Pondsford, M., Streeter, H., Mazza, G., Wraith, D.C., Watts, C. 2002. Destructive processing by asparagine endopeptidase limits presentation of a dominant T cell epitope in MBP. Nat. Immunol. 3 (2), 169.

McCoy, R.C., Johnson, H.K., Stone, W.J., Wilson, C.B. 1982. Absence of nephritogenic GBM antigen(s) in some patients with hereditary nephritis. Kidney Int. 21 (4), 642.

McPhaul, J.J., Jr. Dixon, F.J. 1970. Characterization of human antiglomerular basement membrane antibodies eluted from glomerulonephritic kidneys. J. Clin. Invest. 49, 308.

Meyers, K.E., Allen, J., Gehert, J., Jacobovits, A., Neilson, E.G., Hopfer, H., Kalluri, R., Madaio, M.P. 2002. Human antiglomerular basement membrane autoantibody disease in XenoMouse II. Kidney Int. 61 (5), 1666.

Miner, J.H. 1999. Renal basement membrane components. Kidney Int. 56, 2016.

Netzer, K.O., Leinonen, A., Boutaud, A., Borza, D.B., Todd, P., Gunwar, S., Langeweld, J.P., Hudson, B.G. 1999. The goodpasture autoantigen. Mapping the major conformational epitope(s) of alpha3(IV) collagen to residues 17–31 and 127–141 of the NC1 domain. J. Biol. Chem. 274 (16), 11267.

New Zealand Glomerulonephritis Study Group. 1989. The New Zealand Glomerulonephritis Study: introductory report. Clin. Nephrol. 31, 239.

Ohno, S., Wolf, U., Aitkin, N.B. 1968. Evolution from fish to mammals by gene duplication. Hereditas 59 (1), 169.

Omata, M., Taniguchi, H., Koya, D., Kanasaki, K., Sho, R., Kato, Y., Kojima, R., Haneda, M., Inomata, N. 2006. N-acetyl-seryl-aspartyl-lysyl-proline ameliorates the progression of renal dysfunction and fibrosis in WKY rats with established anti-glomerular basement membrane nephritis. J. Am. Soc. Nephrol. 17 (3), 674.

Pepys, E.O., Rees, A.J., Pepys, M.B. 1982. Enumeration of lymphocyte populations in whole peripheral blood of patients with antibody mediated nephritis during treatment with cyclosporin A. Immunol. Lett. 4, 211.

Perez, G.O., Bjornsson, S., Ross, A.H., Aamato, J., Rothfield, N. 1974. A mini-epidemic of Goodpasture's syndrome—clinical and immunological studies. Nephron. 13, 16173.

Phelps, R.G., Jones, V., Turner, A.N., Rees, A.J. 2000. Properties of HLA class II molecules divergently associated with Goodpasture's disease. Int. Immunol. 12, 1135. Currently the definitive analysis of the association of specific HLA types with Goodpasture disease.

Phelps, R.G., Jones, V.L., Coughlan, M., Turner, A.N., Rees, A.J. 1998. Presentation of the Goodpasture autoantigen to CD4 T cells is influenced more by processing constraints than by HLA class II peptide binding preferences. J. Biol. Chem. 273 (19), 11440.

Phelps, R.G., Turner, A.N., Rees, A.J. 1996. Direct identification of naturally processed autoantigen-derived peptides bound to HLA-DR15. J. Biol. Chem. 271 (31), 18549.

Proskey, A.J., Weatherbee, L., Easterling, R.E., Greene, J.A., Jr. Weller, J.M. 1970. Goodpasture's syndrome. A report of five cases and review of the literature. Am. J. Med. 48, 162.

Querin, S., Schurch, W., Beaulieu, R. 1992. Cyclosporin in Goodpasture's syndrome. Nephron. 60, 353.

Rees, A.J., Lockwood, C.M., Peters, D.K. 1979. Nephritis due to antibodies to GBM. In: P. Kincaid-Smith, A.J.F. d'Apice, R.C. Atkins (Eds.), In Progress in Glomerulonephritis, Wiley, New York, 347.

Rees, A.J., Peters, D.K., Compston, D.A., Batchelor, J.R. 1978. Strong association between HLA-DRW2 and antibody-mediated Goodpasture's syndrome. Lancet i, 966.

Reynolds, J., Cook, P.R., Ryan, J.J., Norsworthy, P.J., Glazier, A.M., Duda, M.A., Evans, D.J., Aitman, T.J., Pusey, C.D. 2002. Segregation of experimental autoimmune glomerulonephritis as a complex genetic trait and exclusion of *COL4A3* as a candidate gene. Exp. Nephrol. 10 (5–6), 402.

Reynolds, J., Prodromidi, E.I., Juggapah, J.K., Abbott, D.S., Holthaus, K.A., Kalluri, R., Pusey, C.D. 2005. Nasal administration of recombinant rat alpha3(IV)NC1 prevents the development of experimental autoimmune glomerulonephritis in the WKY rat. J. Am. Soc. Nephrol. 16 (5), 1350.

Reynolds, J., Tam, F.W., Chandraker, A., Smith, J., Karkar, A.M., Cross, J., Peach, R., Sayegh, M.H., Pusey, C.D. 2000. CD28-B7 blockade prevents the development of experimental autoimmune glomerulonephritis. J. Clin. Invest. 105 (5), 643.

Robertson, J., Wu, J., Arends, J., Glass, W., 2nd Southwood, S., Sette, A., Lou, Y.H. 2005. Characterization of the T-cell epitope that causes anti-GBM glomerulonephritis. Kidney Int. 68 (3), 1061.

Rutgers, A., Meyers, K.E., Canziani, G., Kalluri, R., Lin, J., Nadaio, M.P. 2000. High affinity of anti-GBM antibodies from Goodpasture and transplanted Alport patients to alpha3(IV)NC1 collagen. Kidney Int. 58 (1), 115.

Ryan, J.J., Mason, P.J., Pusey, C.D., Turner, N. 1998. Recombinant alpha-chains of type IV collagen demonstrate that the amino terminal of the Goodpasture autoantigen is crucial for antibody recognition. Clin. Exp. Immunol. 113 (1), 17.

Sado, Y., Boutaud, A., Kagawa, M., Naito, I., Ninomiya, Y., Hudson, B.G. 1998. Induction of anti-GBM nephritis in rats by recombinant alpha 3(IV)NC1 and alpha 4(IV)NC1 of type IV collagenKidney Int. 53 (3), 664. Erratum in Kidney Int. 1998. 54 (1), 311. α4NC1 domains are equally nephritogenic to α3 in this model but other NC1 domains are less nephritogenic. This seems most likely to be related to the security of tolerance to these chains. It leaves open the question of why α3(IV)NC1 is consistently the target in spontaneous Goodpasture's disease.

Sado, Y., Kagawa, M., Rauf, S., Naito, I., Moritoh, C., Okigaki, T. 1992. Isologous monoclonal antibodies can induce anti-GBM glomerulonephritis in ratsJ. Pathol. 168 (2), 221. Antibodies can transfer disease in this remarkable model disease.

Salama, A.D., Chaudhry, A.N., Ryan, J.J., Eren, E., Levy, J.B., Pusey, C.D., Lightstone, L., Lechler, R.I. 2001. In Goodpasture's disease, CD4(+) T cells escape thymic deletion and are reactive with the autoantigen alpha3(IV)NC1. J. Am. Soc. Nephrol. 12 (9), 1908. Evidence that reactivity to Goodpasture antigen is not deleted.

Saus, J., Wieslander, J., Langeveld, J.P., Quinones, S., Hudson, B.G. 1988. Identification of the Goodpasture antigen as the alpha 3(IV) chain of collagen IV. J. Biol. Chem. 263 (26), 13374.

Savage, C.O., Pusey, C.D., Bowman, C., Rees, A.J., Lockwood, C.M. 1986. Anti-GBM antibody mediated disease in the British Isles 19804. Br. Med. J. 292, 301.

Schindler, R., Kahl, A., Lobeck, H., Berweck, S., Kampf, D., Frei, U. 1998. Complete recovery of renal function in a dialysis dependent patient with Goodpasture syndrome. Nephrol. Dial. Transplant. 13, 462.

Schmidt, R.H., Sieh, S., Rohl, D., Geiger, H., Mondorff, U.F., Grone, H.J., Lenz, T. 1999. Spontaneous remission of Goodpasture syndrome in a 21-year-old patient. Dtsch. Med. Wochenschr. 124, 1201.

Segelmark, M., Butowski, R., Wieslander, J. 1990. Antigen restriction and IgG subclasses among anti-GBM autoantibodies. Nephrol. Dial. Transplant 5 (12), 991.

Sharma, S. 1998. Bilateral serous retinal detachments associated with Goodpasture's syndrome. Can. J. Ophthal. 33, 226.

Silverstein, A.M., Rose, N.R. 2000. There is only one immune system! The view from immunopathology. Semin. Immunol. 12 (3), 173, discussion 257.

Simpson, I.J., Doak, P.B., Williams, L.C., Blacklock, H.A., Hill, R.S., Teague, C.A., Herdson, P.B., Wilson, C.B. 1982. Plasma exchange in Goodpasture's syndrome. Am. J. Nephrol. 2, 301.

Stanton, M.C., Tange, J.D. 1958. Goodpasture's syndrome (pulmonary haemorrhage associated with glomerulonephritis). Aust. N.Z.J. Med. 7, 132.

Teague, C.A., Doak, P.B., Simpson, I.J., Rainer, S.P., Herdson, P.B. 1978. Goodpasture's syndrome: an analysis of 29 cases. Kidney Int. 13, 492.

Timoshanko, J.R., Holdsworth, S.R., Kitching, A.R., Tipping, P.G. 2002. IFN-gamma production by intrinsic renal cells and bone marrow-derived cells is required for full expression of crescentic glomerulonephritis in mice. J. Immunol. 168 (8), 4135.

Timoshanko, J.R., Kitching, A.R., Holdsworth, S.R., Tipping, P.G. 2001. Interleukin-12 from intrinsic cells is an effector of renal injury in crescentic glomerulonephritis. J. Am. Soc. Nephrol. 12 (3), 464.

Tipping, P.G., Holdsworth, S.R. 2006. T cells in crescentic glomerulonephritis. J. Am. Soc. Nephrol. 17 (5), 1253.

Tipping, P.G., Kitching, A.R., Huang, X.R., Mutch, D.A., Holdsworth, S.R. 1997. Immune modulation with interleukin-4 and interleukin-10 prevents crescent formation and glomerular injury in experimental glomerulonephritis. Eur. J. Immunol. 27 (2), 530.

Turner, A.N., Rees, A.J. 1998. Anti-GBM disease. In: A.M. Davison, J.S. Cameron, J.-P. Grunfeld, D.N.S. Kerr, E. Ritz C.G. Winearls (Eds.), Oxford Textbook of Clinical Nephrology, 2nd ed., OUP, Oxford, p. 647.

Turner, N., Mason, P.J., Brown, R., Fox, M., Povey, S., Rees, A., Pusey, C.D. 1992. Molecular cloning of the human Goodpasture antigen demonstrates it to be the α3 chain of type IV collagen. J. Clin. Invest. 89, 592.

Walker, R.G., Scheinkestel, C., Becker, G.J., Owen, J.E., Dowling, J.P., Kinncaid-Smith, P. 1985. Clinical and morphological aspects of the management of crescentic anti-GBM antibody (anti-GBM) nephritis/Goodpasture's syndrome. Q. J. Med. 54, 75.

Wieslander, J., Barr, J.F., Butkowski, R.J., Edwards, S.J., Bygren, P., Heinegard, D., Hudson, B.G. 1984. Goodpasture antigen of the GBM: localization to noncollagenous regions of type IV collagen. Proc. Natl. Acad. Sci. USA 81 (12), 3838.

Wieslander, J., Langeveld, J., Butkowski, R., Jodlowski, M., Noelken, M., Hudson, B.G. 1985. Physical and immunochemical studies of the globular domain of type IV collagen. Cryptic properties of the Goodpasture antigen. J. Biol. Chem. 260 (14), 8564.

Williams, P.S., Davenport, A., McDicken, I., Ashby, D., Goldsmith, H.J., Bone, J.M. 1988. Increased incidence of anti-glomerular basement membrane antibody (anti-GBM) nephritis in the Mersey region, September 1984–October 1985. Q. J. Med. 68,727,

Wilson, C.B., Dixon, F.J. 1973. Anti-GBM antibody-induced glomerulonephritis. Kidney Int. 3, 74.

Wilson, C.B., Dixon, F.J. 1981. The renal response to immunological injury. In: B.M. Brenner F.C. Rector (Eds.), The Kidney, W.B. Saunders, Philadelphia, PA, pp. 1237–1350.

Wolf, D., Hochegger, K., Wolf, A.M., Rumpold, H.F., Gastl, G., Tilg, H., Mayer, G., Gunsilius, E., Rosenkranz, A.R. 2005. CD4+ CD25+ regulatory T cells inhibit experimental anti-glomerular basement membrane glomerulonephritis in mice. J. Am. Soc. Nephrol. 16 (5), 1360.

Wong, D., Phelps, R.G., Turner, A.N. 2001. The Goodpasture antigen is expressed in the human thymus. Kidney Int. 60 (5), 1777.

Wu, J., Hicks, J., Borillo, J., Glass, W.F., 2nd Lou, Y.H. 2002. CD4(+) T cells specific to a GBM antigen mediate glomerulonephritis. J. Clin. Invest. 109 (4), 517.

Wucherpfennig, K.W. 2001. Mechanisms for the induction of autoimmunity by infectious agents. J. Clin. Invest. 108, 1097.

Wucherpfennig, K.W., Strominger, J.L. 1995. Molecular mimicry in T cell-mediated autoimmunity: viral peptides activate human T cell clones specific for myelin basic protein. Cell 80 (5), 695.

Yamamoto, T., Wilson, C.B. 1987. Binding of anti-basement membrane antibody to alveolar basement membrane after intratracheal gasoline instillation in rabbits. Am. J. Pathol. 126, 497.

Zou, J., Henderson, L., Thomas, V., Swan, P., Turner, A.N., Phelps, R.G. 2007. Presentation of the Goodpasture autoantigen requires proteolytic unlocking steps that destroy prominent T cell epitopes. J. Am. Soc. Nephrol. 18 (3), 771.

# CHAPTER 12

## Renal Disease in Cryoglobulinemic Vasculitis

Frank Bridoux[a,b], Christophe Sirac[b], Arnaud Jaccard[c], Ramzi Abou Ayache[a], Jean Michel Goujon[d,e], Michel Cogné[b], Guy Touchard[a,e],*

[a]Service de Néphrologie, Hémodialyse et Transplantation Rénale, CHU de Poitiers, Université de Poitiers, 2 rue de la Milétrie, 86021 Poitiers, France
[b]Laboratoire d'Immunologie, CNRS UMR 6101, Faculté de Médecine, Université de Limoges, 2 rue du Dr. Marcland, 87025 Limoges, France
[c]Service d'Hématologie Clinique, CHU de Limoges, Université de Limoges, Avenue Martin Luther King, 87025 Limoges, France
[d]Service d'Anatomie Pathologique, CHU de Poitiers, Université de Poitiers, 2 rue de la Milétrie, 86021 Poitiers, France
[e]INSERM ERM 324, CHU de Poitiers, Université de Poitiers, 2 rue de la Milétrie, 86021 Poitiers, France

## 1. Introduction

Cryoglobulins are immunoglobulins (Ig) that precipitate as serum is cooled below body temperature and dissolve after rewarming at 37°C (Kallemuchikkal and Gorevic, 1999). They are classified into three types, on the basis of their Ig composition, according to Brouet et al. (1974) (Table 1):

- Type I cryoglobulins are entirely made up of a monoclonal Ig (mostly IgM). Type I cryoglobulinemia is usually observed in the context of lymphoplasmacytic proliferation, mainly Waldenström's macroglobulinaemia, chronic lymphocytic leukemia, or multiple myeloma.
- Type II (or mixed) cryoglobulins are composed of two distinct components: a monoclonal Ig (usually IgMκ, less frequently IgG) that displays a specific antibody activity (rheumatoid factor) against the polyclonal component of the cryoglobulin (most commonly IgG).

Although type II mixed cryoglobulinemia (MC) has been considered for a long time as an "essential" condition (Cordonnier et al., 1975, 1983), it has now been established that the disease is associated with chronic hepatitis C virus (HCV) infection in 40–100% of cases, depending on the geographic area (Agnello et al., 1992; Misiani et al., 1992; Sansonno and Dammacco, 2005). Other conditions may feature type II cryoglobulins, such as Sjögren's syndrome, non-Hodgkin B-cell lymphoma, or Waldenström's macroglobulinemia.

- Type III cryoglobulins are composed of one or several classes of polyclonal Ig. They are observed in various pathologic conditions with immune complex formation, including infectious diseases, autoimmune disorders, malignancies, or even in apparently healthy individuals (Brouet et al., 1974; Garin et al., 1980).

With the use of sensitive techniques, such as immunoblotting and two-dimensional electrophoresis, the existence of further types of cryoglobulins has emerged. These cryoglobulins do not correspond to the original classification and probably

*Corresponding author.
Tel.: 33 5 49 44 43 56; Fax: 33 5 49 44 42 36
E-mail address: g.touchard@chu-poitiers.fr

**Table 1**
Classification of cryoglobulins

| Type | Ig composition | Main associated disorders |
|---|---|---|
| I | Monoclonal immunoglobulin (IgG, IgA, IgM) | Multiple myeloma<br>Chronic lymphocytic leukemia<br>Monoclonal gammopathy<br>Waldenström's macroglobulinemia<br>Other B-cell lymphoproliferative disorders |
| II | Monoclonal Ig (mostly IgM) with rheumatoid factor activity, and polyclonal IgG | HCV infection<br>Chronic lymphocytic leukemia<br>B-cell lymphoproliferative disorders<br>Essential |
| III | Polyclonal Ig | Viral infections (hepatitis C, hepatitis B)<br>Epstein–Barr, cytomegalovirus, HIV<br>Bacterial infections (endocarditis, leprosy, post-streptococcal GN, ventriculoatrial shunt infection, brucella, rickettsia)<br>Parasitic infections (echinococcosis, malaria, schistosomiasis, toxoplasmosis, leishmaniasis)<br>Connective tissue diseases (systemic lupus erythematosus, Sjögren's syndrome, rheumatoid arthritis)<br>Lymphoproliferative disorders<br>Paraneoplastic disease<br>Dermatological diseases<br>Inflammatory bowel diseases<br>Chronic liver diseases<br>Essential |

represent transition steps between classical type III and type II cryoglobulins. They are characterized by the association of oligoclonal IgM or IgG and polyclonal IgG (type II/III cryoglobulins) (Tissot et al., 1994), or by the presence of an additional monoclonal IgG component in unusual varieties of type II cryoglobulins (Musset et al., 1994; Trejo et al., 2001).

Renal involvement is frequent during the course of cryoglobulinemia, with an overall prevalence ranging from 21 to 47%, irrespective of cryoglobulin type, in the largest published series (Brouet et al., 1974; Trejo et al., 2001; Bryce et al., 2006b). In type I and type II cryoglobulinemia, renal disease usually manifests as acute glomerulonephritis (GN) with renal impairment, with a typical pattern of membranoproliferative GN (MPGN) on kidney biopsy, often associated with intrarenal vasculitis (Brouet et al., 1974; Cordonnier et al., 1983; Trejo et al., 2001). Strong arguments based on animal model studies support a direct pathogenic role for type I and type II cryoglobulins in the development of glomerular and vascular lesions.

By contrast, various non-specific renal manifestations usually related to the underlying disease, may be observed in patients with type III cryoglobulins. Although experimental data from transgenic mice over-expressing thymic stromal lymphopoeitin suggest that polyclonal (type III) cryoglobulins are involved in the induction of MPGN (Taneda et al., 2001), evidence for a direct pathogenic property of polyclonal cryoglobulins in human renal disease is not established. Only in the particular situation of patients with systemic lupus erythematosus (SLE) and glomerular involvement, do histopathological data support a potential nephrotoxic effect of polyclonal cryoglobulins. In some patients with lupus proliferative GN, glomerular deposits may be focally arranged into crystals, made up of lamellar curvilinear structures that display a periodic striation of 22 nm. These deposits, commonly referred to as "fingerprints", contain a mixture of polyclonal IgG, IgM, and

IgA, together with DNA and complement components, and are almost invariably associated with type III cryoglobulinemia (Su et al., 2002). The present review will focus on renal involvement in type II and type I cryoglobulinemia.

## 2. Detection and identification of circulating cryoglobulins

Both detection and identification of circulating cryoglobulins require careful and meticulous techniques. Common errors result from failure to properly separate serum from whole blood, loss of cryoprecipitate due to cooling before centrifugation, or an inadequate volume of serum for testing cryoglobulins present at low levels. Ten to 20 ml of blood, taken under fasting conditions and without anticoagulant, should be maintained at 37°C and rapidly transported to the laboratory. After separation by centrifugation, serum is kept at 4°C for 7 days. Cryoprecipitation is variable, depending on type, concentration, and thermal amplitude of the cryoglobulin. Type I and type II cryoglobulins generally begin to precipitate within hours of precipitation and are apparent by the next day. By contrast, type III cryoglobulins, usually present at low levels, may require several days to precipitate. The temperature of precipitation is usually between 25 and 30°C. Detailed characterization of cryoglobulins should be performed after repeated (3–6) washing of the cryoprecipitate to remove non-specifically adherent serum proteins, followed by resolubilization by warming at 37°C, to confirm warm solubility.

Concentration of the cryoglobulin is measured as the cryocrit, or as total protein determination. For the cryocrit, a volume of initial warm serum is kept at 4°C until maximal cryoprecipitation has been obtained, centrifuged cold, and the percent total volume occupied by the pellet is determined by visual inspection (Kallemuchikkal and Gorevic, 1999). Cryocrit is generally between 1 and 7% in type II cryoglobulinemia. Cryocrit may vary considerably in the same patient, and is poorly predictive of prognosis and severity of organ involvement (D'Amico, 1998). However, when performed in reference laboratories using standardized techniques, cryoglobulin levels may correlate with response to treatment and disease evolution (Tarantino et al., 1995; Fornasieri and D'Amico, 1996; Kallemuchikkal and Gorevic, 1999; Trejo et al., 2001). Qualitative study of the cryoglobulin is performed after redissolving by warming at 37°C in saline-buffered medium at pH 7. The immunoglobulin composition of the cryoglobulin, and the presence of a monoclonal component, is determined by immunofixation or immunoelectrophoresis using specific antibodies. More sensitive techniques, such as immunoblotting, two-dimensional gel electrophoresis, or capillary zone electrophoresis may be useful to detect low concentrations of monoclonal component (Beaume et al., 1994; Musset et al., 1994; Tissot et al., 1994; Kallemuchikkal and Gorevic, 1999). Monoclonal Igs in type II cryoglobulins are almost invariably IgMκ (Kallemuchikkal and Gorevic, 1999).

## 3. Renal disease in mixed (type II) cryoglobulinemia

### 3.1. Pathophysiology

Cryoglobulinemia induces a systemic vasculitis that predominantly affects small and, to a lesser extent, medium-size arteries and veins, through deposition of immune complexes and subsequent activation of the complement cascade (Sansonno and Dammacco, 2005).

#### 3.1.1. Type II cryoglobulinemia: from viral infection to lymphoid malignancy

The etiological role of HCV infection in type II cryoglobulinemia has emerged with the demonstration of circulating anti-HCV antibodies and active viral replication in most patients (Agnello et al., 1992; Misiani et al., 1992). Studies performed on cryoprecipitates showed that they contained immune complexes made up of monoclonal IgM rheumatoid factor molecules, bearing a specific activity against the immune complex composed of HCV core protein and polyclonal anti-HCV IgG.

The presence of HCV core and other viral proteins in various tissues, including glomerular capillary walls, suggests that immune complexes are formed in situ through binding between the antigen on the surface of endothelial cells and circulating Igs (Sansonno and Dammacco, 2005). Type II mixed cryoglobulinaemia (MC) results from B-cell hyperactivation and expansion, a common feature of connective tissue diseases and chronic HCV infection. Moreover, almost 10% of patients with HCV-related MC develop low-grade lymphoplasmacytic B-cell non-Hodgkin lymphoma (De Vita et al., 1997; Racanelli et al., 2001; Sansonno and Dammacco, 2005). The pathogenetic mechanisms underlying progression from chronic HCV infection to MC and lymphoma remain hypothetical. B-lymphocytes represent an important site for extrahepatic HCV replication (Zignego et al., 1992), via the cell surface protein CD81 (Curry et al., 2003). B-cell repertoire in patients with HCV-associated MC is limited, with variable regions of heavy and light chains of IgM rheumatoid factor molecules being encoded by few germline genes and V$\kappa$III over-representation (Ivanovski et al., 1998). Moreover, MC patients display defective B-cell apoptosis through rearrangement of Bcl-2 (Zignego et al., 2002) and increased levels of soluble tumor necrosis superfamily receptors (Realdon et al., 2001).

These data support the following hypothesis: activation and expansion of rheumatoid factor producing B-cells, particularly by immune complexes with HCV and anti-HCV, result in secretion of polyclonal IgM rheumatoid factor, as illustrated by the high prevalence of type III cryoglobulinemia in HCV infected patients. Through somatic mutations induced by persistent antigenic stimulation, polyclonal B-cell activation may progress to oligoclonal B-cell expansion with production of type II–III cryoglobulins, and then to the selection of a single clone producing a cryoprecipitating monoclonal IgM rheumatoid factor. Finally, triggered by chromosomal abnormalities, B-cell lymphoma may develop (Mariette 2001; Sansonno and Dammacco, 2005). Various factors, including duration of HCV infection, genetic predisposition, hormonal and environmental factors, or co-infection by other viruses, such as Epstein–Barr virus, could participate in this process (D'Amico, 1995; Fornasieri and D'Amico, 1996; Sansonno and Dammacco, 2005).

The mechanisms of cryoprecipitation remain incompletely understood. They involve conformational changes of the protein induced by decrease in the temperature, Ig surface charges that depend on amino acid sequence and carbohydrate composition, and pH of the solution. The high concentration of C1q protein in the cryoprecipitate probably plays a role in specific deposition on endothelial cells, through C1q receptor binding (Sansonno and Dammacco, 2005). A direct nephrotoxic role for circulating type II cryoglobulins has been demonstrated in various experimental models. Injection of soluble type II cryoglobulins purified from patients with typical MPGN into mice, results in similar glomerular lesions in the animals (Fornasieri et al., 1993). These lesions, which initially affect the mesangium, appear to be kidney specific, as they are not induced by the injection of cryoglobulins from patients without renal involvement (Fornasieri et al., 1998). In vitro, monoclonal IgM$\kappa$ cryoglobulins also bind to fibronectin, a component of the mesangial matrix, whereas polyclonal IgM, or monoclonal IgM without cryoglobulin activity, lack affinity for fibronectin (Fornasieri et al., 1996).

The cellular mechanisms of cryoglobulinemic vasculitis remain largely unknown. Decreased hepatosplenic elimination of circulating cryoglobulins (Roccatello et al., 1997), and defective monocyte/macrophage function with impaired capacity to catabolize cryoglobulins in vitro are likely to contribute to renal disease (Roccatello et al., 1993). The extent and severity of glomerular infiltration by monocytes and macrophages, correlates with overexpression of the chemotactic and activating cytokine, monocyte chemotactic protein-1 (MCP-1), following cryoglobulin deposition (Gesualdo et al., 1997). Inflammatory cytokines are probably involved in the induction of vasculitis in MC, as suggested by increased monocyte production of interleukin-1 (IL-1) and IL-6, in vivo and/or in vitro, after incubation with immune complexes derived from patients with type II MC or with HCV core protein (Chantry et al., 1989; Feldmann et al., 2006, Libra et al., 2006). Certain HLA haplotypes, such as B8, DR3, and

DR11 antigens, seem to confer susceptibility to the development of MC in HCV infected patients (Lenzi et al., 1998; Cacoub et al., 2001). As these patients display increased serum production of Th-1 cytokines, a key role for HCV-driven Th-1 cellular immunity in the pathogenesis of HCV-associated MC vasculitis has recently been proposed (Saadoun et al., 2004).

## 3.2. Clinical presentation

The prevalence of renal involvement in type II cryoglobulinemia is highly variable in the different series reported in the literature, ranging from 10 to 60% (Brouet et al., 1974; Cordonnier et al., 1983; Monti et al., 1995; Bryce et al., 2006b). Renal disease generally occurs in the fifth or sixth decade, with a slight female predominance (D'Amico, 1998; Tarantino et al., 1995). Although renal and systemic manifestations may appear simultaneously, in many cases recurrent flares of extra-renal symptoms with spontaneous remission are typically present months or years before the onset and diagnosis of nephropathy (Tarantino et al., 1995). Rarely, isolated renal disease precedes systemic organ involvement (Cordonnier et al., 1983; D'amico, 1998; Tarantino et al., 1981, 1995).

### 3.2.1. Extra-renal disease in type II cryoglobulinemia

At the time of kidney biopsy or renal diagnosis, most patients have non-specific systemic symptoms including fatigue, cutaneous and articular manifestations. The classical Meltzer and Franklin triad (weakness, vasculitic purpura, and polyarthralgia) is present in one third of the cases (Monti et al., 1995; Meltzer et al., 1966). Vasculitic purpura, sometimes necrotic, is observed in 50–70% of the cases. Lesions predominate in the lower limbs and are often triggered by cold exposure, orthostatism, or minimal traumatism (Cordonnier et al., 1983; Monti et al., 1995; Tarantino et al., 1995; Trejo et al., 2001; Bryce et al., 2006b). Twenty five to 50% of the patients have other cutaneous symptoms, such as cold urticaria or Raynaud's phenomenon. Bilateral, symmetrical, inflammatory polyarthralgia, affecting 18% to more than 50% of the patients, most commonly involve ankles, knees, metacarpophalangeal and phalangeal joints, without deformation. True arthritis is rare, whereas myalgias are frequently associated with articular pain (Bryce et al., 2006b).

Severe clinical manifestations related to vasculitis are less common. Although nerve biopsies and electromyographic studies often reveal peripheral nerve involvement, symptomatic peripheral neuropathy is rare. Less than one third of patients have sensory or sensory motor polyneuropathy, or mononeuritis multiplex, that usually predominates in lower limbs. Central nervous system involvement is exceptional. Gastro-intestinal tract vasculitis may be responsible for various symptoms, including abdominal pain, constipation, diarrhea, and hemorrhage. Pulmonary involvement, reported in 2–50% of the patients, is generally clinically mild or manifests as dyspnoea and non-productive cough. Pulmonary function tests usually show small airway disease and impairment of gas exchange. Interstitial infiltrates or pleural effusion may be present on chest CT scan. Less commonly, patients present with dramatic symptoms such as haemoptysis and massive pulmonary hemorrhage with acute respiratory distress syndrome. Cardiac complications have been also described, including pericarditis, valvular disease, coronary disease and myocarditis secondary to vasculitis, or congestive heart failure usually precipitated by uncontrolled hypertension (Cordonnier et al., 1983; Tarantino et al., 1995, Trejo et al., 2001). Hepatic involvement is considered to be frequent in MC, with a 50% prevalence of hepatomegaly, sometimes associated with portal hypertension or cirrhosis with advanced hepatic disease (Cordonnier et al., 1983). In most cases, hepatic dysfunction appears to be related directly to chronic HCV infection (Lunel et al., 1994; Tarantino et al., 1995).

### 3.2.2. Renal manifestations

Renal symptoms at the time of diagnosis are variable. Non-nephrotic range proteinuria with glomerular haematuria is the most frequent clinical presentation, associated with mild to moderate chronic renal failure in more than half of the cases. Hypertension is present in approximately 80% of the patients, often severe and resistant to anti-hypertensive drugs. Severe renal manifestations occur in 25% of the cases, including acute nephritic syndrome, heavy glomerular proteinuria, hypoalbuminemia, frank or gross haematuria, and acute renal failure. Anuria develops in 5% of patients with symptoms of rapidly progressive GN. Fluid retention is often a predominant clinical feature in the more dramatic forms of glomerular involvement, where increased capillary permeability secondary to macrophage and endothelial cell activation by the cryoglobulin adds to renal disease (Cordonnier et al., 1983; Monti et al., 1995; D'Amico 1998; Tarantino et al., 1981, 1995; Fornasieri and D'Amico, 1996).

### 3.2.3. Natural history and prognosis

The course of renal and extra-renal manifestations in type II cryoglobulinemia is unpredictable, with acute disease exacerbations alternating with quiescent phases. Renal flares, which occur in 25% of the cases, usually manifest as nephrotic syndrome or acute nephritic syndrome, often accompanied by general symptoms. Rarely, acute exacerbations of the disease lead to dramatic multi-organ failure, refractory to aggressive therapy. However, irrespective of the severity of initial organ involvement, including renal disease, partial or complete remission is observed in at least one third of the patients, either spontaneously or following therapy (D'Amico 1998; Tarantino et al., 1981, 1995; Fornasieri and D'Amico, 1996). Remission of advanced renal disease is possible, as described in one patient after 6 months on chronic haemodialysis (Dussol et al., 2001). Intravenous administration of polyvalent IgG may trigger disease relapse in patients with MC (Barton et al., 1987), or in those with a serum monoclonal IgMκ component bearing rheumatoid factor activity (Odum et al., 2001).

End-stage renal disease (ESRD) requiring continuous renal replacement therapy is a rare event in type II cryoglobulinemia, even after years of disease with persistence of proteinuria and haematuria, and despite initial moderate impairment in renal function (Cordonnier et al., 1983; D'Amico 1998; Tarantino et al., 1981, 1995). By contrast, control of hypertension is often difficult to achieve, predisposing patients to life-threatening cardiovascular events (Tarantino et al., 1995). In a large series of 105 patients, the prevalence of ESRD was less than 15% over a follow-up period of 11 years. Patient survival was 49% at 10 years after renal biopsy. Forty percent of the patients had died from cardiovascular complications, infection, liver failure, or malignant disease. In those over 50 years, splenomegaly, relapsing purpura, cryocrit over 10%, serum C3 level of less than 0.54 mg/dl, and serum creatinine level above 136 μmol/l, were significantly associated with decreased renal and patient survival (Tarantino et al., 1995). Simultaneous HIV infection also reduces survival in type II cryoglobulinemia (Morales et al., 1997; Cheng et al., 1999); clinical remission of cryoglobulinemic vasculitis may be obtained with anti-HCV therapy, whereas anti-retroviral therapy is usually ineffective (Morales et al., 1997; Saadoun et al., 2006a).

### 3.3. Laboratory findings

High serum levels of C reactive protein are common, reflecting a chronic inflammatory response. Rheumatoid factor activity, which results from the antibody specificity of the monoclonal IgM against polyclonal IgG, is commonly detected, together with other autoantibodies, including antinuclear antibodies. Low serum levels of complement components are nearly constant during flares-up of the disease. Early components, C1q, C2, and C4 are predominantly affected, and are sometimes undetectable. By contrast, CH50 and C3 levels are usually normal, or slightly diminished during disease exacerbations. Levels of late components (C5–C9) and of C1 inhibitor are generally unaffected or moderately elevated (Cordonnier et al., 1983; Fornasieri and D'Amico, 1996; D'Amico 1998; Trejo et al., 2001). The mechanisms by which type II cryoglobulins activate the complement cascade remain to be fully understood. They may involve efficient engagement of C1q protein by cryoglobulin (Sansonno and Dammacco, 2005), reduced synthesis of early components, activation of the classical pathway C3 convertase, or activation of the C4 binding-protein (D'Amico, 2003).

Abnormal liver tests, including raised liver enzymes and cholestasis, are present in 50–70% of the patients with type II cryoglobulinemia, generally resulting from chronic HCV infection. Finally, circulating cryoglobulins may interfere with various laboratory tests, including erythrocyte sedimentation rate and white blood cell measurements (Haeney, 1976).

## 3.4. Renal pathology

Meticulous histopathological study of the kidney biopsy is a key step for accurate diagnosis of renal disease in type II cryoglobulinemia. Exudative MPGN is the characteristic and almost constant pattern of renal involvement, usually referred to as "cryoglobulinemic glomerulonephritis". This peculiar form of MPGN should be distinguished from classical type I MPGN and from proliferative GN in SLE (Cordonnier et al., 1975, 1983; Tarantino et al., 1981, 1995; D'Amico, 1998; Fornasieri and D'Amico, 1996; Mougenot and Ronco, 1996).

Light microscopic examination of kidney biopsy samples typically shows diffuse endocapillary proliferation, related to massive and characteristic infiltration by mononuclear cells, including T- and B-lymphocytes, but mainly CD68+ monocytes. Glomerular inflammation is associated with fibrinoid, eosinophilic, PAS-positive subendothelial deposits. These deposits are often abundant and have the appearance of pseudo-thrombi with narrowing of the glomerular capillary lumens. Although suggestive of the diagnosis, complete and direct obstruction of glomerular capillary lumens by circulating cryoglobulin ("true" glomerular thrombi) is not constant (Fig. 1).

Proliferation of mesangial cells, accompanied by increased mesangial matrix with mesangial interposition, and inflammatory infiltration by mononuclear cells, may result in the "double contour" appearance of glomerular basement membranes, better demonstrated with PAS and silver staining (Fig. 2). Double contour appearance of glomerular capillary walls appears to be less frequent in type II cryoglobulinemic GN than in idiopathic type I MPGN. Typically, extra-capillary proliferation leading to the formation of glomerular crescents is mild or absent. The extent of glomerular deposits and endocapillary proliferation usually correlates with the severity of renal and systemic symptoms. Renal vascular

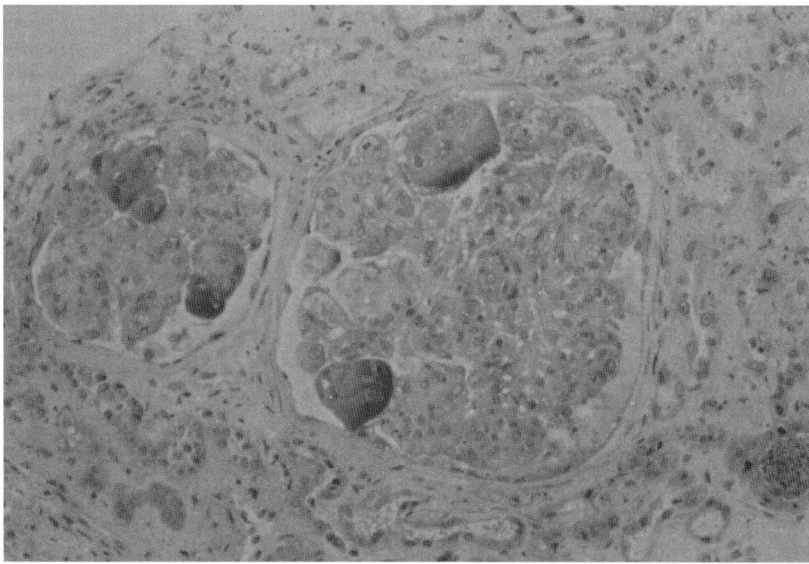

**Figure 1.** Cryoglobulinemic glomerulonephritis (GN). Kidney biopsy. Light microscopy, trichrome staining (original magnification × 400). Voluminous fibrinoid thrombi in glomerular capillary lumens, with exudative membranoproliferative GN (MPGN).

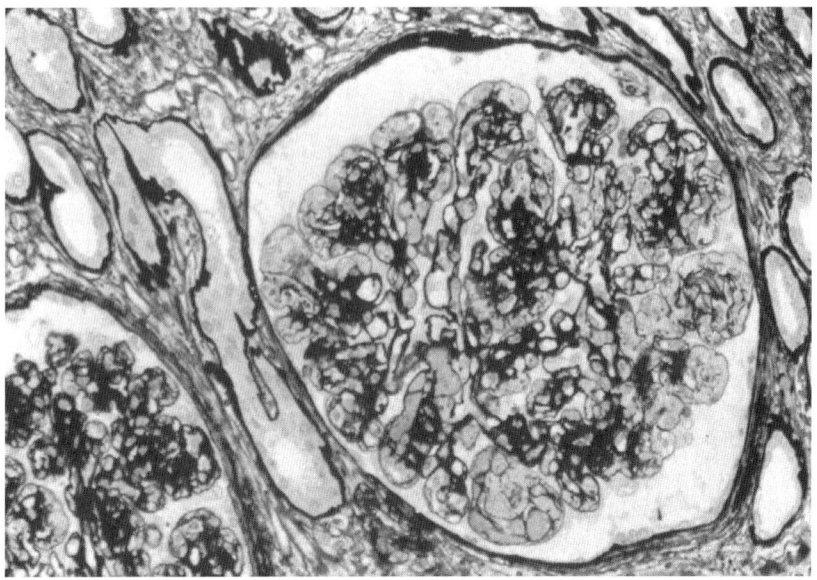

**Figure 2.** Cryoglobulinemic GN. Kidney biopsy. Light microscopy, Marinozzi's silver staining (original magnification × 400). Double contour appearance of glomerular capillary walls with luminal thrombi and parietal subendothelial deposits. Note the accentuation of lobulation secondary to mesangial hyperplasia, and glomerular infiltration by macrophages and neutrophils.

involvement is common, with vasculitic lesions of small to middle-size intrarenal arteries in nearly one third of the cases. They are characterized by endoluminal PAS positive deposits, fibrinoid necrosis of the vessel walls, and perivascular and endoluminal infiltration by monocytes and polymorphonuclear neutrophils. These lesions, commonly found in the most severe forms of the disease, may be isolated or associated with segmental glomerular pathological changes. Lesions of thrombotic microangiopathy affecting renal arterioles have been rarely described (Herzenberg et al., 1998). Interstitial monocyte infiltration is often present, sometimes associated with mild to moderate fibrosis.

By direct immunofluorescence microscopy, vascular and granular glomerular parietal and luminal deposits display the same immunoglobulin composition as the circulating cryoglobulin, as demonstrated by staining with both specific anti-heavy chain $\mu$ (generally intense) and $\gamma$ conjugates, and also with anti-$\kappa$ and $\lambda$ conjugates. Parietal fixation of anti-C3, anti-C1q, anti-C4, and anti-fibrinogen conjugates is often observed. According to the abundance of glomerular deposits, immunofluorescence patterns may vary from isolated segmental granular sub-endothelial deposits, to diffuse sub-endothelial deposits, or capillary thrombi with variable sub-endothelial deposits (Mougenot and Ronco, 1996).

On electron microscopic examination, glomerular infiltration is evident, with monocytes often in close vicinity to sub-endothelial deposits. Dense deposits may be granular, amorphous (immune-complex type), or organized into cylindrical curved and annular spoked-wheel-like sub-structures. The spoked annular sub-structures are 30–60 nm in external diameter, and, in cross section, are found to correspond to the cylinders (Fig. 3). In the latter case, similar patterns of ultrastructural organization of the serum cryoprecipitate is often seen (Cordonnier et al., 1975, 1983; Touchard, 2003).

In patients with moderate renal involvement limited to urine abnormalities, glomerular lesions may be mild and less suggestive of the diagnosis, with a pattern of segmental and focal proliferative GN. Monocyte infiltration is less intense and glomerular thrombi are not found, while sub-endothelial deposits are scanty and weakly stained by specific conjugates. A pattern of type I lobular MPGN has been reported in some patients with

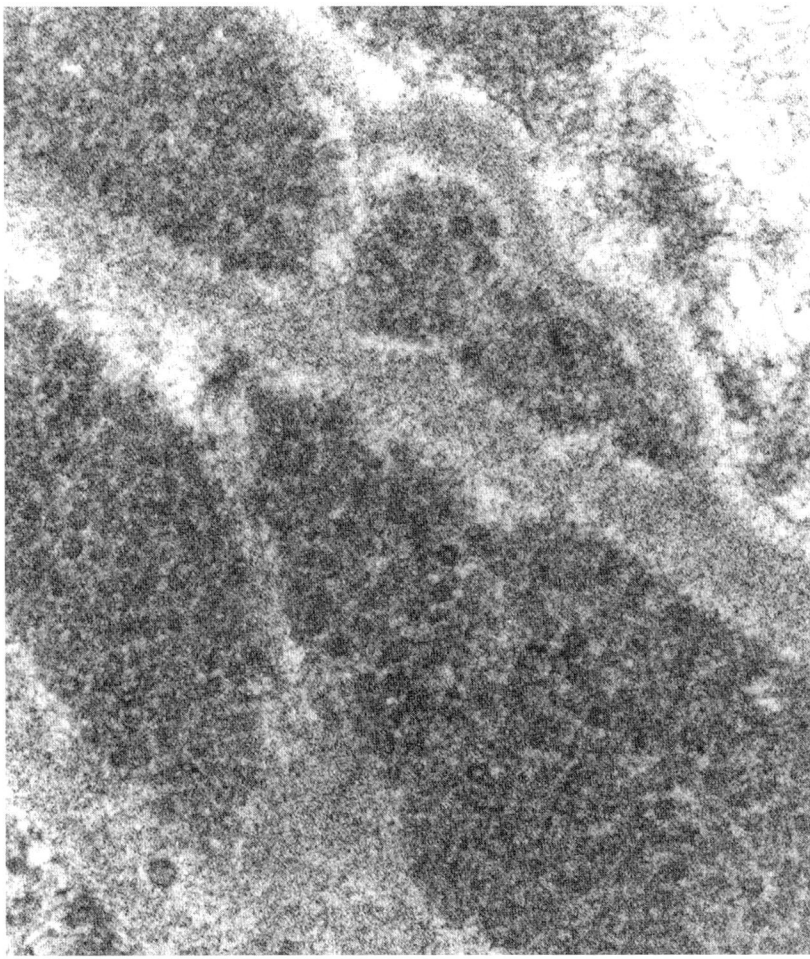

**Figure 3.** Type II cryoglobulinemia (monoclonal IgMκ and polyclonal IgG). Kidney biopsy. Electron microscopy (original magnification × 33,000). Glomerular organized electron dense deposits with cylindrical curved and annular spoked-wheel-like substructures.

heavy proteinuria or nephrotic syndrome, with lesions similar to those observed in idiopathic MPGN, except for mild monocyte infiltration (Tarantino et al., 1981, 1995; D'Amico 1998; Fornasieri and D'Amico, 1996; Mougenot and Ronco, 1996).

## 3.5. Treatment of type II cryoglobulinemia with renal disease

The therapeutic strategy for type II cryoglobulinemia should be carefully evaluated in each patient, after appropriate tests for the detection of HCV infection, including tests for HCV antibodies and HCV RNA in the patient's serum and, if necessary, in the cryoprecipitate. In the most severe forms of the HCV-associated MC with renal involvement, therapeutic advances have been made with combined anti-HCV therapy and/or specific anti-CD20 monoclonal antibody targeting cryoglobulin production by B-lymphocytes.

### 3.5.1. Antiviral therapy

Alfa-interferon (IFN-α) monotherapy has shown limited efficacy in the treatment of HCV-associated

MC, particularly on peripheral nerve and renal symptoms. In an initial randomized crossover-controlled trial including 26 patients, Ferri et al. reported a transient beneficial effect of subcutaneous IFN-α (2 million IU/day subcutaneously for 1 month, then every other day for 5 months) on purpuric lesions, liver enzyme, and serum cryoglobulins, in 20 patients. A rebound phenomenon of clinical and serologic parameters was observed after IFN-α discontinuation. Of note, only one patient had evidence of nephropathy, and patients with serum creatinine level above 1.5 mg/dl were excluded from the trial (Ferri et al., 1993). In a randomized controlled study of 53 patients (40 with renal involvement), a standard regimen of IFN-α (3 million IU three times a week for 24 weeks) in 27 patients, resulted in undetectable serum levels of HCV RNA in 15 cases, with parallel improvement in cutaneous vasculitis and significant decreases in levels of anti-HCV-antibodies, cryoglobulins, rheumatoid factor, and creatinine. Cryoglobulinemia and viremia recurred systematically after treatment withdrawal. Johnson et al. reported similar results in 34 patients with HCV-associated GN, 11 of whom had a diagnosis of MC. Conventional IFN-α therapy (3 million IU three times per week for 6 to 12 months) in 14 patients induced a 60% reduction in proteinuria, without improvement in renal function. Again, clinical response correlated with viral response, but relapse of renal disease and viremia was observed after completing therapy (Johnson et al., 1994). In a randomized study of 65 patients, Dammacco et al., showed that conventional IFN-α therapy (3 million IU, three times a week for 48 weeks) with or without oral methylprednisolone (16 mg/day) was associated with a 50% response rate (as defined by reduction of cryocrit to less than 50% of the initial value, with improvement of cutaneous and/or neurological and/or renal symptoms). Relapse rate after completion of therapy was slightly reduced (from 100 to 75%) with the association of IFN-α and methylprednisolone, compared to those who received IFN-α alone (Dammaco et al., 1994). High pre-treatment viral load (HCV-RNA >2 million copies/ml), persistent viremia 4–12 weeks after the onset of therapy, and viral genotype 1b have been identified as predictive factors of a lack of long-term response to IFN-α therapy (Johnson et al., 1994; Dammaco et al., 1994; D'Amico, 2003).

A prolonged response, as defined by undetectable serum HCV-RNA 6 months after withdrawal of IFN-α therapy is obtained in only 15–20% of patients receiving an initial 12-month course of IFN-α 3 million IU three times a week (D'Amico, 2003). Prolonged clinical remission may be achieved with high-dose IFN-α (up to 10 million IU three times a week) over a short period of time (Campise and Tarantino, 1999). In the series reported by Casato et al., 31 patients with type II MC (17 with renal involvement) received 3 million IU of IFN-α/day for 3 months, and then every other day for 9 months. In 62% of the patients, clinical symptoms regressed and cryocrit level decreased below 10% of the initial value, with simultaneous normalization of serum transaminases and disappearance of circulating HCV-RNA, for a mean period of time of 33 months (and more than 5 years in three cases). Predictive factors for a prolonged response were a cumulative dose of IFN-α >621 million IU and the presence of solitary anti-C22 (HCV core) antibody (Casato et al., 1997). However, the long-term beneficial effects of intensive IFN-α protocols remains to be established (D'Amico, 2003) and their use is limited by potentially severe side effects, neurological disorders including worsening of peripheral neuropathy, arrhythmias, and cytopenias (Misiani et al., 1994). The latter effect may be enhanced by the concomitant use of angiotensin converting enzyme inhibitors (Casato et al., 1995).

More recently, the combination of IFN-α and ribavirin, was shown to improve results in the treatment of HCV-associated MC, although with lower efficiency than in patients with chronic hepatitis C without cryoglobulinemia. Zuckerman et al. reported nine patients with symptomatic MC resistant to conventional IFN-α therapy, who were re-treated with a regimen of IFN-α 2a or IFN-α 2b three times weekly and ribavirin 15 mg/kg daily for 6 months. Arthritis, proteinuria, and cutaneous vasculitis improved in all cases, with a parallel decrease or disappearance of serum cryoglobulins and decrease or normalization of serum transaminases. However, polyneuropathy related symptoms were relatively resistant to treatment and complete virologic and clinical response was achieved in only 25% of the patients (Zuckerman et al., 2000). Similar results were observed by Mazzaro et al. in 27 patients who failed to respond or relapsed after initial IFN-α monotherapy (Mazzaro et al., 2003). In another series of 27 patients with HCV-associated systemic vasculitis (including 22 MC cases), combination of IFN-α (mean duration 20 months) and ribavirin therapy (mean duration 14 months) resulted in a complete clinical response in 59% of the patients, and a partial response in 33%. Sustained virologic responses were observed in 64% of patients with sufficient follow-up after withdrawal of therapy, and paralleled sustained clinical responses. Clinical response rates varied depending on organ involvement (i.e. cutaneous 85–100%, neural 25–50%, renal 25–50%). A prolonged period of therapy (18–24 months) was required to obtain efficacy and to avoid vasculitis relapse. The low incidence of HCV genotype 1 in this series, was likely involved in the high virologic response rates seen (Cacoub et al., 2002).

The main side effects of ribavirin therapy are hyperuricemia and hemolytic anemia. Due to reduced clearance in patients with renal failure, and because it is not removed by dialysis, ribavirin is not recommended when creatinine clearance is below 50 ml/min. However, a combined IFN-α plus ribavirin regimen showed beneficial effects in small series of patients with MC and renal failure, in whom ribavirin dose was adapted to renal function or to a trough plasma concentration of 10–15 mmol/l. Erythropoietin therapy was used to control anemia (Rossi et al., 2003, Bruchfeld et al., 2003, Alric et al., 2004). Alric et al. reported a series of 25 patients with HCV cryoglobulinemic MPGN, initially treated with prednisone, furosemide, and plasmapheresis in over 50% of cases. Eighteen patients (six with a serum creatinine level >150 μmol/l) received additional therapy with IFN-α (four with pegylated IFN) and ribavirin for a mean period of 18 months. With a follow-up of at least 6 months after treatment withdrawal, 12 of the 18 treated patients (67%) (and none of those untreated or non-responders) had a sustained virologic response, with significant decrease in cryoglobulin levels and improvement in proteinuria and purpura. Serum creatinine levels were unchanged, and no effect was observed on polyarthralgia and polyneuropathy. Anemia required a reduction in the ribavirin dose in eight patients (Alric et al., 2004).

The addition of a polyethylene glycol molecule to IFN results in a biologically more active molecule with a longer half-life, allowing a more convenient once weekly dosing. Pegylated IFN has greater efficacy in terms of sustained virologic response and it is currently recommended in combination with ribavirin in the treatment of chronic hepatitis C (Kamar et al., 2006b). In an initial Italian study, 18 patients with MC received pegylated IFN-α 2b (1 μg/kg weekly) plus ribavirin (1 mg daily) for 48 weeks, regardless of the HCV genotype. Whereas clinical symptoms improved and HCV RNA became undetectable in 83% of the patients at the end of therapy, 44% relapsed both clinically and virologically soon after treatment withdrawal and only 44% achieved a sustained virological response (Mazzaro et al., 2005). However, Cacoub et al. showed that a longer duration (mean 13 months) of combined treatment with pegylated IFN-α 2b and ribavirin resulted in sustained virologic and clinical responses in 78% of their patients, including all those with renal involvement and nearly 50% of those with peripheral neuropathy. Serum cryoglobulins disappeared or decreased and complement levels normalized in most cases. Only one patient had clinical and virological relapse after cessation of treatment and responded to a second course of combined therapy (Cacoub et al., 2005).

Recently, in a long-term follow-up single-center study of 72 consecutive patients, the same group compared treatment with IFN-α 2b (3 million IU three times a week, 32 patients) or pegylated IFN-α 2b (1.5 μg/kg/week, 40 patients), both in combination with oral ribavirin (600–1200 mg/day) for at least 6 months. Twenty-two patients had renal involvement, with biopsy proven MPGN and glomerular filtration rate <70 ml/min in 17 and 16 cases, respectively. Nine patients had low-grade B-cell non-Hodgkin's lymphoma. Patients with renal failure, severe polyneuropathy, and/or life-threatening complications additionally received oral corticosteroids ($n=20$), immunosuppressive drugs ($n=4$), and/or plasmapheresis ($n=9$). With a mean follow-up period of 40 months, a complete clinical response occurred in 45 patients (62.5%), with sustained virologic response (as defined by the absence of detectable serum HCV RNA 6 months after stopping antiviral treatment) in 42 patients (58.3%) and disappearance of cryoglobulins in 33 patients (45.8%). Antiviral therapy induced higher response rates for purpura and arthralgia (86.3 and 80% of cases, respectively) than for peripheral neuropathy and renal involvement, which resolved in 68.2 and 40.9% of cases, respectively. A reappearance of HCV RNA was observed in eight patients, a median of 2 months after discontinuing therapy, six of whom experienced a relapse of cryoglobulinemic vasculitis. Eight patients died, mostly of cardiovascular, hepatic, and infectious complications. Adverse events, mostly fatigue, fever, cytopenia, and myalgia, were observed in 39 patients. No therapy interruptions were needed, but reduction of antiviral therapy was required in 11 patients because of hematologic side effects. Patients treated with pegylated IFN-α 2b plus ribavirin showed a higher rate of sustained clinical (67.5 vs. 56.3%), virologic (62.5 vs. 53.1%), and immunologic (57.5 vs. 31.3%) response than those receiving IFN-α 2b plus ribavirin, and required plasmapheresis and immunosuppressive drugs less frequently. In multivariate analyses, complete clinical response positively correlated with an early (within 3 months after starting antiviral treatment) virologic response, and negatively correlated with a glomerular filtration rate <70 ml/min (Saadoun et al., 2006b).

### 3.5.2. Corticosteroids, plasmapheresis, and immunosuppressive drugs

Since the development of antiviral therapy, corticosteroids and cytotoxic drugs (cyclophosphamide, chlorambucil, azathioprin) are no longer used in the treatment of slowly progressive type II MC. These therapies do not protect against renal and extra-renal flares and enhance the risk of infections, cardiovascular disease, and neoplasia, including exacerbation of HCV-related low-grade B-cell lymphoma (Campise and Tarantino, 1999). Short-term aggressive treatment remains indicated in severe flares of the disease, with acute renal failure, skin necrosis, advanced polyneuropathy, and cardiomyopathy. The combination of intravenous methylprednisolone (MP) (0.75–1 g daily for 3 days) followed by oral prednisone (0.5 mg/kg/day for 2 weeks, progressively tapered to 10 mg/day over 2–6 months), with oral cyclophosphamide (2 mg/kg/day, 3–6 months) and plasma exchanges (one plasma volume, 3 times weekly for 2–3 weeks) is generally employed to rapidly eliminate circulating cryoglobulins and reduce their production by B lymphocytes. In uncontrolled studies, intravenous MP pulses have produced dramatic effects on extra-renal manifestations, with rapid disappearance of systemic symptoms and skin manifestations, but a less pronounced effect on peripheral neuropathy. Furthermore, MP pulses rapidly improved renal function (in up to 85% of the patients), while proteinuria and cryocrit levels decreased more slowly (Madore et al., 1996; Campise and Tarantino, 1999; Kamar et al., 2006b). Long-term immunosuppressive therapy should not be considered, because of increased risk of malignancy and infections, including enhanced HCV replication and progression of chronic hepatitis (D'Amico, 2003; Campise and Tarantino, 1999, Kamar et al., 2006b). Plasmapheresis should be performed with warmed replacement fluid in order to prevent cryoprecipitation (Evans et al., 1984). Other techniques, such as double cascade filtration, cryofiltration, or immunoabsorption apheresis, that minimize the need for replacement fluid and selectively remove circulating cryoglobulins, are not widely available (Siami et al., 1995; Russo et al., 1996; Stefanutti et al., 2003).

Rituximab is a chimeric monoclonal antibody that directly and selectively targets B cells by reacting with the transmembrane CD20 protein, present in different maturation steps of B-lymphocytes (from early pre-B to mature lymphocytes), with no direct effect on plasma cells. Rituximab, which proved effective and was well tolerated in B-cell non-Hodgkin lymphomas and various autoantibody-mediated immune diseases, has been successfully used in MC patients with resistant or relapsing disease after antiviral or immunosuppressive therapy, or in those with HCV-related lymphoproliferative disorders (Sansonno et al., 2003; Zaja et al., 2003; Basse et al., 2006; Bryce et al., 2006a; Quartuccio et al., 2006). The two largest reported series included 20 and 15 patients respectively, who were treated with rituximab 375 mg/m$^2$ intravenously weekly for 4 weeks (Sansonno et al., 2003; Zaja et al., 2003). Almost all patients responded to therapy, with a significant decrease in serum cryoglobulin level, rapid improvement in general symptoms, purpura, peripheral neuropathy, and disappearance of B-cell clones in those with associated lymphoproliferative disease. Three patients had renal involvement. Of those, a decrease in proteinuria was observed in only one patient with MPGN of recent onset (Zaja et al., 2003). Response to therapy was not predicted by disease duration, age, or HCV genotype 1 distribution (Sansonno et al., 2003). Remission was maintained throughout follow-up in 75 and 60% of the patients, respectively. Tolerance of therapy was excellent, except for retinal artery thrombosis after two infusions in one case (Zaja et al., 2003). However, rituximab had a deep impact on HCV viremia, with increased in viral load in 25% of the patients (Zaja et al., 2003) and doubling of baseline HCV RNA levels in responders (Sansonno et al., 2003).

Rocatello et al. evaluated the long-term effects of rituximab in six patients with cryoglobulinemic GN and chronic HCV infection genotype 1b (three cases) and 2a2c (three cases). Three patients had bone marrow clonal restriction. All patients received four standard weekly doses, plus two additional monthly infusions in five cases, without other immunosuppressive drugs or antiviral treatment. Improvement or disappearance of constitutional symptoms, and resolution of bone marrow abnormalities was observed in all cases. Renal function remained stable or improved, while proteinuria and cryocrit significantly decreased at months 2, 6, and 12. Rheumatoid factor and IgM levels significantly decreased, whereas C4 levels increased at 6 months. HCV viral load remained stable, and no significant side effects were observed (Rocatello et al., 2004). Although as yet unproven in randomized controlled trials, combined treatment with rituximab followed by pegylated IFN plus ribavirin may be an effective therapy in HCV-associated MC resistant to standard antiviral and immunosuppresive therapy (Lamprecht et al., 2003).

### 3.5.3. Symptomatic and supportive therapy

Due to the frequency and severity of hypertension in patients with cryoglobulinemic GN, aggressive treatment based on angiotensin converting inhibitors and angiotensin receptor antagonists should be initiated promptly to reduce progression of renal insufficiency and mortality from cardiovascular complications (Tarantino et al., 1995). High-dose furosemide is required in patients with fluid retention, which, in the most severe cases, may necessitate prompt hemodialysis or hemofiltration.

Life expectancy of MC patients with ESRD, treated either by hemodialysis or peritoneal dialysis, appears to be similar to that of the general dialysis population. However, patients with severe disease at the beginning of dialysis have a poor prognosis, because of uncontrolled cryoglobulinemic vasculitis or side effects of an aggressive cytotoxic or corticosteroid therapy (Tarantino et al., 1994). In HCV-positive patients on chronic hemodialysis, serum cryoglobulin levels are usually lower than in non-HCV patients, and manifestations of cryoglobulinemic vasculitis are rare (Okuda et al., 1998). In these patients, treatment with standard interferon-α is indicated in the case of symptomatic cryoglobulinemia, significant liver disease (fibrosis score ≥2), and in candidates for renal transplantation, whatever the severity of liver disease. An overall 30–40% rate of sustained viral eradication may be achieved (Pol et al., 2002; Kamar et al., 2006a).

Although cryoglobulinemic GN may recur after renal transplantation (Hiesse et al., 1989), most patients are asymptomatic and cryoglobulinemia does not appear to affect graft function (Sens et al., 2005). However, transplant glomerulopathy (Morales, 2004) and chronic allograft dysfunction might be more frequent in HCV-positive renal transplant recipients, particularly in those with complement activation (Weiner et al., 2004). Antiviral therapy is problematic in HCV-positive renal transplant patients. IFN-α therapy is contraindicated because of a high risk of acute rejection and graft loss. Ribavirin monotherapy, which has shown beneficial but transient effect on proteinuria and nephrotic syndrome in liver transplant patients with HCV-associated MC (Pham et al., 1998), is currently the only available regimen. Basse et al. showed that rituximab is efficient in treating de novo type III cryoglobulinemia-associated MPGN in renal transplant recipients. In seven patients, of whom five were HCV positive, weekly infusions of 375 mg/m$^2$ resulted in remission or improvement of nephrotic syndrome in five cases, with sustained clearance of serum cryoglobulins in six. However, two patients experienced severe infectious complications, probably related to excessive immunosuppression (Basse et al., 2006). Combined ribavirin and rituximab therapy has not been evaluated in renal transplant patients.

### 3.5.4. Current recommendations

Anti-viral therapy appears to be indicated in all patients with HCV-MC and renal involvement. In patients with moderate renal (isolated urine abnormalities) and extra-renal manifestations, immunosuppressive agents are not indicated. Combined pegylated IFN and ribavirin for at least 1 year appears to be the treatment of choice. The ribavirin dose should be adapted according to creatinine clearance in order to prevent hemolytic anemia, which may require supplementary recombinant erythropoietin therapy.

Patients with severe renal (nephrotic syndrome, progressive renal failure) or extra-renal disease should be aggressively treated. Plasmapheresis plus pulsed steroids are commonly used during acute flares of the disease, followed by immunosuppressive therapy with either oral cyclophosphamide (2 mg/kg/day) or rituximab (375 mg/m$^2$, four weekly courses). Corticosteroids and cytotoxic drugs should not be given for more than 6 months, to limit infectious, cardiovascular, and malignant complications (Campise and Tarantino, 1999). Rituximab, which appears as efficient as cyclophosphamide, is better tolerated, and may induce less viral replication, has been proposed as first line therapy (Kamar et al., 2006b). However, tolerance and efficiency of rituximab and cyclophosphamide have not been compared in randomized controlled trials. Whether anti-HCV therapy should be introduced immediately following plasmapheresis, or 2–4 weeks after resumption of immunosuppressive drugs is not established. Although ribavirin has been used safely in patients with renal failure, it is not recommended for patients with a creatinine clearance below 50 ml/min. Similar concerns currently apply to pegylated interferon because of its long half-life, and patients with advanced or end-stage renal failure, should be treated initially with standard interferon.

In patients with non-HCV MC and renal disease, therapy should focus on the underlying disease. A similar regimen of high-dose corticosteroids combined with plasmapheresis, cytotoxic therapy, or rituximab is generally employed to control disease flares with severe renal and systemic manifestations, followed in some cases by low-dose steroid maintenance therapy.

## 4. Renal disease in type I cryoglobulinemia

Although renal manifestations are reported in 25–40% of patients in two large series (Brouet et al., 1974, Trejo et al., 2001), glomerular disease related to type I cryoglobulinemia remains poorly described, with less than 30 biopsy-proven cases to date (Touchard et al., 1994, Touchard 2003). Type I cryoglobulinemic GN, the diagnosis of which requires sensitive techniques for the immunopathologic analysis of the renal biopsy, with simultaneous identification of the underlying and sometimes latent B-cell proliferative disorder, is probably underestimated. Furthermore, glomerular disease in type I cryoglobulinemia may be confused with other forms of glomerulopathy related to the deposition of monoclonal Igs, mainly GN with organized microtubular monoclonal Ig deposits (GOMMID) or immunotactoid glomerulopathy (Touchard et al., 1994; Bridoux et al., 2002) (Table 2 and 3).

**Table 2**
Classification of nephropathies with organized monoclonal Ig deposits

| Microtubular deposits | | | Fibrillary deposits (Congo red+) | | Crystals | |
|---|---|---|---|---|---|---|
| IgG<br>IgA<br>IgM<br>κ > λ | IgMκ<br>anti-IgG | IgG<br>κ > λ | Ig light chain<br>λ > κ | γ heavy chain | Ig light chain | Ig light chain<br>IgGκ<br>IgMκ |
| Type I cryo. | Type II cryo. | GOMMID<br>(immuno-<br>tactoid GN) | AL<br>amyloidosis | AH<br>amyloidosis | Fanconi<br>syndrome<br>(κ > λ).<br>Myeloma cast<br>nephropathy | Crystalcryo.<br>Crystal-<br>storing<br>histiocytosis |

*Abbreviations*: Cryo, cryoglobulin; GOMMID, glomerulonephritis with organized microtubular monoclonal Ig deposits. In type II cryoglobulinemia, deposits appear polyclonal, as the monoclonal component is masked by polyclonal IgG.


**Table 3**
Type I cryoglobulinemic GN and GOMMID: distinctive pathologic features

| Type I cryoglobulinemic GN | GOMMID (immunotactoid GN) |
|---|---|
| Membranoproliferative GN<br>Numerous neutrophils and macrophages<br>Pseudo thrombi + thrombi<br>Subendothelial and mesangial deposits, rarely subepithelial | Atypical membranous GN or MPGN<br>Few neutrophils in capillary loops, no macrophages<br>Pseudo thrombi<br>Subepithelial, intra-membranous, subendothelial, and mesangial deposits |
| Microtubular substructures or crystalline inclusions in deposits and in endothelial cells, mesangial cells, and macrophages<br>Protein aggregates within glomerular and vascular lumens | Microtubular inclusions in glomerular deposits and in malignant lymphocytes, not in glomerular cells |
| Vasculitis (glomerular and extraglomerular) | No vasculitis |

*Abbreviations*: GOMMID, glomerulonephritis with organized microtubular monoclonal Ig deposits.


## 4.1. Pathophysiology

Not all monoclonal Ig in humans and mice exhibit cryoglobulin activity and induce specific glomerular lesions. The prominent role of primary structure and physico-chemical characteristics of nephrotoxic monoclonal cryoglobulins has been illustrated in experimental animal models. Izui et al. isolated hybridomas derived from MRL-Fas(lpr) mice that spontaneously developed a systemic autoimmune disease characterized by proliferative GN, polyathropathy, and diffuse necrotizing vasculitis, with high serum titers of IgG antibodies with rheumatoid factor (anti-IgG) activity and cryoglobulinemia. They first showed that the injection of a hybridoma secreting a monoclonal IgG3 cryoglobulin with anti-IgG2a activity into susceptible mice induces systemic vasculitis and acute cryoglobulinemic GN with mesangial proliferation, glomerular thrombi, and diffuse glomerular IgG3 and C3 deposits (Lemoine et al., 1992; Itoh et al., 1993). The induction of glomerular lesions was independent of the antibody specificity of the monoclonal IgG3, but depended on its property to self-aggregate through Fc–Fc interactions and to cryoprecipitate.

A variable pattern of glomerular lesions was seen depending on the type of IgG3 used in the experiments. Glycosylation and galactosylation in the constant domain of monoclonal IgG3 play a role in self-aggregation and cryoprecipitation, while both cryoprecipitation and nephrotoxicity of monoclonal IgG3 depend on positively charged residues in the constant and variable (particularly in positions 6 and 23) domains of the heavy chain (Panka et al., 1995; Kuroki et al., 2002).

In a transgenic model, Kikuchi et al. demonstrated that the association of heavy and light chains of the monoclonal IgG3 was required for the induction of GN, the pattern of which was influenced by the level of production of the complete monoclonal cryoglobulin (Kikuchi et al., 2002). Infiltrating polymorphonuclear leukocytes and C5 activation through alternative pathway play a crucial role in the induction of glomerular lesions (Trendelenburg et al., 2005). Rengers et al. confirmed the importance of the primary structure of Ig in the pathogenesis of murine monoclonal cryoglobulinemic GN. In an experimental model in mice, they showed that a 3-amino-acid deletion in the V$\kappa$ CDR1 region converted an IgG3$\kappa$ responsible for highly organized glomerular deposits typical of crystalcryoglobulinemic GN, into a more classical serum cryoglobulin. This mutation resulted in isolated amorphous thrombi in glomerular capillaries, reminiscent of those seen in humans with Waldenström's disease and the hyperviscosity syndrome (Rengers et al., 2000). In one patient with chronic lymphocytic leukemia complicated by IgG1$\kappa$ cryoglobulinemic GN characterized by mixed granular and microtubular glomerular deposits, study of the Ig molecular sequence revealed alterations of charge and hydrophobicity in the heavy and light chain variable regions, potentially promoting a crystal-like aggregation into microtubules (Galea et al., 2002).

## 4.2. Clinical presentation

Patients with type I cryoglobulinemic GN present with renal and systemic symptoms close to those of type II MC. Mean age at time of diagnosis is 55 years, with a slight male predominance. Hypertension, sometimes severe but rarely malignant, is present in more than 80% of the cases. Renal manifestations are prominent, characterized by heavy proteinuria in almost all cases, and nephrotic syndrome with marked fluid retention in nearly 60% of the patients. Glomerular hematuria is almost invariably found, which is rarely macroscopic. Most patients have mild to moderate impairment of renal function, with a mean serum creatinine level of 250 µmol/l. More severe presentations have been described, including acute nephritic syndrome, or anuric acute renal failure in 25% of the cases (Provot et al., 2000; Karras et al., 2002). Acute renal failure may be related to the formation of diffuse glomerular thrombi triggered by exposure to a temperature below that of cryoprecipitation, as described in a patient with type I IgM$\kappa$ cryoglobulin following prolonged surgical intervention in a cool operating room (Carloss and Tavassoli, 1980).

The frequency of extra-renal manifestations in patients with type I cryoglobulinemic GN appears lower than that in those with type II MC. A palpable purpura is reported in 30–40%, articular involvement in 30%, and Raynaud's phenomenon in less than 20% of the cases. Other symptoms, such as livedo reticularis, digital ischemia, gangrene, cardiomyopathy, or mononeuritis multiplex are rare and occur in the most severe cases (Provot et al., 2000; Trejo et al., 2001; Karras et al., 2002). Neurological symptoms related to hyperviscosity syndrome or thrombosis, have been described in a few patients (Brouet et al., 1974). An underlying B-cell lymphoproliferative disorder (chronic lymphocytic leukemia, non-Hodgkin's B-cell lymphoma, Waldenström's macroglobulinemia, multiple myeloma, or isolated monoclonal gammopathy) is found in more than 60% of the cases, either simultaneously or months to years before the diagnosis of type I cryoglobulinemic GN (Provot et al., 2000).

Crystalcryoglobulinemia is a rare condition characterized by crystallization of a monoclonal

Ig within plasma cells and various tissues, usually associated with multiple myeloma. The disease, which may be the initial manifestation of the underlying plasma cell disorder, is related to diffuse intravascular precipitation of crystals, consisting of monoclonal IgG or light chain, that damage the endothelium and lead to thrombosis. It typically presents as systemic necrotizing vasculitis with rapidly progressive renal failure, destructive polyarthropathy, peripheral neuropathy, and cutaneous lesions (Papo et al., 1996; Touchard, 2003).

## 4.3. Laboratory findings

In patients with type I cryoglobulinemic GN, cryoglobulins predominantly consist of monoclonal IgG (40%) and less frequently IgM or IgA, associated with a $\kappa$ light chain in 80% of the cases. These findings differ from those of two large series of type I cryoglobulinemia where cryoglobulins were composed of monoclonal IgM in half of the cases. However, whether the frequency of renal involvement varied with the isotype of monoclonal Ig was not determined (Brouet et al., 1974; Trejo et al., 2001). In one third of the cases, circulating cryoglobulins are not detected, despite repeated attempts and the presence of characteristic lesions of cryoglobulinemic MPGN (Provot et al., 2000). This might be related to the lack of sensitivity of the techniques used, but also suggests that there is no correlation between the concentration of serum monoclonal cryoglobulins and the development of related GN (Provot et al., 2000). Similar findings have been observed in AL amyloidosis or light chain deposition disease, where a serum or urine monoclonal component is not detected in 10% of patients (Preud'homme et al., 1994). Although monoclonal IgG and IgA cryoglobulins with an anti-IgG activity have been described, rheumatoid factor antibody activity is found in the serum or cryoprecipitate in a minority of patients (Gilboa et al., 1979; Rollino et al., 1992;

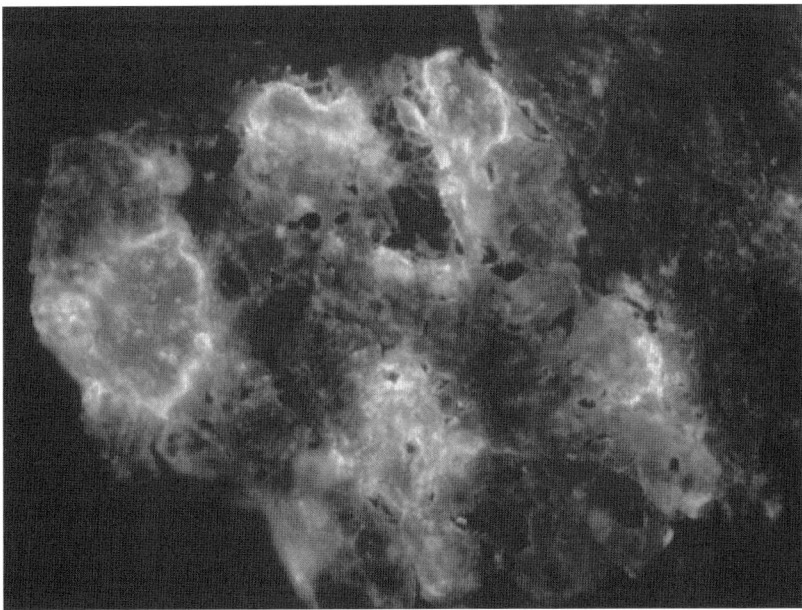

Figure 4. Type I cryoglobulinemic GN. Kidney biopsy. Immunofluorescence microscopy. Anti-gamma FITC-conjugate (original magnification × 400). Note the heavy staining of glomerular thrombi with peripheral reinforcement, contrasting with few anti-gamma positive parietal deposits.

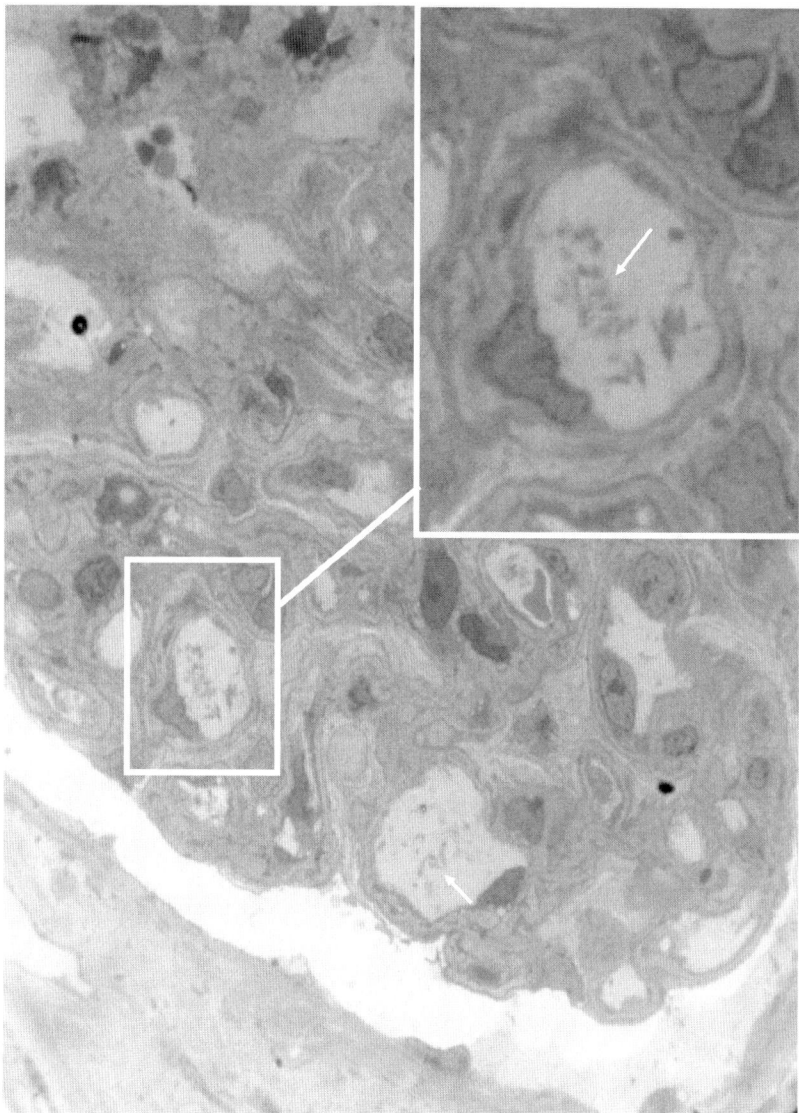

**Figure 5.** IgGκ crystalcryoglobulinemia. Kidney biopsy. Light microscopy, semi-thin sections, toluidine blue staining (original magnification ×400). MPGN. The most striking feature is the presence of needle-like crystals within glomerular capillary lumens, easily detected at a higher magnification (inset).

Touchard, 2003). Activation of complement with decreased serum levels of CH50, C3, and C4 appears to be less frequent than in type II MC (Provot et al., 2000; Karras et al., 2002). Whereas a high prevalence of HCV infection has been reported in type I cryoglobulinemia (Trejo et al., 2001), most reported patients with type I cryoglobulinemic GN are HCV negative (Provot et al., 2000). Hyperviscosity may be present, particularly in patients with high levels of monoclonal IgM cryoglobulin (Brouet et al., 1974).

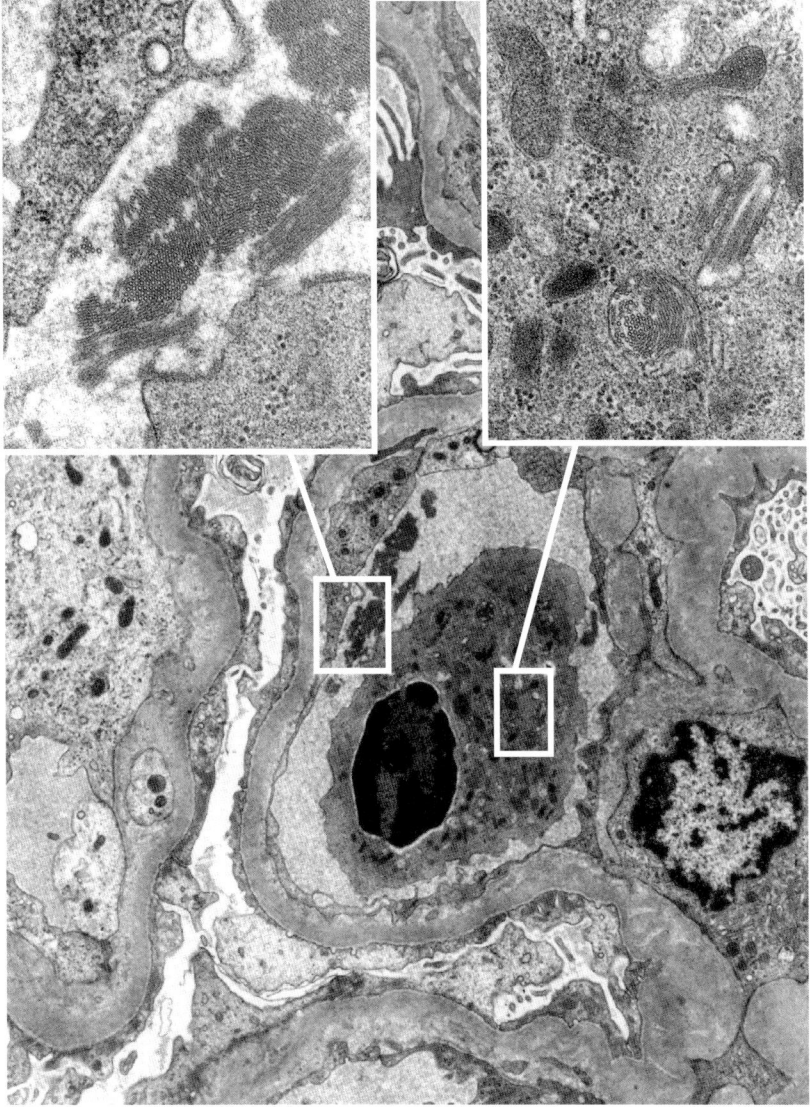

**Figure 6.** IgGκ crystalcryoglobulinemia. Kidney biopsy (same patient). Electron microscopy (original magnification ×3000). Circulating plasmacytoid cell in glomerular capillary lumen. Inset, left (original magnification ×30,000): cytoplasmic inclusions with microtubular substructures 14 nm in external diameter. Inset, right (original magnification ×30,000): same microtubular substructures, freely circulating within glomerular capillary and parallel randomly oriented bundles.

## 4.4. Pathological findings

By light microscopy, the usual pattern of glomerular lesions is that of MPGN, with eosinophilic, PAS positive, predominantly subendothelial deposits that narrow the lumen of the glomerular capillaries. Obstruction of capillary loops by fibrinoid thrombi is observed in more than 80% of the cases. Glomerular inflammatory infiltrates by monocytes and neutrophils is a constant feature in patients with severe renal symptoms. A double contour pattern of capillary walls, secondary to

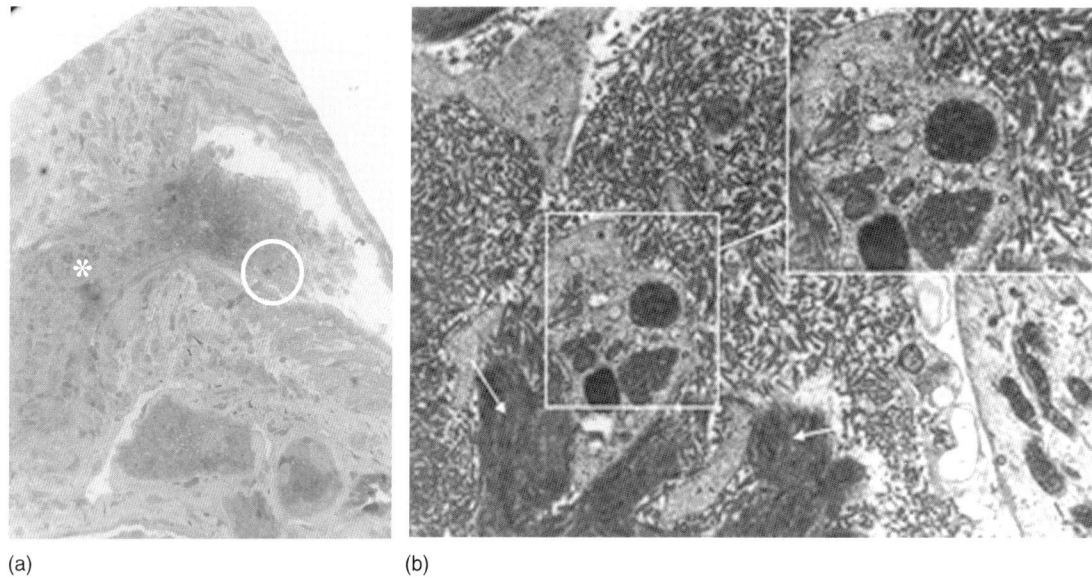

**Figure 7.** Kidney biopsy (same patient as Fig. 6). Arteriolar lesions induced by IgGκ crystalcryoglobulinemia. A: Light microscopy, semi-thin sections, toluidine blue staining (original magnification ×400). Fibrinoid thrombus, with base adherent to the intima, at the bifurcation of arcuate artery into interlobular artery. Tip of the thrombus, surrounded by mononuclear cells, is protruding into the arcuate artery lumen, while the interlobular artery is completely occluded by an inflammatory granuloma (∗). Circle: area of interest for electron microscopic study. B: Electron microscopy (original magnification ×8000). Highly organized arterial thrombus with extracellular microtubular substructures and cytoplasmic inclusions showing the same ultrastructural pattern in a mononuclear cell. Note the presence of osmiophilic fibrillar substructures (arrow) that correspond to fibrin.

mesangial interposition may be present, as well as moderate extra-capillary proliferation with crescents (Hent et al., 1997; Grcevska et al., 1998; Tomiyoshi et al., 1998; Provot et al., 2000; Karras et al., 2002). Patterns of endocapillary GN (Verroust et al., 1971; Provot et al., 2000), diffuse mesangial GN (Ponticelli et al., 1977), or segmental and focal GN (Galea et al., 2002) have been reported in few cases.

Interstitial inflammatory infiltration by lymphocytes and monocytes is common, and massive infiltration by malignant B cells may be prominent in patients with an associated lymphoproliferative disorder (Provot et al., 2000). Rarely, small and medium-size intra-renal arteries display typical lesions of vasculitis, characterized by fibrinoid necrosis and inflammatory infiltration of the vessel wall (Grcevska et al., 1998; Verroust et al., 1971; Provot et al., 2000). Immunofluoresence analysis, which should use conjugates specific for the different heavy chain isotypes and Ig subclasses, confirms the identity between the circulating cryoglobulin and the monoclonal Ig (most commonly IgG) in glomerular deposits and thrombi (Fig. 4). In the rare cases where sub-class composition was studied, glomerular IgG deposits were predominantly composed of IgG1 or IgG3 (Touchard et al., 1994; Provot et al., 2000; Karras et al., 2002).

By electron microscopy, IgG glomerular deposits are commonly organized into tangled or curved bundles of microtubules 10–60 nm in external diameter (Touchard 2003). A finger print pattern has been rarely described (Ogihara et al., 1979). Amorphous and microtubular deposits may coexist in the same area. (Galea et al., 2002). By contrast, monoclonal IgM cryoglobulins usually form amorphous finely granular osmiophilic deposits (Touchard, 2003). In crystalcryoglobulinemia, highly organized Ig crystals in the kidney are intracellular, in the cytoplasm of glomerular endothelial cells (Verroust et al., 1971; Bengtsson et al., 1975), mesangial cells (Provot et al., 2000), or within histiocytes (Tomiyoshi et al., 1998), and/or extracellular, in glomerular subendothelial spaces and within vascular lumens (Papo et al., 1996; Provot et al., 2000) (Figs. 5–7). Extracellular crystalline glomerular deposits and thrombi may display a typical "grid-like" appearance (Provot et al., 2000; Touchard, 2003). Ultrastructural examination of the serum cryoprecipitate usually reveals the same microtubular or crystalline organization as organ deposits (Galea et al., 2002; Touchard, 2003).

## 4.5. Treatment and prognosis

Due to the scarcity of reported cases, the optimal treatment strategy and outcome of type I cryoglobulinemic GN remain poorly described. Therapy targeting the underlying lymphoproliferative disorder, based on alkylating drugs or combination chemotherapy is required. High-dose chemotherapy with autologous stem cell support may be considered in patients with refractory disease. The efficacy of rituximab in type I cryoglobulinemia remains to be established (Nehme-Schuster et al., 2005). Pulsed intravenous steroids and plasma exchange are used in patients with severe systemic or renal manifestations (Provot et al., 2000). The evolution of renal disease in type I cryoglobulinemia is generally favorable, providing that remission of the underlying hematological disease is achieved with chemotherapy. Remission of nephrotic syndrome occurs in half of the cases, with parallel disappearance of glomerular monoclonal Ig deposits. Renal function improves or remains stable in a majority of patients, and less than 10% of patients progress to ESRD. Treatment is associated with significant mortality, with more than one third of patients dying from cardiovascular, infectious, and neoplastic complications. As in type II cryoglobulinemia, serum levels of monoclonal cryoglobulins are not predictive of prognosis (Provot et al., 2000).

**Key points**

- Renal disease is a frequent complication in both type II (composed of monoclonal IgM and polyclonal IgG) and type I (composed of a single monoclonal Ig) cryoglobulins.
- Type II cryoglobulinemia is usually associated with chronic hepatitis C infection, and type I cryoglobulinemia with lymphoproliferative disorders.
- Renal manifestations range from mild proteinuria with microscopic hematuria and moderate renal failure, to nephrotic syndrome, and nephritic syndrome with severe renal failure during flares of the disease. Severe hypertension is common and should be aggressively treated to reduce cardiovascular complications. Progression to end-stage renal disease is rare, providing appropriate therapy is initiated early.
- Extra-renal symptoms are dominated by cutaneous and articular symptoms, but cryoglobulinemic vasculitis may involve almost all organs, with severe peripheral nerve, lung, gastro-intestinal, and heart involvement during disease exacerbations.
- MPGN, associated or not with glomerular thrombi and renal vasculitis, is the usual pattern of glomerular lesions. Renal biopsy with careful immunohistochemical studies using specific anti-heavy and light chain conjugates is mandatory for the diagnosis.
- In hepatitis C-associated type II cryoglobulinemia, combined pegylated interferon, and ribavirin for at least 1 year is the treatment of choice in patients with moderate renal involvement. Patients with severe renal disease should be treated initially with standard interferon. Acute flares with severe renal or extra-renal manifestations should be treated with plasmapheresis and pulse corticosteroids, followed by monoclonal anti-CD20 antibody therapy, or oral cyclophosphamide for up to 6 months. In type I cryoglobulinemia, treatment of the underlying lymphoproliferative disorder is usually effective, associated with pulse steroids and plasmapheresis in the most severe forms.

## Acknowledgments

We are greatly indebted to our colleagues for clinical observations and kidney biopsies particularly Professor H. Nivet and Dr. M.C. Machet, CHU Tours France.

## References

Agnello, V., Chung, R.T., Kaplan, L.M. 1992. A role for hepatitis C virus infection in type II cryoglobulinemia. N. Engl. J. Med. 327, 1490–1495.

Alric, L., Plaisier, E., Thebault, S., et al. 2004. Influence of antiviral therapy in hepatitis C virus-associated cryoglobulinemic MPGN. Am. J. Kidney Dis. 43, 617–623.

Barton, J.C., Herrera, G.A., Galla, J.H., Bertoli, L.F., Work, J., Koopman, W.J. 1987. Acute cryoglobulinemic renal failure after intravenous infusion of gamma globulin. Am. J. Med. 82, 624–629.

Basse, G., Ribes, D., Kamar, N., et al. 2006. Rituximab therapy mixed cryoglobulinemia in seven renal transplant patients. Transplant. Proc. 38, 2308–2310.

Beaume, A., Brizard, A., Dreyfus, B., Preud'homme, J.L. 1994. High incidence of serum monoclonal Igs detected by a sensitive immunoblotting technique in B-cell chronic lymphocytic leukemia. Blood 84, 1216–1219.

Bengtsson, U., Larsson, O., Lindstedt, G., Svalander, C. 1975. Monoclonal IgG cryoglobulinemia with secondary development of glomerulonephritis and nephrotic syndrome. Q. J. Med. 44, 491–503.

Bridoux, F., Hugue, V., Coldefy, O., et al. 2002. Fibrillary glomerulonephritis and immunotactoid (microtubular) glomerulopathy are associated with distinct immunologic features. Kidney Int. 62, 1764–1775.

Brouet, J.C., Clauvel, J.P., Danon, F., Klein, M., Seligmann, M. 1974. Biologic and clinical significance of cryoglobulins. A report of 86 cases. Am. J. Med. 57, 775–788.

Bruchfeld, A., Lindahl, K., Stahle, L., Soderberg, M., Schvarcz, R. 2003. Interferon and ribavirin treatment in patients with hepatitis C-associated renal disease and renal insufficiency. Nephrol. Dial. Transplant. 18, 1573–1580.

Bryce, A.H., Dispenzieri, A., Kyle, R.A., et al. 2006a. Response to rituximab in patients with type II cryoglobulinemia. Clin. Lymphoma Myeloma 7, 140–144.

Bryce, A.H., Kyle, R.A., Dispenzieri, A., Gertz, M.A. 2006b. Natural history and therapy of 66 patients with mixed cryoglobulinemia. Am. J. Hematol. 81, 511–518.

Cacoub, P., Lidove, O., Maisonobe, T., et al. 2002. Interferon alfa and ribavirin treatment in patients with hepatitis C virus-related systemic vasculitis. Arthritis Rheum. 46, 3317–3326.

Cacoub, P., Renou, C., Kerr, G., et al. 2001. Influence of HLA-DR phenotype on the risk of hepatitis C virus-associated mixed cryoglobulinemia. Arthritis Rheum. 44, 2118–2124.

Cacoub, P., Saadoun, D., Limal, N., Sene, D., Lidove, O., Piette, C. 2005. Pegylated interferon alfa-2b and ribavirin treatment in patients with hepatitis C virus-related systemic vasculitis. Arthritis Rheum. 52, 911–915.

Campise, M., Tarantino, A. 1999. Glomerulonephritis in mixed cryoglobulinemia: what treatment? Nephrol. Dial. Transplant. 14, 281–283.

Carloss, H.W., Tavassoli, M. 1980. Acute renal failure from precipitation of cryoglobulins in a cool operating room. J. Am. Med. Assoc. 244, 1472–1473.

Casato, M., Agnello, V., Pucillo, L.P., et al. 1997. Predictors of long-term response to high-dose interferon therapy in type II cryoglobulinemia associated with hepatitis C virus infection. Blood 90, 3865–3873.

Casato, M., Pucillo, L.P., Leoni, M., et al. 1995. Granulocytopenia after combined therapy with interferon and angiotensin-converting enzyme inhibitors: evidence for a synergistic hematologic toxicity. Am. J. Med. 99, 386–391.

Chantry, D., Winearls, C.G., Maini, R.N., Feldmann, M. 1989. Mechanism of immune complex-mediated damage: induction of interleukin 1 by immune complexes and synergy with interferon-gamma and tumor necrosis factor-alpha. Eur. J. Immunol. 19, 189–192.

Cheng, J.T., Anderson, H.L., Markowitz, G.S., Appel, G.B., Pogue, V.A., D'Agati, V.D. 1999. Hepatitis C virus-associated glomerular disease in patients with human immunodeficiency virus coinfection. J. Am. Soc. Nephrol. 10, 1566–1574.

Cordonnier, D., Martin, H., Groslambert, P., et al. 1975. Mixed IgG–IgM cryoglobulinemia with glomerulonephritis. Immunochemical, fluorescent and ultrastructural study of kidney and in vitro cryoprecipitate. Am. J. Med. 59, 867–872.

Cordonnier, D., Vialtel, P., Renversez, J.C., et al. 1983. Renal diseases in 18 patients with mixed type II IgM–IgG cryoglobulinemia: monoclonal lymphoid infiltration (2 cases) and membranoproliferative glomerulonephritis (14 cases). Adv. Nephrol. Necker Hosp. 12, 177–204.

Curry, M.P., Golden-Mason, L., Doherty, D.G., et al. 2003. Expansion of innate CD5pos B cells expressing high levels of CD81 in hepatitis C virus infected liver. J. Hepatol. 38, 642–650.

D'Amico, G. 1995. Is type II mixed cryoglobulinemia an essential part of hepatitis C (HCV)-associated glomerulonephritis? Nephrol. Dial. Transplant. 10, 1279–1282.

D'Amico, G. 1998. Renal involvement in hepatitis C infection: cryoglobulinemic glomerulonephritis. Kidney Int. 54, 650–671.

D'Amico, G. 2003. Monoclonal cryoglobulinemia kidney. In: G. Touchard et al. Monoclonal Gammopathies and the Kidney. Kluwer Academic Publishers, Dordrecht, pp. 145–151.

Dammaco, F., Sansonno, D., Han, J.H., et al. 1994. Natural interferon-alfa versus its combination with 6-methylprednisolone in the therapy of type II mixed cryoglobulinemia: a long-term, randomized, controlled study. Blood 84, 3336–3343.

De Vita, S., Sacco, C., Sansonno, D., et al. 1997. Characterization of overt B-cell lymphomas in patients with hepatitis C virus infection. Blood 90, 776–782.

Dussol, B., Moal, V., Daniel, L., Pain, C., Berland, Y. 2001. Spontaneous remission of HCV-induced cryoglobulinaemic glomerulonephritis. Nephrol. Dial. Transplant. 16, 156–159.

Evans, T.W., Nicholls, A.J., Shortland, J.R., et al. 1984. Acute renal failure in essential mixed cryoglobulinemia: precipitation and reversal by plasma exchange. Clin. Nephrol. 21, 287–293.

Feldmann, G., Nischalke, H.D., Nattermann, J., et al. 2006. Induction of interleukin-6 by hepatitis C virus core protein in hepatitis C-associated mixed cryoglobulinemia and B-cell non-Hodgkin's lymphoma. Clin. Cancer Res. 12, 4491–4498.

Ferri, C., Marzo, E., Longombardo, G., et al. 1993. Interferon-alfa in mixed cryoglobulinemia patients: a randomized, crossover-controlled trial. Blood 81, 1132–1136.

Fornasieri, A., Armelloni, S., Bernasconi, P., et al. 1996. High binding of immunoglobulin M kappa rheumatoid factor from type II cryoglobulins to cellular fibronectin: a mechanism for induction of in situ immune complex glomerulonephritis? Am. J. Kidney Dis. 27, 476–483.

Fornasieri, A., D'Amico, G. 1996. Type II mixed cryoglobulinemia, hepatitis C virus infection, and glomerulonephritis. Nephrol. Dial. Transplant. 11 (Suppl. 4), 25–30.

Fornasieri, A., Li, M., Armelloni, S., et al. 1993. Glomerulonephritis induced by human IgMK–IgG cryoglobulins in mice. Lab. Invest. 69, 531–540.

Fornasieri, A., Tazzari, S., Li, M., et al. 1998. Electron microscopy study of genesis and dynamics of immunodeposition in IgMκ–IgG cryoglobulin-induced glomerulonephritis in mice. Am. J. Kidney Dis. 31, 435–442.

Galea, H.R., Bridoux, F., Aldigier, J.C., et al. 2002. Molecular study of an IgG1κ cryoglobulin yielding organized microtubular deposits and glomerulonephritis in the course of chronic lymphocytic leukemia. Clin. Exp. Immunol. 129, 113–118.

Garin, E.H., Fennell, R.S., Shulman, S.T., Iravani, A., Richard, G.A. 1980. Clinical significance of the presence of cryoglobulins in patients with glomerulopathies not associated with systemic diseases. Clin. Nephrol. 13, 5–11.

Gesualdo, L., Grandaliano, G., Ranieri, E., et al. 1997. Monocyte recruitment in cryoglobulinemic membranoproliferative glomerulonephritis: a pathogenetic role for monocyte chemotactic peptide-1. Kidney Int. 51, 155–163.

Gilboa, N., Durante, D., Guggenheim, S., et al. 1979. Immune deposit nephritis and single component cryoglobulinemia associated with chronic lymphocytic leukemia. Nephron. 24, 223–231.

Grcevska, L., Polenakovik, M., Polenakovik, B. 1998. Renal involvement in essential monoclonal (type 1) IgG cryoglobulinemia. Clin. Nephrol. 50, 200–202.

Haeney, M.R. 1976. Erroneous values for the total white cell count and ESR in patients with cryoglobulinemia. J. Clin. Pathol. 28, 894–897.

Hent, R., Bergkamp, F.J., Weening, J.J., van Dorp, W. 19997. Delayed onset of membranoproliferative glomerulonephritis in a patient with type I cryoglobulinemia. Nephrol. Dial. Transplant. 12, 2155–2158.

Herzenberg, A.M., Telford, J.J., De Luca, L.G., Holden, J.K., Magil, A.B. 1998. Thrombotic microangiopathy associated with cryoglobulin membranoproliferative glomerulonephritis and hepatitis C. Am. J. Kidney Dis. 31, 521–526.

Hiesse, C., Bastuji-Garin, S., Santelli, G., et al. 1989. Recurrent essential mixed cryoglobulinemia in renal allografts. Report of two cases and review of the literature. Am. J. Nephrol. 9, 150–154.

Itoh, J., Nose, M., Takahashi, S., et al. 1993. Induction of different types of glomerulonephritis by monoclonal antibodies derived from an MRL/lpr lupus mouse. Am. J. Pathol. 143, 1436–1443.

Ivanovski, M., Silvestri, F., Pozzato, G., et al. 1998. Somatic hypermutation, clonal diversity, and preferential expression of the VH 51p1/VL kv325 immunoglobulin gene combination in hepatitis C virus-associated immunocytomas. Blood 91, 2433–2442.

Johnson, R.J., Gretch, D.R., Couser, W.G., et al. 1994. Hepatitis C virus-associated glomerulonephritis. Effect of α-interferon therapy. Kidney Int. 46, 1700–1704.

Kallemuchikkal, U., Gorevic, P.D. 1999. Evaluation of cryoglobulins. Arch. Pathol. Lab. Med. 123, 119–124.

Kamar, N., Ribes, D., Izopet, J., Rostaing, L. 2006a. Treatment of hepatitis C virus infection (HCV) after renal transplantation: implications for HCV-positive patients awaiting a kidney transplant. Transplantation 82, 853–856.

Kamar, N., Rostaing, L., Alric, L. 2006b. Treatment of hepatitis C-virus related glomerulonephritis. Kidney Int. 69, 436–439.

Karras, A., Noel, L.H., Droz, D., et al. 2002. Renal involvement in monoclonal (type I) cryoglobulinemia: two cases associated with IgG3k cryoglobulin. Am. J. Kidney Dis. 40, 1091–1096.

Kikuchi, S., Pastore, Y., Fossati-Jimack, L., et al. 2002. A transgenic mouse model of autoimmune glomerulonephritis and necrotizing arteritis associated with cryoglobulinemia. J. Immunol. 169, 4644–4650.

Kuroki, A., Kuroda, Y., Kikuchi, S., et al. 2002. Level of galactosylation determines cryoglobulin activity of murine IgG3 monoclonal rheumatoid factor. Blood 99, 2922–2928.

Lamprecht, P., Lerin-Lozano, C., Merz, H., et al. 2003. Rituximab induces remission in refractory HCV associated cryoglobulinaemic vasculitis. Ann. Rheum. Dis. 62, 1230–1233.

Lemoine, R., Berney, T., Shibata, T., et al. 1992. Induction of "wire-loop" lesions by murine monoclonal IgG3 cryoglobulins. Kidney Int. 41, 65–72.

Lenzi, M., Frisoni, M., Mantovani, V., et al. 1998. Haplotype HLA-B8-DR3 confers susceptibility to hepatitis C virus-related mixed cryoglobulinemia. Blood 91, 2062–2066.

Libra, M., Mangano, K., Anzaldi, M., et al. 2006. Analysis of interleukin (IL)-1beta, IL-1 receptor antagonist, soluble IL-1 receptor type II and IL-1 accessory protein in

HCV-associated lymphoproliferative disorders. Oncol. Rep. 15, 1305–1308.

Lunel, F., Musset, L., Cacoub, P., et al. 1994. Cryoglobulinemia in liver diseases : role of hepatitis C virus and liver damage. Gastroenterology 106, 1291–1300.

Madore, F., Lazarus, J.M., Brady, H.R. 1996. Therapeutic plasma exchange in renal diseases. J. Am. Soc. Nephrol. 7, 367–386.

Mariette, X. 2001. Lymphomas complicating Sjögren's syndrome and hepatitis C virus infection may share a common pathogenesis: chronic stimulation of rheumatoid factors. Ann. Rheum. Dis. 60, 1007–1011.

Mazzaro, C., Zorat, F., Comar, C., et al. 2003. Interferon plus ribavirin in patients with hepatitis C virus positive mixed cryoglobulinemia resistant to interferon. J. Rheumatol. 30, 1775–1781.

Mazzaro, C., Zorat, F., Caizzi, M., et al. 2005. Treatment with peg-interferon alfa-2b and ribavirin of hepatitis C virus-associated mixed cryoglobulinemia: a pilot study. J. Hepatol. 42, 632–638.

Meltzer, M., Franklin, E.C., Elias, K., McCluskey, R.J., Cooper, W. 1966. Cryoglobulinemia. A clinical and laboratory study. II. Cryoglobulins with rheumatoid factor activity. Am. J. Med. 40, 837–856.

Misiani, R., Bellavita, P., Fenili, D., et al. 1992. Hepatitis C virus infection in patients with essential mixed cryoglobulinemia. Am. J. Med. 117, 573–577.

Misiani, R., Bellavita, P., Fenili, D., et al. 1994. Interferon alfa-2a therapy in cryoglobulinemia associated with hepatitis C virus. N. Engl. J. Med. 330, 751–756.

Monti, G., Galli, M., Invernizzi, F., et al. 1995. Cryoglobulinemias: a multi-centre study of the early clinical and laboratory manifestations of primary and secondary disease. GISC. Italian Group for the Study of Cryoglobulinemias. Q. J. Med. 88, 115–126.

Morales, E., Alegre, R., Herrero, J.C., Morales, J.M., Ortuno, T., Praga, M. 1997. Hepatitis-C-virus-associated cryoglobulinaemic membranoproliferative glomerulonephritis in patients infected by HIV. Nephrol. Dial. Transplant. 12, 1980–1984.

Morales, J.M. 2004. Hepatitis C virus infection and renal diseases after renal transplantation. Transplant. Proc. 36, 760–762.

Mougenot, B., Ronco, P. 1996. La biopsie rénale dans les dysprotéinémies et les dysglobulinémies. In: La biopsie rénale. Droz D, Lantz B, eds. Editions INSERM pp. 237–265.

Musset, L., Duarte, F., Gaillard, O., et al. 1994. Immunochemical characterization of monoclonal IgG containing mixed cryoglobulins. Clin. Immunol. Immunopathol. 70, 166–170.

Nehme-Schuster, H., Korganow, A.S., Pasquali, J.L., Martin, T. 2005. Rituximab inefficiency during type I cryoglobulinaemia. Rheumatol. (Oxford) 44, 410–411.

Odum, J., D'Costa, D., Freeth, M., Taylor, D., Smith, N., MacWhannell, A. 2001. Cryoglobulinaemic vasculitis caused by intravenous immunoglobulin treatment. Nephrol. Dial. Transplant. 16, 403–406.

Ogihara, T., Saruta, T., Saito, I., et al. 1979. Finger print deposits of the kidney in pure monoclonal IgG kappa cryoglobulinemia. Clin. Nephrol. 12, 186–190.

Okuda, K., Yokosuka, O., Otake, Y., et al. 1998. Cryoglobulinaemia among maintenance haemodialysis patients and its relation to hepatitis C infection. J. Gastroenterol. Hepatol. 13, 248–252.

Panka, D.J., Salant, D.J., Jacobson, B.A., Minto, A.W., Marshak-Rothstein, A. 1995. The effect of VH residues 6 and 23 on IgG3 cryoprecipitation and glomerular deposition. Eur. J. Immunol. 25, 279–284.

Papo, T., Musset, L., Bardin, T., et al. 1996. Cryocrystalglobulinaemia as a cause of systemic vasculopathy and widespread erosive arthropathy. Arthritis Rheum. 39, 335–340.

Pham, H.P., Feray, C., Samuel, D., et al. 1998. Effects of ribavirin on hepatitis C-associated nephrotic syndrome in four liver recipients. Kidney Int. 54, 1311–1319.

Pol, S., Vallet-Pichard, A., Fontaine, H., Lebray, P. 2002. HCV infection and hemodialysis. Semin. Nephrol. 22, 331–339.

Ponticelli, C., Imbasciati, E., Tarantino, A., Pietrogrande, M. 1977. Acute anuric glomerulonephritis in monoclonal cryoglobulinemia. Br. Med. J. 1, 948.

Preud'homme, J.L., Aucouturier, P., Touchard, G., et al. 1994. Monoclonal immunoglobulin deposition disease (Randall type). Relationship with structural abnormalities of immunoglobulin chains. Kidney Int. 46, 965–972.

Provot, F., Bridoux, F., Vanhille, P., et al. 2000. Spectrum of glomerular disease in type I cryoglobulinemia. J. Am. Soc. Nephrol. 11, 95A.

Quartuccio, L., Soardo, G., Romano, G., et al. 2006. Rituximab treatment for glomerulonephritis in HCV-associated mixed cryoglobulinaemia: efficacy and safety in the absence of steroids. Rheumatol. (Oxford) 45, 842–846.

Racanelli, V., Sansonno, D., Piccoli, C., D'Amore, F.P., Tucci, F.A., Dammacco, F. 2001. Molecular characterization of B cell clonal expansions in the liver of chronically hepatitis C virus-infected patients. J. Immunol. 67, 21–29.

Realdon, S., Pontisso, P., Adami, F., et al. 2001. High levels of soluble tumor necrosis factor superfamily receptors in patients with hepatitis C virus infection and lymphoproliferative disorders. J. Hepatol. 34, 723–729.

Rengers, J.U., Touchard, G., Decourt, C., Deret, S., Hartmut, M., Cogné, M. 2000. Heavy and light chain primary structures control IgG3 nephritogenicity in an experimental model for cryocrystalglobulinemia. Blood 65, 3467–3472.

Rocatello, D., Baldovino, S., Rossi, D., et al. 2004. Long-term effects of an anti-CD20 monoclonal antibody treatment of cryoglobulinaemic glomerulonephritis. Nephrol. Dial. Transplant. 19, 3054–3061.

Roccatello, D., Isidoro, C., Mazzucco, G., et al. 1993. Role of monocytes in cryoglobulinemia-associated nephritis. Kidney Int. 43, 1150–1155.

Roccatello, D., Morsica, G., Picciotto, G., et al. 1997. Impaired hepatosplenic elimination of circulating cryoglobulins in patients with essential mixed cryoglobulinemia and hepatitis C (HCV) virus infection. Clin. Exp. Immunol. 110, 9–14.

Rollino, C., Dieny, A., Le Marc'hadour, F., Renversez, J.C., Pinel, N., Cordonnier, D. 1992. Double monoclonal cryoglobulinemia, glomerulonephritis and lymphoma. Nephron. 62, 459–464.

Rossi, P., Bertani, T., Baio, P., et al. 2003. Hepatitis C virus-related cryoglobulinemic glomerulonephritis: long-term remission after antiviral therapy. Kidney Int. 63, 2236–2241.

Russo, G.E., Caramiello, M.S., Vitaliano, E., et al. 1996. Haemorheological changes in mixed cryoglobulinaemia during apheresis treatment. Transfus. Sci. 17, 499–503.

Saadoun, D., Aaron, L., Resche-Rigon, M., Pialoux, G., Piette, J.C., Cacoub, P. 2006a. GERMIVIC Study Group. Cryoglobulinaemia vasculitis in patients co-infected with HIV and hepatitis C virus. AIDS 20, 871–877.

Saadoun, D., Boyer, O., Trebeden-Negre, H., et al. 2004. Predominance of type 1 (Th1) cytokine production in the liver of patients with HCV-associated mixed cryoglobulinemia vasculitis. J. Hepatol. 41, 1031–1037.

Saadoun, D., Resche-Rigon, M., Thibault, V., Piette, J.C., Cacoub, P. 2006b. Antiviral therapy for hepatitis C virus-associated mixed cryoglobulinemia vasculitis. Arthritis Rheum. 54, 3696–3706.

Sansonno, D., Dammacco, F. 2005. Hepatitis C virus, cryoglobulinaemia, and vasculitis: immune complex relations. Lancet Infect. Dis. 5, 227–236.

Sansonno, D., De Re, V., Lautella, G., Tucci, F.A., Boiocchi, M., Dammaco, F. 2003. Monoclonal antibody treatment of mixed cryoglobulinemia resistant to interferon alfa with an anti-CD20. Blood 101, 3818–3826.

Sens, Y.A., Malafronte, P., Souza, J.F., et al. 2005. Cryoglobulinemia in kidney transplant recipients. Transplant. Proc. 37, 4273–4275.

Siami, G.A., Siami, F.S., Ferguson, P., Stone, W.J., Zborowski, M. 1995. Cryofiltration apheresis for treatment of cryoglobulinemia associated with hepatitis C. ASAIO J. 41, M315–M318.

Stefanutti, C., Di Giacomo, S., Mareri, M., et al. 2003. Immunoadsorption apheresis (Selesorb) in the treatment of chronic hepatitis C virus-related type 2 mixed cryoglobulinemia. Transfus. Apher. Sci. 28, 207–214.

Su, C.C., Chen, H.H., Yeh, J.C., Chen, S.C., Liu, C.C., Tzen, C.Y. 2002. Ultrastructural 'fingerprint' in cyoprecipitates and glomerular deposits: a clinicopathologic analysis of fingerprint deposits. Nephron. 90, 37–42.

Taneda, S., Segerer, S., Hudkins, K.L., et al. 2001. Cryoglobulinemic glomerulonephritis in thymic stromal lymphopoietin transgenic mice. Am. J. Pathol. 159, 2355–2369.

Tarantino, A., De Vecchi, A., Montagnino, G., et al. 1981. Renal disease in essential mixed cryoglobulinemia. Long-term follow-up of 44 patients. Q. J. Med. 50, 1–30.

Tarantino, A., Campise, M., Banfi, G., et al. 1995. Long-term predictors of survival in essential mixed cryoglobulinemic glomerulonephritis. Kidney Int. 47, 618–623.

Tarantino, A., Moroni, G., Banfi, G., Manzoni, C., Segagni, S., Ponticelli, C. 1994. Renal replacement therapy in cryoglobulinaemic nephritis. Nephrol. Dial. Transplant. 9, 1426–1430.

Tissot, J.D., Schifferli, J.A., Hochstrasser, D.F., et al. 1994. Two-dimensional polyacrylamide gel electrophoresis analysis of cryoglobulins and identification of an IgM-associated peptide. J. Immunol. Methods 173, 63–75.

Tomiyoshi, Y., Sakemi, T., Yoshikawa, Y., Shimokama, T., Watanabe, T. 1998. Fibrillar crystal structure in essential monoclonal IgM kappa cryoglobulinemia. Clin. Nephrol. 49, 325–327.

Touchard, G. 2003. Ultrastructural pattern and classification of renal monoclonal immunoglobulin deposits. In: G. Touchard et al. Monoclonal Gammopathies and the Kidney. Kluwer Academic Publishers, Dordrecht, pp. 95–117.

Touchard, G., Bauwens, M., Goujon, J.M., Aucouturier, P., Patte, D., Preud'homme, J.L. 1994. Glomerulonephritis with organized microtubular monoclonal immunoglobulin deposits. Adv. Nephrol. Necker Hosp. 23, 149–175.

Trejo, O., Ramos-Casals, M., Garcia-Carrasco, , et al. 2001. Cryoglobulinemia. Study of etiologic factors and clinical and immunologic features in 443 patients from a single center. Medicine 80, 252–262.

Trendelenburg, M., Fossati-Jimack, L., Cortes-Hernandez, H., et al. 2005. The role of complement in cryoglobulin-induced immune complex glomerulonephritis. J. Immunol. 175, 6909–6914.

Verroust, P., Mery, J.P., Morel-Maroger, L., et al. 1971. Glomerular lesions in monoclonal gammopathies and mixed essential cryoglobulinemias IgG–IgM. Adv. Nephrol. Necker Hosp. 1, 161–194.

Weiner, S.M., Thiel, J., Berg, T., et al. 2004. Impact of in vivo complement activation and cryoglobulins on graft outcome of HCV-infected renal allograft recipients. Clin. Transplant. 18, 7–13.

Zaja, F., De Vita, S., Mazzaro, C., et al. 2003. Efficacy and safety of rituximab in type II mixed cryoglobulinemia. Blood 101, 3827–3834.

Zignego, A.L., Ferri, C., Gianelli, F., et al. 2002. Prevalence of bcl-2 rearrangement in patients with hepatitis C virus-related mixed cryoglobulinemia with or without B-cell lymphomas. Ann. Intern. Med. 137, 571–580.

Zignego, A.L., Macchia, D., Monti, M., et al. 1992. Infection of peripheral mononuclear blood cells by hepatitis C virus. J. Hepatol. 15, 382–386.

Zuckerman, E., Keren, D., Slobodin, G., et al. 2000. Treatment of refractory, symptomatic, hepatitis C virus related mixed cryoglobulinemia with ribavirin and interferon alfa. J. Rheumatol. 27, 2172–2178.

# CHAPTER 13

# Henoch-Schönlein Purpura

Miguel A. Gonzalez-Gay*, Carlos Garcia-Porrua, Jose A. Miranda-Filloy

*Rheumatology Division, Hospital Xeral Calde, c/Dr. Ochoa s/n, 27004, Lugo, Spain*

## 1. Introduction and definition

Henoch-Schönlein purpura (HSP) is a systemic vasculitis characterized by purpuric skin lesions unrelated to any underlying coagulopathy, abdominal pain, and gastrointestinal bleeding, joint manifestations, and renal involvement (Gonzalez-Gay et al., 2005; Saulsbury, 2001). The classic clinical triad of HSP is palpable purpura, joint symptoms, and abdominal pain. However, renal involvement is the most serious complication. HSP is characterized histologically by infiltration of the small blood vessels with polymorphonuclear leukocytes and the presence of leukocytoclasia. Immunofluorescence staining usually reveals the presence of IgA-dominant immune deposits in the walls of the small vessels (capillaries, venules, or arterioles) and in the renal glomeruli (Giancomo and Tsai, 1977; Jennette et al., 1994).

## 2. Epidemiology, pathophysiology, and genetic influence

HSP is the most common vasculitis in children and an infrequent condition in adults. The annual incidence in children ranges between 125 and 180 cases per million (Gonzalez-Gay and Garcia-Porrua, 2001; Trapani et al., 2005), and in adults the annual incidence generally ranges between 8 and 14 cases per million (Gonzalez-Gay and Garcia-Porrua, 2001). The disease is observed predominantly in children between the ages of 2 and 10 years (Saulsbury, 1999) and boys slightly outnumber girls. Peaks in autumn, and winter have been described (Gonzalez-Gay and Garcia-Porrua, 2001). In at least 50% of cases in the pediatric age range an upper respiratory tract infection may precede the onset of the disease. Thus, β-hemolytic streptococcus group A is the organism most frequently isolated (Farley et al., 1989).

Mesangial deposition of nephritis-associated plasmin receptor, a group A streptococcal antigen, has been detected in the glomeruli of children with HSP and nephritis (Masuda et al., 2003). *Helicobacter pylori* has also been implicated in the gastrointestinal and the extra-gastrointestinal manifestations of the disease (Novak et al., 2003). Some drugs, especially penicillin, ampicillin, and erythromycin, paracetamol, and non-steroidal anti-inflammatory drugs have also been considered to precipitate HSP (Garcia-Porrua et al., 1999; Gonzalez-Gay et al., 2004). Exposure to cold, insect bites, food allergens, and pregnancy have also been considered as precipitants for HSP onset or recurrence in susceptible individuals.

HSP is a vasculitis due to IgA-mediated inflammation of small vessels. In HSP, IgA-dominant immune deposits are observed in the walls of the small vessels and in the renal glomeruli. There are two subclasses of IgA, IgA1 and IgA2. Increased IgA may be due to increased production or decreased clearance. Abnormalities involving the

---

*Corresponding author.
Tel.: +34-982-296188/296220; Fax: +34-982-242405
E-mail address: miguelaggay@hotmail.com

© 2008 Elsevier B.V. All rights reserved.
DOI: 10.1016/S1571-5078(07)07013-4

glycosylation of the hinge region of IgA1 may be responsible for the altered clearance and deposition of IgA, leading to clinical and histopathologic features of HSP (Saulsbury, 1999, 2001).

An unknown antigen may stimulate IgA production, activating pathways leading to necrotizing vasculitis, which could include IgA immune complexes and IgA isotype autoantibodies (rheumatoid factor, ANCA, and antiendothelial cell antibodies) (Tizard, 1999). The IgA immune complexes are capable of activating complement, leading to formation of chemotactic factors such as C5a, which in turn recruit polymorphonuclear leukocytes to the site of deposition. The release of lysosomal enzymes due to the ingestion of immune complexes by the polymorphonuclear leukocytes results in vessel damage. The membrane-attack complex (MAC) is also involved in endothelial damage; serum concentration of the C5b-9 complex has been found to be significantly elevated in many patients at the time of disease flare. The MAC has been found along with IgA and C3 on the vessel walls of the skin, and on the capillary walls and mesangium of glomeruli in patients with HSP nephritis (Kawana and Nishiyama, 1992). Hisano et al. (2005) confirmed the presence of complement activation through both the alternative and lectin pathways in patients with HSP nephritis. These authors demonstrated that complement activation is promoted in situ in the glomerulus. Complement activation through the lectin pathway may play a role in the development of advanced glomerular injury and prolonged urinary abnormalities (Hisano et al., 2005). Pro-inflammatory cytokines may also be involved in the pathogenesis of nephritis. In the acute phase of the disease serum TNF-α levels were significantly higher in proteinuric HSP than in patients without renal involvement. These observations suggest that increased TNF-α levels in the serum induce a series of functional and morphological changes in the glomerular cells in the acute phase and may be used as markers for disease activity of HSP in patients with severe renal involvement (Ha, 2005).

The familial occurrence of HSP in different episodes separated by several years supports a genetic predisposition (Lofters et al., 1973). Genetic susceptibility to HSP may be conferred by the interaction of a number of loci, including the major histocompatibility complex (MHC). HSP has been associated with HLA-DRB1*01 (Amoroso et al., 1997; Amoli et al., 2001). Both HSP nephritis and IgA nephropathy have been associated with deficiencies in the second and fourth components of complement (C2 and C4), and with deletion of C4 genes (Ault et al., 1990; Jin et al., 1996; Stefansson Thors et al., 2005). Recent genetic studies in the Lugo region of Northwestern Spain have highlighted the role of non-MHC genes in the susceptibility to (Martin et al., 2005) or the increased risk for the development of gastrointestinal manifestations, and susceptibility to nephritis or increased risk for nephrotic syndrome and/or renal insufficiency in HSP (Amoli et al., 2004; Rueda et al., 2006).

## 3. Clinical features

A rash of erythematous papules or, more rarely, a pruriginous and urticarial rash that is followed by palpable purpura are the most common initial manifestations. The distribution of the purpura is roughly symmetrical, where it typically appears on the lower extremities and then extends to the thighs and buttocks (Gonzalez-Gay et al., 2005) (Fig. 1). The rash does not blanch with pressure. The rash is intermittently progressive and is exacerbated by prolonged standing. In young children, facial involvement and subcutaneous edema of the hands, feet, scalp, and ears may be observed as an early manifestations of the disease (Dillon and Ansell, 1995).

Abdominal pain constitutes the second most frequent clinical manifestation of HSP, occurring in approximately 60–75% of patients (Calviño et al., 2001; Kraft et al., 1998). This is commonly periumbilical, frequently colicky, sometimes severe, and associated with nausea and vomiting. Bowel angina was described in 70% of children from Northwestern Spain (Calviño et al., 2001). The frequency of gastrointestinal bleeding in children with HSP from Northwestern Spain (Calviño et al., 2001) and Charlottesville, VA (Saulsbury, 1999) was 31 and 33%, respectively. In patients with hematemesis or melena, upper

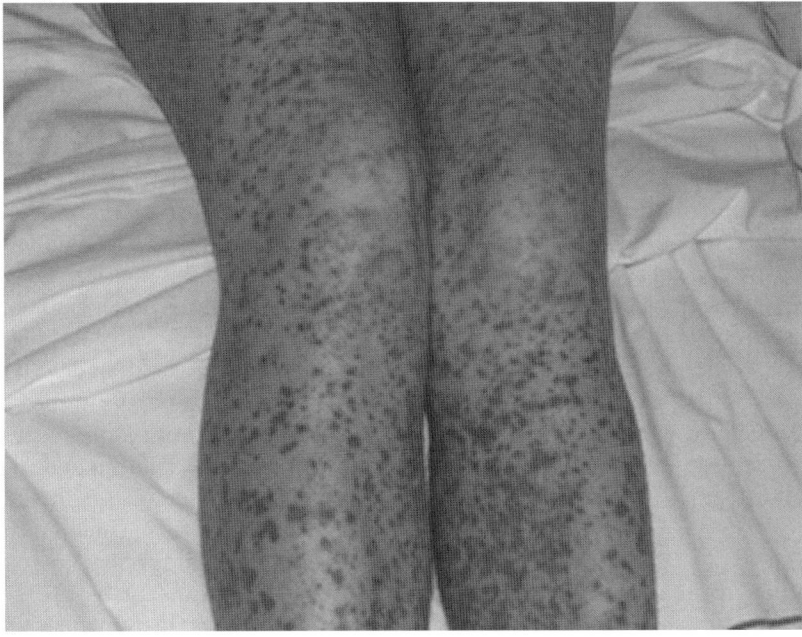

Figure 1. Typical palpable purpura in dependent areas of the lower extremities.

gastrointestinal endoscopy typically reveals redness, petechiae, and mucosal ulcerations and erosions, especially in the second part of duodenum (Kato et al., 1992). Acute intussusception may be observed in 1–5% of children (Robson and Leung, 1994). Perforation is rare. Severe cases may present with hemorrhagic shock, or duodenojejunal stenosis. Hepatosplenomegaly has also been reported in patients with HSP (Kraft et al., 1998).

Joint manifestations are generally transient, and permanent deformities are rarely seen. They may occur in more than 50% of cases and precede the development of palpable purpura by several days. Patients may present with arthralgia without objective signs of synovitis. Arthralgia or arthritis of the knees and ankles (Garcia-Porrua and Gonzalez-Gay, 1999) may be associated with edema. Upper extremity joints, such as elbows and wrists, may also be involved (Garcia-Porrua and Gonzalez-Gay, 1999; Calviño et al., 2001). Other manifestations such as malaise and low-grade fever are observed in half of the patients with HSP (Robson and Leung, 1994).

Renal involvement constitutes the most serious feature of HSP, and occurs in 20–80% of patients (Chang et al., 2005; Garcia-Porrua et al., 2002; Kaku et al., 1998), most commonly in older children and adults. It generally occurs within the first 3 months after clinical onset of the disease (Calviño et al., 2001); however, it may be observed later, generally in the setting of relapses of palpable purpura. In unselected patients with HSP from Northwestern Spain, the incidence of nephritis, manifested by the presence of hematuria with or without proteinuria, was almost similar in children (54%) (Calviño et al., 2001) and adults (around 50%) (Garcia-Porrua and Gonzalez-Gay, 1999). However, renal sequelae, characterized by the presence of nephrotic syndrome or renal insufficiency, were more commonly observed in adults (Garcia-Porrua et al., 2002). Renal disease, however, may be more common than is clinically apparent, as minor degrees of focal mesangial proliferation have been reported in the absence of urinary abnormalities (White, 1994).

Nephropathy in patients with HSP usually presents with macroscopic hematuria lasting a few days (although it may persist for several weeks), followed by microscopic hematuria that may persist for months or even years. Recurrences of macroscopic hematuria may be observed in association with new relapses of skin lesions. Recurrent hematuria, appearing substantially after other manifestations of HSP have resolved, is less common.

Persistent, severe proteinuria accompanied by microscopic hematuria suggests the presence of a mild or moderate glomerulonephritis, and may cause nephrotic syndrome (Niaudet and Habib, 1998). The most severe clinical presentation is that of mixed nephritic and nephrotic syndromes, with hematuria, hypertension, and renal insufficiency, severe proteinuria, and hypoalbuminemia. In patients with nephritis the glomerular filtration rate is moderately reduced early and is lower in patients with severe proteinuria and in those with more advanced morphological changes (Halling et al., 2005).

The long-term morbidity and mortality of HSP are almost completely due to renal involvement. A high frequency of chronic renal failure in children and adults was reported in selected patients, usually sent to referral centers because of kidney dysfunction (Counahan et al., 1977; Fogazzi et al., 1989; Lee et al., 1986; Roth et al., 1985). In contrast, unselected series of HSP (Blanco et al., 1997; Garcia-Porrua et al., 2002) reported a higher frequency of severe renal involvement in adults compared with children. In Northwestern Spain, complete recovery was observed in 65 of 73 children after 6 years' median follow-up. However, almost 40% of 31 adults had persistent hematuria and 3 of them (10%) had renal insufficiency that required hemodialysis (in two cases after 5 years' follow-up) (Garcia-Porrua et al., 2002).

According to a comprehensive review of 12 studies that included 1133 unselected children with HSP (Narchi, 2005), there is no need to undertake long-term periodical urinalysis testing in those cases whose urinalyses did not yield abnormalities within the first 6 months after the diagnosis of the disease.

In most cases, severity of disease at onset appears to predict outcome. The presence of both proteinuria and hematuria at the onset of the disease may be associated with progression to renal insufficiency (Kraft et al., 1998). In 69 unselected children from Northwestern Spain, the development of nephrotic syndrome within the first 3 months after the onset of the disease was the best predictor of renal sequelae during the extended follow-up (Calviño et al., 2001). In a long-term study on 78 children with HSP selected by the presence of nephritis, Goldstein et al. (1992) observed that 44% of those with nephritic syndrome, nephrotic syndrome, or both at the onset of the disease had long-term impairment of renal function. In another study on 114 children with HSP nephritis, a poor outcome at last follow-up was associated with the presence of nephrotic syndrome, decreased factor XIII activity, hypertension, and renal failure at the onset of the disease (Kawasaki et al., 2003).

Based on the morphological classification of HSP glomerulonephritis in the International Study for Kidney Disease in Children (ISKDC), in which renal biopsy findings may be graded from grade I to VI (Counahan et al., 1977), Goldstein et al. (1992) correlated the outcome with the severity of the lesion on the initial renal biopsy. In this study, 58% of the children in whom more than 50% of the glomeruli were affected by crescent formation (corresponding to grades IV and V of the ISKDC classification) had a poor outcome, compared with only 17% of children with less than 50% of glomeruli with crescents (grade III) or with no crescents (grades I and II). Other studies have confirmed that children with glomerular crescents have a high risk of developing end-stage renal disease. Kaku et al. (1998) examined the relationship between the progression of renal involvement in HSP children and various factors. They observed renal disease in 63 of their 194 children between 3 days and 17 months after onset of the disease. An increased risk of developing renal insufficiency was associated with age at onset of more than 7 years, the presence of persistent proteinuria, and decreased activity of coagulation factor XIII. The probability of renal involvement in HSP was influenced by the presence of severe abdominal symptoms, persistent purpura, and decreased activity of coagulation factor XIII. In a series of 28 unselected adults with HSP from Northwestern Spain who had prolonged follow-up, hematuria at the onset of the disease or renal manifestations during the course of the disease, frequently observed in patients with relapses of this vasculitis, were the main risk factors for the development of renal sequelae (Garcia-Porrua et al., 2001). In adults previously selected by the presence of nephritis, Fogazzi et al. (1989) observed a high rate of renal function deterioration (11 of their 16 adults with a mean follow-up of 90.5 months). Although patients who developed renal insufficiency had a higher percentage of crescents at the disease onset, no other clinical features at presentation allowed prediction of the course of the disease in this series (Fogazzi et al., 1989). However, a poor outcome and high frequency of renal insufficiency in adults has not been corroborated by more recent studies that included unselected adults, regardless of the presence or absence of nephritis, within the first months after the onset of the disease (Blanco et al., 1997; Garcia-Porrua and Gonzalez-Gay, 1999; Garcia-Porrua et al., 2002).

Extrarenal genitourinary problems sometimes precede the onset of purpuric lesions. Acute scrotal swelling due to inflammation and hemorrhage was observed in 32% of the series of boys reported by Chamberlain and Greenberg (1992).

Central nervous system involvement usually causes headache. Ostergaard and Storm (1991) reported headache in 31% of 26 cases. Other neurologic problems include behavioral changes due to encephalopathy, changes in mental status, apathy, hyperactivity, mood swings, and seizures (Fielding et al., 1998). Subdural hematomas, intracranial hemorrhage, intraparenchymal bleeding, and non-hemorrhagic vasculitis of the cerebral parenchyma have also been documented (Chiaretti et al., 1995). Peripheral nervous system lesions may appear as mononeuropathy involving the facial, ulnar, femoral, sciatic, or peroneal nerves. Polyneuropathy such as Guillain–Barré syndrome, polyradiculoneuropathy, and brachial plexopathy have also been reported (Robson and Leung, 1994).

Interstitial pulmonary disease is common but generally asymptomatic. Impairment of lung diffusion capacity has been reported in the majority of children during the active phase of the disease (Chaussain et al., 1992). A few cases of pulmonary hemorrhage leading in some cases to death, or interstitial pneumonia, have been described (Olson et al., 1992; Nadrous et al., 2004).

## 4. Laboratory findings

Elevation of acute phase reactants, moderate leukocytosis and thrombocytosis are common during the active phase of disease. Hemoglobin is generally normal unless severe gastrointestinal or pulmonary bleeding occurs.

A pathogenic role for IgA is supported by its presence in cryoprecipitates and the finding of an increased number of circulating IgA-secreting cells in patients with active HSP (Casanueva et al., 1983). IgA-dominant immune deposits can be observed in many cases of HSP (Hené et al., 1986), and its presence has been included in the definition adopted by the Consensus Conference on the Nomenclature of Systemic Vasculitides (Jennette et al., 1994). However, although IgA levels in the serum were reported to be increased in 50% of children in acute phases of disease (Dillon and Ansell, 1995), they were increased in only 5.6% of the tested patients in the American College of Rheumatology (ACR) study database (Mills et al., 1990). In Northwestern Spain, increased values of serum IgA were only observed in 10 of 27 (37%) adults and 20 of 37 (54%) children tested (Garcia-Porrua et al., 2002).

Serum C3, C4, and CH50, are generally normal; however, in a series of patients with HSP and IgA nephropathy the measurement of plasma anaphylatoxins C3a and C4a showed significant correlation with plasma creatinine and urea values (Abou-Ragheb et al., 1992). This suggests a role for plasma anaphylatoxin determination as a sensitive indicator of complement activation and a useful parameter in monitoring HSP activity. Complement activation through both the alternative and lectin pathways has been found in patients with HSP nephritis (Hisano et al., 2005).

Antineutrophil cytoplasmic antibodies (ANCA) have been identified in a wide variety of vasculitic disorders. Van den Wall Bake et al. (1987) suggested a role for ANCA in the pathogenesis of HSP, as they detected IgA ANCA in 55% of their patients. However, O'Donoghue et al. (1992) failed to confirm this, as none of 30 children with early HSP were ANCA-positive. Coppo et al. (1997) suggested that the conflicting reports on IgA ANCA might be due to atypical characteristics of the reaction in some ELISA assays. More recently, Ozaltin et al. (2004) undertook a prospective study to establish the role of IgA subclass ANCA in HSP. IgA ANCA in a cytoplasmic pattern was detected in a higher percentage of children diagnosed with HSP (82% of 35) in the acute phase compared to those in children with other vasculitides (38% of 13). In the resolution phase of HSP, IgA ANCA was negative in 88% of the HSP patients. No relationship was found between disease severity of HSP and IgA ANCA. According to these results (Ozaltin et al., 2004), IgA ANCA testing might be useful to confirm the diagnosis of HSP in children.

High concentrations of von Willebrand factor have been observed (De Mattia et al., 1995), suggesting its possible use as a marker of disease severity. Elevated levels of serum thrombomodulin, derived from damaged endothelium, have been reported in patients with HSP nephritis (Fujieda et al., 1998). The prothrombin time and partial thromboplastin time are typically normal. Reduced factor XIII activity has been found in patients with severe gastrointestinal complications (De Mattia et al., 1995).

## 5. Histology

### 5.1. Skin

Cutaneous lesions of patients with HSP generally involve capillaries, postcapillary venules, and arterioles ($<50\,\mu m$ in diameter) that are found mainly within the superficial papillary dermis (Gonzalez-Gay et al., 2005) (Fig. 2).

Biopsy samples of the cutaneous lesions in patients with HSP show a leukocytoclastic vasculitis of small blood vessels with infiltration of neutrophils within and around vessel walls, leukocytoclasia (degranulation and fragmentation of neutrophils leading to the production of nuclear "dust"), fibrinoid necrosis of the vessel walls, and necrosis, swelling and proliferation of the endothelial cells, and red cell extravasation. Eosinophils

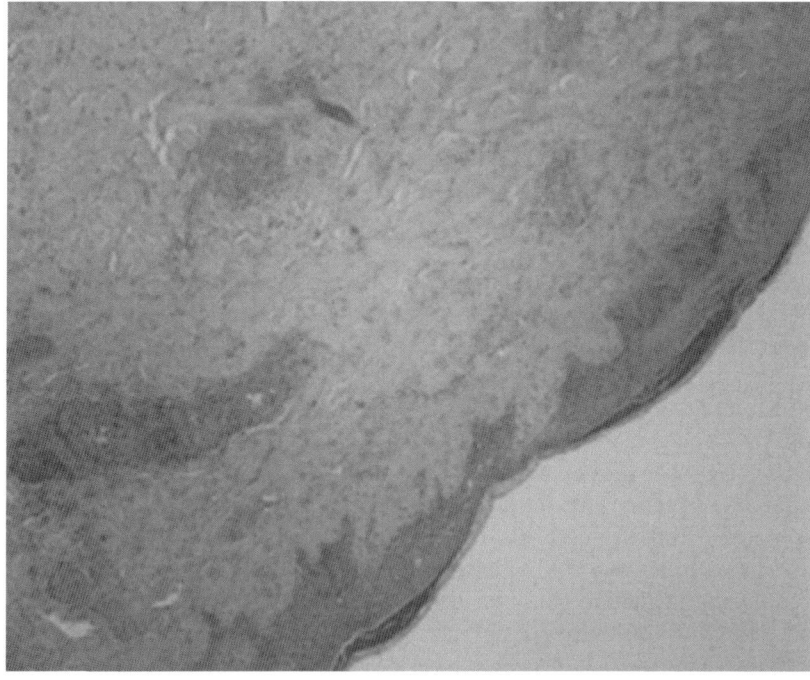

**Figure 2.** Skin biopsy of a patient with HSP showing dermal vascular neutrophilic inflammatory infiltration, leukocytoclasia, vessel wall fibrinoid necrosis, and erythrocyte extravasation (Hematoxylin and Eosin × 100).

may also be present. IgA, C3, and fibrin may deposit within the walls of the dermal vessels, as well as in the connective tissue of the upper dermis, in purpuric skin lesions. IgA deposits have also been found, albeit less often, in biopsy specimens of non-purpuric skin (Giancomo and Tsai, 1977).

## 5.2. Kidney

The early lesion is an endocapillary, focal or diffuse, proliferative glomerulonephritis involving both endothelial and mesangial cells (Robson and Leung, 1994). The glomeruli are infiltrated with polymorphonuclear and mononuclear cells. Proliferation of extracapillary cells, including epithelial cells and infiltrating macrophages, may result in variable degrees of crescent formation, due to adhesion of the proliferating cells to the glomerular tuft (Fig. 3). Interstitial inflammation and tubular changes, with atrophy and tubular casts, are common. Disease of renal arterioles occurs infrequently; therefore the brunt of the disease is borne by the glomeruli, which characteristically shows two basic lesions: mesangial proliferation (Fig. 4) and epithelial crescent formation (White, 1994).

Pathologic studies have reported a great variety in the extent and type of glomerular disease from one patient to another (Duquesnoy, 1991). Renal biopsy findings may be graded according to the classification of the ISKDC, which is based on the percentage of glomeruli showing crescents and segmental lesions (Counahan et al., 1977). Renal biopsies in HSP may disclose minimal to severe glomerulonephritis indistinguishable from IgA nephropathy. When renal involvement is minimal, glomeruli appear normal on light microscopy (Yoshikawa et al., 1981). Mesangial proliferation may be either diffuse or focal and segmental. Associated features include thrombosis and necrosis. Epithelial crescents vary in size from small segmental wedges, affecting one or two lobules, to circumferential forms. Large cellular crescents cause extensive obliteration of the urinary spaces. In the acute phase, crescents are predominantly cellular, but become fibrous after being infiltrated with collagen. Adherent glomerular capillaries become sclerotic. The extent of tubular atrophy,

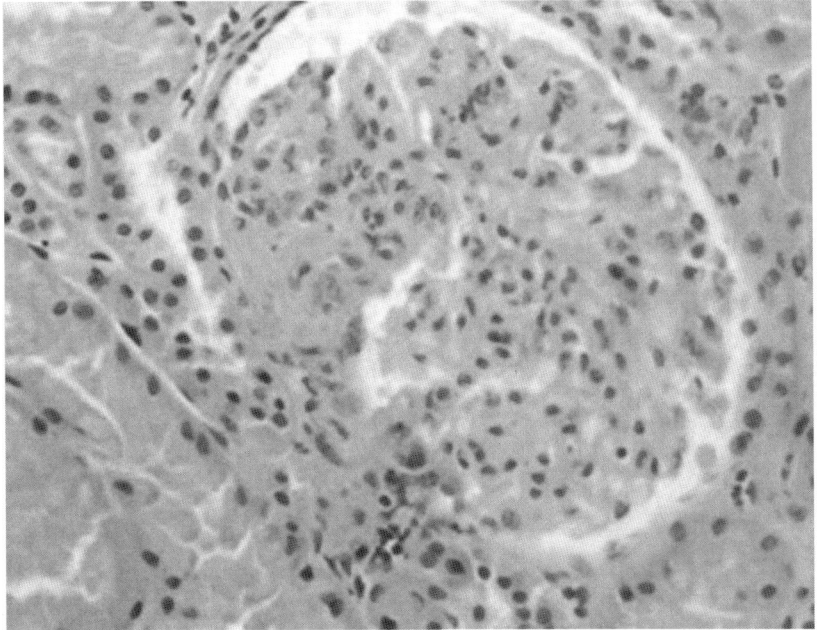

**Figure 3.** Kidney biopsy showing a glomerulus with crescentic formation (Hematoxylin and Eosin × 400).

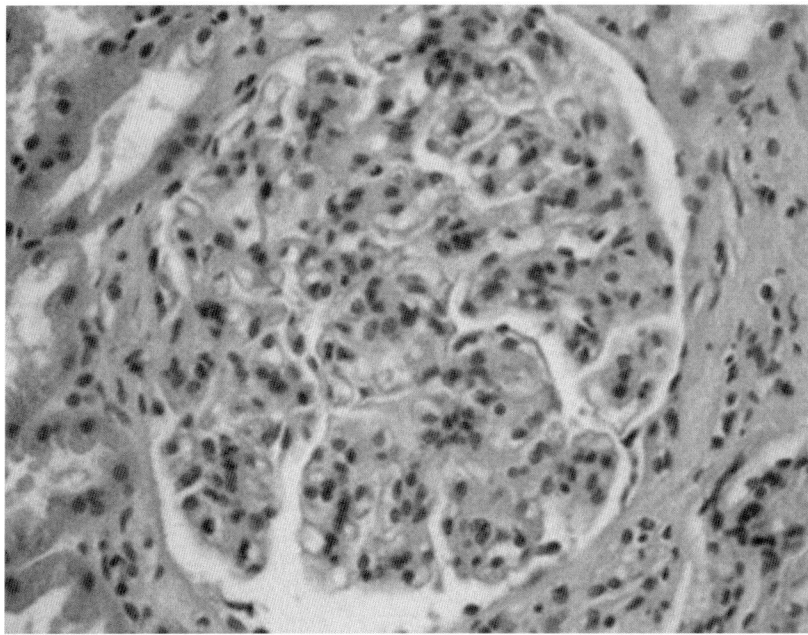

Figure 4. Renal biopsy showing a glomerulus with diffuse mesangial proliferative involvement (Hematoxylin and Eosin × 400).

and interstitial cellular infiltration and fibrosis is a measure of the severity of the glomerular lesions (White, 1994).

Immunofluorescence microscopy almost invariably reveals diffuse distribution of mesangial deposits of IgA (Fig. 5), which may be associated with minimal amounts of IgG, IgM, C3, and properdin. In patients with more severe disease, IgA deposits may extend into the capillary wall and fibrin may be observed (Heaton et al., 1977). Electron microscopy shows mesangial deposits, especially in the perimesangium. Smaller deposits are often observed in the subendothelial zone of the capillary walls adjacent to the mesangiocapillary junction, and to a minor extent in the subepithelial region (White, 1994).

## 6. Diagnosis

The clinical diagnosis of HSP is relatively straightforward in children presenting with the classic picture of palpable purpura, arthritis, and gastrointestinal manifestations or hematuria. An elevation of serum IgA may support the diagnosis. However, the histologic picture is characterized by a leukocytoclastic vasculitis that is indistinguishable from hypersensitivity vasculitis and other systemic vasculitides involving small blood vessels of the skin (Gonzalez-Gay et al., 2003, 2005). The diagnosis of HSP is supported by the presence of IgA immune deposits in small vessels of the skin and in the renal glomeruli.

Although IgA glomerulonephritis is typical of HSP, other conditions such as systemic lupus erythematosus, seronegative spondyloarthropathies, dermatologic diseases (psoriasis or dermatitis herpetiformis), neoplasms, and intestinal disorders (celiac disease or hepatic cirrhosis) have been associated with this type of glomerulonephritis. These conditions can be clearly differentiated from IgA glomerulonephritis in the context of HSP or idiopathic IgA nephropathy by clinical features (Galla, 1995).

As no gold standard test is available, classification criteria and definitions are frequently used to differentiate patients with HSP from other

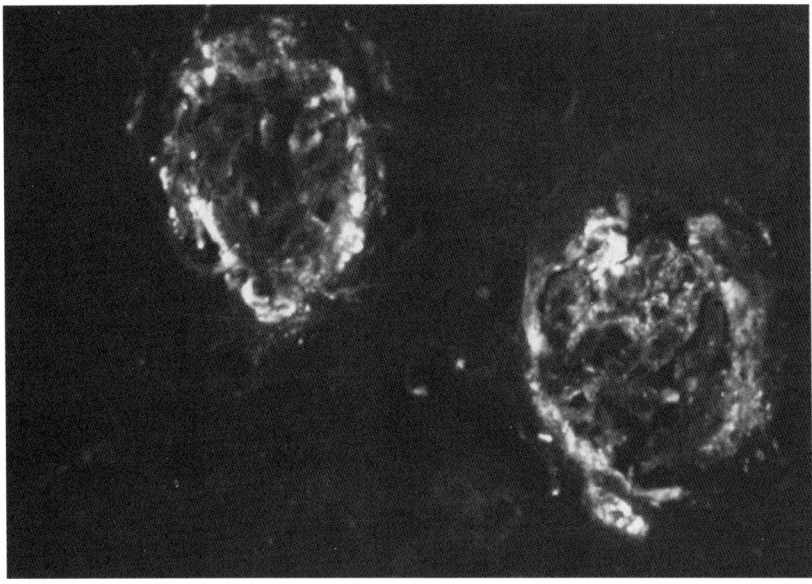

Figure 5. Renal biopsy from a patient with proliferative mesangial glomerulonephritis. Granular mesangial deposits of IgA. (IgA immunofluorescence × 400).

vasculitides. In 1990, the ACR proposed several classification criteria for HSP. These criteria were presented in two forms, a traditional format and a tree format. The traditional format included the following four features: palpable purpura defined by the presence of slightly raised skin lesions unrelated to thrombocytopenia; age at disease onset younger than 20 years old; bowel angina consisting of diffuse abdominal pain or bowel ischemia, with or without bloody diarrhea; and histologic changes showing granulocytes in the walls of arterioles or venules on skin biopsy (Mills et al., 1990). At least two of these four criteria were required for the diagnosis of HSP. However, both HSP and hypersensitivity (leukocytoclastic) vasculitis are small blood vessel vasculitides involving the skin and, due to this, they share many clinicopathologic features, such as the presence of leukocytoclasia and cutaneous involvement with palpable purpura.

To compare the characteristics of leukocytoclastic vasculitis and HSP as separate and definable clinical syndromes, Michel et al. (1992), using the ACR database, investigated which clinical criteria best differentiated between these two vasculitides. The authors reported that the presence of three or more criteria, from a list of six (palpable purpura, bowel angina, gastrointestinal bleeding, hematuria, age at onset less than 20 years, and no medications) yielded correct classification in 87.1% of HSP cases. Two or fewer criteria from the same list of six criteria yielded a percentage of cases correctly classified as leukocytoclastic vasculitis in 74.2% of cases.

In 1994, the Consensus Conference on the Nomenclature of Systemic Vasculitides highlighted the importance of the presence of IgA-dominant immune deposits for the definition of HSP (Jennette et al., 1994). However, the requirement for immunofluorescence data would have underestimated the number of HSP patients reported in previous series (Blanco et al., 1997).

## 7. Treatment

Treatment is largely supportive, including adequate hydration and regular monitoring. Nonsteroidal anti-inflammatory drugs should be avoided in patients with renal insufficiency. Corticosteroids are frequently used in patients with nephritis or gastrointestinal manifestations but without convincing evidence of benefit. They have been prescribed in patients with severe gastrointestinal manifestations, such as abdominal pain (Szer, 1996; Rosenblum and Winter, 1987; Blanco et al., 1997; Calviño et al., 2001; Garcia-Porrua and Gonzalez-Gay, 1999). Controversy still exists on the efficacy of these drugs to prevent the development of severe complications, in particular of nephritis (Gonzalez-Gay and Llorca, 2005).

A retrospective study based on 50 children with HSP, without nephritis at the time of diagnosis, showed a similar frequency of development of nephritis during follow-up regardless of corticosteroid therapy (Saulsbury, 1993). In contrast, in a series of 168 children with HSP without nephritis that were randomized to receive either prednisone (1 mg/kg per day orally for 2 weeks) or not, Mollica et al. (1992) observed that none of the group treated with prednisone ($n = 84$), but 10 from the control group ($n = 84$), developed nephropathy within 6 weeks. Also, Kaku et al. (1998) reported that corticosteroid treatment may reduce the risk of nephritis. According to these authors, patients with risk factors for renal involvement should be treated with corticosteroids to avoid renal impairment. However, in a more recent randomized, placebo-controlled study in 40 children with HSP, aimed at assessing whether early corticosteroid administration within 7 days of disease onset could reduce the rate of renal or gastrointestinal complications, Huber et al. (2004) found that early prednisone therapy did not reduce the risk of renal involvement at 1 year, or the risk of acute gastrointestinal complications.

Patients with severe nephritis have been treated in various ways, including corticosteroids (oral or pulse therapy) alone or in combination with immunosuppressive agents such as cyclophosphamide, azathioprine, chlorambucil, or cyclosporine. Other approached include: plasmapheresis; high-dose intravenous immunoglobulin (IVIG) therapy; danazol; and fish oil (Kawasaki et al., 2004a, b; Szer, 1996; Shin et al., 2005a, b; Tarshish et al., 2004; White, 1994). In most cases the absence of randomized placebo-controlled studies means it is difficult to draw strong conclusions. Based on a series of 20 patients with HSP nephritis, Shin et al. (2005b) suggested that combination therapy with azathioprine and corticosteroids might be beneficial in improving histopathological features and the clinical course of HSP patients with severe nephritis. Niaudet and Habib (1998) evaluated the efficacy of pulsed methylprednisolone therapy on the outcome of nephropathy in 38 children with severe forms of HSP. All their patients were treated with high-dose methylprednisolone for 3 days followed by oral prednisone for 3 months. Based on clinical symptoms and histopathological changes observed after a mean follow-up of 67 months, these authors observed that pulsed methylprednisolone therapy should be limited to HSP patients with nephritis who are at risk of progressive renal disease, especially those with nephrotic syndrome or crescentic glomerulonephritis. They considered this therapy useful when it was started early in the disease, before crescents became fibrosed.

The prognosis is generally poor if patients with HSP present with rapidly progressive glomerulonephritis. Tarshish et al. (2004) found no differences in outcome in 56 patients with histopathologically severe HSP nephritis randomized to receive supportive therapy with or without cyclophosphamide for 42 days. However, in an uncontrolled study of 12 children with HSP and biopsy-proven crescentic glomerulonephritis, Oner et al. (1995) suggested that a combination of methylprednisolone for 3 days (30 mg/kg/day) followed by oral prednisone at 45 mg/m$^2$/day tapered over 2 months, oral cyclophosphamide at 2 mg/kg/day for 2 months, and dipyridamole at 5 mg/kg/day for 6 months, may be effective in normalizing glomerular filtration. Further results from a series of 14 children with 7.5 years mean follow-up supported the use of intensive combination therapy (prednisolone, cyclophosphamide, heparin/warfarin, and dipyridamole) in children with severe nephritis and crescent formation (Iijima et al., 1998). More recently, Kawasaki et al. (2004b) assessed results from a series of 37 patients with HSP who had been diagnosed with glomerulonephritis of at least grade IVb. Twenty were treated with methylprednisolone and urokinase pulse therapy (group A), and the remaining

17 (group B) were treated with methylprednisolone and urokinase pulse therapy combined with cyclophosphamide. After 6 months of treatment, the mean urinary protein excretion in the group treated with methylprednisolone and urokinase pulse therapy combined with cyclophosphamide was significantly decreased compared with the other group. Also, at the second biopsy, the chronicity index was lower in those from Group B. These observations support the use of combined therapy with cyclophosphamide and methylprednisolone in HSP patients with severe nephritis.

Beneficial effects of cyclosporine in HSP children with nephrotic syndrome have been described (Shin et al., 2005a). IVIG therapy may also be considered in the treatment of patients with autoimmune diseases resistant to conventional therapy. Patients with nephrotic syndrome seem to be good candidates for this treatment. Rostoker et al. (1994, 1995) reported that both low- and high-dose IVIG may be effective in treating either moderate or severe nephritis in HSP and IgA nephropathy. However, as nephrotoxicity may occur following IVIG, alternative therapies should be considered in elderly patients or in those with renal insufficiency (Gonzalez-Gay, 2004).

Treatment with plasma exchange in combination with corticosteroids, anticoagulants, and immunosuppressive drugs has been used in children with crescentic glomerulonephritis related to HSP (Jardim et al., 1992). However, despite this combined therapy, progression to end-stage renal failure has been reported in 50% of cases. The interval between the disease onset and the beginning of therapy seemed to be an important prognostic factor. In a retrospective study of plasma exchange in children with rapidly progressive nephritis or cerebral vasculitis associated with HSP, Gianviti et al. (1996) assessed 17 patients. Fourteen had severe glomerulonephritis (30–100% of glomeruli with crescents) or were dialysis-dependent, and three had cerebral vasculitis. Recovery was observed in the three children with cerebral vasculitis. The time of onset of therapy was a determinant of outcome in those with severe nephritis, as all nine with renal vasculitis who started plasma exchange (combined with corticosteroids, cyclophosphamide, or azathioprine) within 1 month of disease onset had significant improvement in renal function. In contrast, five of six children with HSP nephritis treated later in the course of the disease developed end-stage renal failure. No relapses of the disease were observed after treatment with plasma exchange. These results support the use of plasma exchange, together with immunosuppressive therapy, in cases of severe renal or extrarenal HSP.

Renal transplantation may be considered for the small group of patients who progress to end-stage renal insufficiency. Recurrences have been described and they appear to be associated with living related donor transplants (Hasegawa et al., 1989; Nast et al., 1987). When the graft function is seriously impaired by recurrent disease, other systemic manifestations, including purpura, tend to recur.

## 8. Clinical course, and outcome

Most patients with HSP have a self-limiting disease (Garcia-Porrua et al., 2002). In children from Northwestern Spain, Calviño et al. (2001) reported relapses in 15% of children who had a follow-up of at least 12 months. In adults from the same region, relapses occurred in 21% of patients (Gonzalez-Gay and García-Porrua, 1999).

The long-term morbidity and mortality of HSP are predominantly attributable to renal involvement. HSP has been reported to account for between 5 and 15% of children developing end-stage renal failure (Bunchman et al., 1988; Meadow, 1978). Bunchman et al. (1988) observed that failure to reach a creatinine clearance higher than $70 \, ml/min/1.73 \, m^2$ by 3 years after the onset of HSP predicted progression to end-stage renal failure. In an unselected series of 141 children with HSP, Koskimies et al. (1981) reported persistence of abnormal urinary sediment for at least 1 month in 28% of their patients. After a mean follow-up of 7.2 years, only one child progressed to end-stage renal failure (0.7%) and two (1.4%) developed chronic glomerular disease. In another unselected series of 270 children, Stewart et al. (1988) observed initial evidence of renal involvement in 55 (20%). Re-examination at an average of 8.3

years after the onset of the disease yielded a good overall prognosis, with mortality less than 1% overall and long-term morbidity of only 1.1% (Stewart et al., 1988). Unlike adults, none of 73 unselected children with HSP from Northwestern Spain who had a follow-up of at least 1 year developed end-stage renal failure (Garcia-Porrua et al., 2002). All these studies (Garcia-Porrua et al., 2002; Koskimies et al., 1981; Stewart et al., 1988) support a better prognosis for HSP nephritis in children than the majority of published estimates. In a more extensive follow-up of 23.4 years in 78 of 99 children with HSP nephritis (Goldstein et al., 1992), the authors concluded that the severity of the clinical presentation and the initial findings on the renal biopsy correlated well with the outcome. In 16 of 44 girls, subsequent pregnancies were complicated by proteinuria and hypertension, even in the absence of active renal disease. Because of that, Goldstein et al. (1992) suggested that HSP nephritis in children should be followed long-term, especially during pregnancy.

## 9. Conclusions

HSP is an IgA-mediated disease involving small blood vessels. It is the most common vasculitis in children and an infrequent condition in adults. Genetic and environmental factors have been implicated in its pathogenesis. It may be preceded by an infection, generally in the upper respiratory tract. Cutaneous, joint, gastrointestinal, and renal manifestations are commonly observed. In general, it is a benign and self-limited condition, particularly in children. However, a small percentage of cases, generally adults, may progress to end-stage renal failure. Due to this, close follow-up with repeated urinalysis is recommended in the patients who develop renal manifestations during the first 6 months after the onset of the disease. Pharmacological treatments are controversial and so far no management of HSP has been confirmed to be effective in patients with renal disease or severe gastrointestinal complications. Reports on prophylactic corticosteroid therapy to prevent renal disease have yielded contradictory results.

---

**Key points**

- HSP is the most common vasculitis in children and uncommon in adults.
- It involves small-sized blood vessels.
- IgA immune-deposits are commonly observed in skin and kidney biopsies.
- It may be preceded by infections, in particular from the upper respiratory tract.
- Skin, joints, gastrointestinal tract, and kidneys are the organs most commonly involved.
- In most children HSP is a benign and self-limited disease.
- Progression to renal insufficiency may occur in a small percentage of cases, mainly in adults.
- Repeated urinalysis is recommended in those cases presenting with renal manifestations.
- Optimal management of renal involvement and gastrointestinal complications of HSP remains to be determined.
- Reports on prophylactic corticosteroid therapy to prevent renal disease have yielded contradictory results.

---

## References

Abou-Ragheb, H.H.A., Williams, A.J., Brown, C.B., et al. 1992. Plasma levels of the anaphylatoxins C3a and C4a in patients with IgA nephropathy/Henoch-Schönlein nephritis. Nephron. 62, 22.

Amoli, M.M., Calviño, M.C., Garcia-Porrua, C., et al. 2004. Interleukin 1beta gene polymorphism association with severe renal manifestations and renal sequelae in Henoch-Schönlein purpura. J. Rheumatol. 31, 295.

Amoli, M.M., Thomson, W., Hajeer, A.H., et al. 2001. HLA-DRB1*01 association with Henoch-Schönlein purpura in patients from northwest Spain. J. Rheumatol. 28, 1266.

Amoroso, A., Berrino, M., Canale, L., et al. 1997. Immunogenetics of Henoch-Schönlein disease. Eur. J. Immunogenet. 24, 323.

Ault, B.H., Stapleton, F.B., Rivas, M.L., et al. 1990. Association of Henoch-Schönlein purpura glomerulonephritis with C4B deficiency. J. Pediatr. 117, 753.

Blanco, R., Martinez-Taboada, V.M., Rodriguez-Valverde, et al. 1997. Henoch-Schönlein purpura in the adulthood and in the childhood: two different expressions of the same syndrome. Arthritis Rheum. 40, 859.

Bunchman, T.E., Mauer, S.M., Sibley, R.K., et al. 1988. Anaphylactoid purpura: characteristics of 16 patients who progressed to renal failure. Pediatr. Nephrol. 2, 393.

Calviño, M.C., Llorca, J., Garcia-Porrua, C., et al. 2001. Henoch-Schönlein purpura in children from northwestern Spain: a 20-year epidemiologic and clinical study. Medicine (Baltimore) 80, 279.

Casanueva, B., Rodriguez-Valverde, V., Merino, J., et al. 1983. Increased IgA-producing cells in the blood of patients with active Henoch-Schönlein purpura. Arthritis Rheum. 26, 854.

Chamberlain, R.S., Greenberg, L.W. 1992. Scrotal involvement in Henoch-Schönlein purpura. A case report and review of literature. Pediatr. Emerg. Care. 8, 213.

Chang, W.L., Yang, Y.H., Wang, L.C., et al. 2005. Renal manifestations in Henoch-Schönlein purpura: a 10-year clinical study. Pediatr. Nephrol. 20, 1269.

Chaussain, M., De Boissieu, D., Kalifa, G., et al. 1992. Impairment of lung diffusion capacity in Henoch-Schönlein purpura. J. Pediatr. 121, 12.

Chiaretti, A., Scommegna, S., Castorina, M., et al. 1995. Intracranial hemorrhage in Henoch-Schönlein syndrome. Pediatr. Med. Chir. 17, 177.

Coppo, R., Cirina, P., Amore, A., et al. 1997. Properties of circulating IgA molecules in Henoch-Schönlein purpura nephritis with focus on neutrophil cytoplasmic antigen IgA binding (IgA-ANCA): new insight into a debated issue. Italian Group of Renal Immunopathology Collaborative Study on Henoch-Schönlein purpura in adults and children. Nephrol. Dial. Transplant. 12, 2269.

Counahan, R., Winterborn, M.H., White, R.H.R., et al. 1977. Prognosis of Henoch-Schönlein purpura in children. BMJ 2, 11.

De Mattia, D., Penza, R., Giordano, P., et al. 1995. Von Willebrand factor and factor XIII in children with Henoch-Schönlein purpura. Pediatr. Nephrol. 9, 603.

Dillon, M.J., Ansell, B.M. 1995. Vasculitis in children and adolescents Rheum. Dis. Clin. North Am. 21, 1115.

Duquesnoy, B. 1991. Henoch-Schönlein purpura. Bailliers Clin. Rheumatol. 5, 253.

Farley, T.A., Gillespi, S., Rasoulpour, M., et al. 1989. Epidemiology of a cluster of Henoch-Schönlein purpura. Am. J. Dis. Child. 143, 798.

Fielding, R.E., Hawkins, C.P., Hand, M.F., et al. 1998. Seizure complicating Henoch-Schönlein purpura. Nephrol. Dial. Transplant. 13, 761.

Fogazzi, G.B., Pasquali, S., Moriggi, M., et al. 1989. Long-term outcome of Schönlein-Henoch nephritis in the adult. Clin. Nephrol. 31, 60.

Fujieda, M., Oishi, N., Naruse, K., et al. 1998. Soluble thrombomodulin and antibodies to bovine glomerular endothelial cells in patients with Henoch-Schönlein purpura. Arch. Dis. Child. 78, 240.

Galla, J.H. 1995. IgA nephropathy. Kidney Int. 47, 377.

Garcia-Porrua, C., Calviño, M.C., Llorca, et al. 2002. Henoch-Schönlein purpura in children and adults: clinical differences in a defined population. Semin. Arthritis Rheum. 32, 149.

Garcia-Porrua, C., Gonzalez-Gay, M.A. 1999. Comparative clinical and epidemiologic study of hypersensitivity vasculitis versus Henoch-Schönlein purpura in adults. Semin. Arthritis Rheum. 28, 404.

Garcia-Porrua, C., Gonzalez-Gay, M.A., Lopez-Lazaro, L. 1999. Drug-associated cutaneous vasculitis in adulthood. Clinical and epidemiological associations in a defined population of Northwestern Spain. J. Rheumatol. 26, 1942.

Garcia-Porrua, C., Gonzalez-Louzao, C., Llorca, J., et al. 2001. Predictive factors for renal sequelae in adults with Henoch-Schönlein purpura. J. Rheumatol. 28, 1019.

Giancomo, J., Tsai, C.C. 1977. Dermal and glomerular deposition of IgA in anaphylactoid purpura. Am. J. Dis. Child. 131, 981.

Gianviti, A., Trompeter, R.S., Barratt, T.M., et al. 1996. Retrospective study of plasma exchange in patients with idiopathic rapidly progressive glomerulonephritis and vasculitis. Arch. Dis. Child. 75, 186.

Goldstein, A.R., White, R.H., Akuse, R., et al. 1992. Long-term follow-up of childhood Henoch-Schönlein nephritis. Lancet 339, 280.

Gonzalez-Gay, B. 2004. The pros and cons of intravenous immunoglobulin treatment in autoimmune nephropathy. Semin. Arthritis Rheum. 34, 573.

Gonzalez-Gay, M.A., Calviño, M.C., Vazquez-Lopez, M.E., et al. 2004. Implications of upper respiratory tract infections and drugs in the clinical spectrum of Henoch-Schönlein purpura in children. Clin. Exp. Rheumatol. 22, 781.

Gonzalez-Gay, M.A., García-Porrua, C. 1999. Systemic vasculitis in adults in Northwestern Spain, 1988–1997: clinical and epidemiologic aspects. Medicine (Baltimore) 78, 292.

Gonzalez-Gay, M.A., Garcia-Porrua, C. 2001. Epidemiology of the vasculitides. Rheum. Dis. Clin. North Am. 27, 729.

Gonzalez-Gay, M.A., Garcia-Porrua, C., Pujol, R.M. 2005. A clinical approach to cutaneous vasculitis. Curr. Opin. Rheumatol. 17, 56.

Gonzalez-Gay, M.A., Garcia-Porrua, C., Salvarani, C., et al. 2003. Cutaneous vasculitis: a diagnostic approach. Clin. Exp. Rheumatol. 21 (6 Suppl. 32), S85.

Gonzalez-Gay, M.A., Llorca, J. 2005. Controversies on the use of corticosteroid therapy in children with Henoch-Schönlein purpura. Semin. Arthritis Rheum. 35, 135.

Ha, T.S. 2005. The role of tumor necrosis factor-alpha in Henoch-Schönlein purpura. Pediatr. Nephrol. 20, 149.

Halling, S.F., Soderberg, M.P., Berg, U.B. 2005. Henoch Schönlein nephritis: clinical findings related to renal function and morphology. Pediatr. Nephrol. 20, 46.

Hasegawa, A., Kawamura, T., Ito, H., et al. 1989. Fate of renal grafts with recurrent Henoch-Schönlein purpura nephritis in children. Transplant. Proc. 21, 2130.

Heaton, J.M., Turner, D.R., Cameron, J.S. 1977. Localization of glomerular deposits in Henoch-Schönlein nephritis. Histopathology 1, 93.

Hené, R.J., Velthuis, P., van de Wiel, A., et al. 1986. The relevance of IgA deposits in vessel walls of clinically normal skin. Arch. Intern. Med. 146, 745.

Hisano, S., Matsushita, M., Fujita, T., et al. 2005. Activation of the lectin complement pathway in Henoch-Schönlein purpura nephritis. Am. J. Kidney Dis. 45, 295.

Huber, A.M., King, J., McLaine, P., et al. 2004. A randomized, placebo-controlled trial of prednisone in early Henoch Schönlein Purpura. BMC Med. 2, 7.

Iijima, K., Ito-Kariya, S., Nakamura, H., et al. 1998. Multiple combined therapy for severe Henoch-Schönlein nephritis in children. Pediatr. Nephrol. 12, 244.

Jardim, H.M., Leake, J., Risdon, R.A., et al. 1992. Crescentic glomerulonephritis in children. Pediatr. Nephrol. 6, 231.

Jennette, J.C., Falk, R.J., Andrassy, K., et al. 1994. Nomenclature of systemic vasculitides: proposal of an international consensus conference. Arthritis Rheum. 37, 187.

Jin, D.K., Kohsaka, T., Koo, J.W., et al. 1996. Complement 4 locus II gene deletion and DQA1*0301 gene: genetic risk factors for IgA nephropathy and Henoch-Schönlein nephritis. Nephron. 73, 390.

Kaku, Y., Nohara, K., Honda, S. 1998. Renal involvement in Henoch-Schönlein purpura: a multivariate analysis of prognostic factors. Kidney Int. 53, 1755.

Kato, S., Shibuya, H., Naganuma, H., et al. 1992. Gastrointestinal endoscopy in Henoch-Schönlein purpura. Eur. J. Pediatr. 151, 482.

Kawana, S., Nishiyama, S. 1992. Serum SC5b-9 (terminal complement complex) level, a sensitive indicator of disease activity in patients with Henoch-Schönlein purpura. Dermatology 184, 171.

Kawasaki, Y., Suzuki, J., Murai, M., et al. 2004a. Plasmapheresis therapy for rapidly progressive Henoch-Schönlein nephritis. Pediatr. Nephrol. 19, 920.

Kawasaki, Y., Suzuki, J., Sakai, N., et al. 2003. Clinical and pathological features of children with Henoch-Schönlein purpura nephritis: risk factors associated with poor prognosis. Clin. Nephrol. 60, 153.

Kawasaki, Y., Suzuki, J., Suzuki, H. 2004b. Efficacy of methylprednisolone and urokinase pulse therapy combined with or without cyclophosphamide in severe Henoch-Schönlein nephritis: a clinical and histopathological study. Nephrol. Dial. Transplant. 19, 858.

Koskimies, O., Mir, S., Rapola, J., et al. 1981. Henoch-Schönlein nephritis: long-term prognosis of unselected patients. Arch. Dis. Child. 56, 482.

Kraft, D.A., McKee, D., Scott, C. 1998. Henoch-Schönlein purpura: a review. Am. Fam. Physician. 58, 405.

Lee, H.S., Koh, H.I., Kim, M.J., et al. 1986. Henoch-Schönlein nephritis in adults: a clinical and morphological study. Clin. Nephrol. 26, 125.

Lofters, W.S., Pineo, G.F., Luke, K.H., et al. 1973. Henoch-Schönlein purpura occurring in three members of a family. Can. Med. Assoc. J. 109, 46.

Martin, J., Paco, L., Ruiz, M.P., et al. 2005. Inducible nitric oxide synthase polymorphism is associated with susceptibility to Henoch-Schönlein purpura in Northwestern Spain. J. Rheumatol. 32, 1081.

Masuda, M., Nakanishi, K., Yoshizawa, N., et al. 2003. Group A streptococcal antigen in the glomeruli of children with Henoch-Schönlein nephritis. Am. J. Kidney Dis. 41, 366.

Meadow, S.R. 1978. The prognosis of Henoch-Schönlein nephritis. Clin. Nephrol. 9, 87.

Michel, B.A., Hunder, G.G., Bloch, D.A., et al. 1992. Hypersensitivity vasculitis and Henoch-Schönlein purpura: a comparison between the 2 disorders. J. Rheumatol. 19, 721.

Mills, J.A., Michel, B.A., Bloch, D.A., et al. 1990. The ACR 1990 criteria for the classification of Henoch-Schönlein purpura. Arthritis Rheum. 33, 1114.

Mollica, F., Li Volti, S., Garozzo, R., et al. 1992. Effectiveness of early prednisone treatment in preventing the development of nephropathy in anaphylactoid purpura. Eur. J. Pediatr. 15, 140.

Nadrous, H.F., Yu, A.C., Specks, U., et al. 2004. Pulmonary involvement in Henoch-Schönlein purpura. Mayo Clin. Proc. 79, 1151.

Narchi, H. 2005. Risk of long term renal impairment and duration of follow up recommended for Henoch-Schönlein purpura with normal or minimal urinary findings: a systematic review. Arch. Dis. Child. 90, 916.

Nast, C.C., Ward, H.J., Kyole, M.A., et al. 1987. Recurrent Henoch-Schönlein purpura following renal transplantation. Am. J. Kidney Dis. 9, 39.

Niaudet, P., Habib, R. 1998. Methylprednisolone pulse therapy in the treatment of severe forms of Schönlein-Henoch purpura nephritis. Pediatr. Nephrol. 12, 238.

Novak, J., Szekanecz, Z., Sebesi, J., et al. 2003. Elevated levels of anti-*Helicobacter pylori* antibodies in Henoch-Schönlein purpura. Autoimmunity 36, 307.

O'Donoghue, D.J., Nusbaum, P., Noel, L.H., et al. 1992. Antineutrophil cytoplasmic antibodies in IgA nephropathy and Henoch-Schönlein purpura. Nephrol. Dial. Transplant. 7, 534.

Olson, J.C., Kelly, K.J., Pan, C.G., et al. 1992. Pulmonary disease with hemorrhage in Henoch-Schönlein purpura. Pediatrics 89, 1177.

Oner, A., Tinaztepe, K., Erdogan, O. 1995. The effect of triple therapy on rapidly progressive Henoch-Schönlein nephritis. Pediatr. Nephrol. 9, 6.

Ostergaard, J.R., Storm, K. 1991. Neurologic manifestations of Schönlein-Henoch purpura. Acta Paediatr. Scand. 80, 339.

Ozaltin, F., Bakkaloglu, A., Ozen, S., et al. 2004. The significance of IgA class of antineutrophil cytoplasmic antibodies (ANCA) in childhood Henoch-Schönlein purpura. Clin. Rheumatol. 23, 426.

Robson, W.L.M., Leung, A.K.C. 1994. Henoch-Schönlein purpura. Adv. Pediatr. 41, 163.

Rosenblum, N.D., Winter, H.S. 1987. Steroid effects on the course of abdominal pain in children with HSP. Pediatrics 79, 1018.

Rostoker, G., Desvaux-Belghiti, D., Pilatte, Y., et al. 1994. Immunoglobulin therapy for severe IgA nephropathy and Henoch-Schönlein purpura. Ann. Intern. Med. 120, 476.

Rostoker, G., Desvaux-Belghiti, D., Pilatte, Y., et al. 1995. Immuno-modulation with low-dose immunoglobulins for moderate IgA nephropathy and Henoch-Schönlein purpura. Nephron. 69, 327.

Roth, R., Wilz, D.R., Theil, G.B. 1985. Schönlein-Henoch syndrome in adults. Q. J. Med. 55, 145.

Rueda, B., Perez-Armengol, C., Lopez-Lopez, S., et al. 2006. Association between functional haplotypes of vascular endothelial growth factor and renal complications in Henoch-Schönlein purpura. J. Rheumatol. 33, 62.

Saulsbury, F.T. 1993. Corticosteroid therapy does not prevent nephritis in Henoch-Schönlein purpura. Pediatr. Nephrol. 7, 69.

Saulsbury, F.T. 1999. Henoch-Schönlein purpura in children. Report of 100 patients and review of the literature. Medicine (Baltimore) 78, 395.

Saulsbury, F.T. 2001. Henoch-Schönlein purpura. Curr. Opin. Rheumatol. 13, 35.

Shin, J.I., Park, J.M., Shin, Y.H., et al. 2005a. Cyclosporin A therapy for severe Henoch-Schönlein nephritis with nephrotic syndrome. Pediatr. Nephrol. 20, 1093.

Shin, J.I., Park, J.M., Shin, Y.H., et al. 2005b. Can azathioprine and steroids alter the progression of severe Henoch-Schönlein nephritis in children? Pediatr. Nephrol. 20, 1087.

Stefansson Thors, V., Kolka, R., Sigurdardottir, S.L., et al. 2005. Increased frequency of C4B*Q0 alleles in patients with Henoch-Schönlein purpura. Scand. J. Immunol. 61, 274.

Stewart, M., Savage, J.M., Bell, B., et al. 1988. Long term renal prognosis of Henoch-Schönlein purpura in an unselected childhood population. Eur. J. Pediatr. 147, 113.

Szer, I.S. 1996. Henoch-Schönlein purpura: when and how to treat. J. Rheumatol. 23, 1661.

Tarshish, P., Bernstein, J., Edelmann, C.M., Jr. 2004. Henoch-Schönlein purpura nephritis: course of disease and efficacy of cyclophosphamide. Pediatr. Nephrol. 19, 51.

Tizard, E.J. 1999. Henoch-Schönlein purpura. Arch. Dis. Child. 80, 380.

Trapani, S., Micheli, A., Grisolia, F., et al. 2005. Henoch Schönlein Purpura in childhood: epidemiological and clinical analysis of 150 cases over a 5-year period and review of literature. Semin. Arthritis Rheum. 35, 143.

Van den Wall Bake, A., Lobatto, S., Jonges, L. 1987. IgA antibodies directed against cytoplasmic antigens of polymorphonuclear leukocytes in patients with Henoch-Schönlein purpura. Nephrol. Dial. Transplant. 7, 1238.

White, R.H.R. 1994. Henoch-Schönlein nephritis. A disease with significant late sequelae. Nephron. 68, 1.

Yoshikawa, N., White, R.H.R., Cameron, A.H. 1981. Prognostic significance of the glomerular changes in Henoch-Schönlein nephritis. Clin. Nephrol. 16, 223.

# CHAPTER 14

# Hemolytic Uremic Syndrome/Thrombotic Thrombocytopenic Purpura

Marina Noris[a], Giuseppe Remuzzi[a], Timothy H.J. Goodship[b],*

[a]Mario Negri Institute for Pharmacological Research, Clinical Research Centre for Rare Diseases, Aldo e Cele Dacco, Villa Camozzi, Bergamo, Italy
[b]The Institute of Human Genetics and School of Clinical Medical Sciences, Newcastle University, Newcastle upon Tyne NE1 3BZ, UK

## 1. Stx-associated HUS

In children the hemolytic uremic syndrome (HUS) is commonly triggered by certain strains of *Escherichia coli* (*E. coli*) that produce powerful exotoxins, the Shiga-like toxins (Stx1 and Stx2) and manifests with diarrhea, often bloody (D+HUS). Cases of Stx-induced HUS (Stx-HUS) which do not present with diarrhea, ~25% (Noris and Remuzzi, 2005), have also been reported.

### 1.1. Epidemiology

The overall incidence of Stx-HUS is estimated to be 2.1 cases per 100,000 persons/year with a peak incidence in children younger than 5 years of age (6.1/100,000/year) and the lowest rate in adults 50–59 years old (0.5/100,000/year) (Ruggenenti et al., 2001). The incidence of the disease parallels the seasonal fluctuation of Stx-producing *E. coli* (Stx-*E. coli*) infections with a peak in warmer months, between June and September. In the US, ~70,000 disease episodes and 60 deaths have been attributed annually to Stx-HUS (Mead et al., 1999). In Argentina and Uruguay Stx-*E. coli* infections are endemic and Stx-HUS is a common cause of acute renal failure in children (Cleary, 1988; Lopez et al., 1989, 2000), with an estimated incidence rate of 10.5/100,000/year (Meichtri et al., 2004). An association between traditional extensive production of cattle with endemic HUS in Argentina has been proposed, as supported by detection of Stx-*E. coli* strains in stool samples from 39% of Argentine healthy young beef steers (Meichtri et al., 2004).

### 1.2. Etiology

In 70% of cases in North America and Western Europe, Stx-HUS is secondary to infection with the *E. coli* serotype O157:H7 (Karmali et al., 1983; Riley et al., 1983; Caprioli et al., 1992; Ludwig et al., 1996; Varma et al., 2003; Brooks et al., 2004; Thorpe, 2004). This serotype has a unique biochemical property (lack of sorbitol fermentation) which renders it readily distinguishable from other fecal *E. coli* (Farmer and Davis, 1985). However, many other *E. coli* serotypes (O111:H8, O103:H2, O121, O145, O26, and O113 (Lopez et al., 1989; McCarthy et al., 2001; Brooks et al., 2004; Sonntag et al., 2004; Thorpe, 2004)), have been shown to cause Stx-HUS. An outbreak of ten cases of HUS associated with *E. coli* O103 infection has been recently reported in Norway (Schimmer, 2006).

*Corresponding author.
Tel.: 44 191 241 8632; Fax: 44 191 241 866
E-mail address: t.h.j.goodship@ncl.ac.uk

Infection by Stx-producing *Shigella dysenteriae* serotype 1 has been commonly linked to Stx-HUS in developing countries of Asia (Srivastava et al., 1991) and Africa (Guerin et al., 2003), but rarely in industrialized countries (Houdouin et al., 2004).

Stx-producing *E. coli* colonize healthy cattle intestine, but have been also isolated from deer, sheep, goats, horses, dogs, birds, and flies (Griffin and Tauxe, 1991; Ruggenenti et al., 2001). They are found in manure and water troughs in farms, which explains the increased risk of infection in people living in rural areas. Humans can become infected from contaminated milk, meat, or water; water-borne outbreaks have occurred as a result of drinking and swimming in unchlorinated water (McCarthy et al., 2001). Infection also occurs following contact with infected animals or humans, from either's excreta (Mead et al., 1997; Mead and Griffin, 1998; Locking et al., 2001) and occasionally through environmental contamination (Varma et al., 2003). Fruits and vegetables may also be contaminated, including radish sprouts, lettuce, and apple cider. Unpasteurized apple juice has been implicated in several outbreaks (Cody et al., 1999). A multi-state outbreak of *E. coli* O157:H7 infection from fresh spinach was reported in late September 2006 to the Center for Disease Control of Atlanta, USA (www.cdc.gov/foodborne/ecolispinach), which affected 187 persons from 26 USA states. Among infected persons, 29 developed Stx-HUS. The proportion of persons who developed HUS was 29% in children, 7% in persons 18–59 years old, and 14% in persons 60 years old or older. *E. coli* O157:H7 was isolated from nine packages of spinach supplied by patients. All packages were marketed as baby spinach and labeled with the same brand name. Person-to-person transmission has been reported in day-care and chronic-care facilities (Reiss et al., 2006).

### 1.3. Clinical manifestation

Following exposure to Stx-*E. coli*, 38–61% of individuals develop hemorrhagic colitis and 3–9% (in sporadic infections) to 20% (in epidemic forms) progress to overt HUS (Mead and Griffin, 1998; Banatvala et al., 2001). Stx-*E. coli* hemorrhagic colitis not complicated by HUS is self-limiting and is not associated with an increased long-term risk of high blood pressure or renal dysfunction, as shown by a recent 4-year follow-up study in 951 children who were exposed to a drinking water outbreak of *E. coli* O157:H7 (Garg et al., 2006).

Stx-HUS is characterized by prodromal diarrhea followed by acute renal failure. The average interval between *E. coli* exposure and illness is 3 days. Illness typically begins with abdominal cramps and non-bloody diarrhea; diarrhea may become hemorrhagic in 70% of cases usually within 1 or 2 days (Chandler et al., 2002). Vomiting occurs in 30–60% of cases and fever in 30%. The leukocyte count is usually elevated, and a barium enema may demonstrate "thumb-printing," suggestive of edema and submucosal hemorrhage, especially in the region of the ascending and transverse colon. HUS is usually diagnosed 6 days after the onset of diarrhea (Ruggenenti et al., 2001). After infection, Stx-*E. coli* may be shed in the stools for several weeks after the symptoms have resolved, particularly in children <5 years of age (Ruggenenti et al., 2001). Diagnosis rests on detection of Stx-*E. coli* in stool cultures. Serologic tests for antibodies to Stx and O157 lipopolysaccharide can be done in research laboratories and tests are being developed for rapid detection of *E. coli* O157:H7 and Stx in stools.

Bloody diarrhea, fever, vomiting, elevated leukocyte count, extremes of age, and female sex as well as the use of antimotility agents (Beatty et al., 2004), have been associated with an increased risk of HUS following *E. coli* infection (Mead and Griffin, 1998).

Stx-HUS is not a benign disease. Seventy-percent of patients who develop HUS require red blood cell transfusions, 50% need dialysis, and 25% have neurological involvement, including stroke, seizure, and coma (Milford, 1992; Mead and Griffin, 1998; Garg et al., 2003). Although mortality for infants and young children in industrialized countries decreased when dialysis became available, as well as after the introduction of intensive care facilities, still 3–5% of patients die during the acute phase of Stx-HUS (Milford, 1992). A meta-analysis of 49 published studies (3476 patients, mean follow-up of 4.4 years) describing long-term prognosis of patients who survived an episode of Stx-HUS, reported death or permanent ESRD in 12% of patients and GFR below 80 ml/min/1.73 m$^2$ in 25% (Garg et al., 2003). The severity of acute illness, particularly central nervous system symptoms, and the need for initial dialysis and microalbuminuria in the first 6–8 months, were strongly associated with a worse long-term prognosis (Tonshoff et al., 1994; Garg et al., 2003; Lou-Meda et al., 2006).

Stx-HUS precipitated by *S. dysenteriae* infection is almost invariably complicated by bacteremia and septic shock, systemic intravascular coagulation and acute cortical necrosis with renal failure, and has a high mortality rate (about 30%) (Date et al., 1982).

## 1.4. Histopathology

The common microvascular lesion of HUS, defined by the term thrombotic microangiopathy, consists of vessel wall thickening with endothelial swelling, which allows accumulation of proteins and cell debris in the subendothelial layer, creating a space between endothelial cells and the underlying basement membrane of affected microvessels (Ruggenenti et al., 2001; Kaplan et al., 1998) (Fig. 1). Both the widening of the subendothelial space and intraluminal platelet thrombi lead to partial or complete obstruction of the vessel lumina. It is probably because of the partial occlusion of the lumen that erythrocytes are disrupted by mechanical trauma, which explains the Coombs-negative hemolysis and finding of fragmented and distorted erythrocytes in the blood smear.

In children with Stx-HUS, the lesion is mainly confined to the glomerular tuft and is noted in an early phase of the disease (Fig. 1). Glomerular capillary lumina are reduced or occluded. In patent glomerular capillaries packed with red blood cells and fibrin, thrombi occasionally are seen. Examination of biopsies taken several months after the disease onset showed that most glomeruli are normal (an indication of the reversibility of the lesions), whereas 20% eventually became sclerotic (Remuzzi and Ruggenenti, 1994; Taylor et al., 1999). Arterial thrombosis does occur but is uncommon and appears to be a proximal extension of the glomerular lesion (Remuzzi and Ruggenenti, 1994; Taylor et al., 1999).

In the acute phase, tubular changes include foci of necrosis of proximal tubular cells, and the presence of red blood cells and eosinophilic casts in the lumina of distal tubules. Occasionally, in the distal tubular lumina, fragmented red blood cells can be detected.

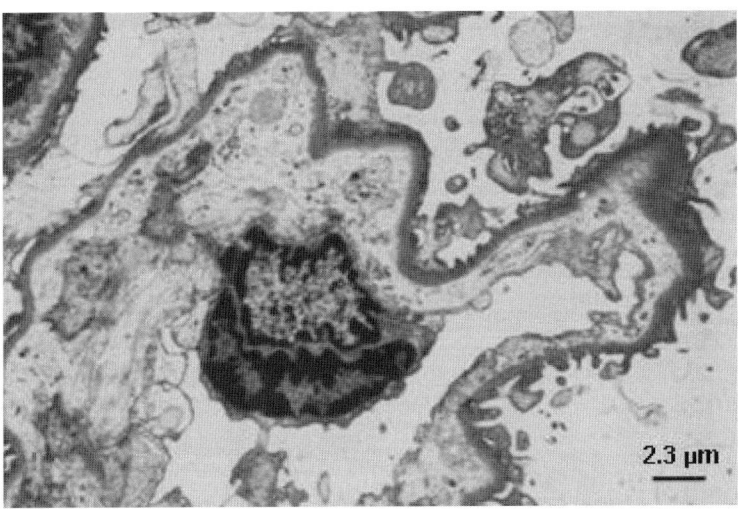

**Figure 1.** Electron micrograph of a glomerular capillary from a patient with hemolytic uremic syndrome. The endothelium is detached from the glomerular basement membrane; the subendothelial space is widened and occupied by electron−lucent fluffy material and cell debris. The capillary lumen is markedly narrowed. Podocyte foot processes are focally effaced. (Magnification ×4400.)

## 1.5. Pathogenesis

The Stxs associated with *E. coli* are designated by a number. Stx-1 is almost identical to Stx from *S. dysenteriae* type 1, differing by a single aminoacid, and is 50% homologous with Stx-2 (Jackson et al., 1987; Tesh et al., 1993; Fraser et al., 2004). Both Stx-1 and -2 are 70-kDa AB5 holotoxins comprised of a single A subunit of 32 kDa and five 7.7-kDa B subunits (Fraser et al., 1994).

Despite their similar sequences, Stx-1 and -2 cause different degrees and types of tissue damage as documented by the higher pathogenicity of strains of *E. coli* that produce only Stx-2 than of those that produce Stx-1 alone (Scotland et al., 1987; Ostroff et al., 1989; Cimolai et al., 1990). In a study in children who become infected by Stx-*E. coli*, *E. coli* strains producing Stx-2 were most commonly associated with HUS, whereas most strains isolated from children with diarrhea alone or remaining asymptomatic only produced Stx-1 (Jenkins et al., 2003).

After oral ingestion, Stx-*E. coli* reaches the gut and closely adheres to the epithelial cells of the gastrointestinal mucosa through a 97 kDa outer membrane protein, intimin (Donnenberg et al., 1993). Stxs are then picked up by polarized gastrointestinal cells via transcellular pathways (Acheson et al., 1996) and translocate into the circulation, probably facilitated by the transmigration of neutrophils (PMN) (Hurley et al., 2001), which increase paracellular permeability. The route of transport of Stxs from the intestine to the kidney has been greatly debated. Circulating human blood cells, such as erythrocytes (Bitzan et al., 1994), platelets (Cooling et al., 1998; Stahl et al., 2006), and monocytes (van Setten et al., 1996) express Stx receptors on their surface and a role for these cells in Stx transport has been hypothesized.

Binding of Stxs to target cells is dependent on B subunits and occurs via the terminal digalactose moiety of the glycolipid cell surface receptor globotriaosylceramide Gb3. Stx-1 and -2 bind to different epitopes on the Gb3 molecule and they also differ in binding affinity and kinetics (Nakajima et al., 2001). Surface plasmon resonance analysis showed that Stx-1 easily binds to and detaches from Gb3, in contrast to Stx-2 which binds slowly but also dissociates very slowly, thus staying on the cells long enough to be incorporated (Nakajima et al., 2001). The latter could explain the fact that Stx-2 is 1000-fold more toxic than Stx-1 on human endothelial cells in vitro (Louise and Obrig, 1995).

Cultured human microvascular endothelial cells are more susceptible to the toxic effects of Stxs than large vessel endothelium (Ohmi et al., 1998). This is consistent with data that the number of Gb3 receptors expressed on human microvascular endothelial cells is 50-fold higher than in endothelial cells from human umbilical veins (Obrig et al., 1987). In human glomerular endothelial cells Gb3 expression and Stx toxicity are further increased on exposure to TNFα (van Setten et al., 1997), in turn released by monocytes in response to Stx binding (van Setten et al., 1996). Together, these data provide the biochemical basis for the preferential localization of microangiopathic lesions to renal vasculature in HUS in humans.

Following internalization by receptor-mediated endocytosis, Stxs are carried by retrograde transport through the Golgi complex to the endoplasmic reticulum, where the A and B subunits likely dissociate. Then the A subunit is translocated to the cytosol and nuclear envelope where it enzymatically blocks protein synthesis (Obrig et al., 1987). Stx-1 and -2 also induce endothelial apoptosis (Pijpers et al., 2001; Brigotti et al., 2002) possibly by inhibiting the expression of the anti-apoptotic Bcl-2 family member, Mcl-1 (Erwert et al., 2003).

For many years, it was assumed that the only relevant biologic activity of Stxs was the block of protein synthesis and destruction of endothelial cells. Recently, however, it has been shown that treatment of endothelial cells with sublethal doses of Stxs, exerting minimal influence on protein synthesis, leads to increased mRNA levels and protein expression of chemokines, such as IL-8, RANTES (Guessous et al., 2005), and monocyte chemoattractant protein-1 (MCP-1), and cell adhesion molecules, a process preceded by NF-κB activation (Zoja et al., 2002). Analysis of genome wide expression patterns of human endothelial cells stimulated with sublethal doses of Stxs evidenced 25 and 24 genes up-regulated by Stx-1 and -2, respectively, mostly encoding for chemokines and cytokines, cell adhesion molecules, including

P-selectin and ICAM-1, and transcription factors (EGR-1, NF-κB2, and NF-κBIA) (Matussek et al., 2003). Chemokines and cytokines are likely involved in the chemoattraction and activation of neutrophils. Adhesion molecules appear to play a critical role in mediating binding of inflammatory cells to the endothelium. This is supported by adhesion experiments under flow showing that Stx-2 treatment enhanced the number of leukocytes adhering and migrating across a monolayer of human endothelial cells (Morigi et al., 1995). Preventing IL-8 and MCP-1 overexpression by adenovirus-mediated blocking of NF-κB inhibited the adhesion and transmigration of leukocytes (Zoja et al., 2002).

Taken together, these findings indicate that Stxs, by altering endothelial cell adhesion properties and metabolism, favor leukocyte-dependent inflammation. The latter activates endothelial cells that lose thromboresistance, which ultimately leads to microvascular thrombosis. Evidence for such a sequence of events has been obtained in experiments of whole blood flowing on human microvascular endothelial cells, pre-exposed to Stx-1, at high shear stress (Morigi et al., 2001). In such circumstances, early platelet activation and adhesion takes place, followed by the formation of organized thrombi dependent on endothelial P-selectin and PECAM-1, offering a plausible patho-physiological pathway for microvascular thrombosis in HUS. In addition, Stx-1 stimulates human monocytes to produce tissue factor, which may also play a role in the acceleration of the inflammation–thrombosis circuit in Stx-HUS (Murata et al., 2006).

## 1.6. Treatment

There is no treatment of proven value, and care during the acute phase of the illness is still merely supportive with no substantial changes as compared to the past. There is no clear consensus on whether antibiotics should be administered to treat Stx-*E. coli* infection. Wong et al. (2000) showed that antibiotic therapy at the stage of gastrointestinal infection with Stx-*E. coli* increases—by about 17-fold—the risk of full-blown HUS. It was postulated that antibiotic induced injury to the bacterial membrane might favor the acute release of large amounts of toxins. On the other hand, a recent meta-analysis of 26 reports failed to show a higher risk of HUS associated with antibiotic administration (Safdar et al., 2002). Of note, in the Wong study none of the patients had bacteremia. While bacteremia is very common in Stx-HUS precipitated by *S. dysenteriae* type 1, and these patients eventually progress to death unless antibiotics are started early enough (Bhimma et al., 1997; Oneko et al., 2001), this complication is exceptionally found in Stx-HUS sustained by *E. coli* O157:H7 infection. However, when it occurs antibiotics should be employed, as indicated by a recent report of an adult patient with *E. coli* O157:H7 induced HUS with bacteremia and urinary tract infection in whom early antibiotic therapy rapidly resolved hematological and renal abnormalities (Chiurchiu et al., 2003).

A study with a Stx binding agent—SYNSORB Pk—composed of particles of silicon linked to the globotriaosylceramide, given orally (Trachtman et al., 2003) failed to find any benefit of SYNSORB over placebo. New agents targeted to prevent organ exposure to Stx are currently under evaluation (MacConnachie and Todd, 2004). In mice, molecular decoys such as orally administered harmless recombinant bacteria that display a Stx receptor on the surface (Paton et al., 2000; Pinyon et al., 2004; Takahashi et al., 2004) have been successfully used. In another study, a plant-based oral vaccination with nicotiana tabacum cells transected with the gene encoding inactivated Stx2, fully protected mice from challenge with a lethal dose of the toxin (Wen et al., 2006). Another approach is to use Stx inhibitors, among them is "STARFISH," an oligobivalent, water-soluble carbohydrate ligand that can simultaneously engage all five B subunits of the toxin, which might help to prevent toxin that already has entered the circulation from destroying kidney microvessels (Mulvey et al., 2003). Others have ameliorated disease in pigs by injection of toxin-neutralizing antibodies (Matise et al., 2001). At present, prevention remains the main approach to decreasing the morbidity and mortality associated with Stx-*E. coli* infection. A multi-faceted approach is required that includes novel ways of decreasing Stx-*E. coli* carrier rate in livestock and implementing a zero-tolerance policy for contaminated foods and beverages.

Most treatments including plasma exchange, intravenous IgG, fibrinolytic agents, antiplatelet drugs, corticosteroids, and antioxidants (Garg et al., 2003), have been shown to be ineffective in controlled clinical trials in the acute phase of the disease (Garg et al., 2003). Careful blood pressure control and renin–angiotensin system blockade may be particularly beneficial in the long term for those patients who suffer chronic renal disease after an episode of Stx-HUS. A study in 45 children with renal sequelae of HUS, followed for 9–11 years, documented that early restriction of proteins and use of ACE inhibitors may have a beneficial effect on long-term renal outcome, as documented by a positive slope of 1/Cr values over time in treated patients (Caletti et al., 2004). In another study, 8–15-year treatment with ACE inhibitors after severe Stx-HUS normalized blood pressure, reduced proteinuria, and improved GFR (Van Dyck and Proesmans, 2004).

Finally, a kidney transplant should be considered as an effective and safe treatment for those children who progress to ESRD. Indeed the outcome of renal transplantation is good in children with Stx-HUS, recurrence rates range from 0 to 10% (Artz et al., 2003; Loirat and Niaudet, 2003) and graft survival at 10 years is even better than in control transplanted children with other diseases (Ferraris et al., 2002).

## 2. Atypical HUS (aHUS, alias non-Stx-HUS)

### 2.1. Epidemiology

aHUS is significantly less common than Stx-HUS, accounting for ~5% of all types of HUS (Noris and Remuzzi, 2005). The incidence in the USA has been reported to be ~2 per million population per year (Constantinescu et al., 2004). Both sporadic and familial forms of aHUS are described (Kavanagh et al., 2006). A variety of precipitating factors have been implicated in the pathogenesis of aHUS including non-enteric infections, drugs, malignancies, transplantation, and pregnancy. A thrombotic microangiopathy indistinguishable from that seen in aHUS is also seen in association with multi-system diseases such as scleroderma, systemic lupus erythematosus (SLE), and the antiphospholipid antibody syndrome. *Streptococcus pneumoniae* infection has been reported to be responsible for ~40% of cases of aHUS in children in the USA (Constantinescu et al., 2004). Neuraminidase produced by *S. pneumoniae* cleaves sialic acid residues from cell surface glycoproteins exposing the Thomsen–Friedenreich antigen (T-antigen). Binding of naturally occurring IgM antibodies to the exposed T-antigen on platelets and endothelial cells may then predispose to a thrombotic microangiopathy (Klein et al., 1977). Previously aHUS was associated with advanced HIV infection. However, the advent of highly active antiretroviral therapy (HAART) has resulted in a decreased incidence (Becker et al., 2004). In ~13% of female patients with aHUS the disease is associated with pregnancy (George, 2003); most episodes occur at term or post-partum. Changes in pregnancy that may predispose to aHUS include increased concentrations of procoagulant factors, decreased fibrinolytic activity and reduced expression of endothelial thrombomodulin.

Many drugs have been associated with aHUS including cytotoxics, immunosuppressants, and antiplatelet agents (Dlott et al., 2004). The mechanism of action is either immune-mediated or direct toxicity. An example of the former is quinine, which is associated with the development of autoantibodies reactive with platelet glycoproteins (Dlott et al., 2004). An example of the latter is mitomycin C, with an incidence of between 4 and 15% in patients receiving it in combination chemotherapy (Valavaara and Nordman, 1985). De novo aHUS is seen post-renal transplantation in association with the use of calcineurin inhibitors (Schriber and Herzig, 1997; Burke et al., 1999). The risk is increased by acute rejection and CMV infection. Metabolic conditions associated with aHUS include cobalamin C disease (cblC) (Geraghty et al., 1992). This is characterized by methylmalonic aciduria and homocystinuria, and is the most common inborn error of cobalamin metabolism. aHUS has been associated with a factor H mutation (Guigonis et al., 2005) and the gene responsible (MMACHC) has recently been identified (Lerner-Ellis et al., 2006).

## 2.2. Genetic factors associated with aHUS

That aHUS could be familial has been recognized for many years (Kaplan et al., 1975; Kaplan and Kaplan, 1992; Berns et al., 1992). The inheritance was thought to be predominantly recessive (Kaplan et al., 1997) but it is now recognized that non-penetrance is a common feature which confounds the interpretation of inheritance; most families are dominant with impaired penetrance. In 1998, Warwicker et al. (1998) published the results of a linkage study in three families with aHUS. This showed segregation of the disease to an area on chromosome 1q32 containing a cluster of genes important in the regulation of complement activation (the RCA cluster). That complement abnormalities were associated with aHUS had been recognized for many years. In particular both low levels of C3 and glomerular deposition of C3 had been reported (Stuhlinger et al., 1974; Hammar et al., 1978; Carreras et al., 1981; Noris et al., 1999). The first candidate gene to be screened in the RCA cluster was factor H (*CFH*) because previous reports had shown an association between CFH deficiency and aHUS (Ohali et al., 1998; Thompson and Winterborn, 1981; Pichette et al., 1994). *CFH* mutation screening of the three families showed that in one of the families all affected members carried a heterozygous missense mutation in the C-terminal exon.

### 2.2.1. Factor H

CFH and other proteins within the RCA cluster share a common basic structure consisting of multiple (contiguous) homologous modules called short complement regulator (SCR) domains or complement control protein (CCP) modules. Factor H has 20 SCRs each comprising ~60 amino acids. Mutations in *CFH* in aHUS patients have been widely described (Richards et al., 2001; Caprioli et al., 2001; Manuelian et al., 2003; Perez-Caballero et al., 2001; Dragon-Durey et al., 2004; Caprioli et al., 2006), are listed at the interactive FH-HUS mutation database (http://www.FH-HUS.org) (Saunders et al., 2006, 2007) and are found in ~30% of patients. This includes both patients with the sporadic and familial forms. To date there are 71 disease-associated mutations (Fig. 2). The majority are heterozygous missense mutations that cluster in the C-terminal exons and are associated with normal factor H levels. A minority are deletions or missense mutations that result in either a severely truncated protein or impaired secretion. This leads to systemic factor H deficiency, usually heterozygous.

The clustering of missense mutations in the C-terminal region of the molecule is remarkable. The alternative pathway is activated by "foreign" surfaces. It exhibits spontaneous activity, which is regulated by factor H in four ways. Factor H acts as a cofactor for factor I-mediated cleavage of C3b (cofactor activity) and accelerates the decay of the C3 convertase C3bBb (decay accelerating activity). It also competes with factor B for binding to C3b and binds to polyanions on cell surfaces. The C-terminal region of factor H where mutations cluster is known to be important in the latter two functions. Structural models of the mutants suggest that it is particularly impairment of the ability to inactivate surface bound C3b that is important. Functional studies have confirmed this finding (Manuelian et al., 2003; Jozsi et al., 2006; Sanchez-Corral et al., 2002, 2004). It has recently been observed that some of the mutations in the C-terminal exons of CFH have arisen by gene conversion (Heinen et al., 2006). This has led to the finding of a hybrid gene (comprising SCRs 1–18 of factor H and SCRs 19–20 of factor H-related protein 1) in association with aHUS (Venables et al., 2006).

There are two animal models of factor H deficiency, the Norwegian Yorkshire pig and a murine model. In both these models, homozygous animals develop membranoproliferative glomerulonephritis (MPGN) rather than HUS (Hogasen et al., 1995; Pickering et al., 2002). This form of glomerulonephritis has also been reported in humans with homozygous factor H deficiency and N-terminal heterozygous *CFH* missense mutations

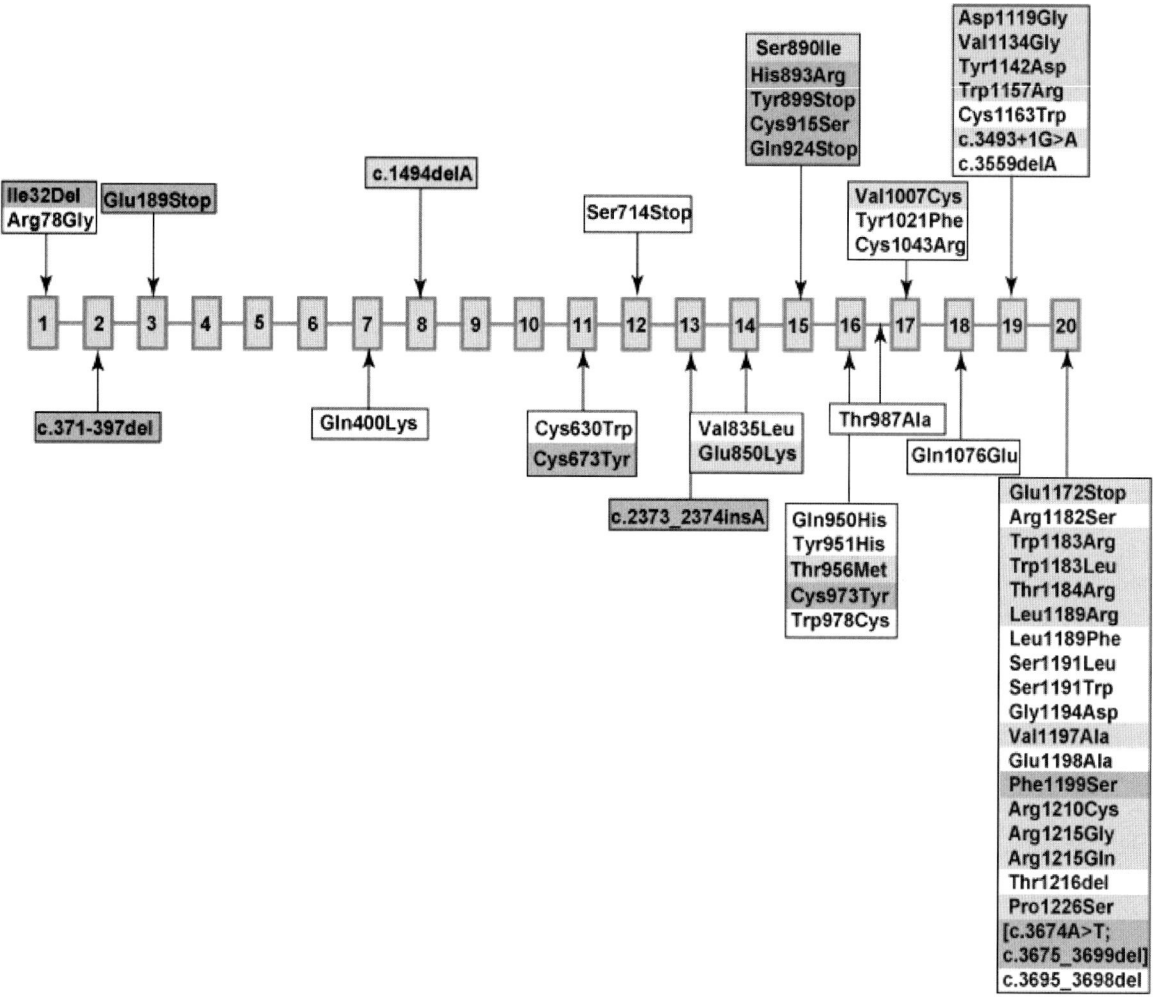

**Figure 2.** Factor H mutations. Those in darker screened area are associated with reduced factor H levels whereas those in lighter screened area have normal levels. The majority of the mutations cluster in the C-terminal region which is important for binding to polyanions and surface bound C3b. (Figure taken from the "FH HUS Mutation Database" with the permission of Prof. Stephen J. Perkins and also reproduced from Saunders et al. (2006) with the permission of Wiley.)

(Dragon-Durey et al., 2004; Licht et al., 2006). It has recently been reported in abstract form that the factor H deficient mouse transgenic for murine factor H lacking the 5 C-terminal SCRs (SCRs 16–20) spontaneously develops HUS. Our current knowledge therefore suggests that factor H deficiency is more commonly, although not exclusively, associated with MPGN rather than HUS. Missense mutations, clustering in the C-terminal exons of *CFH* are usually associated with aHUS, while those found in the N-terminal exons are associated with MPGN. Factor H autoantibodies have also been reported in association with aHUS. To date three patients with IgG antibodies have been described (Dragon-Durey et al., 2005).

### 2.2.2. Membrane cofactor protein

In only one of the three original families reported by Warwicker et al. (1998), there was a mutation found in *CFH*. One of the remaining two families was unusual in that three sibs had all received a renal transplant without evidence of recurrence of

HUS in the allograft. This suggested that an abnormality of the transmembrane complement regulator membrane cofactor protein (MCP) might be implicated in this family. MCP (CD46) is widely expressed on the surface of all cells apart from erythrocytes (Goodship et al., 2004). The extracellular domain comprises 4 SCRs followed by an alternatively spliced region rich in threonine, serine, and proline (the STP region) and a group of 12 amino acids. This is followed by the transmembrane domain and an alternatively spliced cytoplasmic tail, which mediates signaling events. Together with factor I, MCP degrades C3b and C4b bound to the cell surface. Two simultaneous reports (Noris et al., 1992; Richards et al., 2003) showed mutations in *MCP* in association with aHUS. One of these, a 6 bp deletion, was in the aforementioned family. Since then 25 disease-associated *MCP* mutations have been described in aHUS (Caprioli et al., 2006; Esparza-Gordillo et al., 2005; Fremeaux-Bacchi et al., 2006). The functional effect of many of these mutations has been modeled. The majority result in reduced cell surface expression with only two showing reducing C3b binding and cofactor activity.

### 2.2.3. Factor I

Besides abnormalities of soluble and membrane bound regulators of complement activation, mutations in the gene encoding complement factor I (*CFI*) have recently been described in aHUS (Caprioli et al., 2006; Esparza-Gordillo et al., 2005; Kavanagh et al., 2005; Fremeaux-Bacchi et al., 2004). CFI is a soluble regulatory serine protease of the complement system which cleaves three peptide bonds in the α-chain of C3b and two bonds in the α-chain of C4b thereby inactivating these proteins. CFH acts as a cofactor for effects on C3b, C4 binding protein for C4b and MCP for both. CFI is a heterodimer of ~88 kDa which consists of a non-catalytic heavy chain of 50 kDa which is linked to a catalytic light chain of 38 kDa by a disulfide bond. The protein is synthesized as a single chain precursor of 565 amino acids, predominantly in the liver. Four basic amino acids are then excised from the precursor prior to secretion of the heterodimer. Like many of the complement proteins, factor I has a modular structure. The heavy chain contains two low-density lipoprotein receptor (LDLr) domains, a CD5 domain, and a module found only in IF and complement proteins C6 and C7. The *CFI* gene is located on chromosome 4q25 and spans 63 kbp. It comprises 13 exons and there is a strong correlation between the exonic organization of the gene and the modular structure of the protein. The light chain of CFI, which is the serine proteinase region of the molecule, is encoded in five exons. The genomic organization of the enzymic part of CFI is similar to that of trypsin. The gene structure is unusual in that the first exon is small, 86 bp, and is separated from the rest of the gene by a large first intron of 36 kbp (Vyse et al., 1994a). CFI deficiency has been described previously in approximately 30 kindreds and is usually associated with a predisposition to pyogenic infection in homozygous individuals (Vyse et al., 1994b, 1996). The recent reports of *CFI* mutations in aHUS suggest that the prevalence is between 3 and 10%. As with *CFH* and *MCP*, the majority of the mutations are heterozygous and non-penetrance is a common feature. Approximately 40% of the mutations result in partial factor I deficiency, the functional significance of the others remains to be determined.

### 2.2.4. Factor B

Factor B is a zymogen that carries the convertase serine protease domain necessary for amplification of the alternative pathway (Xu et al., 2001). The convertase for this pathway is assembled in two steps. First, C3b associates with factor B and then the C3bB complex is cleaved by the serum protease factor D at a single site in factor B producing Ba and Bb fragments. The Ba fragment dissociates from the complex, while Bb remains bound to C3b to form the active C3 convertase C3bBb. Dissociation of the two components of this complex results in inactivation of the convertase and is promoted by DAF, CR1, and FH. The gene for factor B (*BF*) is located on chromosome 6p21.3 and consists of 18 exons coding for a five-domain glycoprotein. The N-terminal Ba fragment contains three CCP domains. The C-terminal Bb fragment contains two domains. The N-terminal type A domain contains the C3b-binding region and the C-terminal domain is the site of the serine protease. It has been shown in vitro that site directed mutagenesis at the C3b–Bb interface interferes with normal dissociation of C3b from Bb whether spontaneous or promoted by DAF, CR1, or FH (Hourcade et al., 2002). This represents a potential site for human mutations, which would selectively increase activity of the alternative pathway. Two *BF* mutations in association with aHUS have recently been reported (Goicoechea de Jorge et al., 2007). Both alter residues at the C3b–Bb interface in close proximity to the $Mg^{2+}$ binding site and have been shown to be gain-of-function mutations that result in either enhanced formation of the C3bBb convertase or increased resistance to inactivation by complement regulators.

## 2.2.5. C3

C3 is the most abundant soluble complement protein and is composed of $\alpha$ and $\beta$ chains which are connected by a single disulfide bond (Sahu and Lambris, 2001). The gene for C3 is located on chromosome 19 and consists of 41 exons, 16 of which encode the $\beta$ chain and 25 the $\alpha$ chain. C3 undergoes spontaneous hydrolysis to C3b. In contrast to native C3, C3b expresses multiple binding sites for other complement components including C5, properdin (P), factors H, B, and I, CR1, and MCP. Binding of these proteins to C3b leads either to amplification of the C3 convertase (by B and P in the presence of factor D) and hence initiation of the membrane attack complex, or the inactivation of C3b (by factor I in the presence of CFH, CR1, and MCP). The downregulation of C3b by factor I proceeds in three steps and requires one of the cofactor molecules (MCP, CR1, or CFH). Cleavage of the $\alpha$ chain of C3b occurs in two places: first between residues 1281 and 1282 (Arg–Ser) to generate $iC3b_1$ and then between residues 1298 and 1299 (Arg–Ser) to yield $iC3b_2$. Mutations at either of these sites could potentially lead to resistance to the action of factor I and thus increased activity of the alternative pathway. The binding sites for CFH, CR1, and MCP have also been identified. A major binding site for CR1 and CFH is located in the N-terminal region of the $\alpha$ chain of C3b. Again mutations at these sites could impair the cofactor activity of CR1 and CFH.

However, a recent report in abstract (Fremeaux-Bacchi et al., 2007) has shown mutations in C3 in association with aHUS some of which result in impaired secretion of C3. If these findings are replicated then this will challenge the current paradigm for the role of complement in the pathogenesis of aHUS. The abnormalities found in factor H, MCP, and factor I have suggested that it is impairment of complement regulation that is pivotal. However, an alternative hypothesis that takes into account the recent C3 findings is that local levels of C3 are essential for maintaining endothelial integrity.

## 2.2.6. Other complement candidate genes

Abnormalities in CFH, IF, MCP, BF, and C3 account for $\sim 60\%$ of aHUS patients. Other candidate genes that remain to be explored include properdin, CD59, C4 binding protein, and decay-accelerating factor.

## 2.3. Factors affecting the development of aHUS

The aforementioned complement abnormalities are thought to act as susceptibility factors for the development of aHUS rather than being directly causative. A triggering factor is necessary to initiate the disease. In a recent series $\sim 70\%$ of cases associated with a *CFH* mutation were preceded by an "infection." Pregnancy and drugs accounted for 4% (Caprioli et al., 2006).

Screening the relatives of patients known to have a *CFH*, *MCP*, or *IF* mutation has shown that the penetrance of the aHUS is $\sim 50\%$. In addition to aforementioned factors it has been shown that *CFH*, *MCP*, and *IF* act independently as susceptibility factors for the development of the disease (Caprioli et al., 2003; Fremeaux-Bacchi et al., 2005; Esparza-Gordillo et al., 2005). It has recently been shown that one of the genes for the factor H-related proteins (*CFHR5*) is also a susceptibility factor (Monteferrante et al., 2007). Moreover, it has been shown that in families with mutations in both *CFH* and *IF*, the disease segregates with the mutations in combination (Esparza-Gordillo et al., 2006).

## 2.4. Management of aHUS

Plasma exchange (PE) and supportive therapy are the treatment of choice for the acute presentation of aHUS (von Baeyer, 2002). There is good retrospective evidence for the efficacy of PE in patients with *CFH* mutations or anti-CFH antibodies but less so for patients with *MCP* mutations (Stratton and Warwicker, 2002; Caprioli et al., 2006). In some patients with refractory life-threatening disease, bilateral nephrectomy has resulted in a dramatic response (Remuzzi et al., 1996). Despite treatment at least 50% of patients will require long-term renal replacement therapy. Whilst no problems have been reported with the use of hemodialyis and peritoneal dialysis in aHUS, the use of transplantation has been controversial. The risk of recurrence of HUS in an allograft in all patients is $\sim 50\%$ (Conlon et al., 1995, 1996; Miller et al., 1997; Ducloux et al., 1998; Lahlou et al., 2000; Quan et al., 2001; Loirat and Niaudet, 2003; Ruggenenti, 2002) but is significantly greater ($\sim 80\%$) in patients known to have a mutation in either *CFH* or *IF* (Bresin et al., 2006). Whether patients known to have a *CFH* or *IF* mutation should be listed for renal transplantation is debatable. In contrast the outcome for patients known to have only an *MCP* mutation is favorable. It is now recommended that all patients should undergo *CFH*, *IF*, and *MCP* genotyping prior to transplantation. Because both CFH and IF are produced predominantly by the liver, combined liver/kidney transplantation is a logical option. Whilst the outcome in initial reports of this modality was less favorable (Remuzzi et al., 2002b, 2005) a more recent report (Saland et al., 2006) suggested that a favorable long-term outcome was possible. Pivotal to this is the use of prophylactic PE immediately prior to surgery. The increased knowledge of the role of complement in the pathogenesis of aHUS suggests that complement inhibitors could be of therapeutic benefit. The anti-C5 monoclonal antibodies Pexelizumab and Eculizimab have been used in the treatment of paroxysmal nocturnal hemoglobinuria and myocardial infarction (Hillmen et al., 2004; Granger et al., 2003). Agents that mimic the action of factor H such as APT070 and soluble complement receptor 1 (Pratt et al., 1996; Smith and Smith, 2001) may be of benefit in aHUS. Further understanding of the role of complement in the pathogenesis of aHUS will hopefully translate into logical targeted therapeutic agents.

## 3. Thrombotic thrombocytopenic purpura

Thrombotic thrombocytopenic purpura (TTP) is a disseminated form of thrombotic microangiopathy—initially described as a new disease by Moschowitz (1925)—that presents with the development of von Willebrand factor (VWF) and platelet-rich thrombi in the arterioles and capillaries of brain, heart, and other organs. The term TTP should be used when at least two of the major criteria for diagnosis (thrombocytopenia, microangiopathic anemia, and neurological signs) are associated with at least two minor criteria (fever, renal changes, and presence of thrombi in the circulation) (Bukowski, 1982).

## 3.1. Epidemiology and classification

TTP is a rare disease, with an estimated incidence of 2 to 10 cases per million/year in all racial groups. Recently, greater awareness and perhaps improved diagnostic facilities give the impression that incidence is increasing. The disease is more common in women, with a female to male ratio of 3:2. Although the peak incidence occurs in the third decade of life, cases of TTP have been described in patients ranging from 1 to 90 years (Kennedy et al., 1980).

### 3.1.1. Secondary forms of TTP

TTP may occur in pregnancy or may complicate the postpartum period (Ruggenenti and Remuzzi, 1990). Cases of TTP have been discovered in association with neoplastic disorders such as lymphoma, Sjögren's syndrome, rheumatoid arthritis, polyarteritis, and SLE period (Ruggenenti and Remuzzi, 1990). TTP has been recognized in patients with endocarditis. About 200 cases of TTP have been described in the course of neoplastic diseases and appear to depend on the use of some anticancer drugs, such as mitomycin, vinblastine, cisplatin, bleomycin, cytosine arabinoside, and daunorubicin (Ruggenenti and Remuzzi, 1990). TTP has been described in women using oral contraceptives (Ruggenenti and Remuzzi, 1990), but the incidence, prevalence, and strength of this association are not known.

The platelet anti-aggregating agent ticlopidine has been associated with the development of TTP with an estimated incidence of 1 case per 1600–5000 (Bennett et al., 1998). The first occurrence of TTP in association with ticlopidine was recognized seven years after the approval of the drug (Bennett et al., 1998). TTP developed within two weeks of initiation of treatment in 15% of reported cases and within 1 month in 80% of cases. The overall mortality rate for ticlopidine-associated cases of TTP has been estimated as 33%. A new antiplatelet agent, clopidogrel, whose mechanism of action and indications are similar to those of ticlopidine, was associated with 11 cases of TTP (Bennett et al., 2000). Ten of them developed TTP within two weeks of starting treatment with the drug. All were treated with PE, one died and all the others recovered, although for two of them 20 exchanges or more were required before recovery. A very recent report described a case of TTP associated with zoledronic acid, in which an immune-mediated reaction was suspected. The clinical course of a patient who presented with TTP after being started on simvastatin, a HMG-CoA inhibitor, is also described (Galbusera et al., 2006).

Associations between TTP and Coxsackie A, Coxsackie B, other unspecified viruses, *Mycoplasma pneumoniae*, *Legionella pneumophila*, and with recent vaccinations have been described (Ruggenenti and Remuzzi, 1990). Neame hypothesized that viruses may cause the syndrome by producing platelet aggregation, endothelial cell damage, or the production of immune complexes (Neame, 1980). Circulating immune-complexes are probably involved in the pathogenesis of TTP associated with bacterial endocarditis (Ruggenenti and Remuzzi, 1990). TTP may complicate Human Immunodeficiency Virus type 1 infection as well as Acquired Immunodeficiency Syndrome-related complex (Leaf et al., 1988). Elevated platelet-associated levels of IgG and IgM, and of the third and fourth complement component, suggest an immune-mediated pathogenesis of the syndrome (Leaf et al., 1988).

### 3.1.2. Primary forms of TTP

Quite often, patients with TTP have no discernible underlying disease or pathological condition. In these cases the disease is defined as idiopathic TTP. The patients within the idiopathic group are quite heterogeneous; some may have a rapid fatal course with multi-organ failure while others have no neurological or renal manifestations (reviewed in Furlan, 2003).

Recurrent episodes of TTP are not exceptions, but relapses cannot be predicted by any clinical or hematological feature. A congenital chronic relapsing form of TTP was reported by Schulman et al. (1960), who suggested that the disorder was due to hereditary deficiency of a platelet-stimulating factor in the patient's plasma. A similar syndrome was later described in another patient by Upshaw (1978). The chronic relapsing form of TTP has been occasionally described in the literature as Upshaw–Schulman syndrome (reviewed in Furlan, 2003). Based on cases of TTP occurring in siblings, a genetic predisposition has been suggested, and recent genetic studies documented that an autosomal recessive trait underlies this form of TTP (Fuchs et al., 1976). These genetic cases are very rare and represent a small proportion of all TTP ($\sim 10\%$).

## 3.2. The clinical syndrome

As in HUS, the lesions consist of vessel wall thickening (mainly arterioles or capillaries), with endothelial cell swelling and/or detachments from the basement membrane and accumulation of fluffy material in subendothelial space, intraluminal platelet thrombosis, and partial or complete obstruction of the vessel lumina. Thrombocytopenia is the likely consequence of platelet consumption in the microcirculation. The mechanism underlying hemolytic anemia is not as clear, but it may be a consequence of the mechanical fragmentation of erythrocytes during flow through partially occluded microvessels. Peripheral smear shows fragmented red blood cells with the typical picture of burr or helmet cells. Elevations in lactate dehydrogenase (LDH) and low or undetectable haptoglobin levels are markers of hemolysis (Kennedy et al., 1980). The reticulocyte count is almost invariably elevated, Coomb's test is negative. Prothrombin time, partial thromboplastin time (PTT), factor V, factor VIII, and fibrinogen are normal in most cases. In some patients, high levels of fibrin degradation products and prolonged thrombin time have been observed.

The clinical presentation is dominated in most patients by hemorrhage and neurological symptoms (Kennedy et al., 1980). In over 90% of cases, purpura is the initial manifestation, which may or may not be associated with retinal hemorrhage, epistaxis, gingival bleeding, hematuria, gastrointestinal hemorrhage, menorrhagia, and hemoptysis (reviewed in Ruggenenti and Remuzzi, 1990). More rare symptoms are malaise, fatigue, pallor, abdominal pain, arthralgia, myalgia, and jaundice (Ruggenenti and Remuzzi, 1990). Although fever is not frequently seen at onset, it is almost always present during the illness (Ruggenenti and Remuzzi, 1990). Anemia is severe, with average values between 7 and 9 g/dl of hemoglobin (Ruggenenti and Remuzzi, 1990). Transient and fluctuating neurological manifestations are present in almost all patients (Silverstein, 1968). These symptoms include confusion, headache, paresis, aphasia, dysarthria, visual problems, and coma. Angiographic and electroencephalographic studies have not been extensively performed but do not appear to offer major diagnostic contributions. Ocular involvement is frequent, retinal, and choroid hemorrhages being the most common manifestations.

Renal involvement is common, with proteinuria and microhematuria the most constant findings (Kennedy et al., 1980; Ruggenenti and Remuzzi, 1990). Renal function is depressed in 40–80% of patients, although severe renal insufficiency is rare (Ruggenenti and Remuzzi, 1990). For this reason TTP has been closely intertwined with HUS, as evidenced by frequent use of the hybrid term HUS/TTP in the literature (Galbusera et al., 1999; Remuzzi et al., 2002a). Cardiac involvement is infrequent, although congestive heart failure and conduction disturbances have occasionally been reported (Ruggenenti and Remuzzi, 1990). In rare instances, lungs may contain some alveolar and interstitial infiltrates (Ruggenenti and Remuzzi, 1990). Abdominal pain has been reported in 10–30% of cases (Ruggenenti and Remuzzi, 1990) and it has been interpreted as secondary to the involvement of small vessels of the gastrointestinal tract. Pancreatitis has also been described.

Mortality was very high (80–90%) until PE therapy was introduced. When treated with plasma infusion or PE, 70–90% of patients survive the acute episodes. However, relapse occurs in more than one-third of the patients who achieve remission, contributing to further morbidity and mortality. A subset of patients develops chronic TTP, requiring long-term PE (Galbusera et al., 2006).

## 3.3. Pathogenesis

The hypotheses concerning the pathogenesis of TTP are controversial and suggest different mechanisms are responsible for the development of the disorder.

### 3.3.1. Endothelial damage and dysfunction

Endothelial injury has been considered as the central and likely inciting factor that sustains the microangiopathic process. As early as in 1942, Mark Altschule of Harvard Medical School suggested that microvascular endothelial activation was the primary event causing platelet deposition in arterioles and capillaries with secondary clearance of enormous number of platelets from the circulation (Altschule, 1942). Actually, of the agents that have been associated with the disease in subsequent years, all are toxic to microvascular endothelium (Remuzzi and Ruggenenti, 1994). Moreover, plasma from patients with acute TTP induces cytotoxicity (Ruiz-Torres et al., 2005) and apoptosis of human endothelial cells from the microvasculature but not from large vessels.

Antibodies and immune complexes can induce endothelial injury and trigger massive sequestration of platelets and polymorphonuclear leukocytes in the microvasculature, as in acute allograft rejection in humans. It is likely that circulating antibodies or immune-complexes or both play a pathogenetic role in the development of TTP in the course of connective tissue disorders, such as SLE, Sjögren's syndrome, rheumatoid arthritis, and polyarteritis. The most frequent association is with SLE, although the percent incidence varies in the different reports (reviewed in Ruggenenti and Remuzzi, 1990). Occasional patients with idiopathic TTP have cytotoxic antibodies to cultured endothelial cells in vitro (Galbusera et al., 2006). This cytotoxicity is complement-dependent and related to the IgG fraction of immunoglobulins.

Virtually all properties of normal microvascular endothelium are altered in TTP. Endothelial cells synthesize many substances involved in coagulation and fibrinolysis, including prostacyclin, nitric oxide (NO), VWF, thrombomodulin, tissue-type plasminogen activator inhibitor, and protein S. Loss of prostacyclin (Galbusera et al., 2006) and increase in VWF (Galbusera et al., 2006) have been claimed to account for the loss of physiologic thromboresistance and for the consequent widespread platelet aggregation in vascular beds throughout the body, creating a cycle of vasoconstriction with platelet and fibrin deposition and further thrombus formation. Damaged endothelial cells may favor platelet activation and aggregation at the site of endothelial injury.

### 3.3.2. Enhanced platelet aggregation and abnormal von Willebrand factor release and processing

Several groups have attempted to identify platelet-aggregating factors responsible for the formation of disseminated microvascular platelet thrombi in plasma from patients with TTP. These include a 37 kDa protein isolated from plasma of patients with acute TTP (Lian et al., 1992), and a calcium-dependent cysteine protease found in the sera of TTP patients during the acute phase of the disease but not in remission (Murphy et al., 1987). However these results were not confirmed subsequently and this line of research was abandoned. The putative aggregating agent in TTP remained elusive until 1982, when Moake et al. (1982) demonstrated that the plasma of these patients contained highly thrombogenic forms of the multimeric glycoprotein VWF, a major adhesive protein contained in endothelial cells, platelets, and plasma.

In normal individuals, VWF is formed as ultra-large (UL) multimers due to the polymerization in endothelial cells and megakaryocytes of a native subunit with apparent molecular mass of 225 kDa, and is stored as such in Weibel–Palade bodies and platelet α-granules. ULVWF multimers do not normally circulate, since they are rapidly reduced into smaller multimers soon after their secretion by cleavage at position 842 Tyr-843 Met of the mature subunit. In vivo evidence that proteolytic cleavage is involved in the modification of plasma multimers after secretion has been provided by studies showing that circulating VWF multimers are heterogeneous oligomers of a native 225-kDa subunit and of proteolytic fragments with apparent molecular masses of 189–176 and 140 kDa (Dent et al., 1991). In patients with TTP, in contrast to healthy subjects, UL multimers similar to the ones stored in endothelial cells and platelets, were occasionally detected in plasma (Moake and McPherson, 1989). The presence in patients with TTP of circulating UL multimers, which in vitro are capable of supporting platelet aggregation more efficiently than normal multimers, was taken as evidence for their pathogenic role in microvascular thrombi (Moake, 1998). However, direct proof that this was indeed the case was never provided. In patients with TTP who recovered after a single episode, ULVWF multimers were found almost exclusively in the acute phase but no longer in remission, suggesting a massive release from storage sites of acutely injured endothelial cells which possibly transiently overwhelmed the plasma proteolytic capacity (Moake, 1998). In contrast, those cases who had a tendency to recur had circulating ULVWF multimers sometimes in the acute and consistently in the remission phase of the disease, which was taken as evidence of a state of persistent endothelial perturbation (Moake, 1998).

On the other hand, patients with TTP often show increased VWF fragmentation during the acute phase, as indirectly documented by increase of low-molecular weight (LMW) multimers and decrease of high-molecular weight (HMW) multimers and a lower HMW:LMW multimer ratio, than at remission (Galbusera et al., 1999). VWF susceptibility to fragmentation increases in response to rising levels of shear stress (Tsai et al., 1994) that induces protein unfolding and makes VWF proteolytic cleavage sites more accessible to specific plasma protease(s). It is therefore speculated that enhanced shear stress in the severely narrowed damaged microvessels accounts for the abnormal VWF fragmentation observed during the acute phase of TTP. Evidence of increased capacity of fragmented VWF to bind receptors on activated platelets would suggest that shear stress-induced VWF fragmentation may contribute to the maintenance and extension of microvascular thrombosis. Consistent with this possibility in patients with recurrent and sporadic TTP, increased VWF fragmentation normalized after resolution of the microangiopathic process (Galbusera et al., 2006).

### 3.3.3. VWF cleavage by ADAMTS 13

The hypothesis that circulating ULVWF multimers in patients with recurrent TTP may just reflect a condition of endothelial perturbation, has been recently challenged by findings that circulating UL multimers in those patients were associated with a reduced or totally absent activity of the VWF-cleaving protease activity that normally cleaves VWF multimers to smaller molecular forms.

A major contribution to the understanding of VWF processing has been provided by Furlan et al. (1998) and Tsai (Tsai and Lian, 1998), who partially purified and characterized a plasma metalloprotease that physiologically reduces ULVWF multimers by cleaving VWF at the peptide bond between amino acid residues 842Tyr and 843Met in the A2 domain of the subunit. The protease, of ~170 kDa, needs bivalent cations for its activation, is inhibited by calcium-chelating agents and is activated only in conditions of low ionic strength or high shear stress. In 2001, the protease was identified as ADAMTS13, the thirteenth member of the ADAMTS (a disintegrin and metalloprotease with thrombospondin type 1 domains) family (Levy et al., 2001). This metalloprotease is expressed by the homonymous gene restricted on chromosome 9q34 and data are available that suggest that mutations in this gene lead to an inactive enzyme (Levy et al., 2001) and predispose to TTP.

ADAMTS13, expressed predominantly in liver, is one of the largest protein of the ADAMTS family, containing 1427 amino acid residues and consisting of a N-terminal signal peptide, a propeptide, a reprolysin-like metalloprotease domain, a disintegrin-like domain, a first thrombospondin type 1 motif (Tsp1), a cysteine-rich domain, a spacer domain, seven additional Tsp-1 repeats, and two CUB domains (Fig. 3). Hepatic stellate cells have been considered to be the primary source for human plasma ADAMTS13 (Furlan, 2003).

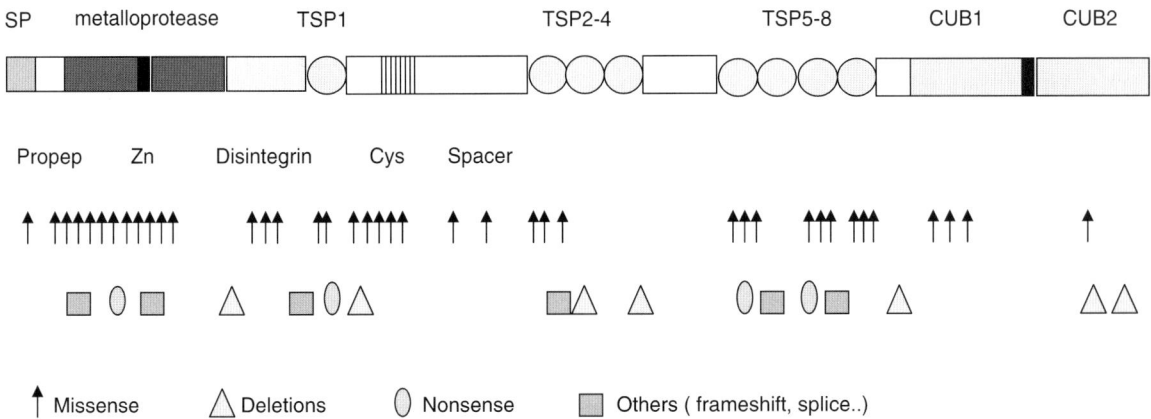

Figure 3. Depiction of the domain structure of ADAMTS13. SP, signal peptide; Cys, cysteine-rich domain; TSP, thrombospondin type 1 motif. The black bar delimits the essential domains for full activity in vitro. Below the ADAMTS13 structure are located the mutations reported to date in patients with TTP.

However recent studies documented that human endothelial cells also synthesize and release ADAMTS13 (Turner et al., 2006). ADAMTS13 was preferentially sorted into the apical compartment of ECV304, an endothelium-derived cell line, and apical sorting depended on the two CUB domains and their association with lipid rafts (Shang et al., 2006). ADAMTS13 was also detected in platelet lysates and on the platelet surface (Liu et al., 2005).

ADAMTS13 is constitutively active in the circulation with a narrow range of activity (70–120%) in normal individuals. Recombinant expression studies revealed that the metalloprotease domain alone is unable to cleave the Tyr–Met bond, but it cleaves the VWF substrate at a different site and with a lower efficiency. The addition of one or more proximal carboxyl-terminal domains (including the disintegrin, the Tsp1-1, the cystein-rich, and the spacer domains) restored substrate specificity. Full proteolytic activity, however was not achieved until all of the proximal carboxyl-terminal domains were added (Ai et al., 2005; Fig. 3). On the other hand, protein truncated after the spacer domain remained proteolytically active toward plasma VWF and appeared to be hyperactive toward unusually large VWF that were newly released from cultured endothelial cells, raising the hypothesis that the C-terminal region—including the Tsp1-2-8 repeats and the two CUB domains—may negatively regulate ADAMTS13 activity (Tao et al., 2005). Physiologic concentrations of chloride ions have been shown to inhibit the hydrolysis of VWF by ADAMTS13. This effect is due to the specific binding of chloride ions to VWF, which stabilizes the folded conformation of the A1–A2–A3 domains (De Cristofaro et al., 2006).

The only known function of ADAMTS13 is the proteolytic processing of VWF but, through its complex structure, ADAMTS13 has the potential to interact with several molecules. In fact, CUB domains are found in developmentally regulated proteins and may have a role in protein–protein interactions (Bork and Beckmann, 1993), the Tsp1 repeats are known to mediate extracellular matrix protein–protein interactions (Bornstein, 2001) and the cystein-rich domain contains an RGD sequence that can interact with integrins (Ruoslahti and Pierschbacher, 1986).

### 3.3.4. ADAMTS 13 deficiency in TTP

Two primary mechanisms for deficiency of the ADAMTS13 activity have been identified in patients with TTP, namely a constitutive deficiency and the presence of a circulating acquired inhibitory antibody (Furlan et al., 1998; Tsai and Lian, 1998).

Patients affected by Upshaw–Schulman syndrome (Upshaw, 1978), which is synonymous with hereditary TTP (Moake, 2002), suffer from severe deficiency of ADAMTS13 caused by heterozygous or homozygous ADAMTS13 gene mutations. In these forms the deficiency is inherited as an autosomal recessive trait. Consistent with this possibility, in the first report on the VWF cleaving protease activity in TTP (Furlan et al., 1997), undetectable ADAMTS13 activity was found in two brothers with chronic relapsing TTP, whereas their parents had about half normal protease activity. Of interest, in both patients with constitutional protease deficiency, disease remission achieved by plasma therapy was concurrent with an almost full recovery of the VWF-cleaving protease activity. Both patients achieved a long lasting remission, although protease activity decreased to less than 20% over 20 days after plasma therapy withdrawal.

To date around 60 ADAMTS13 mutations has been identified in patients with the familial form of TTP (Tsai, 2006; Fig. 3). The mutations have been found along the entire ADAMTS13 gene and no clustering is evident, although more than 70% of them are located from the metalloprotease through the Tsp1-1-2 domains. Studies on secretion and activity of the mutated forms of the protease showed that most of these mutations led to an impaired secretion from the cell, and, when the mutated protein was secreted, the proteolytic activity was greatly reduced (Kokame et al., 2002, 2004; Soejima et al., 2003; Matsumoto et al., 2004; Uchida et al., 2004; Donadelli et al., 2006; Shibagaki et al., 2006; Tsai, 2006).

The patients often present during the neonatal period with periodic episodes of thrombocytopenia and microangiopathic hemolysis that improve quickly on plasma infusion. In patients with less severe disease, TTP may first present later in life and relapse sporadically. Acute renal failure occurs in around 20% of cases (Noris et al., 2005; Tsai, 2006).

In non-familial cases the protease deficiency appears to be a consequence of a specific autoantibody that develops transiently and tends to disappear during remission (Furlan et al., 1998; Tsai and Lian, 1998). These inhibitory anti-ADAMTS13 antibodies, characterized as IgG (Furlan et al., 1998), have been detected in 48–80% of patients with acquired TTP (Veyradier et al., 2001). Recent studies demonstrated that in all the patients with acquired TTP and anti-ADAMTS13 antibodies tested, there were inhibitory anti-protease antibodies reacting against the cystein-rich and spacer domains of recombinant ADAMTS13 (Soejima et al., 2003). In some cases the antibodies were directed only against these epitopes, but in the majority of plasma samples from TTP patients different combinations of antibodies against the propeptide, the Tsp1 and the CUB domains (Klaus et al., 2004) were found, suggesting a polyclonal autoantibody response. The inhibitory IgG autoantibodies, in addition to binding and inhibiting ADAMTS13 proteolytic activity, also accelerate ADAMTS13 clearance (Shelat et al., 2006).

The discovery of deficient ADAMTS13 activity in TTP has been rapidly integrated into the prevailing model of the pathophysiology of VWF-mediated thrombotic microangiopathies. According to this model, congenital or autoimmune dysfunction of ADAMTS13 prevents the normal proteolysis of large VWF multimers as they are secreted from injured endothelial cells (Fig. 4). This event ultimately causes the development of circulating ULVWF. Results of the analysis of the relationship between VWF multimeric pattern and ADAMTS13 activity in TTP patients may offer alternative explanations. On one hand, ULVWF multimers were found in TTP patients with normal ADAMTS13 activity. On the other hand, many TTP patients with complete or severe deficiency of the ADAMTS13 activity did not have ULVWF multimers in their circulation (Galbusera et al., 1999). In addition, patients with deficiency of ADAMTS13 activity showed more VWF fragmentation during the acute phase, than at remission

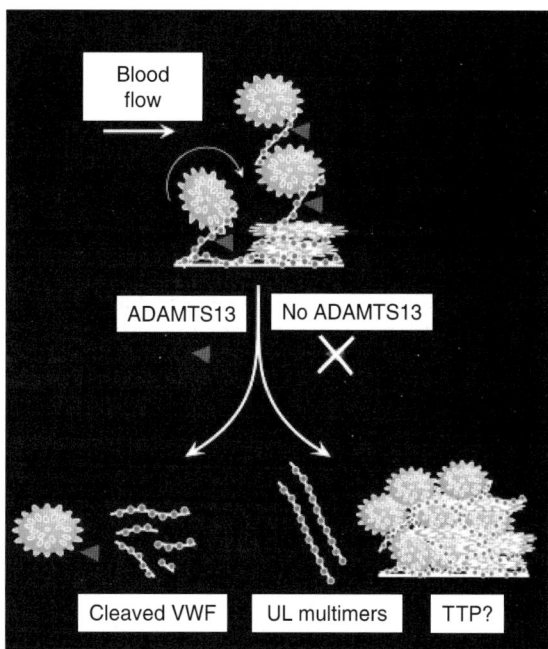

**Figure 4.** Representation of mechanisms leading to microvascular thrombosis in condition of ADAMTS13 deficiency. When a large VWF multimer is attached to an injured vessel, it is conformationally unfolded by high levels of wall shear stress (blood flow) to an elongated form, providing the substrate for platelet adhesion. In the normal circulation VWF and platelets do not interact to form aggregates because ADAMTS13 cleaves the VWF multimers whenever one or more of its cleavage sites are exposed by shear stress. In the absence of ADAMTS13, VWF multimers eventually become fully unfolded by shear stress, causing intravascular platelet thrombosis characteristics of TTP.

(Galbusera et al., 1999). The same results were reported by Veyradier et al. (2001), who found no correlation between ADAMTS13 activity levels and UL multimers in their large series. It was also found that the normal 189-, 176-, and 140-kDa (Galbusera et al., 1999; Remuzzi et al., 2002a) fragments were present in the blood of all patients with deficient ADAMTS13 activity, and the percentage of the native intact VWF subunit was even lower than in healthy subjects, at least in the acute phase. These results indicate that besides ADAMTS13, other protease(s) are present in the blood that cleave VWF to the normal fragments and support the possibility that deficiency of the ADAMTS13 activity is not the only determinant of VWF abnormalities in this disease.

Finally, it is becoming clear that complete loss of ADAMTS13 activity is necessary but not sufficient to initiate an acute episode of TTP. This is supported by data that some subjects with complete ADAMTS13 deficiency may present the first disease symptoms in adulthood or may even never manifest TTP in their life (Noris et al., 2005). Consistently, mice with targeted disruption of the *ADAMTS13* gene do not have any evidence of thrombocytopenia, hemolytic anemia, or microvascular thrombosis, although thrombocytopenia was more readily induced in homozygotes in comparison with wild-type mice after intravenous injection of collagen and epinephrine (Banno et al., 2006). However, challenge of ADAMTS13 deficient mice with Stx resulted in a striking syndrome closely resembling human TTP (Motto et al., 2005). These results may be interpreted as indicating that factors in addition to ADAMTS13 deficiency, such as agents that induce endothelial cell perturbation, may be necessary for development of TTP.

### 3.3.5. Specificity of ADAMTS13 deficiency for TTP

Much debate in recent years has focused on whether it was possible or not to make a differential diagnosis between TTP and HUS. The latter syndrome has in common with TTP microangiopathic hemolytic anemia, consumption thrombocytopenia, and microvascular thrombosis, but differs because of severe renal failure at presentation (Noris and Remuzzi, 2005). However after examination of very large series of patients with HUS and TTP, it has become apparent that a clear distinction between the two syndromes is difficult.

In two large clinical studies (Furlan et al., 1998; Tsai and Lian, 1998), deficiency of ADAMTS13 activity was found in patients with a diagnosis of TTP but not in those with HUS. The observation generated the paradigm that TTP is due to a deficiency of ADAMTS13 activity, which is not involved in the pathogenesis of HUS (Moake, 1998). However, further investigations (Veyradier et al., 2001; Remuzzi et al., 2002a; Vesely et al., 2003) based on a large series of patients with TTP and HUS challenged this hypothesis and has given rise to a debate on whether a severe deficiency of ADAMTS13 activity is enough to distinguish TTP from HUS (Remuzzi, 2003; Tsai, 2003). Indeed not all cases of thrombotic microangiopathy diagnosed as TTP due to the prevalence of neurological symptoms have low or undetectable ADAMTS13 activity. On the other hand, even if most cases of thrombotic microangiopathy diagnosed as HUS for the prevalence of renal symptoms have normal ADAMTS13 there are unequivocal cases of HUS characterized by low or undetectable protease levels (Veyradier et al., 2001; Remuzzi et al., 2002a). A recent report (Noris et al., 2005) on a family with two sisters affected with thrombotic microangiopathy, one presenting with neurological symptoms only and the other one with superimposed severe renal impairment, has offered a genetic explanation for cases with severe ADAMTS13 deficiency and clinical symptoms overlapping those of HUS. The two patients had complete ADAMTS13 deficiency due to two heterozygous gene mutations. However, a heterozygous mutation in the gene encoding for factor H of complement was also found in the patient who developed chronic renal failure but not in her sister with exclusive neurological symptoms (Noris et al., 2005). Since mutations in factor H gene have been found in around 30% of familial cases of HUS, it was hypothesized that in the above patient, factor H haploinsufficiency had a role in determining the renal complications that superimposed on the systemic disease caused by ADAMTS13 deficiency.

### 3.4. Treatment

Differential diagnosis between TTP associated with genetic or immune-mediated ADAMTS13 deficiency is important to predict disease outcome and to guide specific treatments. Disease related to genetic defects may affect different members of the same family and tend to recur more times in the same individual (familial and recurrent TTP). Immune-mediated disease does not cluster in families, may unmask an underlying autoimmune disease, or may follow the exposure to certain drugs. The persistence of anti-ADAMTS13 antibodies during the remission phase may indicate a risk of relapse. The rationale of treatment is also different, replacement with plasma of the defective activity being the key component of treatment of genetic disease and clearance of the autoantibody by PE, or inhibition of its production by immunosuppressive agents, being the main target of treatment in immune-mediated disease (reviewed in George, 2000, 2006). Although a case series suggested that cryosupernatant plasma, which is deficient in VWF, may be superior to fresh-frozen plasma as a replacement product in PE, a small randomized trial failed to confirm this (Rock et al., 1996; Zeigler et al., 2001). Recently, in immune-mediated TTP, the infusion of rituximab, an antibody directed against the B cells, has been proved to be effective in inducing remission in patients refractory to any other treatment (Zeigler et al., 2001) and to maintain patients in remission when used as prophylactic therapy (Galbusera et al., 2005). Longitudinal evaluation of ADAMTS13 activity and of the levels of the autoantibodies is also important to monitor patient response to treatment.

### Key points

- Despite a substantial increase in our understanding of the pathogenesis of Stx-associated HUS there remains no effective treatment apart from supportive measures.
- Recent studies show that at least 50% of patients with aHUS will have an abnormality of one or more of the complement components factor H, MCP, factor I, factor B, and C3. This offers the hope of logical targeted treatment with either recombinant or purified proteins.
- Renal transplantation in aHUS patients with either a factor H or factor I abnormality is associated with a high risk of the disease recurrence post transplant. Combined liver and kidney transplantation has been shown to be an effective treatment in these patients.
- The finding that deficiency of or antibodies against ADAMTS13 antibodies are associated with TTP has led to the introduction of new therapies such as Rituximab for this condition.

## Acknowledgments

This work has been partially supported by grants from Comitato 30 ore per la vita, from Telethon (grant nos. GPP02161 and GPP02162) and from the Foundation for Research in Transplantation. THJG is supported by the Robin Davis Trust and the Foundation for Children with aHUS.

## References

Acheson, D.W., Moore, R., De Breucker, S., et al. 1996. Translocation of Shiga toxin across polarized intestinal cells in tissue culture. Infect. Immun. 64, 3294–3300.

Ai, J., Smith, P., Wang, S., et al. 2005. The proximal carboxyl-terminal domains of ADAMTS13 determine substrate specificity and are all required for cleavage of von Willebrand factor. J. Biol. Chem. 280, 29428–29434.

Altschule, M. 1942. A rare type of acute thrombocytopenic purpura: widespread formation of platelet thrombi in capillaries. N. Engl. J. Med. 227, 477–479.

Artz, M.A., Steenbergen, E.J., Hoitsma, A.J., et al. 2003. Renal transplantation in patients with hemolytic uremic syndrome: high rate of recurrence and increased incidence of acute rejections. Transplantation 76, 821–826.

Banatvala, N., Griffin, P.M., Greene, K.D., et al. 2001. The United States National Prospective Hemolytic Uremic Syndrome Study: microbiologic, serologic, clinical, and epidemiologic findings. J. Infect. Dis. 183, 1063–1070.

Banno, F., Kokame, K., Okuda, T., et al. 2006. Complete deficiency in ADAMTS13 is prothrombotic, but it alone is not sufficient to cause thrombotic thrombocytopenic purpura. Blood 107, 3161–3166.

Beatty, M.E., Griffin, P.M., Tulu, A.N., et al. 2004. Culturing practices and antibiotic use in children with diarrhoea. Pediatrics 113, 628–629.

Becker, S., Fusco, G., Fusco, J., et al. 2004. HIV-associated thrombotic microangiopathy in the era of highly active antiretroviral therapy: an observational study. Clin. Infect. Dis. 39 (Suppl. 5), S267–S275.

Bennett, C.L., Connors, J.M., Carwile, J.M., et al. 2000. Thrombotic thrombocytopenic purpura associated with clopidogrel. N. Engl. J. Med. 342, 1773–1777.

Bennett, C.L., Weinberg, P.D., Rozenberg-Ben-Dror, K., et al. 1998. Thrombotic thrombocytopenic purpura associated with ticlopidine. A review of 60 cases. Ann. Intern. Med. 128, 541–544.

Berns, J.S., Kaplan, B.S., Mackow, R.C., et al. 1992. Inherited hemolytic uremic syndrome in adults. Am. J. Kidney Dis. 19, 331–334.

Bhimma, R., Rollins, N.C., Coovadia, H.M., et al. 1997. Post-dysenteric hemolytic uremic syndrome in children during an epidemic of Shigella dysentery in Kwazulu/Natal. Pediatr. Nephrol. 11, 560–564.

Bitzan, M., Richardson, S., Huang, C., et al. 1994. Evidence that verotoxins (Shiga-like toxins) from *Escherichia coli* bind to P blood group antigens of human erythrocytes in vitro. Infect. Immun. 62, 3337–3347.

Bork, P., Beckmann, G. 1993. The CUB domain. A widespread module in developmentally regulated proteins. J. Mol. Biol. 231, 539–545.

Bornstein, P. 2001. Thrombospondins as matricellular modulators of cell function. J. Clin. Invest. 107, 929–934.

Bresin, E., Daina, E., Noris, M., et al. 2006. Outcome of renal transplantation in patients with non-Shiga toxin-associated hemolytic uremic syndrome: prognostic significance of genetic background. Clin. J. Am. Soc. Nephrol. 1, 88–99.

Brigotti, M., Alfieri, R., Sestili, P., et al. 2002. Damage to nuclear DNA induced by Shiga toxin 1 and ricin in human endothelial cells. FASEB J. 16, 365–372.

Brooks, J.T., Bergmire-Sweat, D., Kennedy, M., et al. 2004. Outbreak of Shiga toxin-producing *Escherichia coli* O111:H8 infections among attendees of a high school cheerleading camp. Clin. Infect. Dis. 38, 190–198.

Bukowski, R.M. 1982. Thrombotic thrombocytopenic purpura: a review. Prog. Hemost. Thromb. 6, 287–337.

Burke, G.W., Ciancio, G., Cirocco, R., et al. 1999. Microangiopathy in kidney and simultaneous pancreas/kidney recipients treated with tacrolimus: evidence of endothelin and cytokine involvement. Transplantation 68, 1336–1342.

Caletti, M.G., Lejarraga, H., Kelmansky, D., et al. 2004. Two different therapeutic regimes in patients with sequelae of hemolytic-uremic syndrome. Pediatr. Nephrol. 19, 1148–1152.

Caprioli, A., Luzzi, I., Rosmini, F., et al. 1992. Hemolytic-uremic syndrome and Vero cytotoxin-producing *Escherichia coli* infection in Italy. The HUS Italian Study Group. J. Infect. Dis. 166, 154–158.

Caprioli, J., Bettinaglio, P., Zipfel, P.F., et al. 2001. The molecular basis of familial hemolytic uremic syndrome: mutation analysis of factor H gene reveals a hot spot in short consensus repeat 20. J. Am. Soc. Nephrol. 12, 297–307.

Caprioli, J., Castelletti, F., Bucchioni, S., et al. 2003. Complement factor H mutations and gene polymorphisms in haemolytic uraemic syndrome: the C-257T, the A2089G and the G2881T polymorphisms are strongly associated with the disease. Hum. Mol. Genet. 12, 3385–3395.

Caprioli, J., Noris, M., Brioschi, S., et al. 2006. Genetics of HUS: the impact of MCP, CFH and IF mutations on clinical presentation, response to treatment, and outcome. Blood 108, 1267–1279.

Carreras, L., Romero, R., Requesens, C., et al. 1981. Familial hypocomplementemic hemolytic uremic syndrome with HLA-A3,B7 haplotype. JAMA 245, 602–604.

Chandler, W.L., Jelacic, S., Boster, D.R., et al. 2002. Prothrombotic coagulation abnormalities preceding the hemolytic-uremic syndrome. N. Engl. J. Med. 346, 23–32.

Chiurchiu, C., Firrincieli, A., Santostefano, M., et al. 2003. Adult nondiarrhoea hemolytic uremic syndrome associated with Shiga toxin *Escherichia coli* O157:H7 bacteremia and urinary tract infection. Am. J. Kidney Dis. 41, E4.

Cimolai, N., Carter, J.E., Morrison, B.J., et al. 1990. Risk factors for the progression of *Escherichia coli* O157:H7 enteritis to hemolytic-uremic syndrome. J. Pediatr. 116, 589–592.

Cleary, T.G. 1988. Cytotoxin-producing *Escherichia coli* and the hemolytic uremic syndrome. Pediatr. Clin. North Am. 35, 485–501.

Cody, S.H., Glynn, M.K., Farrar, J.A., et al. 1999. An outbreak of *Escherichia coli* O157:H7 infection from unpasteurized commercial apple juice. Ann. Intern. Med. 130, 202–209.

Conlon, P.J., Brennan, D.C., Pfaf, W.W., et al. 1996. Renal transplantation in adults with thrombotic thrombocytopenic purpura/haemolytic-uraemic syndrome. Nephrol. Dial. Transplant. 11, 1810–1814.

Conlon, P.J., Howell, D.N., Macik, G., et al. 1995. The renal manifestations and outcome of thrombotic thrombocytopenic purpura hemolytic-uremic syndrome in adults. Nephrol. Dial. Transplant. 10, 1189–1193.

Constantinescu, A.R., Bitzan, M., Weiss, L.S., et al. 2004. Non-enteropathic hemolytic uremic syndrome: causes and short-term course. Am. J. Kidney Dis. 43, 976–982.

Cooling, L.L., Walker, K.E., Gille, T., et al. 1998. Shiga toxin binds human platelets via globotriaosylceramide (Pk antigen) and a novel platelet glycosphingolipid. Infect. Immun. 66, 4355–4366.

Date, A., Raghupathy, P., Jadhav, M., et al. 1982. Outcome of the haemolytic-uraemic syndrome complicating bacillary dysentery. Ann. Trop. Paediatr. 2, 1–6.

De Cristofaro, R., Peyvandi, F., Baronciani, L., et al. 2006. Molecular mapping of the chloride binding site in von Willebrand factor (VWF): energetics and conformational effects on the VWF/ADAMTS-13 interaction. J. Biol. Chem. 288, 30400–30411.

Dent, J.A., Galbusera, M., Ruggeri, Z.M. 1991. Heterogeneity of plasma von Willebrand factor multimers resulting from proteolysis of the constituent subunit. J. Clin. Invest. 88, 774–782.

Dlott, J.S., Danielson, C.F., Blue-Hnidy, D.E., et al. 2004. Drug-induced thrombotic thrombocytopenic purpura/hemolytic uremic syndrome: a concise review. Ther. Apher. Dial. 8, 102–111.

Donadelli, R., Banterla, F., Galbusera, M., et al. 2006. In-vitro and in-vivo consequences of mutations in the von Willebrand factor cleaving protease ADAMTS13 in thrombotic thrombocytopenic purpura. Thromb. Haemost. 96, 454–464.

Donnenberg, M.S., Tzipori, S., McKee, M.L., et al. 1993. The role of the eae gene of enterohemorrhagic *Escherichia coli* in intimate attachment in vitro and in a porcine model. J. Clin. Invest. 92, 1418–1424.

Dragon-Durey, M.A., Fremeaux-Bacchi, V., Loirat, C., et al. 2004. Heterozygous and homozygous factor H deficiencies associated with hemolytic uremic syndrome or membranoproliferative glomerulonephritis: report and genetic analysis of 16 cases. J. Am. Soc. Nephrol. 15, 787–795.

Dragon-Durey, M.A., Loirat, C., Cloarec, S., et al. 2005. Anti-factor H autoantibodies associated with atypical hemolytic uremic syndrome. J. Am. Soc. Nephrol. 16, 555–563.

Ducloux, D., Rebibou, J.M., Semhoun-Ducloux, S., et al. 1998. Recurrence of hemolytic-uremic syndrome in renal transplant recipients: a meta-analysis. Transplantation 65, 1405–1407.

Erwert, R.D., Eiting, K.T., Tupper, J.C., et al. 2003. Shiga toxin induces decreased expression of the anti-apoptotic protein Mcl-1 concomitant with the onset of endothelial apoptosis. Microb. Pathog. 35, 87–93.

Esparza-Gordillo, J., Goicoechea de, J.E., Buil, A., et al. 2005. Predisposition to atypical hemolytic uremic syndrome involves the concurrence of different susceptibility alleles in the regulators of complement activation gene cluster in 1q32. Hum. Mol. Genet. 14, 703–712.

Esparza-Gordillo, J., Goicoechea de Jorge, E., Garrido, C.A., et al. 2006. Insights into hemolytic uremic syndrome: segregation of three independent predisposition factors in a large, multiple affected pedigree. Mol. Immunol. 43, 1769–1775.

Farmer, J.J., III, Davis, B.R. 1985. H7 antiserum-sorbitol fermentation medium: a single tube screening medium for detecting *Escherichia coli* O157:H7 associated with hemorrhagic colitis. J. Clin. Microbiol. 22, 620–625.

Ferraris, J.R., Ramirez, J.A., Ruiz, S., et al. 2002. Shiga toxin-associated hemolytic uremic syndrome: absence of recurrence after renal transplantation. Pediatr. Nephrol. 17, 809–814.

Fraser, M.E., Chernaia, M.M., Kozlov, Y.V., et al. 1994. Crystal structure of the holotoxin from *Shigella dysenteriae* at 2.5 Å resolution. Nat. Struct. Biol. 1, 59–64.

Fraser, M.E., Fujinaga, M., Cherney, M.M., et al. 2004. Structure of Shiga toxin type 2 (Stx2) from *Escherichia coli* O157:H7. J. Biol. Chem. 279, 27511–27517.

Fremeaux-Bacchi, V., Dragon-Durey, M., Blouin, J., et al. 2004. Complement factor I: a susceptibility gene for atypical hemolytic-uremic syndrome. J. Med. Genet. 41, e84.

Fremeaux-Bacchi, V., Kemp, E.J., Goodship, J.A., et al. 2005. The development of atypical haemolytic-uraemic syndrome is influenced by susceptibility factors in factor H and membrane cofactor protein: evidence from two independent cohorts. J. Med. Genet. 42, 852–856.

Fremeaux-Bacchi, V., Moulton, E.A., Kavanagh, D., et al. 2006. Genetic and functional analyses of membrane cofactor protein (CD46) mutations in atypical hemolytic uremic syndrome. J. Am. Soc. Nephrol. 17, 2017–2025.

Fremeaux-Bacchi, V., Regnier, C.H., Blouin, J., et al. 2007. Protective or aggressive: paradoxical role of C3 in atypical hemolytic uremic syndrome. Mol. Immunol. 44, 172.

Fuchs, W.E., George, J.N., Dotin, L.N., et al. 1976. Thrombotic thrombocytopenic purpura. Occurrence two years apart during late pregnancy in two sisters. JAMA 235, 2126–2127.

Furlan, M. 2003. Deficient activity of von Willebrand factor-cleaving protease in thrombotic thrombocytopenic purpura. Expert Rev. Cardiovasc. Ther. 1, 243–255.

Furlan, M., Robles, R., Galbusera, M., et al. 1998. von Willebrand factor-cleaving protease in thrombotic thrombocytopenic purpura and the hemolytic-uremic syndrome. N. Engl. J. Med. 339, 1578–1584.

Furlan, M., Robles, R., Solenthaler, M., et al. 1997. Deficient activity of von Willebrand factor-cleaving protease in chronic relapsing thrombotic thrombocytopenic purpura. Blood 89, 3097–3103.

Galbusera, M., Bresin, E., Noris, M., et al. 2005. Rituximab prevents recurrence of thrombotic thrombocytopenic purpura: a case report. Blood 106, 925–928.

Galbusera, M., Noris, M., Remuzzi, G. 2006. Thrombotic thrombocytopenic purpura—then and now. Semin. Thromb. Hemost. 32, 81–89.

Galbusera, M., Noris, M., Rossi, C., et al. 1999. Increased fragmentation of von Willebrand factor, due to abnormal cleavage of the subunit, parallels disease activity in recurrent hemolytic uremic syndrome and thrombotic thrombocytopenic purpura and discloses predisposition in families. The Italian Registry of Familial and Recurrent HUS/TTP. Blood 94, 610–620.

Garg, A.X., Clark, W.F., Salvadori, M., et al. 2006. Absence of renal sequelae after childhood *Escherichia coli* O157:H7 gastroenteritis. Kidney Int. 70, 807–812.

Garg, A.X., Suri, R.S., Barrowman, N., et al. 2003. Long-term renal prognosis of diarrhoea-associated hemolytic uremic syndrome: a systematic review, meta-analysis, and meta-regression. JAMA 290, 1360–1370.

George, J.N. 2000. How I treat patients with thrombotic thrombocytopenic purpura-hemolytic uremic syndrome. Blood 96, 1223–1229.

George, J.N. 2003. The association of pregnancy with thrombotic thrombocytopenic purpura-hemolytic uremic syndrome. Curr. Opin. Hematol. 10, 339–344.

George, J.N. 2006. Clinical practice. Thrombotic thrombocytopenic purpura. N. Engl. J. Med. 354, 1927–1935.

Geraghty, M.T., Perlman, E.J., Martin, L.S., et al. 1992. Cobalamin C defect associated with hemolytic-uremic syndrome. J. Pediatr. 120, 934–937.

Goicoechea de Jorge, E., Harris, C.L., Esparza-Gordillo, J., et al. 2007. Gain-of-function mutations in complement factor B are associated with atypical hemolytic uremic syndrome. Proc. Natl. Acad. Sci. U.S.A. 104, 240–245.

Goodship, T.H.J., Liszewski, M.K., Kemp, E.J., et al. 2004. Mutations in CD46, a complement regulatory protein, predispose to atypical HUS. Trends Mol. Med. 10, 226–231.

Granger, C.B., Mahaffey, K.W., Weaver, W.D., et al. 2003. Pexelizumab, an anti-C5 complement antibody, as adjunctive therapy to primary percutaneous coronary intervention in acute myocardial infarction: the COMplement inhibition in Myocardial infarction treated with Angioplasty (COMMA) trial. Circulation 108, 1184–1190.

Griffin, P.M., Tauxe, R.V. 1991. The epidemiology of infections caused by *Escherichia coli* O157:H7, other enterohemorrhagic *E. coli*, and the associated hemolytic uremic syndrome. Epidemiol. Rev. 13, 60–98.

Guerin, P.J., Brasher, C., Baron, E., et al. 2003. *Shigella dysenteriae* serotype 1 in west Africa: intervention strategy for an outbreak in Sierra Leone. Lancet 362, 705–706.

Guessous, F., Marcinkiewicz, M., Polanowska-Grabowska, R., et al. 2005. Shiga toxin 2 and lipopolysaccharide induce human microvascular endothelial cells to release chemokines and factors that stimulate platelet function. Infect. Immun. 73, 8306–8316.

Guigonis, V., Fremeaux-Bacchi, V., Giraudier, S., et al. 2005. Late-onset thrombocytic microangiopathy caused by cblC disease: association with a factor H mutation. Am. J. Kidney Dis. 45, 588–595.

Hammar, S.P., Bloomer, H.A., McCloskey, D. 1978. Adult hemolytic uremic syndrome with renal arteriolar deposition of IgM and C3. Am. J. Clin. Pathol. 70, 434–439.

Heinen, S., Sanchez-Corral, P., Jackson, M.S., et al. 2006. De novo gene conversion in the RCA gene cluster (1q32) causes mutations in complement factor H associated with atypical hemolytic uremic syndrome. Hum. Mutat. 27, 292–293.

Hillmen, P., Hall, C., Marsh, J.C., et al. 2004. Effect of eculizumab on hemolysis and transfusion requirements in patients with paroxysmal nocturnal hemoglobinuria. N. Engl. J. Med. 350, 552–559.

Hogasen, K., Jansen, J.H., Mollnes, T.E., et al. 1995. Hereditary porcine membranoproliferative glomerulonephritis type-II is caused by factor-H deficiency. J. Clin. Invest. 95, 1054–1061.

Houdouin, V., Doit, C., Mariani, P., et al. 2004. A pediatric cluster of *Shigella dysenteriae* serotype 1 diarrhoea with hemolytic uremic syndrome in 2 families from France. Clin. Infect. Dis. 38, e96–e99.

Hourcade, D.E., Mitchell, L., Kuttner-Kondo, L.A., et al. 2002. Decay-accelerating factor (DAF), complement receptor 1 (CR1), and factor H dissociate the complement AP C3 convertase (C3bBb) via sites on the type A domain of Bb. J. Biol. Chem. 277, 1107–1112.

Hurley, B.P., Thorpe, C.M., Acheson, D.W. 2001. Shiga toxin translocation across intestinal epithelial cells is enhanced by neutrophil transmigration. Infect. Immun. 69, 6148–6155.

Jackson, M.P., Newland, J.W., Holmes, R.K., et al. 1987. Nucleotide sequence analysis of the structural genes for Shiga-like toxin I encoded by bacteriophage 933J from *Escherichia coli*. Microb. Pathog. 2, 147–153.

Jenkins, C., Willshaw, G.A., Evans, J., et al. 2003. Subtyping of virulence genes in verocytotoxin-producing *Escherichia coli* (VTEC) other than serogroup O157 associated with disease in the United Kingdom. J. Med. Microbiol. 52, 941–947.

Jozsi, M., Heinen, S., Hartmann, A., et al. 2006. Factor H and atypical hemolytic uremic syndrome: mutations in the C-terminus cause structural changes and defective recognition functions. J. Am. Soc. Nephrol. 17, 170–177.

Kaplan, B.S., Chesney, R.W., Drummond, K.N. 1975. Hemolytic uremic syndrome in families. N. Engl. J. Med. 292, 1090–1093.

Kaplan, B.S., Kaplan, P. 1992. Hemolytic uremic syndrome in families. In: B.S. Kaplan, R.S. Trompeter, J.L. Moake (Eds.), Hemolytic Uremic Syndrome and Thrombotic Thrombocytopenic Purpura. Marcel Dekker, New York, pp. 213–225.

Kaplan, B.S., Meyers, K.E., Schulman, S.L. 1998. The pathogenesis and treatment of hemolytic uremic syndrome. J. Am. Soc. Nephrol. 9, 1126–1133.

Kaplan, B.S., Papadimitriou, M., Brezin, J.H., et al. 1997. Renal transplantation in adults with autosomal recessive inheritance of hemolytic uremic syndrome. Am. J. Kidney Dis. 30, 760–765.

Karmali, M.A., Steele, B.T., Petric, M., et al. 1983. Sporadic cases of haemolytic-uraemic syndrome associated with faecal cytotoxin and cytotoxin-producing *Escherichia coli* in stools. Lancet 1, 619–620.

Kavanagh, D., Goodship, T.H.J., Richards, A. 2006. Atypical haemolytic uraemic syndrome. Br. Med. Bull., 77–78.

Kavanagh, D., Kemp, E.J., Mayland, E., et al. 2005. Mutations in complement factor I predispose to development of atypical hemolytic uremic syndrome. J. Am. Soc. Nephrol. 16, 2150–2155.

Kennedy, S.S., Zacharski, L.R., Beck, J.R. 1980. Thrombotic thrombocytopenic purpura: analysis of 48 unselected cases. Semin. Thromb. Hemost. 6, 341–349.

Klaus, C., Plaimauer, B., Studt, J.D., et al. 2004. Epitope mapping of ADAMTS13 autoantibodies in acquired thrombotic thrombocytopenic purpura. Blood 103, 4514–4519.

Klein, P.J., Bulla, M., Newman, R.A., et al. 1977. Thomsen-Friedenreich antigen in haemolytic-uraemic syndrome. Lancet 2, 1024–1025.

Kokame, K., Matsumoto, M., Fujimura, Y., et al. 2004. VWF73, a region from D1596 to R1668 of von Willebrand factor, provides a minimal substrate for ADAMTS-13. Blood 103, 607–612.

Kokame, K., Matsumoto, M., Soejima, K., et al. 2002. Mutations and common polymorphisms in ADAMTS13 gene responsible for von Willebrand factor-cleaving protease activity. Proc. Natl. Acad. Sci. U.S.A. 99, 11902–11907.

Lahlou, A., Lang, P., Charpentier, B., et al. 2000. Hemolytic uremic syndrome—recurrence after renal transplantation. Medicine 79, 90–102.

Leaf, A.N., Laubenstein, L.J., Raphael, B., et al. 1988. Thrombotic thrombocytopenic purpura associated with human immunodeficiency virus type 1 (HIV-1) infection. Ann. Intern. Med. 109, 194–197.

Lerner-Ellis, J.P., Tirone, J.C., Pawelek, P.D., et al. 2006. Identification of the gene responsible for methylmalonic aciduria and homocystinuria, cblC type. Nat. Genet. 38, 93–100.

Levy, G.G., Nichols, W.C., Lian, E.C., et al. 2001. Mutations in a member of the ADAMTS gene family cause thrombotic thrombocytopenic purpura. Nature 413, 488–494.

Lian, E.C., Siddiqui, F.A., Chen, S.H. et al. 1992. Platelet-agglutinating/aggregating proteins from the plasma of patients with thrombotic thrombocytopenic purpura. In: B.S. Kaplan, R.S. Trompeter, J.L. Moake (Eds.), Hemolytic Uremic Syndrome and Thrombotic Thrombocytopenic Purpura. Marcel Dekker, New York, pp. 473–481.

Licht, C., Heinen, S., Jozsi, M., et al. 2006. Deletion of Lys224 in regulatory domain 4 of factor H reveals a novel pathomechanism for dense deposit disease (MPGN II). Kidney Int. 70, 42–50.

Liu, L., Choi, H., Bernardo, A., et al. 2005. Platelet-derived VWF-cleaving metalloprotease ADAMTS-13. J. Thromb. Haemost. 3, 2536–2544.

Locking, M.E., O'Brien, S.J., Reilly, W.J., et al. 2001. Risk factors for sporadic cases of Escherichia coli O157 infection: the importance of contact with animal excreta. Epidemiol. Infect. 127, 215–220.

Loirat, C., Niaudet, P. 2003. The risk of recurrence of hemolytic uremic syndrome after renal transplantation in children. Pediatr. Nephrol. 18, 1095–1101.

Lopez, E.L., Diaz, M., Grinstein, S., et al. 1989. Hemolytic uremic syndrome and diarrhoea in Argentine children: the role of Shiga-like toxins. J. Infect. Dis. 160, 469–475.

Lopez, E.L., Prado-Jimenez, V., O'Ryan-Gallardo, M., et al. 2000. Shigella and Shiga toxin-producing Escherichia coli causing bloody diarrhoea in Latin America. Infect. Dis. Clin. North Am. 14, 41–65.

Louise, C.B., Obrig, T.G. 1995. Specific interaction of Escherichia coli O157:H7-derived Shiga-like toxin II with human renal endothelial cells. J. Infect. Dis. 172, 1397–1401.

Lou-Meda, R., Oakes, R.S., Gilstrap, J.N., et al. 2006. Prognostic significance of microalbuminuria in postdiarrhoeal hemolytic uremic syndrome. Pediatr. Nephrol. 22, 117–120.

Ludwig, K., Bitzan, M., Zimmermann, S., et al. 1996. Immune response to non-O157 Vero toxin-producing Escherichia coli in patients with hemolytic uremic syndrome. J. Infect. Dis. 174, 1028–1039.

MacConnachie, A.A., Todd, W.T. 2004. Potential therapeutic agents for the prevention and treatment of haemolytic uraemic syndrome in Shiga toxin producing Escherichia coli infection. Curr. Opin. Infect. Dis. 17, 479–482.

Manuelian, T., Hellwage, J., Meri, S., et al. 2003. Mutations in factor H reduce binding affinity to C3b and heparin and surface attachment to endothelial cells in hemolytic uremic syndrome. J. Clin. Invest. 111, 1181–1190.

Matise, I., Cornick, N.A., Booher, S.L., et al. 2001. Intervention with Shiga toxin (Stx) antibody after infection by Stx-producing Escherichia coli. J. Infect. Dis. 183, 347–350.

Matsumoto, M., Kokame, K., Soejima, K., et al. 2004. Molecular characterization of ADAMTS13 gene mutations in Japanese patients with Upshaw–Schulman syndrome. Blood 103, 1305–1310.

Matussek, A., Lauber, J., Bergau, A., et al. 2003. Molecular and functional analysis of Shiga toxin-induced response patterns in human vascular endothelial cells. Blood 102, 1323–1332.

McCarthy, T.A., Barrett, N.L., Hadler, J.L., et al. 2001. Hemolytic-uremic syndrome and Escherichia coli O121 at a Lake in Connecticut, 1999. Pediatrics 108, E59.

Mead, P.S., Finelli, L., Lambert-Fair, M.A., et al. 1997. Risk factors for sporadic infection with Escherichia coli O157:H7. Arch. Intern. Med. 157, 204–208.

Mead, P.S., Griffin, P.M. 1998. Escherichia coli O157:H7. Lancet 352, 1207–1212.

Mead, P.S., Slutsker, L., Dietz, V., et al. 1999. Food-related illness and death in the United States. Emerg. Infect. Dis. 5, 607–625.

Meichtri, L., Miliwebsky, E., Gioffre, A., et al. 2004. Shiga toxin-producing Escherichia coli in healthy young beef steers from Argentina: prevalence and virulence properties. Int. J. Food Microbiol. 96, 189–198.

Milford, D. 1992. The hemolytic uremic syndromes in the United Kingdom. In: B.S. Kaplan, R.S. Trompeter, J.L. Moake (Eds.), Hemolytic Uremic Syndrome and Thrombotic Thrombocytopenic Purpura. Marcel Dekker, New York, pp. 39–59.

Miller, R.B., Burke, B.A., Schmidt, W.J., et al. 1997. Recurrence of haemolytic-uraemic syndrome in renal transplants: a single-centre report. Nephrol. Dial. Transplant. 12, 1425–1430.

Moake, J.L. 1998. Moschowitz, multimers and metalloprotease. N. Engl. J. Med. 339, 1631.

Moake, J.L. 2002. Thrombotic microangiopathies. N. Engl. J. Med. 347, 589–600.

Moake, J.L., McPherson, P.D. 1989. Abnormalities of the von Willebrand factor multimers in thrombotic thrombocytopenic purpura and the haemolytic-uraemic syndrome. Am. J. Med. 87, 9N–15N.

Moake, J.L., Rudy, C.K., Troll, J.H. 1982. Unusually large plasma factor VIII: von Willebrand factor multimers in chronic relapsing thrombotic thrombocytopenic purpura. N. Engl. J. Med. 307, 1432–1435.

Monteferrante, G., Brioschi, S., Caprioli, J., et al. 2007. Genetic analysis of the complement factor H related 5 gene in haemolytic uraemic syndrome. Mol. Immunol. 44, 1704–1708.

Morigi, M., Galbusera, M., Binda, E., et al. 2001. Verotoxin-1-induced up-regulation of adhesive molecules renders microvascular endothelial cells thrombogenic at high shear stress. Blood 98, 1828–1835.

Morigi, M., Micheletti, G., Figliuzzi, M., et al. 1995. Verotoxin-1 promotes leukocyte adhesion to cultured endothelial cells under physiologic flow conditions. Blood 86, 4553–4558.

Moschowitz, E. 1925. Acute febrile pleiochromic anemia with hyaline thrombosis of terminal arterioles and capillaries. An undescribed disease. Arch. Intern. Med. 36, 89–93.

Motto, D.G., Chauhan, A.K., Zhu, G., et al. 2005. Shigatoxin triggers thrombotic thrombocytopenic purpura in genetically susceptible ADAMTS13-deficient mice. J. Clin. Invest. 115, 2752–2761.

Mulvey, G.L., Marcato, P., Kitov, P.I., et al. 2003. Assessment in mice of the therapeutic potential of tailored, multivalent Shiga toxin carbohydrate ligands. J. Infect. Dis. 187, 640–649.

Murata, K., Higuchi, T., Takada, K., et al. 2006. Verotoxin-1 stimulation of macrophage-like THP-1 cells up-regulates tissue factor expression through activation of c-Yes tyrosine kinase: possible signal transduction in tissue factor up-regulation. Biochim. Biophys. Acta 1762, 835–843.

Murphy, W.G., Moore, J.C., Kelton, J.G. 1987. Calcium-dependent cysteine protease activity in the sera of patients with thrombotic thrombocytopenic purpura. Blood 70, 1683–1687.

Nakajima, H., Kiyokawa, N., Katagiri, Y.U., et al. 2001. Kinetic analysis of binding between Shiga toxin and receptor glycolipid Gb3Cer by surface plasmon resonance. J. Biol. Chem. 276, 42915–42922.

Neame, P.B. 1980. Immunologic and other factors in thrombotic thrombocytopenic purpura (TTP). Semin. Thromb. Hemost. 6, 416–429.

Noris, M., Benigni, A., Siegler, R. 1992. Renal prostacyclin biosynthesis is reduced in children with haemolytic uraemic syndrome in context of systemic platelet activation. Am. J. Kidney Dis. 20, 144–149.

Noris, M., Bucchioni, S., Galbusera, M., et al., 2005. Complement factor H mutation in familial thrombotic thrombocytopenic purpura with ADAMTS13 deficiency and renal involvement. J. Am. Soc. Nephrol. 16, 1177–1183.

Noris, M., Remuzzi, G. 2005. Hemolytic uremic syndrome. J. Am. Soc. Nephrol. 16, 1035–1050.

Noris, M., Ruggenenti, P., Perna, A., et al. 1999. Hypocomplementemia discloses genetic predisposition to hemolytic uremic syndrome and thrombotic thrombocytopenic purpura: role of factor H abnormalities. J. Am. Soc. Nephrol. 10, 281–293.

Obrig, T.G., Moran, T.P., Brown, J.E. 1987. The mode of action of Shiga toxin on peptide elongation of eukaryotic protein synthesis. Biochem. J. 244, 287–294.

Ohali, M., Shalev, H., Schlesinger, M., et al. 1998. Hypocomplementemic autosomal recessive hemolytic uremic syndrome with decreased factor H—original article. Pediatr. Nephrol. 12, 619–624.

Ohmi, K., Kiyokawa, N., Takeda, T., et al. 1998. Human microvascular endothelial cells are strongly sensitive to Shiga toxins. Biochem. Biophys. Res. Commun. 251, 137–141.

Oneko, M., Nyathi, M.N., Doehring, E. 2001. Post-dysenteric hemolytic uremic syndrome in Bulawayo, Zimbabwe. Pediatr. Nephrol. 16, 1142–1145.

Ostroff, S.M., Kobayashi, J.M., Lewis, J.H. 1989. Infections with Escherichia coli O157:H7 in Washington State. The first year of statewide disease surveillance. JAMA 262, 355–359.

Paton, A.W., Morona, R., Paton, J.C. 2000. A new biological agent for treatment of Shiga toxigenic Escherichia coli infections and dysentery in humans. Nat. Med. 6, 265–270.

Perez-Caballero, D., Gonzalez-Rubio, C., Gallardo, M.E., et al. 2001. Clustering of missense mutations in the C-terminal region of factor H in atypical hemolytic uremic syndrome. Am. J. Hum. Genet. 68, 478–484.

Pichette, V., Querin, S., Schurch, W., et al. 1994. Familial hemolytic-uremic syndrome and homozygous factor-H deficiency. Am. J. Kidney Dis. 24, 936–941.

Pickering, M.C., Cook, H.T., Warren, J., et al. 2002. Uncontrolled C3 activation causes membranoproliferative glomerulonephritis in mice deficient in complement factor H. Nat. Genet. 31, 424–428.

Pijpers, A.H., van Setten, P.A., van den Heuvel, L.P., et al. 2001. Verocytotoxin-induced apoptosis of human microvascular endothelial cells. J. Am. Soc. Nephrol. 12, 767–778.

Pinyon, R.A., Paton, J.C., Paton, A.W., et al. 2004. Refinement of a therapeutic Shiga toxin-binding probiotic for human trials. J. Infect. Dis. 189, 1547–1555.

Pratt, J.R., Hibbs, M.J., Laver, A.J., et al. 1996. Effects of complement inhibition with soluble complement receptor-1 on vascular injury and inflammation during renal-allograft rejection in the rat. Am. J. Pathol. 149, 2055–2066.

Quan, A., Sullivan, E.K., Alexander, S.R. 2001. Recurrence of hemolytic uremic syndrome after renal transplantation in children: a report of the North American Pediatric Renal Transplant Cooperative Study. Transplantation 72, 742–745.

Reiss, G., Kunz, P., Koin, D., et al. 2006. Escherichia coli O157:H7 infection in nursing homes: review of literature and report of recent outbreak. J. Am. Geriatr. Soc. 54, 680–684.

Remuzzi, G. 2003. Is ADAMTS-13 deficiency specific for thrombotic thrombocytopenic purpura? No. J. Thromb. Haemost. 1, 632–634.

Remuzzi, G., Galbusera, M., Noris, M., et al. 2002a. von Willebrand factor cleaving protease (ADAMTS13) is deficient in recurrent and familial thrombotic thrombocytopenic purpura and hemolytic uremic syndrome. Blood 100, 778–785.

Remuzzi, G., Galbusera, M., Salvadori, M., et al. 1996. Bilateral nephrectomy stopped disease progression in plasma-resistant hemolytic uremic syndrome with neurological signs and coma. Kidney Int. 49, 282–286.

Remuzzi, G., Ruggenenti, P. 1994. Thrombotic microangiopathies. In: C. Tisher, B. Brenner (Eds.), Renal Pathology. J. B. Lippincott, Philadelphia, pp. 1154–1184.

Remuzzi, G., Ruggenenti, P., Codazzi, D., et al., 2002b. Combined kidney and liver transplantation for familial haemolytic uraemic syndrome. Lancet 359, 1671–1672.

Remuzzi, G., Ruggenenti, P., Colledan, M., et al. 2005. Hemolytic uremic syndrome: a fatal outcome after kidney and liver transplantation performed to correct factor H gene mutation. Am. J. Transplant. 5, 1146–1150.

Richards, A., Buddles, M.R., Donne, R.L., et al. 2001. Factor H mutations in hemolytic uremic syndrome cluster in exons 18-20, a domain important for host cell recognition. Am. J. Hum. Genet. 68, 485–490.

Richards, A., Kemp, E.J., Liszewski, M.K., et al. 2003. Mutations in human complement regulator, membrane cofactor protein (CD46), predispose to development of familial hemolytic uremic syndrome. Proc. Natl. Acad. Sci. U.S.A. 100, 12966–12971.

Riley, L.W., Remis, R.S., Helgerson, S.D., et al. 1983. Hemorrhagic colitis associated with a rare Escherichia coli serotype. N. Engl. J. Med. 308, 681–685.

Rock, G., Shumak, K.H., Sutton, D.M.C., et al. 1996. Cryosupernatant as replacement fluid for plasma exchange

in thrombotic thrombocytopenic purpura. Br. J. Haematol. 94, 383–386.
Ruggenenti, P. 2002. Post-transplant hemolytic-uremic syndrome. Kidney Int. 62, 1093–1104.
Ruggenenti, P., Noris, M., Remuzzi, G. 2001. Thrombotic microangiopathy, hemolytic uremic syndrome, and thrombotic thrombocytopenic purpura. Kidney Int. 60, 831–846.
Ruggenenti, P., Remuzzi, G. 1990. Thrombotic thrombocytopenic purpura and related disorders. Hematol. Oncol. Clin. North Am. 4, 219–241.
Ruiz-Torres, M.P., Casiraghi, F., Galbusera, M., et al. 2005. Complement activation: the missing link between ADAMTS-13 deficiency and microvascular thrombosis of thrombotic microangiopathies. Thromb. Haemost. 93, 443–452.
Ruoslahti, E., Pierschbacher, M.D. 1986. Arg-Gly-Asp: a versatile cell recognition signal. Cell 44, 517–518.
Safdar, N., Said, A., Gangnon, R.E., et al. 2002. Risk of hemolytic uremic syndrome after antibiotic treatment of Escherichia coli O157:H7 enteritis: a meta-analysis. JAMA 288, 996–1001.
Sahu, A., Lambris, J.D. 2001. Structure and biology of complement protein C3, a connecting link between innate and acquired immunity. Immunol. Rev. 180, 35–48.
Saland, J.M., Emre, S.H., Shneider, B.L., et al. 2006. Favorable long-term outcome after liver-kidney transplant for recurrent hemolytic uremic syndrome associated with a factor H mutation. Am. J. Transplant. 6, 1948–1952.
Sanchez-Corral, P., Gonzalez-Rubio, C., Rodriguez de Cordoba, S., et al. 2004. Functional analysis in serum from atypical hemolytic uremic syndrome patients reveals impaired protection of host cells associated with mutations in factor H. Mol. Immunol. 41, 81–84.
Sanchez-Corral, P., Perez-Caballero, D., Huarte, O., et al. 2002. Structural and functional characterization of factor H mutations associated with atypical hemolytic uremic syndrome. Am. J. Hum. Genet. 71, 1285–1295.
Saunders, R.E., Abarrategui-Garrido, C., Fremeaux-Bacchi, V., et al. 2007. The interactive factor H-atypical haemolytic uraemic syndrome mutation database and website: update and integration of membrane cofactor protein and factor I mutations with structural models. Hum. Mutat. 28, 222–234.
Saunders, R.E., Goodship, T.H.J., Zipfel, P.F., et al. 2006. An interactive web database of factor H-associated hemolytic uremic syndrome mutations: insights into the structural consequences of disease-associated mutations. Hum. Mutat. 27, 21–30.
Schimmer, B. 2006. Outbreak of haemolytic uraemic syndrome in Norway: update. Euro Surveill. 11, E060406.2.
Schriber, J.R., Herzig, G.P. 1997. Transplantation-associated thrombotic thrombocytopenic purpura and hemolytic uremic syndrome. Semin. Hematol. 34, 126–133.
Schulman, I., Pierce, M., Lukens, A., et al. 1960. Studies on thrombopoiesis. I. A factor in normal human plasma required for platelet production; chronic thrombocytopenia due to its deficiency. Blood 16, 943–957.
Scotland, S.M., Willshaw, G.A., Smith, H.R., et al. 1987. Properties of strains of Escherichia coli belonging to serogroup O157 with special reference to production of Vero cytotoxins VT1 and VT2. Epidemiol. Infect. 99, 613–624.
Shang, D., Zheng, X.W., Niiya, M., et al. 2006. Apical sorting of ADAMTS13 in vascular endothelial cells and Madin–Darby canine kidney cells depends on the CUB domains and their association with lipid rafts. Blood 108, 2207–2215.
Shelat, S.G., Smith, P., Ai, J., et al. 2006. Inhibitory autoantibodies against ADAMTS-13 in patients with thrombotic thrombocytopenic purpura bind ADAMTS-13 protease and may accelerate its clearance in vivo. J. Thromb. Haemost. 4, 1707–1717.
Shibagaki, Y., Matsumoto, M., Kokame, K., et al. 2006. Novel compound heterozygote mutations (H234Q/R1206X) of the ADAMTS13 gene in an adult patient with Upshaw–Schulman syndrome showing predominant episodes of repeated acute renal failure. Nephrol. Dial. Transplant. 21, 1289–1292.
Silverstein, A. 1968. Thrombotic thrombocytopenic purpura. The initial neurologic manifestations. Arch. Neurol. 18, 358–362.
Smith, G.P., Smith, R.A. 2001. Membrane-targeted complement inhibitors. Mol. Immunol. 38, 249–255.
Soejima, K., Matsumoto, M., Kokame, K., et al. 2003. ADAMTS-13 cysteine-rich/spacer domains are functionally essential for von Willebrand factor cleavage. Blood 102, 3232–3237.
Sonntag, A.K., Prager, R., Bielaszewska, M., et al. 2004. Phenotypic and genotypic analyses of enterohemorrhagic Escherichia coli O145 strains from patients in Germany. J. Clin. Microbiol. 42, 954–962.
Srivastava, R.N., Moudgil, A., Bagga, A., et al. 1991. Hemolytic uremic syndrome in children in northern India. Pediatr. Nephrol. 5, 284–288.
Stahl, A.L., Svensson, M., Morgelin, M., et al. 2006. Lipopolysaccharide from enterohemorrhagic Escherichia coli binds to platelets through TLR4 and CD62 and is detected on circulating platelets in patients with hemolytic uremic syndrome. Blood 108, 167–176.
Stratton, J.D., Warwicker, P. 2002. Successful treatment of factor H-related haemolytic uraemic syndrome. Nephrol. Dial. Transplant. 17, 684–685.
Stuhlinger, W., Kourilsky, O., Kanfer, A., et al. 1974. Haemolytic-uraemic syndrome: evidence for intravascular C3 activation [Letter]. Lancet 2, 788–789.
Takahashi, M., Taguchi, H., Yamaguchi, H., et al. 2004. The effect of probiotic treatment with Clostridium butyricum on enterohemorrhagic Escherichia coli O157:H7 infection in mice. FEMS Immunol. Med. Microbiol. 41, 219–226.
Tao, Z., Wang, Y., Choi, H., et al. 2005. Cleavage of ultralarge multimers of von Willebrand factor by C-terminal-truncated mutants of ADAMTS-13 under flow. Blood 106, 141–143.
Taylor, C.M., Howie, A.J., Williams, J.M. 1999. No common final pathogenetic pathway in haemolytic uraemic syndromes. Nephrol. Dial. Transplant. 14, 1100–1102.

Tesh, V.L., Burris, J.A., Owens, J.W., et al. 1993. Comparison of the relative toxicities of Shiga-like toxins type I and type II for mice. Infect. Immun. 61, 3392–3402.

Thompson, R.A., Winterborn, M.H. 1981. Hypocomplementaemia due to a genetic deficiency of beta-1 H globulin. Clin. Exp. Immunol. 46, 110–119.

Thorpe, C.M. 2004. Shiga toxin-producing *Escherichia coli* infection. Clin. Infect. Dis. 38, 1298–1303.

Tonshoff, B., Sammet, A., Sanden, I., et al. 1994. Outcome and prognostic determinants in the hemolytic uremic syndrome of children. Nephron. 68, 63–70.

Trachtman, H., Cnaan, A., Christen, E., et al. 2003. Effect of an oral Shiga toxin-binding agent on diarrhoea-associated hemolytic uremic syndrome in children: a randomized controlled trial. JAMA 290, 1337–1344.

Tsai, H.M. 2003. Is severe deficiency of ADAMTS-13 specific for thrombotic thrombocytopenic purpura? Yes. J. Thromb. Haemost. 1, 625–631.

Tsai, H.M. 2006. The molecular biology of thrombotic microangiopathy. Kidney Int. 70, 16–23.

Tsai, H.M., Lian, E.C. 1998. Antibodies to von Willebrand factor-cleaving protease in acute thrombotic thrombocytopenic purpura. N. Engl. J. Med. 339, 1585–1594.

Tsai, H.M., Sussman, B., II, Nagel, R.L. 1994. Shear stress enhances the proteolysis of von Willebrand factor in normal plasma. Blood 83, 2171–2179.

Turner, N., Nolasco, L., Tao, Z., et al. 2006. Human endothelial cells synthesize and release ADAMTS-13. J. Thromb. Haemost. 4, 1396–1404.

Uchida, T., Wada, H., Mizutani, M., et al. 2004. Identification of novel mutations in ADAMTS13 in an adult patient with congenital thrombotic thrombocytopenic purpura. Blood 104, 2081–2083.

Upshaw, J.D., Jr. 1978. Congenital deficiency of a factor in normal plasma that reverses microangiopathic hemolysis and thrombocytopenia. N. Engl. J. Med. 298, 1350–1352.

Valavaara, R., Nordman, E. 1985. Renal complications of mitomycin C therapy with special reference to the total dose. Cancer 55, 47–50.

Van Dyck, M., Proesmans, W. 2004. Renoprotection by ACE inhibitors after severe hemolytic uremic syndrome. Pediatr. Nephrol. 19, 688–690.

van Setten, P.A., Monnens, L.A., Verstraten, R.G., et al. 1996. Effects of verocytotoxin-1 on nonadherent human monocytes: binding characteristics, protein synthesis, and induction of cytokine release. Blood 88, 174–183.

van Setten, P.A., van Hinsbergh, V.W., van der Velden, T.J., et al. 1997. Effects of TNF alpha on verocytotoxin cytotoxicity in purified human glomerular microvascular endothelial cells. Kidney Int. 51, 1245–1256.

Varma, J.K., Greene, K.D., Reller, M.E., et al. 2003. An outbreak of *Escherichia coli* O157 infection following exposure to a contaminated building. JAMA 290, 2709–2712.

Venables, J.P., Strain, L., Routledge, D., et al. 2006. Atypical hemolytic uremic syndrome associated with a hybrid complement gene. PLoS Med. 3, e431.

Vesely, S.K., George, J.N., Lammle, B., et al. 2003. ADAMTS13 activity in thrombotic thrombocytopenic purpura-hemolytic uremic syndrome: relation to presenting features and clinical outcomes in a prospective cohort of 142 patients. Blood 102, 60–68.

Veyradier, A., Obert, B., Houllier, A., et al. 2001. Specific von Willebrand factor-cleaving protease in thrombotic microangiopathies: a study of 111 cases. Blood 98, 1765–1772.

von Baeyer, H. 2002. Plasmapheresis in thrombotic microangiopathy-associated syndromes: review of outcome data derived from clinical trials and open studies. Ther. Apher. Dial. 6, 320–328.

Vyse, T.J., Bates, G.P., Walport, M.J., et al. 1994a. The organization of the human complement factor I gene (IF): a member of the serine protease gene family. Genomics 24, 90–98.

Vyse, T.J., Morley, B.J., Bartok, I., et al. 1996. The molecular basis of hereditary complement factor I deficiency. J. Clin. Invest. 97, 925–933.

Vyse, T.J., Spath, P.J., Davies, K.A., et al. 1994b. Hereditary complement factor I deficiency. QJM 87, 385–401.

Warwicker, P., Goodship, T.H.J., Donne, R.L., et al. 1998. Genetic studies into inherited and sporadic haemolytic uraemic syndrome. Kidney Int. 53, 836–844.

Wen, S.X., Teel, L.D., Judge, N.A., et al. 2006. A plant-based oral vaccine to protect against systemic intoxication by Shiga toxin type 2. Proc. Natl. Acad. Sci. U.S.A. 103, 7082–7087.

Wong, C.S., Jelacic, S., Habeeb, R.L., et al. 2000. The risk of the hemolytic-uremic syndrome after antibiotic treatment of *Escherichia coli* O157:H7 infections. N. Engl. J. Med. 342, 1930–1936.

Xu, Y., Narayana, S.V., Volanakis, J.E. 2001. Structural biology of the alternative pathway convertase. Immunol. Rev. 180, 123–135.

Zeigler, Z.R., Shadduck, R.K., Gryn, J.F., et al. 2001. Cryoprecipitate poor plasma does not improve early response in primary adult thrombotic thrombocytopenic purpura (TTP). J. Clin. Apher. 16, 19–22.

Zoja, C., Angioletti, S., Donadelli, R., et al. 2002. Shiga toxin-2 triggers endothelial leukocyte adhesion and transmigration via NF-kappaB dependent up-regulation of IL-8 and MCP-1. Kidney Int. 62, 846–856.

# PART IV:

# The Connective Tissue Diseases

CHAPTER 15

# Systemic Lupus Erythematosus: Mechanisms

Menna R. Clatworthy, Kenneth G.C. Smith*

*Cambridge Institute for Medical Research and the Department of Medicine, University of Cambridge School of Clinical Medicine, Addenbrooke's Hospital, Hills Road, Cambridge CB2 2XY, UK*

## 1. Introduction

Systemic lupus erythematosus (SLE) is the prototypic systemic autoimmune disease. In contrast to organ-specific autoimmune diseases such as type I diabetes, disease involvement in SLE is extremely diverse and variable. The most commonly affected organs are skin, joints, and kidneys, but any organ may be involved. Immunological abnormalities include the presence of autoantibodies (particularly anti-nuclear antibodies (ANAs) and anti-double stranded DNA antibodies (dsDNA)), hypergammaglobulinaemia, and hypocomplementaemia. Histopathological examination of affected tissues demonstrates immune complex and complement deposition (Kotzin, 1996). Evidence suggests that multiple genes interact to produce a predisposition to SLE and lupus susceptibility genes may well be different in different individuals with the disease. SLE is more common in females than in males suggesting that hormonal factors may influence pathogenesis. Disease flares can be also be triggered by environmental stimuli such as ultraviolet (UV) light or certain drugs. Thus an individual may be genetically predisposed to the development of SLE but will only develop disease if they encounter the correct environmental triggers. Once initiated, other genetic, environmental, and hormonal factors act to modify the spectrum and severity of clinical manifestations.

## 2. Genetic, environmental, and hormonal factors in SLE

### 2.1. Genetic factors

There is strong epidemiological evidence to suggest genetic factors are important in the pathogenesis of SLE. There is a marked racial difference in susceptibility to lupus; African-Americans and Hispanics have a 3–6 fold increased risk of developing disease compared with Caucasians (Reveille et al., 1998). Furthermore, twin studies show a ten-fold higher concordance rate in monozygotic twins (34%) compared with dizygotic twins (3%), and the concordance rate for the presence of ANAs in serum is even higher in monzygotic twins at around 90% (Deapen et al., 1992; Wakeland et al., 2001). The siblings of patients with lupus have a 15–20 fold increased relative risk of developing disease compared with the population as a whole (Block et al., 1975). Together, these epidemiological data point towards an important genetic component in disease pathogenesis in lupus. In a small proportion of patients (<5%), a single gene deletion may be associated with lupus, for example patients with homozygous deficiencies of the early complement components (Slingsby et al., 1996) but in the majority of patients, SLE occurs as a complex

---

*Corresponding author
Tel.: 44-1223-762645; Fax: 44-1223-762640
E-mail address: kgcs2@cam.ac.uk

polygenic disease. Genome wide linkage studies of SLE affected families have identified 48 distinct chromosomal loci that show at least nominal evidence of linkage in human SLE, and seven regions which meet the criteria for significant linkage (LOD score >3.3) (Gaffney et al., 1998; Gray-McGuire et al., 2000; Moser et al., 1998; Shai et al., 1999), specifically 1q23-24, 1q41-42, 2q37, 4p15-16, 6p11-22, 16q12-13, and 17p13. Case-control studies have also provided useful information on immune polymorphisms associated with disease susceptibility.

There are a number of spontaneous and inducible murine models of SLE which have proved useful in genetic studies. Spontaneous models include the NZB/W F1 mouse, the BXSB/*yaa* mouse, and the MRL/*lpr* mouse. Linkage studies in both spontaneous and inducible murine models of lupus have implicated around 50 loci affecting susceptibility to lupus, and have also been useful in identifying loci responsible for mediating susceptibility to particular phenotypes such as ANA production (Wakeland et al., 2001). Some of these loci co-localize with regions linked to other autoimmune diseases, for example insulin-dependent diabetes and collagen-induced arthritis, suggesting that these loci may affect autoimmune susceptibility to many autoimmune diseases by modulating common pathogenic pathways. Linkage analysis has been followed by congenic dissection, for example, using the NZM2410 mouse derived from the NZB/WF1 mouse, allowing susceptibility loci to be narrowed down, facilitating the identification of specific susceptibility and suppressor genes (Morel et al., 1999). Together these genetic studies in humans and mice have implicated, with varying degrees of confidence, a large number of genes in the pathogenesis of lupus, in particular, human leukocyte antigen (HLA), complement, and Fc$\gamma$ receptor genes.

The importance of polymorphisms in HLA molecules centers on their influence upon antigen presentation to, and activation of autoreactive T-cells. The genetic association of SLE with major histocompatibility complex HLA class II gene polymorphisms was identified more than 30 years ago. The DR-B1 alleles DR2 and DR3 have shown consistent association with disease in the Caucasian population with a threefold increase in the frequency of the two alleles compared with controls (Graham et al., 2002). The DR2 and DR3 genes have also been associated with the presence of certain autoantibodies, such as anti-Sm (small nuclear ribonuclear protein), anti-Ro, anti-La, and anti-DNA antibodies (Schur, 1995). However, there do not appear to be very convincing or reproducible associations in non-Caucasian populations (Wakeland et al., 2001). A major problem with the interpretation of these results is the effect of linkage disequilibrium (LD) across this region. The reported associations with SLE of several MHC class III genes, including TNF$\alpha$, the TAP genes and HSP70, may reflect LD with other genes in the HLA region or epistatic effects of several genes on extended haplotypes (Wakeland et al., 2001).

The complement system plays an important physiological role in the disposal of immune complexes and apoptotic cells. Inherited deficiencies in the early classical pathway components (C1q, C2, C4) can lead to SLE (Carroll, 1998; Schur, 1995; Slingsby et al., 1996). C1q deficiency is a very rare disorder and produces a severe form of disease (Slingsby et al., 1996). C1q-deficient mice have reduced splenic immune complex uptake (Nash et al., 2001), accumulation of apoptotic debris within glomeruli, and a predisposition to autoimmunity (Botto et al., 1998), although this may be related to genes in the surrounding area of chromosome 1 derived from the 129 mouse (Bygrave et al., 2004). C2 and C4 deficiencies are also rare and predispose to a milder form of the disease (Schur, 1995). Genes in the HLA class III region encode both these proteins. C4 deficiency can be difficult to detect since there are two isotypes of C4 (C4A and C4B) and each isotype has numerous allelic variants, with null alleles having been identified for each. A C4A null allele is transmitted as part of the extended HLA-A7, B8, DR3 haplotype, which is associated with SLE in Caucasians (Schur, 1995; Schur et al., 1990). Association in African-American and Asian populations, where the null alleles are carried on different class II haplotypes, indicate that these C4 alleles are independent risk factors for SLE (Howard et al., 1986). C4-deficient mice also develop a lupus-like illness (Chen et al., 2000). A number of polymorphisms of CR1 have been identified in humans, one of which has reduced binding for its ligand C3b and has an increased prevalence amongst patients with SLE (Van Dyne et al., 1987).

A plethora of autoantibodies has been identified in patients with lupus including ANAs, anti-dsDNA antibodies, anti-RNP antibodies, anti-phospholipid antibodies, and anti-C1q antibodies (Sherer et al. 2004). Fc$\gamma$ receptors bind to the Fc portion of IgG and may be activatory (Fc$\gamma$RI, IIa, IIIa, IIIb, and IV) or inhibitory (Fc$\gamma$RIIb) (Nimmerjahn and Ravetch, 2006). Linkage studies in mice and humans have also implicated loci containing Fc$\gamma$R genes. *Nba2* and *sle1* are two key linkage intervals for murine lupus, both of which contain Fc$\gamma$RII and Fc$\gamma$RIII genes (Kono et al., 1994; Drake et al., 1995). The human orthologues of these Fc$\gamma$R genes are located within the 1q23-24 linkage region on chromosome 1 described above (Moser et al., 1998). These studies, together with the realization of their importance in mediating the effector functions of antibody and their role in immune complex clearance, led to a number of case-control studies examining possible correlations between Fc receptor polymorphisms and the development of SLE. Overall, these studies suggest that allelic variants of activatory Fc$\gamma$R genes that reduce binding affinity to IgG increase susceptibility to SLE (Lehrnbecher et al., 1999) (see Section 3.2.2). A more recent study has suggested that copy number of the *Fc$\gamma$RIIIb* gene may also influence susceptibility to disease (Aitman et al., 2006) (see Section 3.2.2). A de-functioning polymorphism of the inhibitory Fc$\gamma$R, Fc$\gamma$RIIb has also been described at increased frequency in patients with SLE (Floto et al., 2005), (see Section 3.1.4).

## 2.2. Environmental factors

Although genetic factors and the hormonal milieu may create a predisposition to SLE, the initiation of disease probably results from several environmental triggers and exogenous factors (Table 1). Exposure to sunlight is a well-known trigger of both cutaneous and systemic manifestations of lupus. UV light, particularly UVB, has been shown to exacerbate disease. It has been suggested that skin exposure to UV light alters the location of DNA and other nuclear antigens, including Ro, by the induction of apoptosis (Casciola-Rosen and Rosen, 1997). These previously inaccessible nuclear self-antigens may be internalized by autoreactive cells and lead to activation and proliferation following recognition by Toll-like receptors (TLRs). TLRs are innate immune receptors which have evolved to facilitate a rapid immune response to invading microorganisms by recognition of pathogen associated molecular patterns (PAMPs). TLR7 and TLR9 detect microbial RNA and DNA respectively, and are located within intracellular compartments (Akira et al., 2001; Beutler, 2004). Mammalian nuclear antigens exposed during UV-induced apoptosis may potentially trigger immunogenic antigen presentation through the activation of TLR7 and TLR9 (see Section 3.1.4).

Some drugs, including hydralazine and procainamide, can cause disease, particularly in people who are slow acetylators of drugs that are a substrate for hepatic acetyltransferase (Woosley et al., 1978). Compounds such as aromatic amines and hydralazines are found in a wide variety of compounds in agriculture and industry and have been associated with the development of lupus (Reidenberg et al., 1993). In addition, tobacco also

**Table 1**
Environmental factors which may contribute to the pathogenesis of SLE

Chemical/physical factors
   Aromatic amines
   Drugs: hydralazine, procainamide, chlorpromazine, isoniazid, penicillamine
   Tobacco
   Hair dyes
   Ultraviolet light
Dietary factors
   High intake of saturated fats
   L-canavanin (alfalfa sprouts)
Infectious agents
   Bacterial DNA
   Endotoxin
   Viruses

contains hydralazine. Foodstuffs such as alfalfa sprouts (containing L-canavanine) have been shown to cause SLE-like illnesses (Prete, 1985). Some of these previously mysterious observations may be explained by the effects of these agents on DNA methylation or on RNA structure which may enhance TLR activation.

A potential role for viruses in pathogenesis has been long been suspected, given that disease flares are often preceded by viral infections and that SLE patients have significantly higher rates of Epstein–Barr virus infection compared with controls (Vaughan, 1997). It has been proposed that autoantibody production might begin as a monospecific response to an epitope shared by a microbial antigen and a self-antigen. This auto-antigen may then be processed and presented by B-cells, thus priming autoreactive T-cells (so called molecular mimicry) (Vaughan, 1997; von Herrath and Oldstone, 1996). Using a transgenic mouse model it has been shown that challenge with a self-mimicking foreign antigen can release B-cells from peripheral tolerance independent of T-cell help (Kouskoff et al., 2000). Alternatively, viruses may directly stimulate TLRs initiating the production of type 1 interferons (IFNs) and an inappropriate inflammatory response. There are a number of lines of evidence implicating type I IFNs (IFN-$\alpha$ and IFN-$\beta$) in the pathogenesis of SLE which are discussed in Section 3.1.4.

## 2.3. Hormonal factors

SLE occurs predominantly in females (9:1 female:male ratio) and this may relate to hormonal differences between male and female. Furthermore, first onset of disease before puberty or after the menopause is uncommon, and patients with Klinefelter's syndrome, characterized by hypergonadotrophic hypogonadism, are prone to the development of SLE (French and Hughes, 1983; Kotzin, 1996). Epidemiological studies also reveal an association between the use of exogenous oestrogens and the onset of lupus (Sanchez-Guerrero et al., 1997). Oestrogen has been shown to have a disease accelerating effect in the NZBW/F1

Table 2
Hormonal factors and SLE

Susceptibility to SLE
  Low endogenous oestrogen concentrations are protective
  Low androgen levels and use of exogenous oestrogens increase risk
Disease activity
  Reduced after the menopause
  Cyclical fluctuation of disease during pregnancy and the menstrual cycle
  Oestrogens have disease-accelerating effects in mouse models of SLE
  Androgen levels correlate inversely with disease activity
  Hyperprolactinaemia correlates with disease in some studies

and MRL-*lpr/lpr* murine models of lupus and causes the development of autoantibodies (Carlsten et al., 1991; Carlsten et al., 1990). Similar studies have demonstrated a protective effect of testosterone (Melez et al., 1978). This is of interest since both physiological and supra-physiological levels of oestrogens facilitate humoral responses, leading to increased B-cell proliferation and antibody production in vitro and, in patients with lupus, increased autoantibody production (Kanda and Tamaki, 1999; Kanda et al., 1999).

Prolactin is another hormonal candidate, which has been shown to be elevated in both males and females with SLE (Jara et al., 1992). Non-SLE patients with hyperprolactinaemia tend to develop ANAs and altered IL-2 responses that return to normal when hyperprolactinaemia is corrected (Vidaller et al., 1986). The relationship between several hormones and SLE is summarized in Table 2.

## 3. Mechanisms of disease

In order to develop SLE, an individual may possess a variety of susceptibility genes which lead to abnormalities in a number of biological pathways. We will attempt to outline each pathway involved but it is important to appreciate that dysfunction in multiple processes occurs simultaneously. Thus a genetic polymorphisms leading to a variety of immunological abnormalities will be molded by environmental and hormonal factors to produce a particular clinical disease phenotype.

The precise way in which these factors interact in the development of SLE is far from clear, but the pathogenesis can be divided into 2 stages, each of which contain a number of pathogenic processes which we will consider in turn (summarized in Figs. 1 and 2):-

Stage 1: Loss of tolerance to self-antigens and the generation of autoantibodies

- Failure to remove or silence autoreactive B and T-cells
- Abnormal exposure of self-antigen
- Abnormal presentation of self-antigen
- T-cell hyperactivity
- B-cell hyperactivity

Stage 2: Pathogenic autoantibodies and immune complexes cause inflammation and disease (Fig. 1)

- Directly pathogenic autoantibodies
- Failure of immune complex clearance
- Abnormal inflammatory response following immune complex deposition
- Tissue damage and fibrosis

## 3.1. Stage 1: loss of tolerance to self-antigens and the generation of autoantibodies

During B- and T-cell development, within the vast array of B- and T-cell receptors randomly generated by gene recombination, there will inevitably be those that bind self-antigens. However, the immune system has developed a number of mechanisms to remove or silence such autoreactive cells (tolerance). Failure of these mechanisms can lead to the persistence of self-reactive cells and the development of autoimmunity. SLE is characterized by the production of autoantibodies, particularly to nuclear components. This phenomenon implies the presence of autoreactive B- and T-cells, and a failure of mechanisms imposing self-tolerance. Given the importance of B-cells as auto-antibody producers and the central role of the immune complex in the pathogenesis of lupus, much emphasis has been placed on mechanisms leading to the breakdown of B-cell tolerance. By the provision of help to B-cells, autoreactive CD4 T-cells also contribute to the development of disease.

### 3.1.1. B-cell tolerance

There are a number of "checkpoints" at which autoreactive B-cells are eliminated or neutralized, thus ensuring B-cell tolerance. These occur both during B-cell development (central tolerance) and following antigen encounter in the periphery (peripheral tolerance).

During development in the bone marrow, immature B-cells (at the stage of light chain gene rearrangement) encountering antigen capable of cross-linking their B-cell receptor are either eliminated (clonal deletion), become unresponsive and short lived (anergic) or undergo revision of their B-cell receptor to eliminate self-reactivity (receptor editing). High-affinity interactions with membrane bound antigen result in deletion, whereas lower-affinity interactions and encounter with soluble antigen allows editing or anergy (the latter is characterized by expression of IgD and down-regulation of IgM). Immature cells that do not encounter antigen mature normally and migrate from the bone marrow to the peripheral lymphoid tissue (Goodnow, 1997; Goodnow et al., 1995; Nossal and Pike, 1980).

Despite these mechanisms of central tolerance, some autoreactive B-cells escape deletion or anergy. Thus a number of mechanisms exist to preserve tolerance in the periphery. In many cases B-cells fail to undergo T-dependent activation due to the absence of appropriate T-cell help. T-cell tolerance can thus, by depriving the B-cell of help, impose tolerance on the B-cell repertoire (Fulcher and Basten, 1997). It is also possible that autoreactive B-cells presenting antigen to CD4 + T-cells can be eliminated by delivery of a death signal from Fas ligand on T-cells. Naïve B-cells binding antigen become activated, resistant to apoptosis, and capable of clonal expansion whereas self-reactive B-cells, "desensitized" by chronic binding of autoantigen, down-regulate CD86/80 and remain sensitive to apoptosis.

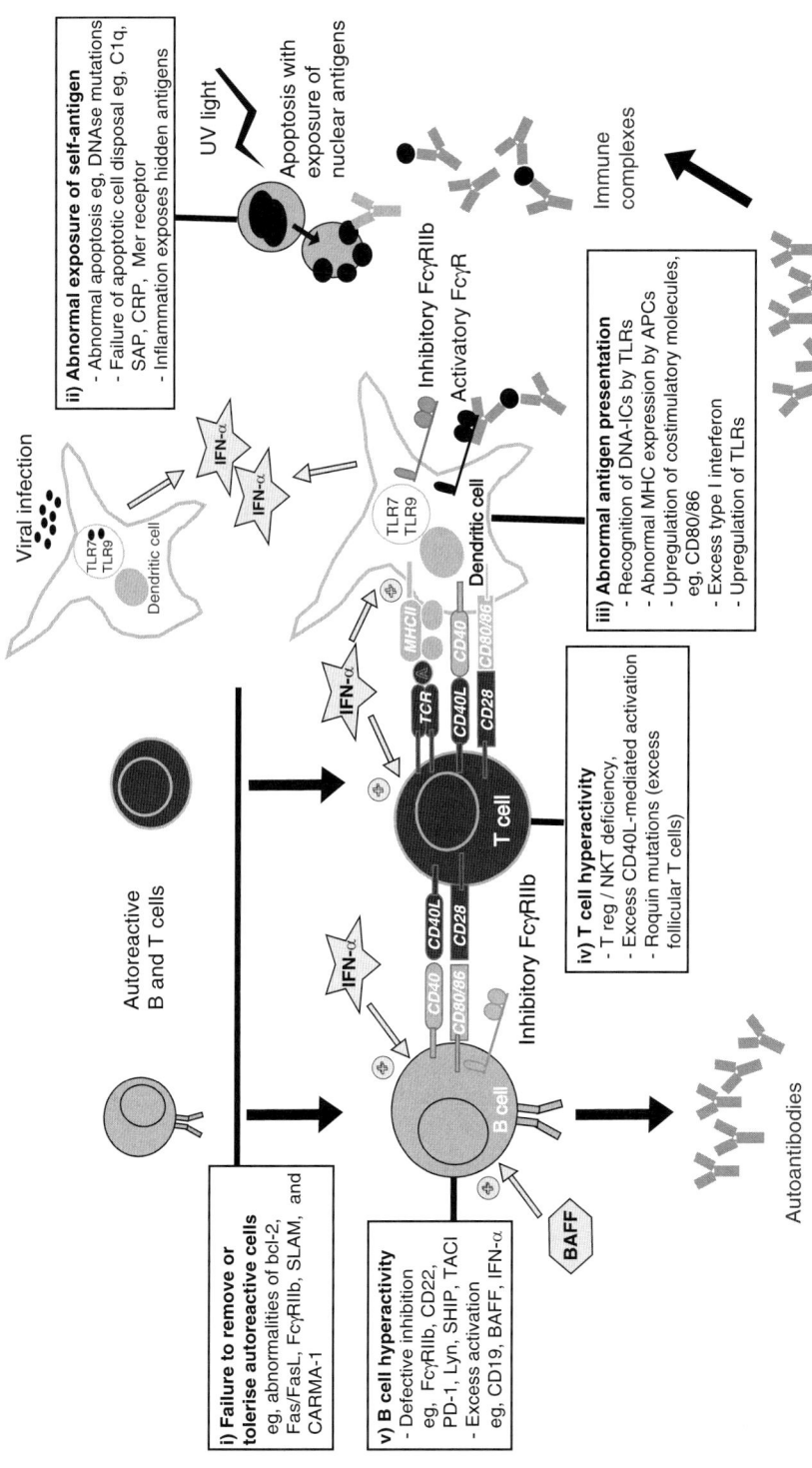

**Figure 1.** Disease mechanisms stage 1: loss of tolerance to self-antigen and the generation of autoantibodies. A failure of mechanisms to remove or tolerize autoreactive B- and T-cells allows their persistence. Abnormal exposure of self-antigen, for example, during apoptosis, facilitates the presentation of self-antigen by APCs to autoreactive, hyperactive T-cells. TLRs play a critical role through the recognition of DNA-immune complexes or viral nucleic acids stimulating APC maturation and the production of type 1 interferons. Hyperactive, autoreactive B-cells are activated by T-cells to produce autoantibodies, which in turn form immune complexes which can be internalized by APCs, further propagating disease.

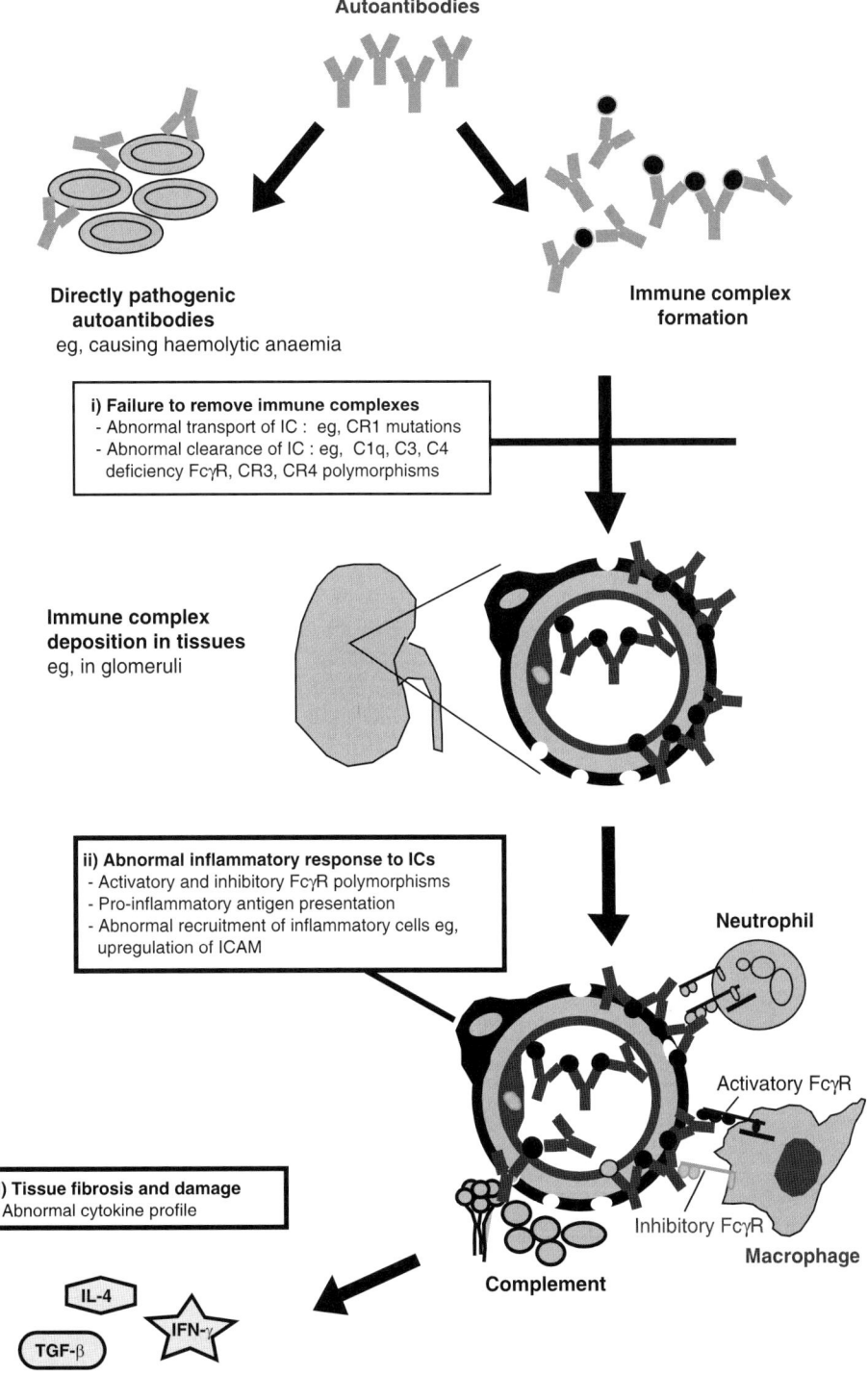

**Figure 2.** Disease mechanisms stage 2: autoantibodies and immune complexes cause inflammation and disease. Autoantibodies produced by B-cells may be directly pathogenic, e.g., those causing haemolytic anemia, or may form immune complexes which are not adequately disposed of, and therefore become deposited in tissues causing inflammation. Further abnormalities in the inflammatory response and in cytokine production lead to fibrosis and irreversible damage.

They may thus be eliminated in the T-cell zone (Goodnow, 1996).

Once in germinal centers, unwanted autoreactive B-cell clones may be produced as a result of somatic hypermutation. Those binding foreign antigen immobilized on follicular dendritic cells are selected for survival, whereas those binding soluble antigen undergo apoptosis, perhaps providing a mechanism for the deletion of autoreactive germinal centre B-cells (Pulendran et al., 1995; Shokat and Goodnow, 1995). B-cell activity is also kept in check by a number of negative regulatory molecules for example, Fc$\gamma$RIIb, CD22, CD72 and PIR-B. These molecules maintain a tonic inhibition of B-cell responsiveness and play a role in enforcing tolerance (Pritchard and Smith, 2003) (see also Section 3.1.6).

Finally, some self-antigens are sequestered inside cells or within native protein folds, or exist in sites of immunological privilege (for example, the eye) and are thus hidden from B-cells. Tolerance to them is therefore never developed in normal circumstances, as they are not exposed to the immune system, a state termed "immunological ignorance" (Chen, 1998). Similarly, it is possible that subsets of autoreactive B-cells may persist within compartments where they do not encounter self-antigen. Honjo and colleagues developed an anti-red blood cell autoantibody transgenic mouse line, in which almost all B-cells were deleted in the periphery. A small number of B-1 cells, however, escaped deletion, survived and expanded in the peritoneal cavity and the gut, because of the absence of red blood cells. Subsequent activation of B-1 cells by enteric bacteria induced autoimmune hemolytic anemia which was cured by elimination of peritoneal B-1 cells (Okamoto et al., 1992).

### 3.1.2. Failure to remove or silence autoreactive B- and T-cells

As described above, in order to enforce central and peripheral tolerance, autoreactive B- and T-cells must be removed. This is achieved by mechanisms of programmed cell death, apoptosis. Abnormalities of the apoptotic process allow the persistence of autoreactive cells, which may subsequently become activated leading to a breakdown in self-tolerance.

The proto-oncogene *bcl-2* was originally identified as the result of its chromosomal translocation in follicular lymphoma (Tsujimoto et al., 1985) and encodes a 24-kDa membrane-associated protein which protects cells from apoptosis (Vaux et al., 1988). Transgenic overexpression of Bcl-2 in B-cells prevents apoptosis, blocks peripheral self-tolerance and can predispose to autoantibody production and immune-mediated glomerulonephritis (Strasser et al., 1991). Thus breakdown of pathways of programmed cell death may well lead to the survival of autoreactive cells and to autoimmune disease.

CD95 (Fas) is a member of the nerve growth factor/tumor necrosis factor receptor superfamily and can initiate a signal transduction cascade leading to apoptosis. It is expressed at high levels in activated lymphocytes and acts as a major pathway for the peripheral deletion of antigen-primed lymphocytes (Nagata, 1997; Nagata and Golstein, 1995). Humans with Fas mutations develop an autoimmune lymphoproliferative syndrome (ALPS), which is characterized by massive lymphadenopathy and autoimmune disease (Fisher et al., 1995). Mice homozygous for the *lpr* or *gdl* mutation (leading to non-functional Fas or FasL proteins, respectively) have increased numbers of B- and T-cells (the latter are CD4$^-$ CD8$^-$B220$^+$), autoantibodies and develop lymphadenopathy and immune complex-mediated glomerulonephritis (Bossu et al., 1993; Russell and Wang, 1993). Furthermore, mice heterozygous for PTEN, a phosphatase involved in apoptosis, have impaired Fas response and develop a disease comparable to Fas mutants (Di Cristofano et al., 1999).

As mentioned previously, it has been proposed that antigen in the germinal centre is retained in the form of immune complexes bound to FDCs and hence B-cell stimulation can occur either through Fc$\gamma$RIIb alone resulting in apoptosis, or through both Fc$\gamma$RIIb and the BCR producing survival (Pearse et al., 1999). Therefore, a failure of Fc$\gamma$RIIb function might allow the persistence of autoimmune B-cells. Recent work suggests that Fc$\gamma$RIIb may additionally contribute to the maintenance of peripheral tolerance via receptor editing

(Fukuyama et al., 2005). In addition to its controlling role in peripheral tolerance, FcγRIIb may also play a role in central B-cell tolerance (Brauweiler and Cambier, 2004). FcγRIIb is expressed on pre-B-cells, and ligation (in the absence of B-cell aggregation) can induce cell death and inhibit migration (Brauweiler and Cambier, 2004). However, if the pre-B-cell receptor is crosslinked, then FcγRIIb can inhibit apoptosis (Kato et al., 2002).

Linkage and congenic studies in murine lupus models have identified a susceptibility locus on chromosome 1, *sle1b*, which impairs B-cell anergy, receptor revision and deletion. Recent evidence suggests that differences in splicing of mRNA encoding a member of the SLAM family of lymphocyte adhesions receptor, Ly108, are sufficient to alter B-cell receptor signaling and lead to the persistence of self-reactive B-cells in the lymph nodes and spleen (Kumar et al., 2006).

Cross-linking the BCR can lead to an immunogenic or tolerogenic response depending on the circumstances. A number of studies have identified key scaffolding molecules, including CARMA-1 (also known as CARD-11) and the Cbl family of ubiquitin ligases. These scaffolding proteins may determine the polarity of response by promoting assembly of particular signaling complexes around receptors (Jun and Goodnow, 2003). CARMA-1 may promote a breakdown in tolerance by assembling molecules which enhance cellular activation (Jun et al., 2003). In contrast, Cbl proteins may encourage a tolerogenic response by facilitating the safe disposal of internalized self-antigens (Bachmaier et al., 2000).

### 3.1.3. Abnormal exposure of self-antigen

In humans with lupus, the evidence of down regulation of apoptosis is much less clear. Only a quarter of patients with Fas or FasL mutations develop ANAs (Vaishnaw et al., 1999). In addition, increased levels of apoptotic cells have been found in SLE patients, although this did not correlate with disease activity (Courtney et al., 1999). The importance of this lies in the observation that nuclear autoantigens cluster in blebs on the surface of apoptotic cells after exposure to UV light (Casciola-Rosen et al., 1994). Post-translational modifications, such as ubiquitination, citrullination, phosphorylation, and methylation, during apoptosis may also result in the presentation of cryptic self-antigens to which tolerance has not been established (Utz and Anderson, 1998). Normally apoptotic cells are swiftly removed by neighboring cells or professional phagocytes, in a process which is not thought to generate a significant inflammatory response (Savill et al., 2002). This rapid removal prevents the release of potential autoantigens from apoptotic blebs, which might then initiate a pro-inflammatory immune response and generate autoantibodies to nuclear components. Apoptotic cells express a number of "eat me" signals, for example phosphatidylserine, which facilitate uptake and are recognized by receptors on phagocytic cells, including the phosphatidylserine receptor, CD14, the C1q receptor, the vitronectin receptor and the MER receptor (Savill et al., 2002; Scott et al., 2001). Bridging molecules such as C1q, C-reactive protein, serum amyloid P protein (SAP), pentraxin-3, thrombospondin, and prothrombin "opsonize" apoptotic cells and can mediate uptake by phagocytes or mask autoantigens (D'Agnillo et al., 2003).

Exposure of normal mice to syngeneic apoptotic thymocytes can induce transient anti-DNA and anti-phospholipid antibodies (Mevorach et al., 1998). Therefore, either an increased production or reduced disposal of apoptotic cells might lead to a breakdown of tolerance. Monocytes from patients with SLE show accelerated apoptosis in vitro (Shoshan et al., 2001). In the NZB/W F1 mouse there is a higher spontaneous apoptotic rate in splenic cells compared with BALB/c, suggesting an increased rate of production. However, it has also been noted that patients with SLE have impaired macrophage-uptake of apoptotic neutrophils (Ren et al., 2003). Furthermore, in NZB/W F1 and MRL mice there is defective uptake of thioglycollate-induced apoptotic neutrophils by peritoneal macrophages (Potter et al., 2003). C1q-deficient mice show high levels of ANAs and increased numbers of apoptotic bodies within glomeruli, suggesting a defect in clearance of apoptotic debris (Botto et al., 1998). As mentioned previously, most patients with C1q-deficiency develop a lupus-like illness (Slingsby et al., 1996). Deficiency of C4 (Chen et al., 2000), SAP (Paul and Carroll, 1999), and MER (Cohen et al., 2002) in mice results in an anti-nuclear autoimmune response and a glomerulonephritis. Prothrombin binds to apoptotic cells and appears to be a target of lupus anticoagulant antibodies (D'Agnillo et al., 2003). Deficiency of DNAse 1, an enzyme which digests chromatin-derived autoantigens, leads to an enhanced susceptibility to autoimmunity in mice and mutations of *DNASE1* have been identified in humans with SLE (Yasutomo et al., 2001). To summarize, there is evidence to suggest that the display of nuclear antigens on the cell surface during apoptosis may facilitate the activation of autoreactive B-cells and the presentation of these antigens to autoreactive T-cells. Thus impaired apoptotic cell clearance may contribute to the breakdown of tolerance to nuclear antigens.

## 3.1.4. Abnormal presentation of self-antigen to autoreactive T-cells

In order to activate autoreactive T-cells, antigen presenting cells (APCs) such as dendritic cells (DCs), macrophages, and B-cells must recognize, bind, internalize, process, and present antigen to autoreactive T-cells. A number of studies in murine models of lupus suggest that abnormalities of antigen processing and presentation may lead to an excessive or inappropriate activation of T-cells. Lupus-like disease is ameliorated in NZB/W-F1 mice treated with an agent which reduces MHC class I expression, suggesting that MHC class I expression confers susceptibility to disease through presentation of self-peptides (Mozes et al., 2005). Other studies show increased maturation of macrophages and DCs (as evidenced by upregulation of costimulatory molecules such as CD40, CD80 and CD86) in a murine lupus model (C57BL/6.*sle3*). Importantly, APCs from these mice were better at stimulating T-cell proliferation in vitro (Zhu et al., 2005).

The situation in humans with SLE is less clear. Some studies have shown reduced numbers of circulating CD11c+ DCs with a diminished T-cell stimulatory capacity (Scheinecker et al., 2001). In vitro-generated, monocyte-derived DCs from SLE patients have a reduced up-regulation of MHC class II molecules on activation, which correlated with disease activity scores (Koller et al., 2004). These findings may well be confounded by the immunosuppressive treatments used in patients with lupus. However, a more recent study of monocyte-derived DCs from lupus patients has shown spontaneous over-expression of CD86 and an increase in activation-induced secretion of IL-6 by DCs (Decker et al., 2006). In humans, the inhibitory Fc$\gamma$R, Fc$\gamma$RIIb plays an important role in regulating macrophage and DC activation. A single nucleotide polymorphism in the *Fc$\gamma$RIIb* gene encodes a threonine (T) for isoleucine (I) substitution at position 232, within the transmembrane domain. Fc$\gamma$RIIb$^{T232}$ has been found at increased frequency in patients with SLE (Kyogoku et al., 2002; Li et al., 2003, Siriboonrit et al., 2003; Chu et al., 2004) and has defective inhibitory function (Floto et al., 2005). This is associated with an increased upregulation of MHC and co-stimulatory molecules in monocyte-derived macrophages following activation (Floto et al., 2005).

Antigen presentation by B-cells may be important in the pathogenesis of SLE. J$_H$D-MRL/*lpr* mice (a B-cell deficient version of the lupus-prone MRL/*lpr* mouse) fail to develop nephritis and dermatitis, emphasizing the importance of B-cells in disease (Chan et al., 1999a). However, mIgM · MRL/*lpr* transgenic mice which have B-cells but are unable to secrete antibody, develop substantial nephritis and vasculitis, suggesting pathogenic B-cell activity independent of antibody production (Chan et al., 1999a, b). It maybe that, in this model, B-cell autoantigen presentation may play a more important role than the production of autoantibody in the development of lupus (Chan et al., 1997).

Nuclear antigens contain motifs which can potentially trigger immunogenic antigen presentation via interactions with intracellular TLRs. TLRs are innate immune receptors which discriminate microbe from self. TLR7 and TLR9 detect microbial RNA and DNA respectively, within intracellular compartments, but mammalian nuclear antigens contain motifs which can potentially trigger these receptors. TLR9 is expressed in macrophages, B-cells, and DCs, and recognizes bacterial DNA with multiple CpG nucleotides. Mammalian DNA is a less potent stimulator of TLR9 because many CpG motifs are masked by methylation. However, studies have shown that internalization of mammalian DNA-containing immune complexes in DCs can be mediated by Fc$\gamma$RIIa, delivering the antigen into intracellular lysosomes containing TLR9, which subsequently initiates DC activation and the production of type I interferons (Means and Luster, 2005). More recently TLR7 has also been implicated in the breakdown of tolerance through genetic studies on the murine lupus Y-linked autoimmune accelerator (*Yaa*) locus. This locus was found to contain a duplication of a segment of X chromosomal DNA containing the *TLR7* gene, which was transposed to the Y-chromosome (Pisitkun et al., 2006; Subramanian et al., 2006). This transposition effectively doubled *TLR7* gene expression within B-cells enhancing responsiveness to TLR7 ligands including self nucleic acids, thus promoting proliferation of autoreactive B-cells. Similarly DCs may be co-activated via surface Fc receptors binding antibody–nucleic acid immune complexes and TLR7 binding of internalized nucleic acids.

There is increasing evidence to suggest that type I IFNs (IFN-$\alpha$ and IFN-$\beta$) may play a role in the pathogenesis of lupus by activating tolerogenic immature myeloid dendritic cells (mDCs). It has long been recognized that some patients with SLE have elevated IFN activity in serum (Preble et al., 1982). More recently DNA microarray studies have identified an upregulation of IFN-induced genes in peripheral blood mononuclear cells (PBMCs) in patients with lupus (Bennett et al., 2003). Furthermore, IFN therapy and viral infections can induce autoantibody formation in patients, some of which become symptomatic (Ronnblom et al., 1991). The study of DCs and the effects of type I IFNs on DC maturation have begun to shed some light on these observations. Two main DC differentiation pathways have been identified, producing tissue resident mDCs and circulating plasmacytoid dendritic cells (pDCs). Immature mDCs appear to play an important role in the maintenance of peripheral tolerance, possibly through the maintenance and induction of regulatory T-cells (Banchereau and Pascual, 2006) and can be activated and matured by type I IFNs to form mature mDCs which act as potent APC and activators of T-cells. pDCs produce vast quantities of IFNs upon viral exposure and express both TLR7 and TLR9 (Siegal et al., 1999). Both types of DC can internalize IC-containing nuclear autoantigens via Fc$\gamma$RIIa. Once internalized into endosomes, these autoantigens stimulate TLR7, further increasing IFN production. Exposure of mDCs to type I IFNs leads to upregulation of TLR7, potentially enhancing the response to self-antigen (Banchereau et al., 2000, 2004; Blanco et al., 2001; Steinman et al., 2003). Treatment of patients with SLE with steroids induces remission and abrogates the type I IFN signature in PBMCs, possibly as a result of pDC depletion (Bennett et al., 2003). Type I IFNs also induce the production of B-cell activity factor (BAFF), which may stimulate autoreactive B-cell proliferation (Litinskiy et al., 2002) (see Section 3.1.6) and enhance the ability of CD4 T-cell to provide B-cell help (Le Bon et al., 2006).

## 3.1.5. T-cell hyperactivity

In order to fully activate autoreactive B-cells, there must be a cognate interaction with, and provision of help by, CD4 T-cells. The maintenance of T-cell tolerance appears to play an important role in imposing tolerance on autoreactive B-cells. Non-autoimmune mice can be induced to develop autoantibodies to dsDNA and glomerulonephritis by immunization with anti-dsDNA antibodies or peptides derived from the $V_H$ region of these antibodies. This immunization stimulates the expansion of autoreactive T-cells, which in turn drive B-cell proliferation and the production of anti-dsDNA antibodies and an associated immune complex mediated nephritis (Singh et al., 2002). This breakdown in self-tolerance does not persist and despite repeated immunizations, mice spontaneously achieve a full recovery from the episode of autoimmunity. The appearance of CD4+, CD25+ T-cells, so-called regulatory T-cells, which decrease the production of anti-dsDNA antibodies in vitro, appears to play an important role in the re-establishment of self-tolerance (Singh et al., 2002). Furthermore, in a number of mouse models of lupus, immunization with nucleosomal peptides can induce the expansion of both CD8+ and CD4+ CD25+ regulatory T-cells (Hahn et al., 2005; Kang et al., 2005). These regulatory T-cells reduce autoantibody production and disease progression via a TGF$\beta$-dependent mechanism. Impaired CD8+ regulatory T-cell function has also been described in humans with active SLE (Filaci et al., 2001). CD8+ T-cells were isolated from patients with active disease and cultured in vitro to generate suppressor lymphocytes. In contrast to cells derived from healthy controls, SLE-derived CD8+ T suppressors failed to inhibit PBMC proliferation in vitro.

NKT cells are a unique subset of T lymphocytes that express both the NK receptor and invariant T-cell receptor. Some murine lupus models such as MRL-lpr mice, have reduced numbers and impaired function of NKT cells (Mieza et al., 1996; Yang et al., 2003a). Indeed, activation of NKT cells by repeated treatment with the NKT cell ligand $\alpha$-galactosylceramide can suppress the development of autoimmunity in both spontaneous and inducible murine models of SLE (Yang et al., 2003a; Singh et al., 2005). In contrast NKT cell deficiency exacerbates lupus nephritis (Yang et al., 2003b). NKT cell deficiency has also been described in humans with SLE (Oishi et al., 2001; Bennett et al., 2003), and NKT cell number seems to correlate inversely with disease activity (Oishi et al., 2001).

As well as a failure of T-cell regulatory mechanisms, there is also evidence to suggest that T-cells from patients and mice with SLE have diminished activation thresholds. TCR-CD3-mediated stimulation of T-cells from patients with SLE show aberrant calcium fluxes and increased intracellular phosphorylation (Liossis et al., 1998; Hoffman, 2004). Furthermore, there also appears to be an excess provision of help to B-cells, particularly via the CD40–CD40L pathway (Yi et al., 2000; Crow and Kirou, 2001). This has led to the idea that blockade of T-cell costimulation may provide a therapeutic target in SLE.

Goodnow and colleagues have used chemical mutagenesis to identify autoimmune regulators in mice. They treated control C57BL/6 mice with ethylnitrosourea and isolated a mouse strain, *sanroque*, with severe autoimmune disease resulting from a single recessive defect affecting mature T-cells, causing the formation of excessive numbers of follicular helper T-cells and germinal centers. The mutation disrupts a repressor of ICOS, an essential co-stimulatory receptor for follicular T-cells. *Sanroque* mice fail to repress diabetes-causing T-cells, and develop high titres of autoantibodies and a pattern of pathology consistent with lupus. The causative mutation is in a gene known as roquin (*Rc3h1*), which encodes a highly conserved member of the RING-type ubiquitin ligase protein family (Vinuesa et al., 2005a). It is proposed that roquin may repress autoantibody production by setting an inhibitory threshold in T-cells that prevents extrafollicular T-cells from assuming a follicular helper phenotype which promotes B-cell antibody production (Vinuesa et al., 2005b).

### 3.1.6. B-cell hyperactvity

Upon antigen binding to the BCR, B-cell activation thresholds are determined by the net effects of positive and negative regulatory molecules. If the balance between these inputs is disturbed then autoimmunity can result. A reduction of inhibitory signals due to dysfunction of negative regulatory molecules such as Fc$\gamma$RIIb, CD22, and PD-1, or an excess of activatory signaling due to abnormalities of CD19, can both lead to a breakdown in tolerance.

Fc$\gamma$ receptors bind IgG and may be activatory (Fc$\gamma$RI, IIa, IIIa, IIIb, and IV) or inhibitory (Fc$\gamma$RIIb) (Nimmerjahn and Ravetch, 2006). Fc$\gamma$RIIb inhibits many features of the immune response, including Fc$\gamma$R-mediated phagocytosis, pro-inflammatory cytokine production, antigen presentation, and antibody responses (Nimmerjahn and Ravetch, 2006; Takai, 2002). Fc$\gamma$RIIb is the only Fc receptor present on B-cells and co-ligation with the BCR during immune complex binding initiates a downstream signaling cascade which culminates in the neutralization of BCR-mediated activation. There is increasing evidence to suggest that defective Fc$\gamma$RIIb inhibition is important in the pathogenesis of SLE. Polygenic murine SLE models such as MRL, NZB, and BXSB, have a deletion in the FcγRIIb promoter associated with reduced receptor expression on macrophages and activated B-cells (Pritchard et al., 2000; Jiang et al., 2000; Xiu et al., 2002). FcγRIIb-deficient mice have augmented humoral responses following immunization with both T-dependent and independent antigens (Takai et al., 1996) and are susceptible to a number of antibody- or immune complex-dependent inducible models of autoimmunity, including collagen-induced arthritis (Yuasa et al., 1999; Kagari et al., 2003), Goodpasture's syndrome (Nakamura et al., 2000), and immune complex mediated alveolitis (Clynes et al., 1999). In addition, FcγRIIb−/− mice derived on a 129/Sv/C57BL/6 background and backcrossed for 10 generations onto a C57BL/6 background, develop hypergammaglobulinaemia, autoantibodies (to antigens such as chromatin and dsDNA), and an immune complex-mediated autoimmune disease resembling SLE (Bolland and Ravetch, 2000). Transfer studies show that the disease is fully transferable and dependent on B-cells. In NZB, BXSB, and FcγRIIb-deficient mice, normalization of bone marrow FcγRIIb expression by retroviral transduction of bone marrow cells leads to a reduction in levels of ANAs, antibodies to dsDNA, and chromatin and renal immune complex deposition, together with improved survival compared with mice reconstituted with control transfected bone marrow (McGaha et al., 2005). Furthermore, mice heterozygous for FcγRIIb-deficiency exhibit only a modest reduction in receptor expression, but have a definite predisposition to autoimmunity (Bolland et al., 2002); thus even small alterations in FcγRIIb expression or function may have a profound effect on maintenance of self-tolerance. Interestingly, a combined deficiency of FcγRIIb together with a Fas mutation (C57BL/6 FcγRIIb−/−Fas$^{lpr/lpr}$ mice) enhances the development of autoimmunity (Yajima et al., 2003). In humans, a lupus-associated FcγRIIb polymorphism (FcγRIIb$^{T232}$) has defective inhibitory function, which is associated with B-cell hyperactivity (Floto et al., 2005; Kono et al., 2005).

CD22 is a B-cell-specific negative regulator (O'Keefe et al., 1996). CD22-deficient mice show B-cell hyperresponsiveness which correlates with the development of autoantibodies directed against double stranded DNA (O'Keefe et al., 1999). Mice deficient in other molecules involved in the inhibitory pathway, such as Lyn and SHP-1, also display B-cell hyperresponsiveness and autoimmune disease (Hibbs et al., 1995).

Programmed cell death gene-1 (*PDCD1*) (or PD-1 as it is known in mice), is a 55 kDa transmembrane protein of the immunoglobulin superfamily which contains an ITIM in its cytoplasmic domain. Mice lacking PD-1 develop a lupus-like disease with arthritis and glomerulonephritis (Nishimura et al., 1999). A polymorphism in PDCD1 has also been identified in humans. An intronic SNP in PDCD1 is associated with the development of SLE in Europeans (found in 12% of affected individuals vs. 5% of controls). The SNP alters a binding site for the runt-related transcription factor 1 (RUNX1) located in an intronic enhancer. Disruption of RUNX1 binding by the SNP may lead to aberrant regulation of PDCD1 expression, and a release of autoreactive cells from inhibitory restraint (Prokunina et al., 2002). Thus defective negative regulation of B-cell activation can lead to B-cell hyperactivity and autoimmunity.

CD19 is a cell surface glycoprotein expressed exclusively on B-cells, in a complex with CD21 (complement receptor 2), CD81, and Leu 13 (Smith and Fearon, 2000). CD19 modulates the proliferation and activation signals delivered to the B-cell by immunoglobulin. Coligation of the CD19/CD21/CD81 complex to the BCR results in a massive decrease in the activation threshold of B-cells stimulated through surface IgM (Carter and Fearon, 1992). Overexpression of human CD19 in mice leads to elevated levels of immunoglobulin and hyperactive B-cells (Sato et al., 1996). Transgenic mice which express a model autoantigen, sHEL (soluble hen egg lysosyme) and high affinity HEL-specific antigen receptors are functionally anergic and do not produce autoantibodies. However, overexpression of CD19 in these mice results in the breakdown of peripheral tolerance and the production of anti-HEL antibodies (Inaoki et al., 1997). In addition, upregulation of CD19 has been noted in patients with systemic sclerosis (Sato et al., 2000). Thus by lowering the activation threshold on B-cells, CD19 overexpression may contribute to the breakdown of tolerance and the development of autoimmune disease.

BAFF (also known as BLyS, TALL-1, and THANK) is a member of the TNF ligand superfamily and an important co-stimulator of B-cell survival and expansion (Moore et al., 1999). Transgenic animals overexpressing BAFF in lymphoid cells develop symptoms characteristic of SLE and expand a rare population of splenic lymphocytes (Mackay et al., 1999). In addition, circulating BAFF is more abundant in NZB/W-F1 and MRL*lpr* mice during the onset and progression of SLE (Gross et al., 2000). High levels of BAFF have also been found in patients with lupus and appear to be associated with autoantibody production (Zhang et al., 2001; Pers et al., 2005). TACI is a TNF receptor family member that binds BAFF. Loss of TACI in mice results in the formation of autoantibodies to nuclear antigens and immune complex deposition in the kidneys (Khare et al., 2000; Seshasayee et al., 2003). Furthermore, treatment of NZB/W-F1 mice with soluble TACI–Ig fusion protein inhibits the development of proteinuria and prolongs survival of the animals (Gross et al., 2000). These studies have identified TACI–Ig as a possible treatment for SLE in humans.

## 3.2. Stage 2: pathogenic autoantibodies and immune complexes cause inflammation and disease

In patients with SLE, autoantibodies can be directed against a large number of autoantigens (Tan, 1989). Some autoantibodies appear to be directly pathogenic, such as those causing haemolytic anemia (Fig. 2). The majority are thought to form immune complexes which, if inadequately cleared, may become deposited in tissues initiating inflammation.

### 3.2.1. Directly pathogenic antibodies
Autoimmune haemolytic anemia is an initial feature in 5% of patients with SLE, and occurs in up to a third of patients. Autoantibodies (usually IgG) bind to red cell membrane components, causing autoagglutination of erythrocytes within the splenic pulp and subsequent removal by phagocytes (warm autoimmune haemolytic anemia) (Kotzin, 1996). Similarly, autoantibody-mediated thrombocytopaenia, neutropaenia, and lymphopaenia may occur in SLE.

Anti-phospholipid antibodies, which recognize a variety of phospholipids including cardiolipin, phosphatidylserine, and $\beta_2$ glycoprotein I ($\beta_2$-GPI), are strongly associated with recurrent episodes of arterial and venous thrombosis, spontaneous fetal loss, and thrombocytopaenia. This triad, termed anti-phospholipid syndrome, is seen in the presence of anti-phospholipid antibodies in patients with and without SLE. A number of pathogenic mechanisms have been proposed for this association. Anti-$\beta_2$-GPI antibodies are thought to interfere with the $\beta_2$ GPI-inhibition of factor Xa production by activated platelets. In addition, autoantibody binding to $\beta_2$-GPI on the endothelial cell surface induces the expression of a number of adhesion molecules, for example, VCAM-1 and E-selectin, thus enhancing monocyte adhesion to endothelial cells (Myones and McCurdy, 2000).

### 3.2.2. Failure of immune complex clearance
Although many individuals develop ANAs (approximately 5% of the population, Kotzin, 1996) most do not go on to get immune complex deposition and disease. Similarly in animal models the presence of antibody does not necessarily lead to disease; B6.NZMc1 congenic mice develop IgG anti-nuclear autoantibody in the absence of nephritis (Morel et al., 1997) as do CD22-deficient mice (O'Keefe et al., 1996). In a recent case-control study 88% of individuals who go on to develop SLE were found to have an autoantibody several years before diagnosis (Arbuckle et al., 2003). The development of disease may require persistent exposure to self-antigen, or defective immune complex clearance or processing. Immune complex formation is a physiological consequence of an adaptive humoral response. Binding of antibody to antigen is designed to promote the removal of

foreign antigens and this task is largely undertaken by the mononuclear phagocytic system of the spleen and liver. Complement components frequently become incorporated into immune complexes and facilitate their transport via binding to CR1 on erythrocytes (Fearon, 1980). Tissue macrophages in the liver and spleen bear both FcγR and complement receptors, CR3 and CR4, whilst follicular dendritic cells also express CR2. The FcγRs involved in immune complex clearance by these cells are thought to be the low-affinity FcγRII and FcγRIII (Frank et al., 1983; Kimberly and Ralph, 1983). Several studies have also shown that clearance of IgG-coated erythrocytes is delayed in patients with SLE compared with controls (Frank et al., 1979; Hamburger et al., 1982). The clearance of soluble immune complexes is also abnormal in lupus patients, with reduced complement- and Fc-mediated uptake by the splenic mononuclear phagocytic system (Davies et al., 1992, 2002).

As mentioned previously, inherited deficiencies in the early classical pathway components (C1q, C2, C4) can lead to SLE (Carroll, 1998; Schur, 1995; Slingsby et al., 1996). Complement components are likely to be important in the disposal of apoptotic cells (see Section 3.1.3) and in the removal of immune complexes. In support of this hypothesis, C1q-deficient mice have reduced splenic immune complex uptake (Botto et al., 1998; Cortes-Hernandez et al., 2004; Nash et al., 2001).

Fcγ receptors bind IgG-containing immune complexes and allow internalization and clearance by cells of the reticuloendothelial system. FcγRII and FcγRIII are thought to play a particularly important role in this function (Frank et al., 1983; Kimberly and Ralph, 1983). FcγRIIa is a single chain activatory receptor which is unique to humans (van de Winkel and Capel, 1993). A G > A point mutation has been identified in the *FcγRIIA* gene, which leads to either an arginine (R131) or histidine (H131) at amino acid position 131. These alleles are co-dominantly expressed, thus an individual might express RR, HR, or HH. FcγRIIa is the only FcγR that significantly binds IgG2 containing ICs, and the affinity of this interaction varies between the polymorphic forms of the receptor, in that FcγRIIa-H131 has a much higher affinity for both IgG2 and IgG3 (Parren et al., 1992). This increased affinity for complexed IgG2 has functional consequences, in that IgG2-opsonised particles (and to a lesser extent, IgG3-opsonised particles) are more readily internalized by phagocytes isolated from FcγRIIa-H131 homozygous individuals compared with FcγRIIa-R131 homozygotes (Salmon et al., 1992). A large number of studies have documented the frequency of FcγRIIa polymorphisms in patients with lupus (Lehrnbecher et al., 1999). Overall, it appears that the FcγRIIa-R/R131 allotype (which binds IgG2 and IgG3 containing IC less well) occurs with increased frequency in patients with SLE, and in lupus nephritis (particularly in patients with IgG2 anti-C1q antibodies) (Haseley et al., 1997; Norsworthy et al., 1999), suggesting that reduced Fc-mediated IC clearance may contribute to disease pathogenesis.

FcγRIII is another activatory Fc receptor which plays an important role in the disposal of ICs. There are two isotypes, FcγRIIIa and FcγRIIIb. The latter is found only in humans on neutrophils and has no cytoplasmic domain and therefore no signaling capacity. FcγRIIIb is linked to the outer leaflet of the plasma membrane by a glycosyl phosphatidylinositol (GPI) anchor and is thought to mediate neutrophil recruitment (Coxon et al., 2001). The major polymorphism of FcγRIIIa is a point mutation (T > G) at nucleotide 559, which results in either a valine (V158) or phenylalanine (F158) at amino acid position 158. These alleles are also co-dominantly expressed and again, the alteration in an extracellular amino acid results in a change in binding to its principle ligands. It has been shown that the FcγRIIIa-V158 allele has a higher affinity for IgG1 and IgG3 and can also interact with IgG4 (Wu et al., 1997). As with FcγRIIa, it is the lower affinity FcγRIIIa-F158 allele or F/F158 genotype, which has been associated with SLE or lupus nephritis in several (particularly Caucasian) populations.

Expression of FcγRIIIb is limited to neutrophils, and two main isoforms exist, varying in their expression of the human neutrophil antigen (HNA). The first two isoforms HNA1a and HNA1b are encoded by genes which differ by five nucleotides (141, 147, 227, 277, and 349) within exon 3, resulting in a four amino acid substitution in its membrane-distal immunoglobulin-like extracellular domain. These are termed HNA1a and HNA1b (previously FγRIIIb-NA1 and FcγRIIIb-NA2). Due to differential glycosylation, they vary in their interaction with IgG, in that FcγRIIIb-HNA1a has a higher affinity for IgG1 and IgG3 and can mediate phagocytosis of IgG1/3-complexed particles (Salmon et al., 1995). Studies of FcγRIIIb polymorphisms in patients with lupus have been conflicting but most demonstrate an association of the HNA1b allotype with disease susceptibility (Gonzalez-Escribano et al., 2002; Kyogoku et al., 2002; Siriboonrit et al., 2003).

About 0.1% of central Europeans do not express FcγRIIIb on neutrophils due to gene deletion. Interestingly, Aitman and colleagues have recently shown that copy number variation in the human *FcγRIIIb* gene and the orthologous rat gene determines susceptibility to immune complex-mediated glomerulonephritis. In rat strains susceptible to glomerulonephritis there was a loss of Fcgr3-related sequence which was associated with macrophage hyperactivity. In humans, there were between zero and four copies to the *FcγRIIIb* gene present and a low copy number was associated with lupus nephritis (Aitman et al., 2006). It may be that reduced neutrophil expression of FcγRIIIb or the expression of the lower affinity FcγRIIIb-HNA1b receptor leads to impaired glomerular clearance of immune complexes thus precipitating glomerular inflammation. This is supported by our own unpublished studies of neutrophil IC binding in an FcγRIIIb-null patient.

### 3.2.3. Abnormal inflammatory response following immune complex deposition

The association of ANAs with SLE is remarkably strong, although they may not be directly pathogenic. The development of inflammatory lesions is thought to require the formation and deposition of immune complexes within tissues. These in turn, initiate an inflammatory response activating complement, and triggering the influx of inflammatory cells such as neutrophils and macrophages.

In a number of animal models of SLE, anti-DNA antibodies have been shown to cause some pathological features of disease, particularly renal manifestations, via the formation of circulating immune complexes which subsequently become deposited in the kidneys (Lefkowith et al., 1996). Infusion of anti-DNA antibodies, obtained from lupus-prone mouse strains such as MRL, into normal mice prompts the development of a proliferative glomerulonephritis (Vlahakos et al., 1992). Intra-peritoneal administration of a monoclonal anti-DNA antibody-secreting hybridoma into control mice can also induce glomerulonephritis, proteinuria, and a dermal vasculitis (Vlahakos et al., 1992). In addition, mouse and human anti-DNA IgG applied to the isolated perfused rat kidney binds avidly to glomeruli and is associated with proteinuria and a reduction in inulin clearance (Raz et al., 1989).

It may be that the renal injury is induced not only through deposition of circulating immune complexes, but also by immune complex formation in tissues. The latter might occur by two different mechanisms; firstly, it has been suggested that DNA could become bound to the glomerulus and subsequently recognized by anti-DNA antibodies, leading to in-situ immune complex formation (Bernstein et al., 1995). Secondly, a sub-set of pathogenic antibodies could cross-react with non-DNA glomerular structures. For example, autoantibodies to the endogenous retroviral glycoprotein gp70 and gp70–anti-gp70 immune complexes have been identified in diseased glomeruli of lupus-prone BXSB mice (Haywood et al., 2001; Izui et al., 1981).

Once deposited, immune complexes then induce tissue injury through complement or FcR-mediated mechanisms on phagocytes (type III hypersensitivity). Deletion of activatory FcγRs protects mice from antibody-mediated spontaneous or induced autoimmune disease without altering expression of autoantibodies. This was demonstrated in the FcRγ deficient NZB/NZW F1 mice which develop autoantibodies and have significant immune complex deposition, but do not develop glomerulonephritis (Clynes et al., 1998). Processing of immune complexes internalized by FcγRs on antigen presenting cells initiates an inflammatory response thus propagating tissue damage. In addition, local deposition of immune complexes can initiate tissue damage via direct complement activation (Walport, 2001). In addition to antibody-mediated mechanisms of tissue injury, there is some evidence that effector T-cells can play a role. In a subset of SLE patients (Alexopoulos et al., 1990) and also in the MRL murine model (Hewicker and Trautwein, 1987) interstitial nephritis with T-cell infiltrates has been documented, indicating that there may be direct T-cell-mediated tissue damage. However, T-cell-targeted therapies have had limited success in the treatment of SLE.

Intracellular adhesion molecule-1 (ICAM-1) is a member of the immunoglobulin superfamily of adhesion receptors and may be involved in the recruitment of lymphocytes to the kidney during inflammation. ICAM-1 is upregulated in the kidneys of MRL/*lpr* and NZB/W F1 mice (Wuthrich et al., 1990). Furthermore MRL/*lpr* mice deficient in ICAM-1 show a reduction in renal disease and a significantly reduced mortality (Bullard et al., 1997) suggesting that abnormalities of ICAM expression may play a role in lymphocyte recruitment.

### 3.2.4. Tissue damage and fibrosis

Disease severity and manifestations in SLE are extremely variable, none more so than lupus nephritis. Renal biopsies show that some patients have only localized inflammation, others diffuse proliferative inflammation with little fibrosis, whilst others have a marked fibrosis or glomerulosclerosis with little inflammation, and some a membranous glomerulonephritis (Bajaj et al., 2000). This may represent the progression of disease with time, but some murine models suggest that specific factors may accelerate or promote chronic damage. Studies in NZM mice demonstrate that certain congenic strains harbor susceptibility loci for acute glomerulonephritis whilst other congenics develop chronic, fibrosing renal lesions (Waters et al., 2004). The action of cytokines may well be responsible for such differences. MRL/*lpr* mice develop predominantly acute inflammatory lesions and have high levels of IFN-γ. In contrast, renal lesions in NZM.2410 mice and NZB/W-F1 mice demonstrate a more fibrotic phenotype and have high in vivo levels of IL-4 and TGF-β respectively (Singh et al., 2003). Treatment of these mice with angiotensin converting enzyme inhibitors (which reduce type 2 cytokines, including IL-4 and TGF-β), or direct blockade of IL-4 or TGF-β with monoclonal antibodies, suppresses the development of fibrotic renal lesions, without altering glomerular inflammation (Singh et al., 2003; De Albuquerque et al., 2004). In humans with SLE an upregulation of the B-cell activating cytokine IL-10, and reduction in Th1 cytokines such as IL-12 and interferon-γ, have been demonstrated (Hagiwara et al., 1996; Horwitz et al., 1998). It may therefore be that a skewing of the cytokine profile from a Th1 to a Th2 response may promote chronic renal lesions.

## 4. Conclusion

Unraveling the pathogenic mechanisms underlying this complex, polygenic, autoimmune disease is proving a long and difficult process. New data emerging on the role of different immunological players and their interactions in SLE is not only of interest as we try to comprehend disease pathogenesis, but provides information which can guide therapeutic approaches. Novel agents targeting hyperactive B-cells (for example, anti-CD20 antibodies, anti-CD22 antibodies, and BAFF-inhibitors), B-cell–T-cell interactions (for example, CTLA-4 blockade and anti-CD40L antibodies), and downstream inflammatory cytokine production (for example, IL-6 and IL-10 blockade) are all emerging as useful treatments in SLE. Their development has been underpinned by advances in the understanding of immunological abnormalities observed in lupus. Future efforts to increase our insight into the immunopathogenesis of this disease should allow the development of even more specific and less toxic therapies for patients affected by this difficult disease.

## Key points

- SLE is a systemic autoimmune disease characterized by autoantibody production and immune complex deposition in many different tissues.
- Multiple genetic, environmental, and hormonal factors contribute to disease pathogenesis.
- There are two stages in the development of disease; firstly, a breakdown in self-tolerance with autoantibody production, and secondly, the deposition of immune complexes, leading to inflammation and disease.
- A breakdown in self-tolerance is facilitated by a failure of apoptotic mechanisms which remove autoreactive cells, the abnormal exposure of self-antigen, inappropriate presentation of self-antigen to T-cells, and abnormal B- and T-cell hyperactivity.
- Defects in mechanisms of immune complex clearance and an excessive inflammatory response following immune complex deposition result in tissue damage.
- A better understanding of disease mechanisms will allow the generation of targeted therapies.

## References

Aitman, T.J., Dong, R., Vyse, T.J., Norsworthy, P.J., Johnson, M.D., Smith, J., Mangion, J., Roberton-Lowe, C., Marshall, A.J., Petretto, E., et al. 2006. Copy number polymorphism in Fcgr3 predisposes to glomerulonephritis in rats and humans. Nature 439, 851–855.

Akira, S., Takeda, K., Kaisho, T. 2001. Toll-like receptors: critical proteins linking innate and acquired immunity. Nat. Immunol. 2, 675–680.

Alexopoulos, E., Seron, D., Hartley, R.B., Cameron, J.S. 1990. Lupus nephritis: correlation of interstitial cells with glomerular function. Kidney Int. 37, 100–109.

Arbuckle, M.R., McClain, M.T., Rubertone, M.V., Scofield, R.H., Dennis, G.J., James, J.A., Harley, J.B. 2003. Development of autoantibodies before the clinical onset of systemic lupus erythematosus. N. Engl. J. Med. 349, 1526–1533.

Bachmaier, K., Krawczyk, C., Kozieradzki, I., Kong, Y.Y., Sasaki, T., Oliveira-dos-Santos, A., Mariathasan, S., Bouchard, D., Wakeham, A., Itie, A., et al. 2000. Negative regulation of lymphocyte activation and autoimmunity by the molecular adaptor Cbl-b. Nature 403, 211–216.

Bajaj, S., Albert, L., Gladman, D.D., Urowitz, M.B., Hallett, D.C., Ritchie, S. 2000. Serial renal biopsy in systemic lupus erythematosus. J. Rheumatol. 27, 2822–2826.

Banchereau, J., Briere, F., Caux, C., Davoust, J., Lebecque, S., Liu, Y.J., Pulendran, B., Palucka, K. 2000. Immunobiology of dendritic cells. Annu. Rev. Immunol. 18, 767–811.

Banchereau, J., Pascual, V. 2006. Type I interferon in systemic lupus erythematosus and other autoimmune diseases. Immunity 25, 383–392.

Banchereau, J., Pascual, V., Palucka, A.K. 2004. Autoimmunity through cytokine-induced dendritic cell activation. Immunity 20, 539–550.

Bennett, L., Palucka, A.K., Arce, E., Cantrell, V., Borvak, J., Banchereau, J., Pascual, V. 2003. Interferon and granulopoiesis signatures in systemic lupus erythematosus blood. J. Exp. Med. 197, 711–723.

Bernstein, K.A., Valerio, R.D., Lefkowith, J.B. 1995. Glomerular binding activity in MRL lpr serum consists of antibodies that bind to a DNA/histone/type IV collagen complex. J. Immunol. 154, 2424–2433.

Beutler, B. 2004. Inferences, questions and possibilities in Toll-like receptor signalling. Nature 430, 257–263.

Blanco, P., Palucka, A.K., Gill, M., Pascual, V., Banchereau, J. 2001. Induction of dendritic cell differentiation by IFN-alpha in systemic lupus erythematosus. Science 294, 1540–1543.

Block, S.R., Winfield, J.B., Lockshin, M.D., D'Angelo, W.A., Christian, C.L. 1975. Studies of twins with systemic lupus erythematosus. A review of the literature and presentation of 12 additional sets. Am. J. Med. 59, 533–552.

Bolland, S., Ravetch, J.V. 2000. Spontaneous autoimmune disease in Fc(gamma)RIIB-deficient mice results from strain-specific epistasis. Immunity 13, 277–285.

Bolland, S., Yim, Y.S., Tus, K., Wakeland, E.K., Ravetch, J.V. 2002. Genetic modifiers of systemic lupus erythematosus in FcgammaRIIB(−/−) mice. J. Exp. Med. 195, 1167–1174.

Bossu, P., Singer, G.G., Andres, P., Ettinger, R., Marshak-Rothstein, A., Abbas, A.K. 1993. Mature CD4+ T lymphocytes from MRL/lpr mice are resistant to receptor-mediated tolerance and apoptosis. J. Immunol. 151, 7233–7239.

Botto, M., Dell'Agnola, C., Bygrave, A.E., Thompson, E.M., Cook, H.T., Petry, F., Loos, M., Pandolfi, P.P., Walport, M.J. 1998. Homozygous C1q deficiency causes glomerulonephritis associated with multiple apoptotic bodies. Nat. Genet. 19, 56–59.

Brauweiler, A.M., Cambier, J.C. 2004. Autonomous SHIP-dependent FcgammaR signaling in pre-B cells leads to inhibition of cell migration and induction of cell death. Immunol. Lett. 92, 75–81.

Bullard, D.C., King, P.D., Hicks, M.J., Dupont, B., Beaudet, A.L., Elkon, K.B. 1997. Intercellular adhesion molecule-1 deficiency protects MRL/MpJ-Fas(lpr) mice from early lethality. J. Immunol. 159, 2058–2067.

Bygrave, A.E., Rose, K.L., Cortes-Hernandez, J., Warren, J., Rigby, R.J., Cook, H.T., Walport, M.J., Vyse, T.J., Botto, M. 2004. Spontaneous autoimmunity in 129 and C57BL/6 mice-implications for autoimmunity described in gene-targeted mice. PLoS Biol. 2, E243.

Carlsten, H., Nilsson, N., Jonsson, R., Tarkowski, A. 1991. Differential effects of oestrogen in murine lupus: acceleration of glomerulonephritis and amelioration of T cell-mediated lesions. J. Autoimmun. 4, 845–856.

Carlsten, H., Tarkowski, A., Holmdahl, R., Nilsson, L.A. 1990. Oestrogen is a potent disease accelerator in SLE-prone MRL lpr/lpr mice. Clin. Exp. Immunol. 80, 467–473.

Carroll, M.C. 1998. The role of complement and complement receptors in induction and regulation of immunity. Annu. Rev. Immunol. 16, 545–568.

Carter, R.H., Fearon, D.T. 1992. CD19: lowering the threshold for antigen receptor stimulation of B lymphocytes. Science 256, 105–107.

Casciola-Rosen, L., Rosen, A. 1997. Ultraviolet light-induced keratinocyte apoptosis: a potential mechanism for the induction of skin lesions and autoantibody production in LE. Lupus 6, 175–180.

Casciola-Rosen, L.A., Anhalt, G., Rosen, A. 1994. Autoantigens targeted in systemic lupus erythematosus are clustered in two populations of surface structures on apoptotic keratinocytes. J. Exp. Med. 179, 1317–1330.

Chan, O., Madaio, M.P., Shlomchik, M.J. 1997. The roles of B cells in MRL/lpr murine lupus. Ann. N. Y. Acad. Sci. 815, 75–87.

Chan, O.T., Hannum, L.G., Haberman, A.M., Madaio, M.P., Shlomchik, M.J. 1999a. A novel mouse with B cells but lacking serum antibody reveals an antibody-independent role for B cells in murine lupus. J. Exp. Med. 189, 1639–1648.

Chan, O.T., Madaio, M.P., Shlomchik, M.J. 1999b. B cells are required for lupus nephritis in the polygenic, Fas-intact MRL model of systemic autoimmunity. J. Immunol. 163, 3592–3596.

Chen, L. 1998. Immunological ignorance of silent antigens as an explanation of tumor evasion. Immunol. Today 19, 27–30.

Chen, Z., Koralov, S.B., Kelsoe, G. 2000. Complement C4 inhibits systemic autoimmunity through a mechanism independent of complement receptors CR1 and CR2. J. Exp. Med. 192, 1339–1352.

Chu, Z.T., Tsuchiya, N., Kyogoku, C., Ohashi, J., Qian, Y.P., Xu, S.B., Mao, C.Z., Chu, J.Y., Tokunaga, K. 2004. Association of Fcgamma receptor IIb polymorphism with susceptibility to systemic lupus erythematosus in Chinese: a common susceptibility gene in the Asian populations. Tissue Antigens 63, 21–27.

Clynes, R., Dumitru, C., Ravetch, J.V. 1998. Uncoupling of immune complex formation and kidney damage in autoimmune glomerulonephritis. Science 279, 1052–1054.

Clynes, R., Maizes, J.S., Guinamard, R., Ono, M., Takai, T., Ravetch, J.V. 1999. Modulation of immune complex-induced inflammation in vivo by the coordinate expression of activation and inhibitory Fc receptors. J. Exp. Med. 189, 179–185.

Cohen, P.L., Caricchio, R., Abraham, V., Camenisch, T.D., Jennette, J.C., Roubey, R.A., Earp, H.S., Matsushima, G., Reap, E.A. 2002. Delayed apoptotic cell clearance and lupus-like autoimmunity in mice lacking the c-mer membrane tyrosine kinase. J. Exp. Med. 196, 135–140.

Cortes-Hernandez, J., Fossati-Jimack, L., Petry, F., Loos, M., Izui, S., Walport, M.J., Cook, H.T., Botto, M. 2004. Restoration of C1q levels by bone marrow transplantation attenuates autoimmune disease associated with C1q deficiency in mice. Eur. J. Immunol. 34, 3713–3722.

Courtney, P.A., Crockard, A.D., Williamson, K., Irvine, A.E., Kennedy, R.J., Bell, A.L. 1999. Increased apoptotic peripheral blood neutrophils in systemic lupus erythematosus: relations with disease activity, antibodies to double stranded DNA, and neutropenia. Ann. Rheum. Dis. 58, 309–314.

Coxon, A., Cullere, X., Knight, S., Sethi, S., Wakelin, M.W., Stavrakis, G., Luscinskas, F.W., Mayadas, T.N. 2001. Fc gamma RIII mediates neutrophil recruitment to immune complexes: a mechanism for neutrophil accumulation in immune-mediated inflammation. Immunity 14, 693–704.

Crow, M.K., Kirou, K.A. 2001. Regulation of CD40 ligand expression in systemic lupus erythematosus. Curr. Opin. Rheumatol. 13, 361–369.

D'Agnillo, P., Levine, J.S., Subang, R., Rauch, J. 2003. Prothrombin binds to the surface of apoptotic, but not viable, cells and serves as a target of lupus anticoagulant autoantibodies. J. Immunol. 170, 3408–3422.

Davies, K.A., Peters, A.M., Beynon, H.L., Walport, M.J. 1992. Immune complex processing in patients with systemic lupus erythematosus. In vivo imaging and clearance studies. J. Clin. Invest. 90, 2075–2083.

Davies, K.A., Robson, M.G., Peters, A.M., Norsworthy, P., Nash, J.T., Walport, M.J. 2002. Defective Fc-dependent processing of immune complexes in patients with systemic lupus erythematosus. Arthritis Rheum. 46, 1028–1038.

De Albuquerque, D.A., Saxena, V., Adams, D.E., Boivin, G.P., Brunner, H.I., Witte, D.P., Singh, R.R. 2004. An ACE inhibitor reduces Th2 cytokines and TGF-beta1 and TGF-beta2 isoforms in murine lupus nephritis. Kidney Int. 65, 846–859.

Deapen, D., Escalante, A., Weinrib, L., Horwitz, D., Bachman, B., Roy-Burman, P., Walker, A., Mack, T.M. 1992. A revised estimate of twin concordance in systemic lupus erythematosus. Arthritis Rheum. 35, 311–318.

Decker, P., Kotter, I., Klein, R., Berner, B., Rammensee, H.G. 2006. Monocyte-derived dendritic cells over-express CD86 in patients with systemic lupus erythematosus. Rheumatology (Oxford) 45, 1087–1095.

Di Cristofano, A., Kotsi, P., Peng, Y.F., Cordon-Cardo, C., Elkon, K.B., Pandolfi, P.P. 1999. Impaired Fas response and autoimmunity in Pten+/− mice. Science 285, 2122–2125.

Drake, C.G., Rozzo, S.J., Hirschfeld, H.F., Smarnworawong, N.P., Palmer, E., Kotzin, B.L. 1995. Analysis of the

New Zealand Black contribution to lupus-like renal disease. Multiple genes that operate in a threshold manner. J. Immunol. 154, 2441–2447.

Fearon, D.T. 1980. Identification of the membrane glycoprotein that is the C3b receptor of the human erythrocyte, polymorphonuclear leukocyte, B lymphocyte, and monocyte. J. Exp. Med. 152, 20–30.

Filaci, G., Bacilieri, S., Fravega, M., Monetti, M., Contini, P., Ghio, M., Setti, M., Puppo, F., Indiveri, F. 2001. Impairment of CD8+ T suppressor cell function in patients with active systemic lupus erythematosus. J. Immunol. 166, 6452–6457.

Fisher, G.H., Rosenberg, F.J., Straus, S.E., Dale, J.K., Middleton, L.A., Lin, A.Y., Strober, W., Lenardo, M.J., Puck, J.M. 1995. Dominant interfering Fas gene mutations impair apoptosis in a human autoimmune lymphoproliferative syndrome. Cell 81, 935–946.

Floto, R.A., Clatworthy, M.R., Heilbronn, K.R., Rosner, D.R., MacAry, P.A., Rankin, A., Lehner, P.J., Ouwehand, W.H., Allen, J.M., Watkins, N.A., Smith, K.G. 2005. Loss of function of a lupus-associated FcgammaRIIb polymorphism through exclusion from lipid rafts. Nat. Med. 11, 1056–1058.

Frank, M.M., Hamburger, M.I., Lawley, T.J., Kimberly, R.P., Plotz, P.H. 1979. Defective reticuloendothelial system Fc-receptor function in systemic lupus erythematosus. N. Engl. J. Med. 300, 518–523.

Frank, M.M., Lawley, T.J., Hamburger, M.I., Brown, E.J. 1983. NIH Conference: Immunoglobulin G Fc receptor-mediated clearance in autoimmune diseases. Ann. Intern. Med. 98, 206–218.

French, M.A., Hughes, P. 1983. Systemic lupus erythematosus and Klinefelter's syndrome. Ann. Rheum. Dis. 42, 471–473.

Fukuyama, H., Nimmerjahn, F., Ravetch, J.V. 2005. The inhibitory Fcgamma receptor modulates autoimmunity by limiting the accumulation of immunoglobulin G+ anti-DNA plasma cells. Nat. Immunol. 6, 99–106.

Fulcher, D.A., Basten, A. 1997. B-cell activation versus tolerance—the central role of immunoglobulin receptor engagement and T-cell help. Int. Rev. Immunol. 15, 33–52.

Gaffney, P.M., Kearns, G.M., Shark, K.B., Ortmann, W.A., Selby, S.A., Malmgren, M.L., Rohlf, K.E., Ockenden, T.C., Messner, R.P., King, R.A., et al. 1998. A genome-wide search for susceptibility genes in human systemic lupus erythematosus sib-pair families. Proc. Natl. Acad. Sci. U.S.A. 95, 14875–14879.

Gonzalez-Escribano, M.F., Aguilar, F., Sanchez-Roman, J., Nunez-Roldan, A. 2002. FcgammaRIIA, FcgammaRIIIA and FcgammaRIIIB polymorphisms in Spanish patients with systemic lupus erythematosus. Eur. J. Immunogenet. 29, 301–306.

Goodnow, C.C. 1996. Balancing immunity and tolerance: deleting and tuning lymphocyte repertoires. Proc. Natl. Acad. Sci. U.S.A. 93, 2264–2271.

Goodnow, C.C. 1997. Balancing immunity, autoimmunity, and self-tolerance. Ann. N. Y. Acad. Sci. 815, 55–66.

Goodnow, C.C., Cyster, J.G., Hartley, S.B., Bell, S.E., Cooke, M.P., Healy, J.I., Akkaraju, S., Rathmell, J.C., Pogue, S.L., Shokat, K.P. 1995. Self-tolerance checkpoints in B lymphocyte development. Adv. Immunol. 59, 279–368.

Graham, R.R., Ortmann, W.A., Langefeld, C.D., Jawaheer, D., Selby, S.A., Rodine, P.R., Baechler, E.C., Rohlf, K.E., Shark, K.B., Espe, K.J., et al. 2002. Visualizing human leukocyte antigen class II risk haplotypes in human systemic lupus erythematosus. Am. J. Hum. Genet. 71, 543–553.

Gray-McGuire, C., Moser, K.L., Gaffney, P.M., Kelly, J., Yu, H., Olson, J.M., Jedrey, C.M., Jacobs, K.B., Kimberly, R.P., Neas, B.R., et al. 2000. Genome scan of human systemic lupus erythematosus by regression modeling: evidence of linkage and epistasis at 4p16-15.2. Am. J. Hum. Genet. 67, 1460–1469.

Gross, J.A., Johnston, J., Mudri, S., Enselman, R., Dillon, S.R., Madden, K., Xu, W., Parrish-Novak, J., Foster, D., Lofton-Day, C., et al. 2000. TACI and BCMA are receptors for a TNF homologue implicated in B-cell autoimmune disease. Nature 404, 995–999.

Hagiwara, E., Gourley, M.F., Lee, S., Klinman, D.K. 1996. Disease severity in patients with systemic lupus erythematosus correlates with an increased ratio of interleukin-10:interferon-gamma-secreting cells in the peripheral blood. Arthritis Rheum. 39, 379–385.

Hahn, B.H., Singh, R.P., La Cava, A., Ebling, F.M. 2005. Tolerogenic treatment of lupus mice with consensus peptide induces Foxp3-expressing, apoptosis-resistant, TGFbeta-secreting CD8+ T cell suppressors. J. Immunol. 175, 7728–7737.

Hamburger, M.I., Lawley, T.J., Kimberly, R.P., Plotz, P.H., Frank, M.M. 1982. A serial study of splenic reticuloendothelial system Fc receptor functional activity in systemic lupus erythematosus. Arthritis Rheum. 25, 48–54.

Haseley, L.A., Wisnieski, J.J., Denburg, M.R., Michael-Grossman, A.R., Ginzler, E.M., Gourley, M.F., Hoffman, J.H., Kimberly, R.P., Salmon, J.E. 1997. Antibodies to C1q in systemic lupus erythematosus: characteristics and relation to Fc gamma RIIA alleles. Kidney Int. 52, 1375–1380.

Haywood, M.E., Vyse, T.J., McDermott, A., Thompson, E.M., Ida, A., Walport, M.J., Izui, S., Morley, B.J. 2001. Autoantigen glycoprotein 70 expression is regulated by a single locus, which acts as a checkpoint for pathogenic anti-glycoprotein 70 autoantibody production and hence for the corresponding development of severe nephritis, in lupus-prone BXSB mice. J. Immunol. 167, 1728–1733.

Hewicker, M., Trautwein, G. 1987. Sequential study of vasculitis in MRL mice. Lab. Anim. 21, 335–341.

Hibbs, M.L., Tarlinton, D.M., Armes, J., Grail, D., Hodgson, G., Maglitto, R., Stacker, S.A., Dunn, A.R. 1995. Multiple defects in the immune system of Lyn-deficient mice, culminating in autoimmune disease. Cell 83, 301–311.

Hoffman, R.W. 2004. T cells in the pathogenesis of systemic lupus erythematosus. Clin. Immunol. 113, 4–13.

Horwitz, D.A., Gray, J.D., Behrendsen, S.C., Kubin, M., Rengaraju, M., Ohtsuka, K., Trinchieri, G. 1998. Decreased production of interleukin-12 and other Th1-type cytokines in patients with recent-onset systemic lupus erythematosus. Arthritis Rheum. 41, 838–844.

Howard, P.F., Hochberg, M.C., Bias, W.B., Arnett, F.C., Jr., McLean, R.H. 1986. Relationship between C4 null genes, HLA-D region antigens, and genetic susceptibility to systemic lupus erythematosus in Caucasian and black Americans. Am. J. Med. 81, 187–193.

Inaoki, M., Sato, S., Weintraub, B.C., Goodnow, C.C., Tedder, T.F. 1997. CD19-regulated signaling thresholds control peripheral tolerance and autoantibody production in B lymphocytes. J. Exp. Med. 186, 1923–1931.

Izui, S., Elder, J.H., McConahey, P.J., Dixon, F.J. 1981. Identification of retroviral gp70 and anti-gp70 antibodies involved in circulating immune complexes in NZB × NZW mice. J. Exp. Med. 153, 1151–1160.

Jara, L.J., Gomez-Sanchez, C., Silveira, L.H., Martinez-Osuna, P., Vasey, F.B., Espinoza, L.R. 1992. Hyperprolactinemia in systemic lupus erythematosus: association with disease activity. Am. J. Med. Sci. 303, 222–226.

Jiang, Y., Hirose, S., Abe, M., Sanokawa-Akakura, R., Ohtsuji, M., Mi, X., Li, N., Xiu, Y., Zhang, D., Shirai, J., et al. 2000. Polymorphisms in IgG Fc receptor IIB regulatory regions associated with autoimmune susceptibility. Immunogenetics 51, 429–435.

Jun, J.E., Goodnow, C.C. 2003. Scaffolding of antigen receptors for immunogenic versus tolerogenic signaling. Nat. Immunol. 4, 1057–1064.

Jun, J.E., Wilson, L.E., Vinuesa, C.G., Lesage, S., Blery, M., Miosge, L.A., Cook, M.C., Kucharska, E.M., Hara, H., Penninger, J.M., et al. 2003. Identifying the MAGUK protein Carma-1 as a central regulator of humoral immune responses and atopy by genome-wide mouse mutagenesis. Immunity 18, 751–762.

Kagari, T., Tanaka, D., Doi, H., Shimozato, T. 2003. Essential role of Fc gamma receptors in anti-type II collagen antibody-induced arthritis. J. Immunol. 170, 4318–4324.

Kanda, N., Tamaki, K. 1999. Estrogen enhances immunoglobulin production by human PBMCs. J. Allergy Clin. Immunol. 103, 282–288.

Kanda, N., Tsuchida, T., Tamaki, K. 1999. Estrogen enhancement of anti-double-stranded DNA antibody and immunoglobulin G production in peripheral blood mononuclear cells from patients with systemic lupus erythematosus. Arthritis Rheum. 42, 328–337.

Kang, H.K., Michaels, M.A., Berner, B.R., Datta, S.K. 2005. Very low-dose tolerance with nucleosomal peptides controls lupus and induces potent regulatory T cell subsets. J. Immunol. 174, 3247–3255.

Kato, I., Takai, T., Kudo, A. 2002. The pre-B cell receptor signaling for apoptosis is negatively regulated by Fc gamma RIIB. J. Immunol. 168, 629–634.

Khare, S.D., Sarosi, I., Xia, X.Z., McCabe, S., Miner, K., Solovyev, I., Hawkins, N., Kelley, M., Chang, D., Van, G., et al. 2000. Severe B cell hyperplasia and autoimmune disease in TALL-1 transgenic mice. Proc. Natl. Acad. Sci. U.S.A. 97, 3370–3375.

Kimberly, R.P., Ralph, P. 1983. Endocytosis by the mononuclear phagocyte system and autoimmune disease. Am. J. Med. 74, 481–493.

Koller, M., Zwolfer, B., Steiner, G., Smolen, J.S., Scheinecker, C. 2004. Phenotypic and functional deficiencies of monocyte-derived dendritic cells in systemic lupus erythematosus (SLE) patients. Int. Immunol. 16, 1595–1604.

Kono, D.H., Burlingame, R.W., Owens, D.G., Kuramochi, A., Balderas, R.S., Balomenos, D., Theofilopoulos, A.N. 1994. Lupus susceptibility loci in New Zealand mice. Proc. Natl. Acad. Sci. U.S.A. 91, 10168–10172.

Kono, H., Kyogoku, C., Suzuki, T., Tsuchiya, N., Honda, H., Yamamoto, K., Tokunaga, K., Honda, Z. 2005. FcgammaRIIB Ile232Thr transmembrane polymorphism associated with human systemic lupus erythematosus decreases affinity to lipid rafts and attenuates inhibitory effects on B cell receptor signaling. Hum. Mol. Genet. 14, 2881–2892.

Kotzin, B.L. 1996. Systemic lupus erythematosus. Cell 85, 303–306.

Kouskoff, V., Lacaud, G., Nemazee, D. 2000. T cell-independent rescue of B lymphocytes from peripheral immune tolerance. Science 287, 2501–2503.

Kumar, K.R., Li, L., Yan, M., Bhaskarabhatla, M., Mobley, A.B., Nguyen, C., Mooney, J.M., Schatzle, J.D., Wakeland, E.K., Mohan, C. 2006. Regulation of B cell tolerance by the lupus susceptibility gene Ly108. Science 312, 1665–1669.

Kyogoku, C., Dijstelbloem, H.M., Tsuchiya, N., Hatta, Y., Kato, H., Yamaguchi, A., Fukazawa, T., Jansen, M.D., Hashimoto, H., van de Winkel, J.G., et al. 2002. Fcgamma receptor gene polymorphisms in Japanese patients with systemic lupus erythematosus: contribution of FCGR2B to genetic susceptibility. Arthritis Rheum. 46, 1242–1254.

Le Bon, A., Thompson, C., Kamphuis, E., Durand, V., Rossmann, C., Kalinke, U., Tough, D.F. 2006. Cutting edge: enhancement of antibody responses through direct stimulation of B and T cells by type I interferon. J. Immunol. 176, 2074–2078.

Lefkowith, J.B., Kiehl, M., Rubenstein, J., DiValerio, R., Bernstein, K., Kahl, L., Rubin, R.L., Gourley, M. 1996. Heterogeneity and clinical significance of glomerular-binding antibodies in systemic lupus erythematosus. J. Clin. Invest. 98, 1373–1380.

Lehrnbecher, T., Foster, C.B., Zhu, S., Leitman, S.F., Goldin, L.R., Huppi, K., Chanock, S.J. 1999. Variant genotypes of the low-affinity Fcgamma receptors in two control populations and a review of low-affinity Fcgamma receptor polymorphisms in control and disease populations. Blood 94, 4220–4232.

Li, X., Wu, J., Carter, R.H., Edberg, J.C., Su, K., Cooper, G.S., Kimberly, R.P. 2003. A novel polymorphism in the Fcgamma receptor IIB (CD32B) transmembrane region alters receptor signaling. Arthritis Rheum. 48, 3242–3252.

Liossis, S.N., Ding, X.Z., Dennis, G.J., Tsokos, G.C. 1998. Altered pattern of TCR/CD3-mediated protein-tyrosyl phosphorylation in T cells from patients with systemic lupus erythematosus. Deficient expression of the T cell receptor zeta chain. J. Clin. Invest. 101, 1448–1457.

Litinskiy, M.B., Nardelli, B., Hilbert, D.M., He, B., Schaffer, A., Casali, P., Cerutti, A. 2002. DCs induce CD40-independent immunoglobulin class switching through BLyS and APRIL. Nat. Immunol. 3, 822–829.

Mackay, F., Woodcock, S.A., Lawton, P., Ambrose, C., Baetscher, M., Schneider, P., Tschopp, J., Browning, J.L. 1999. Mice transgenic for BAFF develop lymphocytic disorders along with autoimmune manifestations. J. Exp. Med. 190, 1697–1710.

McGaha, T.L., Sorrentino, B., Ravetch, J.V. 2005. Restoration of tolerance in lupus by targeted inhibitory receptor expression. Science 307, 590–593.

Means, T.K., Luster, A.D. 2005. Toll-like receptor activation in the pathogenesis of systemic lupus erythematosus. Ann. N. Y. Acad. Sci. 1062, 242–251.

Melez, K.A., Reeves, J.P., Steinberg, A.D. 1978. Modification of murine lupus by sex hormones. Ann. Immunol. (Paris) 129 C, 707–714.

Mevorach, D., Zhou, J.L., Song, X., Elkon, K.B. 1998. Systemic exposure to irradiated apoptotic cells induces autoantibody production. J. Exp. Med. 188, 387–392.

Mieza, M.A., Itoh, T., Cui, J.Q., Makino, Y., Kawano, T., Tsuchida, K., Koike, T., Shirai, T., Yagita, H., Matsuzawa, A., et al. 1996. Selective reduction of V alpha 14+ NK T cells associated with disease development in autoimmune-prone mice. J. Immunol. 156, 4035–4040.

Moore, P.A., Belvedere, O., Orr, A., Pieri, K., LaFleur, D.W., Feng, P., Soppet, D., Charters, M., Gentz, R., Parmelee, D., et al. 1999. BLyS: member of the tumor necrosis factor family and B lymphocyte stimulator. Science 285, 260–263.

Morel, L., Mohan, C., Yu, Y., Croker, B.P., Tian, N., Deng, A., Wakeland, E.K. 1997. Functional dissection of systemic lupus erythematosus using congenic mouse strains. J. Immunol. 158, 6019–6028.

Morel, L., Tian, X.H., Croker, B.P., Wakeland, E.K. 1999. Epistatic modifiers of autoimmunity in a murine model of lupus nephritis. Immunity 11, 131–139.

Moser, K.L., Neas, B.R., Salmon, J.E., Yu, H., Gray-McGuire, C., Asundi, N., Bruner, G.R., Fox, J., Kelly, J., Henshall, S., et al. 1998. Genome scan of human systemic lupus erythematosus: evidence for linkage on chromosome 1q in African-American pedigrees. Proc. Natl. Acad. Sci. U.S.A. 95, 14869–14874.

Mozes, E., Lovchik, J., Zinger, H., Singer, D.S. 2005. MHC class I expression regulates susceptibility to spontaneous autoimmune disease in (NZBxNZW)F1 mice. Lupus 14, 308–314.

Myones, B.L., McCurdy, D. 2000. The antiphospholipid syndrome: immunologic and clinical aspects. Clinical spectrum and treatment. J. Rheumatol. (Suppl. 58), 20–28.

Nagata, S. 1997. Apoptosis by death factor. Cell 88, 355–365.

Nagata, S., Golstein, P. 1995. The Fas death factor. Science 267, 1449–1456.

Nakamura, A., Yuasa, T., Ujike, A., Ono, M., Nukiwa, T., Ravetch, J.V., Takai, T. 2000. Fcgamma receptor IIB-deficient mice develop Goodpasture's syndrome upon immunization with type IV collagen: a novel murine model for autoimmune glomerular basement membrane disease. J. Exp. Med. 191, 899–906.

Nash, J.T., Taylor, P.R., Botto, M., Norsworthy, P.J., Davies, K.A., Walport, M.J. 2001. Immune complex processing in C1q-deficient mice. Clin. Exp. Immunol. 123, 196–202.

Nimmerjahn, F., Ravetch, J.V. 2006. Fcgamma receptors: old friends and new family members. Immunity 24, 19–28.

Nishimura, H., Nose, M., Hiai, H., Minato, N., Honjo, T. 1999. Development of lupus-like autoimmune diseases by disruption of the PD-1 gene encoding an ITIM motif-carrying immunoreceptor. Immunity 11, 141–151.

Norsworthy, P., Theodoridis, E., Botto, M., Athanassiou, P., Beynon, H., Gordon, C., Isenberg, D., Walport, M.J., Davies, K.A. 1999. Overrepresentation of the Fcgamma receptor type IIA R131/R131 genotype in caucasoid systemic lupus erythematosus patients with autoantibodies to C1q and glomerulonephritis. Arthritis Rheum. 42, 1828–1832.

Nossal, G.J., Pike, B.L. 1980. Clonal anergy: persistence in tolerant mice of antigen-binding B lymphocytes incapable of responding to antigen or mitogen. Proc. Natl. Acad. Sci. U.S.A. 77, 1602–1606.

Oishi, Y., Sumida, T., Sakamoto, A., Kita, Y., Kurasawa, K., Nawata, Y., Takabayashi, K., Takahashi, H., Yoshida, S., Taniguchi, M., et al. 2001. Selective reduction and recovery of invariant Valpha24JalphaQ T cell receptor T cells in correlation with disease activity in patients with systemic lupus erythematosus. J. Rheumatol. 28, 275–283.

Okamoto, M., Murakami, M., Shimizu, A., Ozaki, S., Tsubata, T., Kumagai, S., Honjo, T. 1992. A transgenic model of autoimmune hemolytic anemia. J. Exp. Med. 175, 71–79.

O'Keefe, T.L., Williams, G.T., Batista, F.D., Neuberger, M.S. 1999. Deficiency in CD22, a B cell-specific inhibitory receptor, is sufficient to predispose to development of high affinity autoantibodies. J. Exp. Med. 189, 1307–1313.

O'Keefe, T.L., Williams, G.T., Davies, S.L., Neuberger, M.S. 1996. Hyperresponsive B cells in CD22-deficient mice. Science 274, 798–801.

Parren, P.W., Warmerdam, P.A., Boeije, L.C., Arts, J., Westerdaal, N.A., Vlug, A., Capel, P.J., Aarden, L.A., van de Winkel, J.G. 1992. On the interaction of IgG subclasses with the low affinity Fc gamma RIIa (CD32) on human monocytes, neutrophils, and platelets. Analysis of a functional polymorphism to human IgG2. J. Clin. Invest. 90, 1537–1546.

Paul, E., Carroll, M.C. 1999. SAP-less chromatin triggers systemic lupus erythematosus. Nat. Med. 5, 607–608.

Pearse, R.N., Kawabe, T., Bolland, S., Guinamard, R., Kurosaki, T., Ravetch, J.V. 1999. SHIP recruitment attenuates Fc gamma RIIB-induced B cell apoptosis. Immunity 10, 753–760.

Pers, J.O., Daridon, C., Devauchelle, V., Jousse, S., Saraux, A., Jamin, C., Youinou, P. 2005. BAFF overexpression is associated with autoantibody production in autoimmune diseases. Ann. N. Y. Acad. Sci. 1050, 34–39.

Pisitkun, P., Deane, J.A., Difilippantonio, M.J., Tarasenko, T., Satterthwaite, A.B., Bolland, S. 2006. Autoreactive B cell responses to RNA-related antigens due to *TLR7* gene duplication. Science 312, 1669–1672.

Potter, P.K., Cortes-Hernandez, J., Quartier, P., Botto, M., Walport, M.J. 2003. Lupus-prone mice have an abnormal response to thioglycolate and an impaired clearance of apoptotic cells. J. Immunol. 170, 3223–3232.

Preble, O.T., Black, R.J., Friedman, R.M., Klippel, J.H., Vilcek, J. 1982. Systemic lupus erythematosus: presence in human serum of an unusual acid-labile leukocyte interferon. Science 216, 429–431.

Prete, P.E. 1985. The mechanism of action of L-canavanine in inducing autoimmune phenomena. Arthritis Rheum. 28, 1198–1200.

Pritchard, N.R., Cutler, A.J., Uribe, S., Chadban, S.J., Morley, B.J., Smith, K.G.C. 2000. Autoimmune-prone mice share a promoter haplotype associated with reduced expression and function of the Fc receptor FcgammaRII. Curr. Biol. 10, 227–230.

Pritchard, N.R., Smith, K.G. 2003. B cell inhibitory receptors and autoimmunity. Immunology 108, 263–273.

Prokunina, L., Castillejo-Lopez, C., Oberg, F., Gunnarsson, I., Berg, L., Magnusson, V., Brookes, A.J., Tentler, D., Kristjansdottir, H., Grondal, G., et al. 2002. A regulatory polymorphism in PDCD1 is associated with susceptibility to systemic lupus erythematosus in humans. Nat. Genet. 32, 666–669.

Pulendran, B., Kannourakis, G., Nouri, S., Smith, K.G.C., Nossal, G.J.V. 1995. Soluble antigen can cause enhanced apoptosis of germinal-centre B cells. Nature 375, 331–334.

Raz, E., Brezis, M., Rosenmann, E., Eilat, D. 1989. Anti-DNA antibodies bind directly to renal antigens and induce kidney dysfunction in the isolated perfused rat kidney. J. Immunol. 142, 3076–3082.

Reidenberg, M.M., Drayer, D.E., Lorenzo, B., Strom, B.L., West, S.L., Snyder, E.S., Freundlich, B., Stolley, P.D. 1993. Acetylation phenotypes and environmental chemical exposure of people with idiopathic systemic lupus erythematosus. Arthritis Rheum. 36, 971–973.

Ren, Y., Tang, J., Mok, M.Y., Chan, A.W., Wu, A., Lau, C.S. 2003. Increased apoptotic neutrophils and macrophages and impaired macrophage phagocytic clearance of apoptotic neutrophils in systemic lupus erythematosus. Arthritis Rheum. 48, 2888–2897.

Reveille, J.D., Moulds, J.M., Ahn, C., Friedman, A.W., Baethge, B., Roseman, J., Straaton, K.V., Alarcon, G.S. 1998. Systemic lupus erythematosus in three ethnic groups: I. The effects of HLA class II, C4, and CR1 alleles, socioeconomic factors, and ethnicity at disease onset. LUMINA Study Group. Lupus in minority populations, nature versus nurture. Arthritis Rheum. 41, 1161–1172.

Ronnblom, L.E., Alm, G.V., Oberg, K. 1991. Autoimmune phenomena in patients with malignant carcinoid tumors during interferon-alpha treatment. Acta Oncol. 30, 537–540.

Russell, J.H., Wang, R. 1993. Autoimmune gld mutation uncouples suicide and cytokine/proliferation pathways in activated, mature T cells. Eur. J. Immunol. 23, 2379–2382.

Salmon, J.E., Edberg, J.C., Brogle, N.L., Kimberly, R.P. 1992. Allelic polymorphisms of human Fc gamma receptor IIA and Fc gamma receptor IIIB. Independent mechanisms for differences in human phagocyte function. J. Clin. Invest. 89, 1274–1281.

Salmon, J.E., Millard, S.S., Brogle, N.L., Kimberly, R.P. 1995. Fc gamma receptor IIIb enhances Fc gamma receptor IIa function in an oxidant-dependent and allele-sensitive manner. J. Clin. Invest. 95, 2877–2885.

Sanchez-Guerrero, J., Karlson, E.W., Liang, M.H., Hunter, D.J., Speizer, F.E., Colditz, G.A. 1997. Past use of oral contraceptives and the risk of developing systemic lupus erythematosus. Arthritis Rheum. 40, 804–808.

Sato, S., Hasegawa, M., Fujimoto, M., Tedder, T.F., Takehara, K. 2000. Quantitative genetic variation in CD19 expression correlates with autoimmunity. J. Immunol. 165, 6635–6643.

Sato, S., Ono, N., Steeber, D.A., Pisetsky, D.S., Tedder, T.F. 1996. CD19 regulates B lymphocyte signaling thresholds critical for the development of B-1 lineage cells and autoimmunity. J. Immunol. 157, 4371–4378.

Savill, J., Dransfield, I., Gregory, C., Haslett, C. 2002. A blast from the past: clearance of apoptotic cells regulates immune responses. Nat. Rev. Immunol. 2, 965–975.

Scheinecker, C., Zwolfer, B., Koller, M., Manner, G., Smolen, J.S. 2001. Alterations of dendritic cells in systemic lupus erythematosus: phenotypic and functional deficiencies. Arthritis Rheum. 44, 856–865.

Schur, P.H. 1995. Genetics of systemic lupus erythematosus. Lupus 4, 425–437.

Schur, P.H., Marcus-Bagley, D., Awdeh, Z., Yunis, E.J., Alper, C.A. 1990. The effect of ethnicity on major histocompatibility complex complement allotypes and extended haplotypes in patients with systemic lupus erythematosus. Arthritis Rheum. 33, 985–992.

Scott, R.S., McMahon, E.J., Pop, S.M., Reap, E.A., Caricchio, R., Cohen, P.L., Earp, H.S., Matsushima, G.K. 2001. Phagocytosis and clearance of apoptotic cells is mediated by MER. Nature 411, 207–211.

Seshasayee, D., Valdez, P., Yan, M., Dixit, V.M., Tumas, D., Grewal, I.S. 2003. Loss of TACI causes fatal lymphoproliferation and autoimmunity, establishing TACI as an inhibitory BLyS receptor. Immunity 18, 279–288.

Shai, R., Quismorio, F.P., Jr., Li, L., Kwon, O.J., Morrison, J., Wallace, D.J., Neuwelt, C.M., Brautbar, C., Gauderman, W.J., Jacob, C.O. 1999. Genome-wide screen for systemic lupus erythematosus susceptibility genes in multiplex families. Hum. Mol. Genet. 8, 639–644.

Sherer, Y., Gorstein, A., Fritzler, M.J., Shoenfeld, Y. 2004. Autoantibody explosion in systemic lupus erythematosus: more than a hundred different antibodies found in SLE patients. Semin. Arthritis Rheum. 34, 501–537.

Shokat, K.M., Goodnow, C.C. 1995. Antigen-induced B-cell death and elimination during germinal-centre immune responses. Nature 375, 334–338.

Shoshan, Y., Shapira, I., Toubi, E., Frolkis, I., Yaron, M., Mevorach, D. 2001. Accelerated Fas-mediated apoptosis of monocytes and maturing macrophages from patients with systemic lupus erythematosus: relevance to in vitro impairment of interaction with iC3b-opsonized apoptotic cells. J. Immunol. 167, 5963–5969.

Siegal, F.P., Kadowaki, N., Shodell, M., Fitzgerald-Bocarsly, P.A., Shah, K., Ho, S., Antonenko, S., Liu, Y.J. 1999. The nature of the principal type 1 interferon-producing cells in human blood. Science 284, 1835–1837.

Singh, A.K., Yang, J.Q., Parekh, V.V., Wei, J., Wang, C.R., Joyce, S., Singh, R.R., Van Kaer, L. 2005. The natural killer T cell ligand alpha-galactosylceramide prevents or promotes pristane-induced lupus in mice. Eur. J. Immunol. 35, 1143–1154.

Singh, R.R., Ebling, F.M., Albuquerque, D.A., Saxena, V., Kumar, V., Giannini, E.H., Marion, T.N., Finkelman, F.D., Hahn, B.H. 2002. Induction of autoantibody production is limited in nonautoimmune mice. J. Immunol. 169, 587–594.

Singh, R.R., Saxena, V., Zang, S., Li, L., Finkelman, F.D., Witte, D.P., Jacob, C.O. 2003. Differential contribution of IL-4 and STAT6 vs STAT4 to the development of lupus nephritis. J. Immunol. 170, 4818–4825.

Siriboonrit, U., Tsuchiya, N., Sirikong, M., Kyogoku, C., Bejrachandra, S., Suthipinittharm, P., Luangtrakool, K., Srinak, D., Thongpradit, R., Fujiwara, K., et al. 2003. Association of Fcgamma receptor IIb and IIIb polymorphisms with susceptibility to systemic lupus erythematosus in Thais. Tissue Antigens 61, 374–383.

Slingsby, J.H., Norsworthy, P., Pearce, G., Vaishnaw, A.K., Issler, H., Morley, B.J., Walport, M.J. 1996. Homozygous hereditary C1q deficiency and systemic lupus erythematosus. A new family and the molecular basis of C1q deficiency in three families. Arthritis Rheum. 39, 663–670.

Smith, K.G., Fearon, D.T. 2000. Receptor modulators of B-cell receptor signaling—CD19/CD22. Curr. Top. Microbiol. Immunol. 245, 195–212.

Steinman, R.M., Hawiger, D., Nussenzweig, M.C. 2003. Tolerogenic dendritic cells. Annu. Rev. Immunol. 21, 685–711.

Strasser, A., Whittingham, S., Vaux, D.L., Bath, M.L., Adams, J.M., Cory, S., Harris, A.W. 1991. Enforced BCL2 expression in B-lymphoid cells prolongs antibody responses and elicits autoimmune disease. Proc. Natl. Acad. Sci. U.S.A. 88, 8661–8665.

Subramanian, S., Tus, K., Li, Q.Z., Wang, A., Tian, X.H., Zhou, J., Liang, C., Bartov, G., McDaniel, L.D., Zhou, X.J., et al. 2006. A Tlr7 translocation accelerates systemic autoimmunity in murine lupus. Proc. Natl. Acad. Sci. U.S.A. 103, 9970–9975.

Takai, T. 2002. Roles of Fc receptors in autoimmunity. Nat. Rev. Immunol. 2, 580–592.

Takai, T., Ono, M., Hikida, M., Ohmori, H., Ravetch, J.V. 1996. Augmented humoral and anaphylactic responses in Fc gamma RII-deficient mice. Nature 379, 346–349.

Tan, E.M. 1989. Antinuclear antibodies: diagnostic markers for autoimmune diseases and probes for cell biology. Adv. Immunol. 44, 93–151.

Tsujimoto, Y., Cossman, J., Jaffe, E., Croce, C.M. 1985. Involvement of the bcl-2 gene in human follicular lymphoma. Science 228, 1440–1443.

Utz, P.J., Anderson, P. 1998. Posttranslational protein modifications, apoptosis, and the bypass of tolerance to autoantigens. Arthritis Rheum. 41, 1152–1160.

Vaishnaw, A.K., Toubi, E., Ohsako, S., Drappa, J., Buys, S., Estrada, J., Sitarz, A., Zemel, L., Chu, J.L., Elkon, K.B. 1999. The spectrum of apoptotic defects and clinical manifestations, including systemic lupus erythematosus, in humans with CD95 (Fas/APO-1) mutations. Arthritis Rheum. 42, 1833–1842.

van de Winkel, J.G., Capel, P.J. 1993. Human IgG Fc receptor heterogeneity: molecular aspects and clinical implications. Immunol. Today 14, 215–221.

Van Dyne, S., Holers, V.M., Lublin, D.M., Atkinson, J.P. 1987. The polymorphism of the C3b/C4b receptor in the normal population and in patients with systemic lupus erythematosus. Clin. Exp. Immunol. 68, 570–579.

Vaughan, J.H. 1997. The Epstein–Barr virus and systemic lupus erythematosus. J. Clin. Invest. 100, 2939–2940.

Vaux, D.L., Cory, S., Adams, J.M. 1988. *Bcl-2* gene promotes haemopoietic cell survival and cooperates with c-myc to immortalize pre-B cells. Nature 335, 440–442.

Vidaller, A., Llorente, L., Larrea, F., Mendez, J.P., Alcocer-Varela, J., Alarcon-Segovia, D. 1986. T-cell dysregulation in patients with hyperprolactinemia: effect of bromocriptine treatment. Clin. Immunol. Immunopathol. 38, 337–343.

Vinuesa, C.G., Cook, M.C., Angelucci, C., Athanasopoulos, V., Rui, L., Hill, K.M., Yu, D., Domaschenz, H., Whittle, B., Lambe, T., et al. 2005a. A RING-type ubiquitin ligase family member required to repress follicular helper T cells and autoimmunity. Nature 435, 452–458.

Vinuesa, C.G., Tangye, S.G., Moser, B., Mackay, C.R. 2005b. Follicular B helper T cells in antibody responses and autoimmunity. Nat. Rev. Immunol. 5, 853–865.

Vlahakos, D.V., Foster, M.H., Adams, S., Katz, M., Ucci, A.A., Barrett, K.J., Datta, S.K., Madaio, M.P. 1992. Anti-DNA antibodies form immune deposits at distinct glomerular and vascular sites. Kidney Int. 41, 1690–1700.

von Herrath, M.G., Oldstone, M.B. 1996. Virus-induced autoimmune disease. Curr. Opin. Immunol. 8, 878–885.

Wakeland, E.K., Liu, K., Graham, R.R., Behrens, T.W. 2001. Delineating the genetic basis of systemic lupus erythematosus. Immunity 15, 397–408.

Walport, M.J. 2001. Complement. First of two parts. N. Engl. J. Med. 344, 1058–1066.

Waters, S.T., McDuffie, M., Bagavant, H., Deshmukh, U.S., Gaskin, F., Jiang, C., Tung, K.S., Fu, S.M. 2004. Breaking tolerance to double stranded DNA, nucleosome, and other nuclear antigens is not required for the pathogenesis of lupus glomerulonephritis. J. Exp. Med. 199, 255–264.

Woosley, R.L., Drayer, D.E., Reidenberg, M.M., Nies, A.S., Carr, K., Oates, J.A. 1978. Effect of acetylator phenotype on the rate at which procainamide induces antinuclear antibodies and the lupus syndrome. N. Engl. J. Med. 298, 1157–1159.

Wu, J., Edberg, J.C., Redecha, P.B., Bansal, V., Guyre, P.M., Coleman, K., Salmon, J.E., Kimberly, R.P. 1997. A novel polymorphism of FcgammaRIIIa (CD16) alters receptor function and predisposes to autoimmune disease. J. Clin. Invest. 100, 1059–1070.

Wuthrich, R.P., Jevnikar, A.M., Takei, F., Glimcher, L.H., Kelley, V.E. 1990. Intercellular adhesion molecule-1 (ICAM-1) expression is upregulated in autoimmune murine lupus nephritis. Am. J. Pathol. 136, 441–450.

Xiu, Y., Nakamura, K., Abe, M., Li, N., Wen, X.S., Jiang, Y., Zhang, D., Tsurui, H., Matsuoka, S., Hamano, Y., et al. 2002. Transcriptional regulation of *Fcgr2b* gene by polymorphic promoter region and its contribution to humoral immune responses. J. Immunol. 169, 4340–4346.

Yajima, K., Nakamura, A., Sugahara, A., Takai, T. 2003. FcgammaRIIB deficiency with Fas mutation is sufficient for the development of systemic autoimmune disease. Eur. J. Immunol. 33, 1020–1029.

Yang, J.Q., Saxena, V., Xu, H., Van Kaer, L., Wang, C.R., Singh, R.R. 2003a. Repeated alpha-galactosylceramide administration results in expansion of NK T cells and alleviates inflammatory dermatitis in MRL-lpr/lpr mice. J. Immunol. 171, 4439–4446.

Yang, J.Q., Singh, A.K., Wilson, M.T., Satoh, M., Stanic, A.K., Park, J.J., Hong, S., Gadola, S.D., Mizutani, A., Kakumanu, S.R., et al. 2003b. Immunoregulatory role of CD1d in the hydrocarbon oil-induced model of lupus nephritis. J. Immunol. 171, 2142–2153.

Yasutomo, K., Horiuchi, T., Kagami, S., Tsukamoto, H., Hashimura, C., Urushihara, M., Kuroda, Y. 2001. Mutation of DNASE1 in people with systemic lupus erythematosus. Nat. Genet. 28, 313–314.

Yi, Y., McNerney, M., Datta, S.K. 2000. Regulatory defects in Cbl and mitogen-activated protein kinase (extracellular signal-related kinase) pathways cause persistent hyperexpression of CD40 ligand in human lupus T cells. J. Immunol. 165, 6627–6634.

Yuasa, T., Kubo, S., Yoshino, T., Ujike, A., Matsumura, K., Ono, M., Ravetch, J.V., Takai, T. 1999. Deletion of fcgamma receptor IIB renders H-2(b) mice susceptible to collagen-induced arthritis. J. Exp. Med. 189, 187–194.

Zhang, J., Roschke, V., Baker, K.P., Wang, Z., Alarcon, G.S., Fessler, B.J., Bastian, H., Kimberly, R.P., Zhou, T. 2001. Cutting edge: a role for B lymphocyte stimulator in systemic lupus erythematosus. J. Immunol. 166, 6–10.

Zhu, J., Liu, X., Xie, C., Yan, M., Yu, Y., Sobel, E.S., Wakeland, E.K., Mohan, C. 2005. T cell hyperactivity in lupus as a consequence of hyperstimulatory antigen-presenting cells. J. Clin. Invest. 115, 1869–1878.

# CHAPTER 16

# Systemic Lupus Erythematosus: Renal Involvement

H. Terence Cook[a],*, Liz Lightstone[b]

[a]Department of Histopathology, Faculty of Medicine, Imperial College, London W12 ONN, UK
[b]West London Renal and Transplantation Centre, Imperial College London, Hammersmith Hospital, London W12 ONN, UK

## 1. Introduction

The kidney is commonly involved in systemic lupus erythematosus (SLE) with 60–80% of patients developing abnormalities of urine or renal function at some time during their clinical course (Cameron, 1999). Pathological changes in the kidney in SLE may involve the glomeruli, tubules and interstitium, or blood vessels. In most cases the glomerular involvement dominates the picture and, for that reason, the classification of lupus nephritis has been mainly based on the pattern of glomerular disease. In this chapter, we will discuss the pathological changes that are seen in each of the compartments of the kidney and how renal biopsy findings are related to clinical presentation and outcome.

## 2. Renal pathologic changes

### 2.1. Glomeruli

Almost all biopsies from patients with renal involvement in SLE will show deposition of immune complexes in glomeruli and the site of deposition of the immune complexes is closely related to the type of structural and inflammatory changes seen within the glomerulus. The site where the immune complexes deposit is of primary concern in the pathogenesis of the disease because different glomerular localizations of complexes initiate different pathogenic pathways. The localization of the complexes is determined by the specificity, affinity, and avidity of the antibodies formed, their class and subclass, and the size and valence of the complexes. In general, when an immune reaction is characterized by the presence of relatively small amounts of stable, intermediate sized complexes formed with high affinity antibodies, it is likely to result in mesangial glomerulonephritis. These complexes accumulate in the mesangium as part of filtration, and may be cleared adequately by the mesangial clearing system, resulting in mild glomerular lesions. With larger complexes formed by high-avidity antibodies, or with larger numbers of complexes, the capacity of the mesangium to handle macromolecules becomes overloaded, resulting in a subendothelial accumulation of these complexes as well. The subendothelial complexes are able to activate circulating inflammatory mediators, especially the complement system and the Fc receptors in leukocytes. Adhesion molecules are then upregulated and inflammatory cells arrested and activated. This leads to a more severe histopathologic lesion with cell proliferation and, possibly, necrosis. Alternatively, an immune response may lead to the formation of small, unstable immune complexes formed by low-avidity or low-affinity antibodies in the presence of antigen excess.

---

*Corresponding author.
Tel.:44-20-8383-1000; Fax: 44-20-8383-8141
E-mail address: t.h.cook@imperial.ac.uk

© 2008 Elsevier B.V. All rights reserved.
DOI: 10.1016/S1571-5078(07)07016-X

These complexes may dissociate, followed by re-association subepithelially and the development of a membranous type of glomerulopathy. Subepithelial complexes can activate complement, but chemotaxis is frustrated by the inability of inflammatory cells to pass the glomerular basement membrane. Thus a prolonged, chronic inflammation occurs, eventually leading to abnormal basement membrane production, increased basement membrane permeability, proteinuria, and a nephrotic syndrome. Thus, in simple terms, immune complexes that are restricted to the mesangium lead to mesangial hypercellularity without significant inflammation involving the capillary lumens. Patients with mesangial-limited lesions may have overt renal manifestations or minor proteinuria only. Immune complexes on the outside of the glomerular basement membrane beneath the podocytes—subepithelial deposits—lead to podocyte dysfunction with proteinuria and also to structural changes to the glomerular basement membrane giving the morphological appearance of membranous glomerulonephritis. This classically presents with nephrotic range proteinuria but without hematuria. Most serious in terms of glomerular inflammation and progression to scarring is when the immune complexes are found between the endothelium and the glomerular basement membrane—subendothelial deposits. At this site the immune complexes are able to activate complement and other inflammatory mediators leading to leukocyte influx and activation and consequent damage to the glomerular structure with tuft necrosis and progression to glomerular scarring. Patients with proliferative lesions will have proteinuria, hematuria, and varying degrees of renal dysfunction. The recognition of these patterns of immune complex deposition and the associated morphological features forms the basis for the classification system for lupus glomerulonephritis.

Immune complexes in lupus glomerulonephritis are most easily detected by immunohistochemistry and by electron microscopy, although when they are large they may be readily seen by light microscopy. Typically immunohistochemistry will show the presence of IgA, IgG, IgM, and complement activation products within the deposits. Characteristically the complement products will include those that are activated by the classical pathway of complement activation including C1q and C4 as well as C3 and the presence of significant deposits of these early classical components in a renal biopsy should always raise the possibility of SLE. In most cases, it is not possible to be sure what antigens are present in the immune deposits but it is likely that dsDNA and histones are involved. Immune complexes are also easily seen by electron microscopy where they appear as discrete areas of electron dense material.

### 2.1.1. Classification of lupus glomerulonephritis

As discussed above, the site of immune complex deposition in the glomerulus is a major determinant of glomerular morphological changes and of clinical presentation. It is possible to recognize three distinct patterns—mesangial proliferation, membranous glomerulonephritis, and proliferative glomerulonephritis involving the capillary loops, although in any particular biopsy these patterns may overlap. These morphological changes provide the basis for histological classification. We shall first briefly discuss some historical aspects of the classification of lupus glomerulonephritis and then describe the current classification.

One of the first studies to demonstrate the importance of glomerular morphology in determining outcome was published by 1964 (Pollak et al., 1964). They studied 87 patients with SLE for up to 8 years. They classified the renal histology as: normal, lupus glomerulitis, active lupus glomerulonephritis, or membranous glomerulonephritis. Broadly their category of glomerulitis corresponded to a mesangial pattern of disease whereas active lupus glomerulonephritis showed the lesions discussed later (Table 3) that are typically seen with subendothelial deposits. They found a dramatic effect of histology on outcome with 26 of 47 patients with active glomerulonephritis dying of renal failure during the course of the study as opposed to 2 of 40 in the other groups. The first World Health Organization classification of lupus nephritis was formulated by Pirani and Pollak in 1974 and was used in a clinicopathological study in

**Table 1**
2003 ISN/RPS classification of lupus glomerulonephritis

Class I: minimal mesangial lupus nephritis (LN)
  Normal glomeruli by LM, but mesangial immune deposits by IF

Class II: mesangial proliferative lupus nephritis
  Purely mesangial hypercellularity of any degree or mesangial matrix expansion by LM with mesangial immune deposits
  May be a few isolated subepithelial or subendothelial deposits visible by IF or EM but not by LM

Class III: focal lupus nephritis (involving <50% of the total number of glomeruli)
  Active or inactive focal, segmental, or global endo- or extra-capillary GN, typically with focal, subendothelial immune deposits, with or without focal or diffuse mesangial alterations
    III(A) Purely active lesions: *focal proliferative lupus nephritis*
    III(A/C) Active and chronic lesions: *focal proliferative and sclerosing lupus nephritis*
    III(C) Chronic inactive with glomerular scars: *focal sclerosing lupus nephritis*
  Indicate the proportion of glomeruli with active and with sclerotic lesions
  Indicate the proportion of glomeruli with fibrinoid necrosis and/or cellular crescents

Class IV: diffuse lupus nephritis (involving 50% or more of the total number of glomeruli either segmentally or globally)
  Active or inactive diffuse, segmental or global endo- or extra-capillary GN, typically with diffuse subendothelial immune deposits, with or without mesangial alterations. This class is divided into diffuse segmental (IV-S) when >50% of the involved glomeruli have segmental lesions, and diffuse global (IV-G) when >50% of the involved glomeruli have global lesions. Segmental is defined as a lesion that involves less than half of the glomerular tuft
    IV(A) Active lesions: *diffuse segmental or global proliferative lupus nephritis*
    IV(A/C) Active and chronic lesions: *diffuse segmental or global proliferative and sclerosing lupus nephritis*
    IV(C) Inactive with glomerular scars: *diffuse segmental or global sclerosing lupus nephritis*
  Indicate the proportion of glomeruli with active and with sclerotic lesions
  Indicate the proportion of glomeruli with fibrinoid necrosis and/or cellular crescents

Class V: membranous lupus nephritis
  Global or segmental subepithelial immune deposits or their morphologic sequelae by LM and by IF or EM with or without mesangial alterations
  May occur in combination with III or IV in which case both will be diagnosed

Class VI: advanced sclerosing lupus nephritis ≥90% of glomeruli globally sclerosed without residual activity

1978 (Appel et al., 1978). The WHO classification was modified in 1982 and again in 1995. In 2004, a working party set up by the International Society of Nephrology and the Renal Pathology Society (ISN/RPS) proposed a revised classification which aimed to clarify the definitions of glomerular lesions and to standardize the reporting of renal biopsies in lupus nephritis (Weening et al., 2004) and it is this version of the classification that will be described here. The classification is shown in Tables 1 and 2 and we shall consider the classes in detail below. It should be noted that the classification is based on light microscopy and immunohistochemistry and does not depend on access to electron microscopy although electron microscopy is often very helpful in defining the glomerular morphology.

**Table 2**
Abbreviated ISN/RPS classification of lupus nephritis (2003)

| | |
|---|---|
| Class I | Minimal mesangial lupus nephritis (LN) |
| Class II | Mesangial proliferative LN |
| Class III | Focal LN[a] |
| Class IV | Diffuse segmental (IV-S) or global (IV-G) LN[a] |
| Class V | Membranous LN |
| Class VI | Advanced sclerosing LN |

*Note*: Indicate and grade (mild, moderate, severe) of tubular atrophy, interstitial inflammation, and fibrosis, severity of arteriosclerosis or other vascular lesions. Class V may occur in combination with Class III or IV in which case both will be diagnosed.
[a] Indicate the proportion of glomeruli with active and with sclerotic lesions.
[a] Indicate the proportion of glomeruli with fibrinoid necrosis and cellular crescents.

*2.1.1.1. Class I: minimal mesangial lupus nephritis.* An anomaly of the original and subsequent WHO classifications of lupus nephritis was that Class I was defined as having normal glomeruli by light microscopy, immunohistochemistry, and electron microscopy. The ISN/RPS working group felt that it was illogical to include normal glomeruli with lupus glomerulonephritis and therefore defined Class I as showing the deposition of immune complexes within the mesangium but with no changes by light microscopy. It should be rare to diagnose this histologically unless patients are having routine biopsies—they are very unlikely to have hematuria, proteinuria, or abnormal renal function.

*2.1.1.2. Class II: mesangial proliferative lupus nephritis.* Class II lupus nephritis is characterized by the presence of immune deposits within the glomerular mesangium which is associated with expansion of mesangial areas and mesangial hypercellularity. Sometimes scanty immune deposits may also be found by immunohistochemistry or electron microscopy on capillary walls but unless this leads to changes, which are seen at the light microscopic level the biopsy should still be placed in Class II. Patients with Class II may have low-level proteinuria but should not have hematuria or renal impairment unless the patient has had previous episodes of proliferative nephritis.

*2.1.1.3. Classes III and IV.* These two classes can be considered together since the morphological features seen in glomeruli are common to each and the distinction between the classes is made on the basis of the amount of glomerular involvement—if fewer than 50% of glomeruli are involved then the biopsy is placed in Class III and if 50% or more are involved then it is placed in Class IV. The major difference between these classes and the mesangial proliferative lesions considered above is that there is involvement of capillary lumens by inflammation or scarring. The defining feature of these classes is the presence of one or more "active" or "sclerotic" lesions as defined in Table 3. The active lesions represent either the light microscopic features of

**Table 3**
Definition of active and sclerosing lesions according to the 2003 ISN/RPS classification of lupus glomerulonephritis

Active lesions
   Endocapillary hypercellularity with or without leukocyte infiltration and with substantial luminal reduction
   Karyorrhexis
   Fibrinoid necrosis
   Rupture of glomerular basement membrane
   Crescents, cellular or fibrocellular
   Subendothelial deposits identifiable by LM (wireloops)
   Intraluminal immune aggregates (hyaline thrombi)

Sclerosing lesions
   Glomerular sclerosis (segmental, global)
   Fibrous adhesions fibrous crescents

subendothelial immune complexes or their inflammatory consequences whereas the chronic lesions represent the long-term consequences of inflammation which involves capillary lumens and which leads to obliteration of capillary lumens with loss of glomerular filtration surface. Subendothelial immune deposits may often be recognized at the light microscopic level as prominent eosinophilic thickening of the capillary walls sometimes referred to as "wire loop" lesions. In silver stains, these thickened loops show a double contour appearance with the original basement membrane lying outside the deposits and a new layer of basement membrane formed between the deposit and the endothelium. If subendothelial deposits are very large then they may bulge into the capillary lumen with the appearance of a hyaline thrombus. Subendothelial immune complex deposition leads to glomerular inflammation and so typically there are areas of hypercellularity within capillary lumens caused by influx of leukocytes, particularly macrophages, and endothelial cell swelling. If the inflammation is severe there may be necrosis of glomerular cells often accompanied by the presence of eosinophilic fibrin-rich material—so-called fibrinoid necrosis. There may also be capillary wall rupture that allows fibrin and inflammatory cells to spill out into Bowman's space with the formation of a cellular crescent. It is also common to see nuclear fragments in area of necrosis in proliferative lupus nephritis, a phenomenon termed karyorrhexis. Fibrinoid necrosis and GBM rupture have particularly serious implications since they are

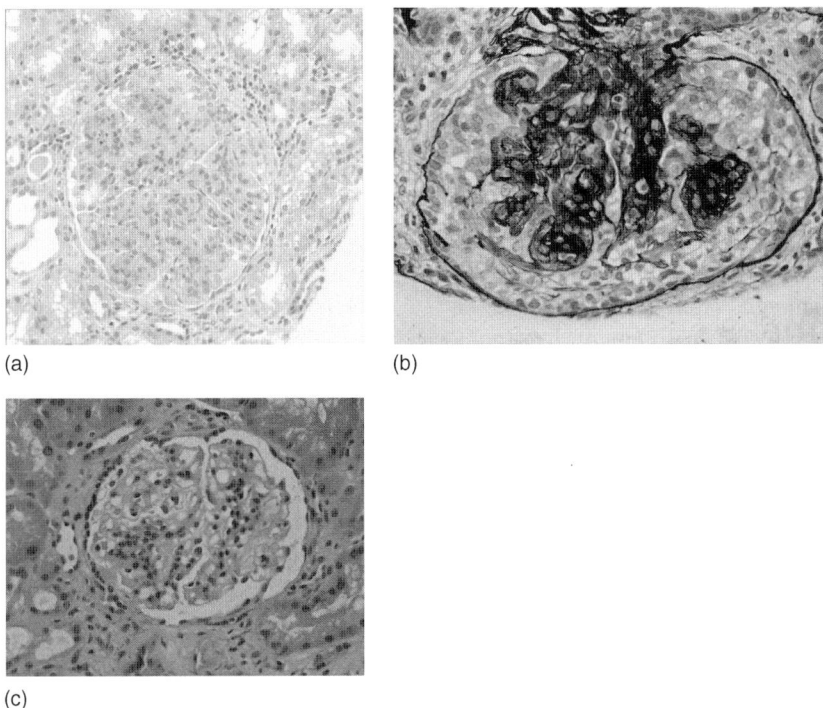

**Figure 1.** A 19-year-old Indian Asian girl, usual weight 45 kg, presents with brief history of arthralgias, hair loss, malaise, and gross peripheral edema. She is found to have gross pitting edema to the thighs, ascites, hypertension, an active urinary sediment with blood 3+, protein 4+, serum albumin 10 g/l, serum creatinine 160 μmol/l, 10 g proteinuria, high anti-dsDNA antibodies and low serum complements. Renal biopsy showed a severe Class IV nephritis with a small percentage of chronic damage. The glomeruli showed marked endocapillary hypercellularity (a) and crescent formation (b). She was treated aggressively with the Eurolupus regime and responded well. Her proteinuria diminished, serum albumin and albumin normalized and her dsDNA antibodies fell into the normal range. Her creatinine fell but to 100 μmol/l—leaving her with an estimated GFR of 66 ml/min/1.73 m². She was keen to know how her kidneys had healed and was rebiopsied. This demonstrated remarkable resolution within 6 months of treatment. The glomeruli show mesangial hypercellularity (c) but no active lesions were seen. Twelve months post treatment she has no proteinuria, stable serum creatinine, and no sign of renal or systemic activity. She is maintained on low dose prednisolone and MMF.

unlikely to heal with restitution of the normal capillary architecture but generally progress to the formation of an area of scarring with obliteration of the capillary lumen. Similarly cellular crescents eventually evolve into fibrous crescents with loss of filtration surface.

Patients with Class III and Class IV can present very similarly and it is this group of patients in whom diagnostic renal biopsy is so important. The classical presentation would be a nephritic pattern—i.e., an active urinary sediment with red cells, red cell casts, severe but not necessarily nephrotic range, proteinuria, and hypertension. Renal function may be completely normal in the early stages but can rapidly deteriorate. Patients can present de novo with severe nephritis or may have a long history of extra renal lupus. They may have florid or no systemic features at the time of renal flare—hence the importance of seeing known patients frequently and always checking renal function, blood pressure, and urine dip (Fig. 1).

*2.1.1.4. Class III: focal lupus nephritis.* In Class III lupus fewer than 50% of glomeruli show active or sclerotic lesions as defined in Table 3. Typically there will also be a background of mesangial expansion and hypercellularity. Further subclassification, with obvious implications for therapy, is on the basis of whether the lesions are all active,

Class III(A), all sclerotic, Class III(C), or a mixture of the two (A/C).

*2.1.1.5. Class IV: diffuse lupus nephritis.* In Class IV, 50% or more of the glomeruli show active or sclerotic lesions as defined in Table 3. Typically there will be a background of mesangial expansion and hypercellularity. Subendothelial immune deposits are usual and may be extensive. In addition there are usually prominent mesangial immune deposits and there may be scattered subepithelial deposits. Even when almost all the glomeruli are involved Class IV lupus is generally characterized by considerable variability in histological changes from glomerulus to glomerulus and even from segment to segment within the same glomerulus. Even allowing for this variability it is apparent that some biopsies show a predominant proliferative pattern whereas in others the principle lesion is segmental fibrinoid necrosis resembling that seen in ANCA-associated vasculitis. It has been suggested that this difference in pattern may have prognostic significance with a worse outcome in those biopsies with predominantly segmental lesions (Najafi et al., 2001). In order to allow further assessment of the possible significance of this distinction the ISN/RPS classification divides Class IV nephritis into Class IV-S where the predominant pattern of glomerular involvement by active or sclerotic lesions is segmental (i.e., involving less than half of the glomerular tuft) and IV-G where the predominant pattern is global. Hill et al. (2005) have examined the validity of this distinction. They concluded that the distinction between these patterns was possible on morphological grounds and suggested that there are differences in clinical features and probably in pathogenesis. At one end of the spectrum they could recognize biopsies with mainly global lesions that were characterized by prominent capillary wall immune deposits with a clear relationship between the extent of the deposits and the morphological changes. This pattern seems to represent the typical immune-complex mediated type of lupus proliferative glomerulonephritis. At the other end of the spectrum were biopsies showing mainly segmental lesions, often with fibrinoid necrosis but with far fewer subendothelial deposits and often with fibrinoid necrosis in the absence of hypercellularity. They suggest that the morphologic findings cast doubt on whether immune complexes are the cause of these segmental lesions and suggest that ANCA or antiendothelial antibodies should be considered as possible etiological factors. In many patients it appeared that there was a mixture of the two different patterns of glomerular disease suggesting that there is actually a continuous spectrum. Unlike Najafi they did not find a difference in renal survival between the two patterns on the presenting biopsy. However, when they examined biopsies taken 6 months after treatment was started they found that patients with persistence of a diffuse pattern of glomerular involvement had a very poor prognosis compared with those with a segmental pattern. Further studies will be needed to define fully the implications of the IV-G and IV-S patterns of glomerular involvement.

As with Class III, Class IV can be subclassified depending on whether only active (A), active and sclerotic (A/C), or only sclerotic (C) lesions are present (Fig. 2).

*2.1.1.6. Class V: membranous lupus nephritis.* Class V disease is defined by the presence of conspicuous immune deposits on the outside of the GBM beneath the podocytes. These deposits lead to thickening of the glomerular basement membrane, which begins with projections of the GBM surrounding the deposits giving rise to the typical pattern of spikes seen on silver staining. Later the deposits become covered by new basement membrane and so incorporated within the membrane. In most cases there is also mesangial expansion and hypercellularity with mesangial deposits. It is not uncommon to see a membranous pattern of disease together with active lesions of Class III or IV. In the second revision of the WHO classification (Churg and Sobin, 1982), these biopsies were classified as subtypes of Class IV; for example membranous together with diffuse proliferative glomerulonephritis was classified as Class Vd. The ISN/RPS group felt that this had the potential to lead to clinical misunderstandings and also

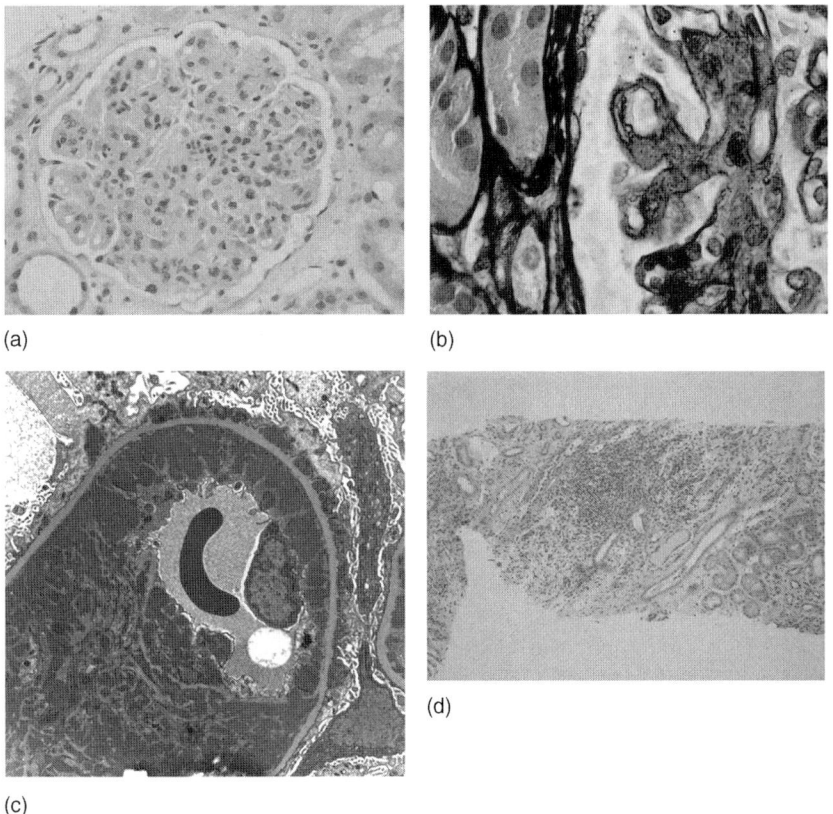

**Figure 2.** A 19-year-old Indian Asian man who had first presented with cerebral and renal lupus age 13. At that time he had required acute dialysis. He developed Class IV lupus nephritis aged 18 and failed to respond (as judged by persistent proteinuria and hematuria) to conventional treatment with either MMF or pulsed cyclophosphamide. At presentation to the tertiary center he had preserved renal function but active urinary sediment and 2 g proteinuria. Biopsy showed very active Class IV nephritis with glomeruli showing endocapillary hypercellularity (a) and capillary wall double contours on silver staining (b). Electron microscopy showed large mesangial, subendothelial and subepithelial electron dense deposits (c). There was no chronic damage. He went into a complete sustained remission with Rituximab. He relapsed 2 years later with modest proteinuria and a slight rise in his creatinine. Biopsy once again showed active disease but he now had some chronic damage with areas of tubulointerstitial scarring and chronic inflammatory cell infiltrate (d).

fails to emphasize the active lesions that are most likely to require treatment. The current recommendation is that when Class III or Class IV disease occurs together with Class V then both should be reported. Since subepithelial deposits are not uncommon in Classes III and IV the diagnosis of Class V in that case requires that subepithelial deposits are present in more than half of the tuft in more than half of the glomeruli. Patients with isolated Class V classically have no hematuria but present with nephrotic syndrome that can be extremely severe. However, renal function is usually preserved, at least in the early stages, unless intravascularly deplete due to hypoalbuminaemia. Class V in combination with Class III or IV should be suspected in the patient with a nephritic sediment, impaired function, and surprisingly heavy proteinuria. The other relatively common clinical presentation is in the setting of the patient with Class III or IV who appears to have responded by most measures but has significant persistent proteinuria. Repeat biopsy often shows transition to a Class V lesion (Fig. 3).

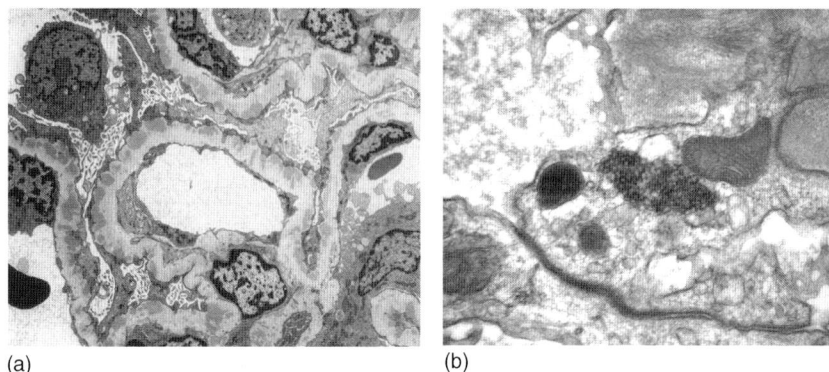

**Figure 3.** A 35-year-old Indian Asian woman with long history of severe lupus who presented with nephrotic syndrome in pregnancy 11 years previously. She had a severe relapse about 6 years ago and had been treated with a prolonged NIH pulsed cyclophosphamide regime. This had induced remission and she had excellent renal function (serum creatinine 60 μmol/l). She then relapsed with isolated proteinuria. Biopsy revealed an isolated Class V lesion and no chronic damage. Electron microscopy shows multiple subepithelial electron dense deposits (a). Tubuloreticular inclusions were seen in endothelial cells (b).

*2.1.1.7. Class VI: advanced sclerotic lupus nephritis.* Class VI is reserved for those cases in which there is more than global glomerulosclerosis due to SLE but with no active glomerular disease.

## 2.2. Tubules and interstitium

The tubules in a kidney affected by SLE may show acute or chronic changes. Acute changes are common in the presence of the nephrotic syndrome when many proximal tubular epithelial cells may contain protein resorption droplets. The nephrotic syndrome may sometimes be associated with more severe acute tubular damage with epithelial cell dedifferentiation. In cases with longstanding proteinuria there may be accumulation of foam cells—lipid-containing macrophages—in the interstitium. Tubules may also be involved by an acute inflammatory process—acute tubulointerstitial nephritis. This is characterized by an interstitial infiltrate of mononuclear inflammatory cells with tubulitis—that is, infiltration of the inflammatory cells through the tubular basement membrane with damage to the epithelial cells. Immunophenotyping shows that the majority of the cells are T-cells with smaller numbers of macrophages and T-cells. It is common to see tubulointerstitial nephritis in the presence of active glomerular inflammation but, in our experience, it is unusual in the absence of significant glomerular disease. The possibility of superimposed drug-induced tubulointerstitial nephritis should always be considered. Many patients with acute tubulointerstitial nephritis will have immune deposits on tubular basement membranes, which can be recognized by immunohistochemistry or electron microscopy. Patients with severe tubulointerstitial nephritis may well present like those with Class III or IV as they can have proteinuria, hematuria, hypertension, and will commonly have impaired function. Urinary microscopy will demonstrate sterile pyuria (as well as hematuria) which may be the only manifestation of milder tubulointerstitial nephritis (Fig. 4).

Chronic damage to the tubules leads to tubular atrophy and tubulointerstitial fibrosis with non-specific chronic inflammation. In general the degree of chronic tubulointerstitial damage parallels the chronic glomerular damage but because of the problems with glomerular sampling in small needle biopsies the amount of tubular atrophy usually provides the best overall estimate of the amount of chronic irreversible damage in a biopsy.

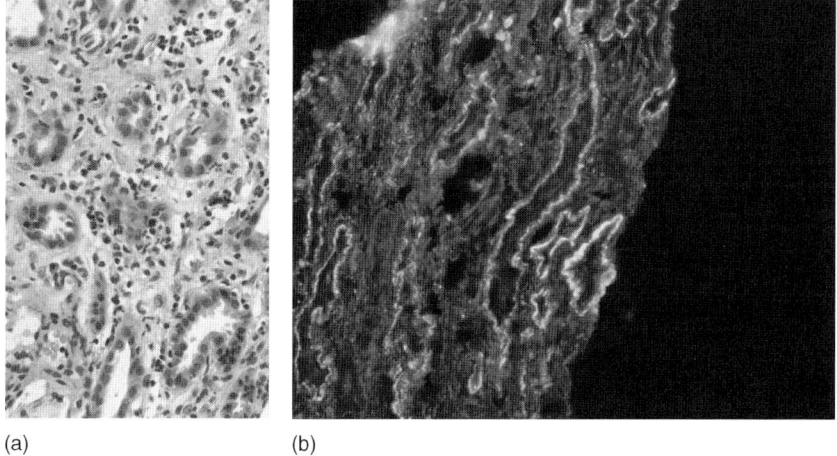

Figure 4. A 24-year-old African-Caribbean woman with a short history of systemic lupus, presented with increasing proteinuria and rapidly rising creatinine. Her urine sediment showed heavy pyuria and hematuria. Renal biopsy showed minor glomerular changes but very severe active tubular interstitial nephritis (a) with immunoglobulin deposition on tubular basement membranes (b). At presentation her creatinine was 400 μmol/l and despite aggressive treatment with cyclophosphamide she rapidly became dialysis dependent. However, her pyuria and proteinuria diminished remarkably. Rebiopsy within 1 month showed no active inflammation but gross irreversible scarring. Immunosuppression was reduced and she remains dialysis dependent.

## 2.3. Vessels

A number of distinct vascular lesions are described in the kidney in patients with SLE (Table 4). In a large Italian study renal vascular lesions were found in 28% of cases and were associated with a higher rate of progression to renal failure (Banfi et al., 1991).

**Table 4**
Vascular lesions in lupus nephritis

Uncomplicated vascular immune deposits
Noninflammatory necrotizing vasculopathy (lupus vasculopathy)
Thrombotic microangiopathy
Necrotizing vasculitis

### 2.3.1. Uncomplicated vascular immune deposits

This is characterized by the deposition of immune complexes in the walls of small arteries and arterioles without significant inflammatory response. Often the vessels appear normal by light microscopy although there may be subendothelial eosinophilic material. Immunohistochemistry demonstrates the presence of immunoglobulins and complement components in the vessels wall. Finding IgM or C3 alone is not diagnostic as these are common in other causes of arteriolar hyalinosis. These immune deposits do not appear to carry a higher risk of progressive renal disease.

### 2.3.2. Noninflammatory necrotizing vasculopathy (lupus vasculopathy)

This is usually seen in the setting of Class IV lupus glomerulonephritis. It affects afferent arterioles and interlobular arteries, which show prominent luminal and intimal deposits of eosinophilic material with swelling of the endothelium and degeneration of the smooth muscle cells of the media without inflammatory cell infiltration. Immunohistochemistry shows variable staining of the involved vessels for immunoglobulins and complement components. Severe hypertension is often, although not always, present and almost certainly exacerbates the vascular damage.

## 2.3.3. Thrombotic microangiopathy

The histological changes in thrombotic microangiopathy overlap those seen in lupus vasculopathy and these appearances may represent part of a spectrum of the same pathological process. Thrombotic microangiopathy may occur in association with a distinct clinical syndrome of Hemolytic Uremic Syndrome or Thrombotic Thrombocytopenic Purpura. Histologically the lesions are similar to those seen with other causes of thrombotic microangiopathy and affect interlobular arteries, afferent arterioles, and glomeruli. Glomeruli show intraluminal thrombi and mesangiolysis and in more chronic cases there may be a double contour appearance to the glomerular capillary walls on light microscopy. By electron microscopy this double contour is seen to be associated with the accumulation of subendothelial flocculent material. The affected arterioles show intraluminal fibrin thrombi and there may be fibrin and fragmented red blood cells in the intima. Interlobular arteries typically show loose intimal expansion. This pattern of disease may be seen superimposed on any class of lupus glomerulonephritis. Many patients with thrombotic microangiopathy will have antiphospholipid antibodies. These patients may present as nephritic if they have an underlying Class III or IV but may simply develop acute severe renal dysfunction if a the thrombotic microangiopathy is the prime lesion. This is important to diagnose since treatment would include plasma exchange—however an associated thrombocytopenia often makes biopsy difficult to undertake acutely.

## 2.3.4. Necrotizing vasculitis

Rarely the kidney in patients with SLE may show a true inflammatory necrotizing arteritis with leukocyte infiltration of vessel walls. The morphology is identical to that seen in classical polyarteritis nodosa or ANCA-associated vasculitis and it is possible that ANCA play a role in the pathogenesis when this lesion is seen in SLE. It is important to recognize true necrotizing vasculitis as the prognosis is poor and it requires aggressive immunosuppressive therapy. These patients will classically present with an RPGN like picture—i.e. an active urinary sediment and rapidly deteriorating renal function. Even with aggressive treatment there may not be full recovery of renal function.

## 3. The renal biopsy in SLE: practical considerations

The ISN/RPS classification (Weening et al., 2004) made a number of recommendations to ensure reliable classification of renal biopsy changes and also to ensure that reports are prepared in a standard format. For light microscopy it is essential that sections are cut at 3 microns or less and examined at multiple levels. In order to exclude focal lesions the biopsy should include at least 10 glomeruli. Immunohistochemistry is essential and should include staining for IgA, IgG, IgM, kappa and lambda light chains, and complement components C1q and C3. Electron microscopy is not essential for the classification of lupus glomerulonephritis but may be very helpful. Under the electron microscope immune deposits may be recognized as typical electron dense areas and in some cases may have an organized substructure, for example microtubular deposits or resembling fingerprints. In many cases tubuloreticular inclusions will be seen within endothelial cells. These are intracellular structures that form in response to interferon alpha.

The renal biopsy report should be presented in a structured fashion and should include a full description of the morphological appearances by light microscopy, immunohistochemistry, and electron microscopy. This should be followed by a summary including the class of lupus nephritis percentage of glomeruli with severe active lesions (fibrinoid necrosis, crescents), and of glomeruli with other active and chronic lesions. The extent, severity, and type of tubulointerstitial and vascular disease should also be documented and graded in the diagnostic line. A more formal numerical assessment of the degree of activity and chronicity may be included in the report by using a scoring system for activity index and chronicity index as described by Austin et al. (1983).

## Key points

- Kidney involvement is common in SLE and in most cases affects glomeruli with deposition of immune complexes.
- The severity of glomerular involvement and hence the clinical presentation is critically influenced by the site of immune complex deposition in the glomerulus.
- Immune complex glomerulonephritis is classified according to the 2004 International Society of Nephrology/Renal Pathology Society revision of the WHO classification.
- For clinical assessment, it is necessary to have measures of the activity and chronicity of glomerular disease in addition to the class.
- SLE may also affect the vessels and the tubulointerstitium in the kidney and in some patients such involvement may dominate the clinical presentation.

## References

Appel, G.B., Silva, F.G., Pirani, C.L., et al. 1978. Renal involvement in systemic lupus erythematosus (SLE): a study of 56 patients emphasizing histologic classification. Medicine 75, 371.

Austin, H.A., III, Muenz, L.R., Joyce, K.M., et al. 1983. Prognostic factors in lupus nephritis. Contribution of renal histological data. Am. J. Med. 75, 382.

Banfi, G., Bertani, T., Boeri, V., et al. 1991. Renal vascular lesions as a marker of poor prognosis in patients with lupus nephritis. Gruppo Italiano per lo Studio della Nefrite Lupica (GISNEL). Am. J. Kidney Dis. 18, 240.

Cameron, J.S. 1999. Lupus nephritis. J. Am. Soc. Nephrol. 10, 413.

Churg, J., Sobin, L.H. 1982. Renal disease: classification and atlas of glomerular disease. Igaku-Shoin, Tokyo.

Hill, G.S., Delahousse, M., Nochy, D., et al. 2005. Class IV-S versus class IV-G lupus nephritis: clinical and morphologic differences suggesting different pathogenesis. Kidney Int. 68, 2288.

Najafi, C.C., Korbet, S.M., Lewis, E.J., et al. 2001. Significance of histologic patterns of glomerular injury upon long-term prognosis in severe lupus glomerulonephrits. Kidney Int. 59, 2156.

Pollak, V.E., Pirani, C.L., Schwartz, F.D. 1964. The natural history of the renal manifestations of systemic lupus erythematosus. J. Lab. Clin. Med. 63, 537.

Weening, J.J., D'Agati, V.D., Schwartz, M.M. 2004. The classification of glomerulonephritis in systemic lupus erythematosus revisited. J. Am. Soc. Nephrol. 15, 241.

# CHAPTER 17

# Systemic Lupus Erythematosus: Treatment

Marianne Monahan, Gerald B. Appel*

*Professor of Clinical Medicine, Columbia University, College of Physicians and Surgeons, Director of Clinical Nephrology, Columbia University Medical Center, New York, NY 10032, USA*

## 1. Introduction

Lupus nephritis (LN) is serious complication of systemic lupus erythematosis (SLE). As many as two-thirds of patients with SLE will develop renal disease during their illness (Mok and Tang, 2004; Waldman and Appel, 2006). Studies have shown that delay in treatment results in poorer long-term renal survival making early recognition of renal disease and initiation of therapy important (Esdaile et al., 1995). The goals of therapy include induction of remission, prevention of relapse, and prevention of progression to end-stage renal disease (ESRD). Both the induction of remission and prevention of relapse have been shown to improve outcome. Achieving remission is associated with improved long-term renal survival and each relapse contributes to poorer renal outcome (Moroni et al., 1996; Korbet et al., 2000). Ideally, both induction of remission and maintenance free of relapse should be achieved while minimizing the toxicity burden that accompanies most immunosuppressive regimens.

When treating LN patients, it is important to recognize that LN is a heterogeneous disease both in the pattern and the severity of renal involvement. Therefore, treatment must be individualized. Decision making by the physician should incorporate evaluation of the patient's overall clinical picture including co-existing infection, cytopenias, and extra-renal lupus involvement, as well as evaluation of the renal histology, prior therapies, the patient's tolerability of potential side effects, and compliance. Clear differences exist in different ethnic groups in both response to therapy and long-term outcome. In many studies, African Americans have a poorer initial response and ultimate renal outcome when compared to non-Blacks (Dooley et al., 1997; Illei et al., 2002; Barr et al., 2003; Contreras et al., 2006).

Over the years many studies have used a variety of classification systems of the renal biopsy as a guide to prognosis and ultimate therapy. It is often difficult to reliably predict renal histology on the basis of clinical and laboratory manifestations of LN and the renal histology remains an excellent predictor of long-term outcome. Although there is considerable controversy regarding the accuracy and reproducibility of many such schema, the WHO classification and more recently the International Society of Nephrology (ISN) Classification, have proven valuable as prognostic and therapeutic guides (Weening et al., 2004). The ISN classification has modified the older WHO classification to make it more useful to both pathologists and clinicians dealing with biopsies from LN patients.

Patients with mild mesangial disease (ISN Class I and II) do not require immunosuppressive therapy directed at the kidney. They have an excellent renal prognosis. Although mild LN may transform to

*Corresponding author.
Tel.: 212-305-3273; Fax: 212-305-6692
E-mail address: gba2@columbia.edu

more severe proliferative disease (Class III or IV) over time, this is usually heralded by increased proteinuria and manifestations of renal involvement. At this point, repeat biopsy may be indicated. Patients with ISN Class III and IV, focal and diffuse proliferative LN, require therapy to prevent progressive renal damage. While the treatment may be much more vigorous for a patient with crescentic global involvement by proliferative lesions than one with only mild areas of endocapillary proliferation, in many cases the difference between focal and diffuse proliferative disease is a quantitative rather than qualitative difference in lesions. Indeed, in some series patients with segmental focal lesions have actually fared worse than others with diffuse proliferative lesions. Patients with Class V, membranous lupus, although typically presenting with the nephrotic syndrome, often have only a slowly progressive course as long as there are no superimposed proliferative lesions. Finally, patients with Class VI, sclerosing LN, have kidneys approaching ESRD and should not receive immunosuppressives directed at trying to save moribund kidneys at the expense of potential medication related toxicity.

Fortunately, the prognosis of LN has improved over past decades (Cervera et al., 1999; Mok, 2005). Factors contributing to improved outcomes include a better understanding of the pathogenesis and natural history of disease, and improved treatment regimens and the use of adjunctive therapy. Despite improvements in therapy and reduced morbidity and mortality, the optimal treatment for many individuals with LN remains controversial.

## 2. Induction therapy with cyclophosphamide

Despite a number of controlled randomized trials, at present there is still no universal protocol for the treatment of severe LN. However, for over two decades treatment regimens using intravenous (IV) pulse cyclophosphamide and corticosteroids have been considered the most effective and have been the mainstay of treatment. A series of randomized controlled trials performed at the National Institutes of Health, and subsequent studies elsewhere, demonstrated improved patient and renal survival with cyclophosphamide-based therapy (Boumpas et al., 1992; Valeri et al., 1994; Illei et al., 2002).

In 1996, Gourley et al. reported results from a randomized controlled trial comparing three regimens for biopsy proven proliferative nephritis conducted at the NIH. Patients were randomized to one of three groups: pulse therapy with methylprednisolone ($1\,g/m^2$ body surface area) monthly for at least 1 year; pulse IV cyclophosphamide ($0.5\,g–1.0\,g/m^2$ body surface area) every month for 6 months and then quarterly; or pulse therapy with both methylprednisolone and cyclophosphamide. Renal remission, defined as $<10$ dysmorphic red blood cells per high power field, absence of cellular casts, proteinuria of $<1.0\,g/day$, and absence of doubling of serum creatinine, was achieved in 85% of the combination group, 62% of the cyclophosphamide group, and 29% of the methylprednisolone group ($P=0.028$). Infections and amenorrhea were more common in the patients receiving cyclophosphamide. When analyzed at longer follow-up in 2001, the group receiving combined therapy fared even better when compared to the two other groups, especially in terms of renal outcome. Far fewer patients in the combined group had doubling of the serum creatinine, 50% decline in GFR, or reached ESRD. Moreover, the long-term side effects of the combined cyclophosphamide with methylprednisolone group were no different from those of the isolated cyclophosphamide group. Nonetheless, toxicity in the combination treatment group was significant with hypertension in 50%, hyperlipidemia in 42%, aseptic bone necrosis in 30%, premature menopause in 56%, Herpes zoster in 25%, and major infections in 45% of patients. Although more prolonged therapy with cyclophosphamide is associated with fewer renal relapses, the risks of therapy in terms of malignancy, infertility, and other side effects are cumulative. Thus, although cyclophosphamide-based regimens appeared highly effective, the high potential for major toxicity remains. This has led to induction studies attempting to minimize cyclophosphamide exposure.

The European Lupus Nephritis Trial, a prospective multi-center study published in 2002, was designed to compare the efficacy of low-dose IV cyclophosphamide to conventional high-dose IV cyclophosphamide in the treatment of severe LN. Ninety patients with severe LN were randomized to either standard high-dose IV pulse cyclophosphamide ($0.5-1\,g/m^2$) monthly for six doses followed by pulses at 9 and 12 months or to low-dose therapy (500 mg IV every 2 weeks for six doses only). Following the above induction therapy, both groups received oral azathioprine for maintenance. At a median follow up of 41 months, there were no statistically significant differences in achievement of remission or incidence of renal flares. Notably, infections were more frequent in the high-dose group but this did not reach statistical significance (Houssiau et al., 2002). Although these results demonstrate efficacy of lower doses of the alkylating agent in this population, the findings may not be applicable to all patients. Eighty-four percent of the patients in this study were White and based on serum creatinine and level of proteinuria many had milder disease than many previous studies. Whether these results can be reproduced in high-risk patients, including African Americans is unclear. Therefore, this regimen cannot currently be recommended for all patients.

## 3. Induction therapy with mycophenolate mofetil

Mycophenolate mofetil (MMF), introduced into clinical transplantation in 1995, is a reversible inhibitor of the enzyme inosine monophosphate dehydrogenase, a rate-limiting enzyme in de novo purine synthesis (Allison and Eugui, 2000). Lymphocytes do not have a salvage pathway for purine synthesis, are dependent on de novo synthesis, and thus are selectively damaged by MMF. In vitro, MMF blocks the proliferation of B- and T-cells, inhibits antibody production and cytotoxic T-cell generation, inhibits mesangial cell proliferation, and inhibits expression of adhesion molecules on endothelial cells. MMF is an efficacious and well-tolerated immunosuppressant in transplant patients, and has been used in numerous other autoimmune disorders including rheumatoid arthritis, autoimmune hemolytic anemia, and autoimmune thrombocytopenia.

In murine models of LN, MMF has been shown to both attenuate renal disease and improve animal survival (Corna et al., 1997; Van Bruggen et al., 1998). Initial anecdotal reports described successful short-term treatment with MMF in patients with LN who had failed other regimens or were unable to tolerate the significant side effects of other immunosuppressive medications. Dooley et al. published results of a series of 13 patients with relapsing or resistant proliferative nephritis, 12 of whom had previously been treated with IV cyclophosphamide. Proteinuria declined in 10 patients and serum creatinine either improved or remained stable in 11 patients (Dooley et al., 1999). Others have reported patients with diffuse proliferative LN who had failed treatment with steroids and cyclophosphamide (Kingdon et al., 2001; Karim et al., 2002). Reductions in proteinuria and serum creatinine were achieved. Numerous other small and uncontrolled series confirmed successful therapy of LN using MMF (Buratti et al., 2001).

Based on these encouraging results, a number of controlled trials were conducted to compare MMF to cyclophosphamide for induction therapy of LN. In 2000, Chan et al. published results of a study comparing MMF and prednisolone with cyclophosphamide and prednisolone for induction of remission of severe diffuse proliferative LN. Forty-two patients were randomized to either oral MMF at a dose of 2 g/day for 6 months followed by MMF at a dose of 1 g/day for an additional 6 months, or oral cytoxan at a dose of 2.5 mg/kg/day for 6 months followed by azathioprine at a dose of 1.5 mg/kg/day for 6 months. Both groups also received prednisolone and were followed for 12 months. The primary endpoint was complete remission defined as urinary protein excretion of $<0.3\,g/24\,h$, with normal urinary sediment, normal serum albumin, and a creatinine clearance and serum creatinine that were $<15\%$ above the baseline values. Partial remission was defined by 24 h urine protein excretion 0.3–2.9 g, with a serum albumin $>3.0$ and stable serum creatinine. The incidence of complete (81% of MMF patients and 76% of cyclophosphamide patients) and partial

(14% of each group) remissions was similar in the two groups. Moreover, relapse rates were similar: 15% in the MMF group and 11% in the cyclophosphamide group. Infections (13% MMF vs. 40% cyclophosphamide) and amenorrhea (4% MMF vs. 36% cyclophosphamide) were significantly less common in the MMF group and all of the mortality was in the cyclophosphamide group (Chan et al., 2000).

Although encouraging, this study was conducted in Hong Kong, and it is unclear if the results are applicable to other patient populations especially African Americans. In addition, the duration of follow-up was short. Subsequently, this study extended follow-up of patients to a median of 63 months and added 22 more patients. Over 90% of patients responded to induction with complete or partial remission. During follow-up, seven patients exhibited progressive renal dysfunction (four in the MMF group and three in the cyclophosphamide group). Two patients in the cyclophosphamide group reached ESRD. Relapse of renal disease occurred in 11 MMF patients and nine cyclophosphamide patients ($P=0.08$). Relapse-free survival was similar in both groups. MMF treated patients developed significantly fewer infections, and no mortality versus two deaths in the cyclophosphamide group (Chan et al., 2005). Another randomized trial in China compared oral MMF (1.0–1.5 g/day for 6 months, then 0.5–1 g/day) with IV cyclophosphamide (0.75–1.0 g/m$^2$ monthly for 6 months, then quarterly) for Class IV LN. The study concluded that MMF was more effective in reducing proteinuria, hematuria, and autoantibody production (Hu et al., 2002).

A recent US multi-center, randomized, controlled trial compared oral MMF with IV cyclophosphamide for induction therapy in lupus patients with biopsy proven, WHO Class III, IV or V disease. One hundred forty patients were randomized to receive either MMF or IV cyclophosphamide. The baseline characteristics of the two groups were similar, and both groups had over 50% African Americans. Mean proteinuria was over 4 g daily, with an active urinary sediment. MMF was initiated at 500 mg orally BID and was increased to a maximum dose of 3 g per day (mean dose MMF 2.7 g/day). IV cytoxan was administered as monthly pulses based on the National Institutes of Health protocol. All patients received prednisone at an initial dose of 1 mg/kg, which was tapered based on clinical improvement. The primary endpoint was complete remission defined as a return to within 10% of normal values of serum creatinine, proteinuria, and urinary sediment at 24 weeks. Partial remission was defined by a 50% improvement in all renal measurement and no worsening renal measurements. 16 of 71 patients in the mycophenolate group (23%) and 4 of 69 patients in the cyclophosphamide group (6%) had a complete remission ($P=0.005$). Partial remission was demonstrated in 21 patients (30%) in the mycophenolate group and 17 patients (25%) in the cyclophosphamide group. ($P=NS$). The combined rate of complete and partial remission was 52% in the mycophenolate group and 30% of the cyclophosphamide group ($P=0.009$). There was no difference in renal flares, renal failure, or ESRD at 3 years follow-up although all were less frequent in the MMF group. Side effects appeared less severe and frequent in the MMF group (Ginzler et al., 2005).

Despite these results, questions regarding dosage and duration of treatment with MMF remain unanswered. It is important to remember that prolonged observation has confirmed that treatment with cyclophosphamide preserves renal function and truly long-term data are simply not yet available for newer treatment modalities. Fortunately, studies with long-term follow-up are currently underway. The ALMS (Aspreva Lupus Management Study) trial, an international multi-center, randomized, controlled trial comparing MMF and cyclophosphamide for induction and MMF versus azathioprine for long-term maintenance has currently enrolled 370 patients (Appel et al., 2005). Initial analysis after 6 months shows no significant difference in remission rate or toxicity between MMF and IV cyclophosphamide (Appel et al., 2007).

## 4. Maintenance therapy

Despite successful induction of remission, relapses occur in from 37 to 59% of patients depending on severity of the initial renal disease, immunosuppressive regimen used, and duration of follow-up (Illei et al., 2002; El Hachmi et al., 2003). The goal of maintenance therapy is to administer the minimal dose of immunosuppressant required to prevent relapses. Although studies have demonstrated that long-term administration of cyclophosphamide is associated with a low incidence of renal relapse, the toxicity, including infertility and malignancy, increases with an increased cumulative dose (Mok et al., 1998; Medeiros et al., 2001; Yang et al., 2005). The significant toxicity burden has lead researchers and clinicians to search for regimens that are not only effective but also better tolerated over a long time interval.

A recent randomized, open-label-controlled trial compared cyclophosphamide, MMF, and azathioprine for maintenance therapy in patients who had achieved clinical remission with monthly boluses of IV cyclophosphamide plus steroids. Fifty-nine patients with LN (46 with WHO Class IV, 12 with Class III, and 1 with Class Vb), including 46% African American and many Hispanics, received induction therapy. After induction, patients were randomly assigned to oral MMF (dose 500–3000 mg/day), oral azathioprine (1–3 mg/kg), or quarterly IV cyclophosphamide. At the beginning of the maintenance phase, the three groups were similar. The primary endpoints were patient and renal survival. Secondary endpoints included renal relapse, hospitalization, infection, and amenorrhea for 12 months.

Initial remission was achieved during induction in 49 patients (16 in the azathioprine group, 17 in the cyclophosphamide group, and 16 in the mycophenolate group). Five patients died during maintenance therapy: four from the cyclophosphamide group and one from the mycophenolate group. Chronic renal failure developed in five patients: three from the cyclophosphamide group and one each from the mycophenolate and azathioprine group. Event-free survival rate for the composite end point of death or chronic renal failure was higher in the mycophenolate and azathioprine groups than in the cyclophosphamide group ($P=0.05$ and 0.09). The rate of relapse-free survival was higher in the mycophenolate group than the cyclophosphamide group and this difference was statistically significant ($P=0.02$). The hospitalization rate, infection rate, and rate of amenorrhea were all higher in the cyclophosphamide group. Thus, short-term therapy with IV cyclophosphamide followed by maintenance with oral MMF or azathioprine was not only more efficacious but also safer than long-term therapy with IV cyclophosphamide (Contreras et al., 2004). The European Working Party on Systemic Lupus Erythematosus is currently conducting a randomized multi-center trial (MAINTAIN Nephritis Trial) to compare the efficacy and safety of MMF and azathioprine for maintenance after induction with a short course of IV cyclophosphamide.

Other immunosuppressives have also proven effective in maintaining remission in LN following cyclophosphamide induction therapy. A recent Italian study compared maintenance with cyclosporine to azathioprine in 69 patients with diffuse proliferative LN (Moroni, 2006). Results with both treatment regimens were highly effective and there were few discontinuations due to side effects. Long-term tacrolimus therapy has also been used for maintenance treatment (Lei-Shi et al., 2005) (see Table 1).

## 5. Newer therapies

There is good evidence that B-cells play an important role in the pathogenesis of SLE (Madaio, 1998, 2003; Looney et al., 2004; Anolik and Aringer, 2005; Waldman and Madaio, 2005) and agents specifically targeting B-cells have shown promise in the treatment of LN. The most promising of these is rituximab; a mouse–human chimeric monoclonal anti-CD20 antibody, which allows for the selective elimination of peripheral B-cells. It was first approved by the United States Food and Drug Administration in 1997 for the treatment of refractory or relapsed B-cell non-Hodgkin's lymphoma (Grillo-Lopez et al., 1999). In this group of patients, it was noted that B-cell depletion could be sustained for 6–9 months and was not associated with an increased risk of infection. Subsequently, B lymphocyte depletion using rituximab was used in the treatment of

**Table 1**
Treatment recommendations

| | |
|---|---|
| Class III, IV | |
|   Induction | |
|     Cyclophosphamide | High risk: standard dose IV pulse cyclophosphamide (0.5–1 g/m$^2$) monthly for 6 months with steroids |
| | Low risk: low-dose (500 mg) IV pulse cyclophosphamide, every 2 weeks for six doses with steroids |
| | Or |
|     Mycophenolate mofetil | Orally at a target dose of 2–3 g/day |
|   Maintenance | |
|     Mycophenolate mofetil | 500–1000 mg orally BID |
|     Azathioprine | 50–100 mg orally daily |
|     Cyclosporine | Orally, twice daily, target trough level of 100–150 ng/ml |
|     Tacrolimus | Orally, twice daily, target trough level of 5–10 ng/ml |
| Class V | |
|   Nephrotic | IV pulse cyclophosphamide, oral cyclosporine, oral mycophenolate mofetil, or azathioprine |
|   Non-nephrotic | ACE-inhibitor or angiotensin receptor blocker |

several autoimmune disorders with encouraging results (Leandro et al., 2002a, b; Zaja et al., 2002; Edwards et al., 2004).

A number of uncontrolled case series have reported efficacy of rituximab in LN (Leandro et al., 2002a, b; Fra et al., 2003; van Vollenhoven et al., 2004). These have included patients with severe nephritis and some patients resistant to other standard therapies. An example is a recent study of 10 patients with LN including six with diffuse proliferative disease who were treated with rituximab 375 mg/m$^2$ weekly for four doses. Complete remissions with normal creatinines, urinalysis, and proteinuria <500 mg daily were achieved in five patients (with partial remissions in eight patients) which were sustained in four for 12 months (Sfikakis et al., 2005). In our experience similar results have been achieved with a regimen of 1000 mg IV followed by a similar dose 2 weeks later. The percent of patients who will respond to this treatment is unclear and it is also unknown what other therapy must be given concurrently to achieve remission. A current trial (LUNAR) compares MMF to a regimen of MMF plus IV rituximab for induction therapy in severe LN. (Appel et al., 2006). Allergic reactions may occur during administration and rare reports of viral brain infection (progressive multifocal leukoencephalopathy) have been noted. It is unclear how many patients will require repeat dosing at periodic intervals as B-cell populations return. It is also uncertain whether the development of human anti-chimeric antibodies to the medication will render it less effective with repeat administration.

LJP-934 (Riquent, Abetimus) is a small polyglycol platform with four DNA side chains designed to reduce B-cell production of anti-DNA antibodies (Abetimus, 2003; Wallace and Tumlin, 2004). It effectively does this and reduces renal injury in murine models of SLE. In initial human blinded-controlled trials, the drug reduced anti-DNA antibody titers, as well as reducing flares of the disease and decreasing the need for corticosteroids (Alarcon-Segovia et al., 2003). Subsequent studies have not been able to confirm a significant reduction in renal flares or time to renal flare, perhaps due to more effective background immunosuppressive therapy. Studies with this agent do show the value of randomized blinded trials to demonstrate the benefits of newer agents in the treatment of LN patients.

Intravenous gamma globulin (IVGG) infusion has been used to treat a variety of autoimmune diseases including SLE and LN (De Vita et al., 1996). Most studies are small and uncontrolled (Levy et al., 2000). One small randomized trial did show benefit (Boletis et al., 1999). The precise indications, treatment regimen, and role for this therapy remains unclear in the absence of controlled randomized trials. Likewise, autologous stem cell transplantation has been used in small numbers of severely ill lupus patients with varied results (Traynor and Burt, 1999; Traynor et al., 2000). Again any usage should be considered experimental until there is more data on safety and efficacy.

Several new medications used to treat LN have focused on blockade of the necessary co-stimulatory pathways between T- and B-cells in the immune response. Studies with a monoclonal antibody, anti-CD40 ligand, designed to interrupt the co-stimulation between CD40 on B-cells and CD154 on T-cells, although showing powerful immunosuppressive properties, have not been successful in humans. One formulation of the medication led to thrombotic events in a human trial (Boumpas et al., 2003), and the second proved ineffective (Kalunian et al., 2002). CTLA-4Ig (Abatacept) competes with CD28 for B7 ligands and interrupts T- and B-cell co-stimulation. It has proven effective in rheumatoid arthritis and is currently under study in SLE (Kremer et al., 2003; Emery et al., 2006). Other potential targets for new treatments for LN include blockers or inhibitors of cytokines, interferons, BAFF (B-cell activation factor), complement components, and Toll-like receptors.

## 6. Membranous lupus nephritis (MLN)

Approximately 20% of biopsied patients with LN are found to have pure membranous disease (Illei et al., 2002). The optimal treatment of pure MLN is unknown, in part due to the variability in the natural history of the disease and in part due to a lack of prospective, randomized clinical trials.

A prospective trial conducted by the NIH compared prednisone, cyclosporine, and intermittent IV cyclophosphamide in 42 patients with lupus membranous nephropathy, with mean proteinuria of 5.8 g/day and mean GFR of 85 ml/min. Patients were followed for 75 months. More complete and partial remissions were achieved in the patients receiving IV cyclophosphamide or cyclosporine compared to patients receiving oral prednisone. Cyclosporine treated patients remitted faster than patients treated with IV cyclophosphamide but relapses were more frequent with cyclosporine than with cyclophosphamide. The authors concluded that IV cyclophosphamide and oral cyclosporine were more effective than prednisone in inducing remission and that IV cyclophosphamide led to more sustained remissions. Azathioprine may also be efficacious for the treatment of MLN. Mok et al. conducted an open-label trial of prednisone and azathioprine in 38 patients with pure MLN. At 12 months of follow up, the complete and partial remission rates were 67 and 22%. Treatment was well tolerated (Mok et al., 2004).

The role of MMF in patients with MLN remains to be defined. Positive results have been reported in small numbers of patients in uncontrolled and retrospective series. For example, in one study 13 patients with MLN (mean urinary protein to creatinine ratio of 5:1) were treated with prednisone, MMF and ACE-inhibitors or angiotensin receptor blockers (Spetie et al., 2004). At follow up of 16 months, nine patients had achieved complete remission and two had partial remission. In all patients, the serum creatinine either remained stable or improved. Further evidence for efficacy of MMF in pure MLN comes from sub-group analysis of patients enrolled in the 140 patient multi-center study comparing cyclophosphamide to MMF. Of the 140 patients, 27 had pure Class V LN. Sixteen of these patients (eight each with MMF or cyclophosphamide) completed 6 months of therapy. There were no differences between the two groups in the rate of partial or complete remission, or change in serum creatinine or albumin, and proteinuria decreased equally over 6 months in both groups (Radhakrishnan et al. 2005).

In summary, treatment of MLN should be based on disease severity. Patients with sub-nephrotic proteinuria and normal renal function should be treated with ACE-inhibitors or angiotensin receptor blockers, statins as needed and possibly a short course of low-dose corticosteroids. Options for higher risk patients with nephrotic syndrome include cyclosporine, pulsed intermittent cyclophosphamide, MMF or azathioprine, and corticosteroids. Patients who have findings of proliferative LN and membranous nephritis should be treated based on the severity of their proliferative LN.

## 7. Adjunctive therapy

As patient survival has improved, cardiovascular disease has become a major cause of morbidity and mortality. Thus, cardiovascular risk factors should be treated aggressively. Blood pressure control to a target of $<130/80$ and treatment of hyperlipidemia are important aspects of risk modification. Although there are no specific data in LN patients, the use of ACE inhibitors and angiotensin receptor blockers to reduce proteinuria and slow progression of chronic renal disease is strongly recommended. Use of HMG CoA reductase inhibitors to optimally control elevated cholesterol and LDL levels is also advisable.

Corticosteroids are included in almost all LN treatment regimens, and significant adverse effects including infection, diabetes, cosmetic, and neuropsychiatric changes, osteoporosis, and cataracts may all occur. Therefore, steroids must be tapered and maintained at as low a dose as feasible to minimize long-term toxicity. The risk of glucocorticoid-induced osteoporosis should be attenuated with calcium, vitamin D and bisphosphonates, and weight bearing exercise when appropriate.

## 8. Conclusion

Although the pathogenesis of LN remains incompletely understood, advances in this area have identified new treatment options that appear at least as effective as older regimens. As long-term outcomes continue to improve, the toxicity of treatment becomes increasingly important. Newer therapeutic regimens will focus not only on preventing flares of renal disease and ESRD, but also in preventing the long-term complications of immunosuppressive medications.

### Key points

- The treatment of Lupus and Lupus nephritis is rapidly changing.
- Older therapies such as corticosteroids and cyclophosphamide are effective, but potentially highly toxic.
- Mycophenolate mofetil is now being more widely used for induction and maintenance therapy fo severe SLE.
- Newer agents such as rituximab, abetimus, and co-stimulatory molecule blockade are being developed, but need more study.
- Current therapy needs to be individualized as therapeutic options have broadened.

## Acknowledgment

This work has been supported in part by The Glomerular Center at Columbia University and "Zo's Fund for Life."

## References

Abetimus. 2003. Abetimus: Abetimus sodium, LJP 394. BioDrugs 17 (3), 212–215.

Alarcon-Segovia, D., Tumlin, J.A., Furie, R.A., et al. 2003. LJP 394 for the prevention of renal flare in patients with systemic lupus erythematosus: results from a randomized, double-blind, placebo-controlled study. Arthritis Rheum. 48 (2), 442–454.

Allison, A.C., Eugui, E.M. 2000. Mycophenolate mofetil and its mechanisms of action. Immunopharmacology 47 (2–3), 85–118.

Anolik, J.H., Aringer, M. 2005. New treatments for SLE: cell-depleting and anti-cytokine therapies. Best Pract. Res. Clin. Rheumatol. 19 (5), 859–878.

Appel, G.B., Dooley, M.A., Ginzler, E.M., Isenberg, D., Jayne, D., Solomons, N., Wofsy, D. 2007. Mycophenolate mofetil compared with intravenous cyclophosphamide as induction therapy for lupus nephritis: Aspreva Luypus Management Study (ALMS) results [ASN abst 2007].

Appel, G.B., Looney, R.G., Eisenberg, R.A., et al. 2006. Protocol for the LN assessment with rituximab (LUNAR) study. J. Am. Soc. Nephrol. 17, 573A.

Barr, R.G., Seliger, S., Appel, G.B., et al. 2003. Prognosis in proliferative lupus nephritis: the role of socio-economic status and race/ethnicity. Nephrol. Dial .Transplant. 18 (10), 2039–2046.

Boletis, J.N., Ioannidis, J.P., et al. 1999. Intravenous immunoglobulin compared with cyclophosphamide for proliferative lupus nephritis. Lancet 354 (9178), 569–570.

Boumpas, D.T., Austin, H.A., Vaughn, E.M., et al. 1992. Controlled trial of pulse methylprednisolone versus two regimens of pulse cyclophosphamide in severe lupus nephritis. Lancet 340 (8822), 741–745.

Boumpas, D.T., Furie, R., Manzi, S., et al. 2003. A short course of BG9588 (anti-CD40 ligand antibody) improves serologic activity and decreases hematuria in patients with proliferative lupus glomerulonephritis. Arthritis Rheum. 48 (3), 719–727.

Buratti, S., Szer, I.S., Spencer, C.H. 2001. Mycophenolate mofetil treatment for severe renal disease in pediatric SLE. J. Rheum. 28, 2103–2108.

Cervera, R., Khamashta, M.A., Font, J., et al. 1999. Morbidity and mortality in systemic lupus erythematosus during a 5-year period. A multicenter prospective study of 1,000 patients. European Working Party on Systemic Lupus Erythematosus. Medicine (Baltimore) 78 (3), 167–175.

Chan, T.M., Li, F.K., Tang, C.S., et al. 2000. Efficacy of mycophenolate mofetil in patients with diffuse proliferative lupus nephritis. Hong Kong-Guangzhou Nephrology Study Group. N. Engl. J. Med. 343 (16), 1156–1162.

Chan, T.M., Tse, K.C., Tang, C.S., et al. 2005. Long-term study of mycophenolate mofetil as continuous induction and maintenance treatment for diffuse proliferative lupus nephritis. J. Am. Soc. Nephrol. 16 (4), 1076–1084.

Contreras, G., Lenz, O., Pardo, V., et al. 2006. Outcomes in African Americans and Hispanics with lupus nephritis. Kidney Int. 69 (10), 1846–1851.

Contreras, G., Pardo, V., Leclercq, B., et al. 2004. Sequential therapies for proliferative lupus nephritis. [See comment]. N. Engl. J. Med. 350 (10), 971–980.

Corna, D., Morigi, M., Facchinetti, D., et al. 1997. Mycophenolate mofetil limits renal damage and prolongs life in murine lupus autoimmune disease. Kidney Int. 51 (5), 1583–1589.

De Vita, S., Ferraccioli, G.F., et al. 1996. High dose intravenous immunoglobulin therapy for rheumatic diseases: clinical relevance and personal experience. Clin. Exp. Rheumatol. 14 (Suppl. 15), S85–S92.

Dooley, M.A., Cosio, F.G., Nachman, P.H., et al. 1999. Mycophenolate mofetil therapy in lupus nephritis: clinical observations. J. Am. Soc. Nephrol. 10 (4), 833–839.

Dooley, M.A., Hogan, S., Jennett, C., Falk, R., et al. 1997. Cyclophosphamide therapy for lupus nephritis: poor renal survival in black Americans. Glomerular Disease Collaborative Network. Kidney Int. 51 (4), 1188–1195.

Edwards, J.C., Szczepanski, L., Szechinski, J., et al. 2004. Efficacy of B-cell-targeted therapy with rituximab in patients with rheumatoid arthritis. N. Engl. J. Med. 350 (25), 2572–2581.

El Hachmi, M., Jadoul, M., Lefebvre, C., et al. 2003. Relapses of lupus nephritis: incidence, risk factors, serology and impact on outcome. Lupus 12 (9), 692–696.

Emery, P., Kosinski, M., et al. 2006. Treatment of rheumatoid arthritis patients with abatacept and methotrexate significantly improved health-related quality of life. J. Rheumatol. 33 (4), 681–689.

Esdaile, J.M., Joseph, L., et al. 1995. The benefit of early treatment with immunosuppressive drugs in lupus nephritis. J. Rheumatol. 22 (6), 1211.

Fra, G.P., Avanzi, G.C., et al. 2003. Remission of refractory lupus nephritis with a protocol including rituximab. Lupus 12 (10), 783–787.

Ginzler, E.M., Dooley, M.A., Aranow, C., et al. 2005. Mycophenolate mofetil or intravenous cyclophosphamide for lupus nephritis. [See comment]. N. Engl.J. Med. 353 (21), 2219–2228.

Grillo-Lopez, A.J., White, C.A., Varns, C., et al. 1999. Overview of the clinical development of rituximab: first monoclonal antibody approved for the treatment of lymphoma. Semin. Oncol. 26 (5 Suppl. 14), 66–73.

Houssiau, F.A., Vasconcelos, C., D'Cruz, D., et al. 2002. Immunosuppressive therapy in lupus nephritis: the Euro-Lupus Nephritis Trial, a randomized trial of low-dose versus high-dose intravenous cyclophosphamide. Arthritis Rheum. 46 (8), 2121–2131.

Hu, W., Liu, Z., Chen, H., et al. 2002. Mycophenolate mofetil vs. cyclophosphamide therapy for patients with diffuse proliferative lupus nephritis. Chin. Med. J. (Engl.) 115 (5), 705–709.

Illei, G.G., Takada, K., Parkin, D., et al. 2002. Renal flares are common in patients with severe proliferative lupus nephritis treated with pulse immunosuppressive therapy: long-term followup of a cohort of 145 patients participating in randomized controlled studies. Arthritis Rheum. 46 (4), 995–1002.

Kalunian, K.C., Davis, J.C., Merrill, J.T., et al. 2002. Treatment of systemic lupus erythematosus by inhibition of T cell costimulation with anti-CD154: a randomized, double-blind, placebo-controlled trial. Arthritis Rheum. 46 (12), 3251–3258.

Karim, M.Y., Alba, P., Cuadrado, M.S., et al. 2002. Mycophenolate mofetil for systemic lupus erythematosus refractory to other immunosuppressive agents. Rheumatology (Oxford) 41 (8), 876–882.

Kingdon, E.J., McLean, A.G., Psimenon, E., et al. 2001. The safety and efficacy of MMF in lupus nephritis: a pilot study. Lupus 10 (9), 606–611.

Korbet, S.M., Lewis, E.J., Schwartz, M.M., et al. 2000. Factors predictive of outcome in severe lupus nephritis. Lupus Nephritis Collaborative Study Group. Am. J. Kidney Dis. 35 (5), 904–914.

Kremer, J.M., Westhovens, R., Leon, M., et al. 2003. Treatment of rheumatoid arthritis by selective inhibition of T-cell activation with fusion protein CTLA4Ig. N. Engl. J. Med. 349 (20), 1907–1915.

Leandro, M.J., Edwards, J.C., et al. 2002a. Clinical outcome in 22 patients with rheumatoid arthritis treated with B lymphocyte depletion. Ann. Rheum. Dis. 61 (10), 883–888.

Leandro, M.J., Edwards, J.C., Cambridge, G., et al. 2002b. An open study of B lymphocyte depletion in systemic lupus erythematosus. Arthritis Rheum. 46 (10), 2673–2677.

Levy, Y., Sherer, Y., et al. 2000. Intravenous immunoglobulin treatment of lupus nephritis. Semin. Arthritis Rheum. 29 (5), 321–327.

Lei-Shi, L., Zhang, H-T., et al. 2005. Controlled trial of tacrolimus vs. indensive cyclophosphamide as induction therapy of severe lupus nephritis. J. Am. Soc. Nephrol. 16, 556A.

Looney, R.J., Anolik, J., Campbell, D., et al. 2004. B cells as therapeutic targets for rheumatic diseases. Curr. Opin. Rheumatol. 16 (3), 180–185.

Madaio, M.P. 1998. B cells and autoantibodies in the pathogenesis of lupus nephritis. Immunol. Res. 17 (1–2), 123–132.

Madaio, M.P. 2003. Lupus autoantibodies 101: one size does not fit all; however, specificity influences pathogenicity. Clin. Exp. Immunol. 131 (3), 396–397.

Medeiros, M.M., Silveira, V.A., et al. 2001. Risk factors for ovarian failure in patients with systemic lupus erythematosus. Braz. J. Med. Biol. Res. 34 (12), 1561–1568.

Mok, C.C. 2005. Prognostic factors in lupus nephritis. Lupus 14 (1), 39–44.

Mok, C.C., Lau, C.S., Wong, R.W., et al. 1998. Risk factors for ovarian failure in patients with systemic lupus erythematosus receiving cyclophosphamide therapy. Arthritis Rheum. 41 (5), 831–837.

Mok, C.C., Tang, S.S. 2004. Incidence and predictors of renal disease in Chinese patients with systemic lupus erythematosus. Am. J. Med. 117 (10), 791–795.

Mok, C.C., Ying, K.Y., Lau, C.S., et al. 2004. Treatment of pure membranous lupus nephropathy with prednisone and azathioprine: an open-label trial. Am. J. Kidney Dis. 43 (2), 269–276.

Moroni, G. 2006. A randomized pilot trial comparing cyclosporine and azathioprine for maintenance therapy in diffuse lupus nephritis over four years. Clin. J. Am. Soc. Nephrol. 1 (No. 5), 925–932.

Moroni, G., Quaglini, S., Maccario, M., et al. 1996. "Nephritic flares" are predictors of bad long-term renal outcome in lupus nephritis. Kidney Int. 50 (6), 2047–2053.

Radhakrishnan, J., Ginzler, E., Appel, G.B. 2005. Mycophenolate mofetil vs. intravenous cyclophosphamide for severe lupus nephritis: subgroup analysis of patients with membranous nephropathy (SLE V). J. Am. Soc. Nephrol. 16, 8A.

Sfikakis, P.P., Boletis, J.N., Lionakis, S., et al. 2005. Remission of proliferative lupus nephritis following B cell depletion therapy is preceded by down-regulation of the T cell costimulatory molecule CD40 ligand: an open-label trial. Arthritis Rheum. 52 (2), 501–513.

Spetie, D.N., Tang, Y., Rovin, B., et al. 2004. Mycophenolate therapy of SLE membranous nephropathy. Kidney Int. 66 (6), 2411–2415.

Traynor, A., Burt, R.K. 1999. Haematopoietic stem cell transplantation for active systemic lupus erythematosus. Rheumatology (Oxford) 38 (8), 767–772.

Traynor, A.E., Schroeder, J., Burt, R.K., et al. 2000. Treatment of severe systemic lupus erythematosus with high-dose chemotherapy and haemopoietic stem-cell transplantation: a phase I study. Lancet 356 (9231), 701–707.

Valeri, A., Radhakrishnan, J., Estes, D., et al. 1994. Intravenous pulse cyclophosphamide treatment of severe lupus nephritis: a prospective five-year study. Clin. Nephrol. 42 (2), 71–78.

Van Bruggen, M.C., Walgreen, B., Rijke, T.P., Berden, J.H., et al. 1998. Attenuation of murine lupus nephritis by mycophenolate mofetil. J. Am. Soc. Nephrol. 9 (8), 1407–1415.

van Vollenhoven, R.F., Gunnarsson, I., et al. 2004. Biopsy-verified response of severe lupus nephritis to treatment with rituximab (anti-CD20 monoclonal antibody) plus cyclophosphamide after biopsy-documented failure to respond to cyclophosphamide alone. Scand. J. Rheumatol. 33 (6), 423–427.

Waldman, M., Appel, G.B. 2006. Update on the treatment of lupus nephritis. Kidney Int. 70 (8), 1403–1412.

Waldman, M., Madaio, M.P. 2005. Pathogenic autoantibodies in lupus nephritis. Lupus 14 (1), 19–24.

Wallace, D.J., Tumlin, J.A. 2004. LJP 394 (Abetimus sodium, Riquent) in the management of systemic lupus erythematosus. Lupus 13 (5), 323–327.

Weening, J.J., D'Agati, V.D., Schwartz, M.M., et al. 2004. The classification of glomerulonephritis in systemic lupus erythematosus revisited. Kidney Int. 65 (2), 521–530.

Yang, X.Y., Zhu, X., et al. 2005. Risk factors of ovarian failure in the patients with systemic lupus erythematosus receiving cyclophosphamide therapy. Zhonghua Yi Xue Za Zhi 85 (14), 960–962.

Zaja, F., Iacona, I., Masolini, P., et al. 2002. B-cell depletion with rituximab as treatment for immune hemolytic anemia and chronic thrombocytopenia. Haematologica 87 (2), 189–195.

# CHAPTER 18

# The Antiphospholipid Syndrome

David D'Cruz*

*The Lupus Research Unit, The Rayne Institute, St. Thomas' Hospital, London SE1 7EH, UK*

## 1. Introduction

The cardinal features of the antiphospholipid syndrome (APS) or Hughes syndrome, first described in 1983 by Dr. Graham Hughes and his team at the Hammersmith Hospital, included recurrent arterial and venous thromboses, fetal losses, and thrombocytopenia (Hughes, 1983). Although a wide variety of clinical features have been added over the last two decades these major features have stood the test of time. The description of the APS has been a pivotal advance in the management of lupus and the ramifications of the syndrome extend to all disciplines of medicine. APS is now recognized as a common disorder and certainly not a "small print" disease. Its importance lies in the fact that once diagnosed, this is a treatable condition. However, for many patients diagnosis is often delayed, sometimes for years, with consequent disability, loss of livelihood, inability to start a family, or even death.

## 2. Laboratory diagnosis

The presence of antiphospholipid antibodies (aPL) is central to the diagnosis of APS and the two characteristic autoantibodies are the lupus anticoagulant (LA) and anticardiolipin antibodies (aCL). aPL are a heterogeneous group of immunoglobulins directed at phospholipid binding proteins. aCL are detected by an enzyme linked immunosorbent assay (ELISA) which was first described by Harris and colleagues at the Hammersmith Hospital (Harris et al., 1983). The LA is a misnomer—it may occur in patients without lupus and it is in fact a prothrombotic autoantibody. It is commonly detected by the Dilute Russell Viper Venom Test although there are several other methods available for detection. Plasma is required and it is difficult to measure the LA in patients on warfarin, though tests such as the Taipan Snake Venom Tests are used in some laboratories. LA is measured according to the International Society for Thrombosis and Hemostasis criteria (Brandt et al., 1995).

The prevalence of aPL in otherwise healthy populations is less than 1%, and up to 5% in older healthy populations. In autoimmune diseases, especially SLE, the prevalence is much higher. There have been several large studies of the prevalence of aPL in SLE patients. Perhaps the largest is the Euro-Lupus study which found a prevalence of 24% IgG aCL, 13% IgM aCL, and 15% LA respectively in a cohort of 1000 patients with SLE (Cervera et al., 1993). The prevalence of aPL and definite APS may increase with longer follow-up, further pregnancies, and repeat testing for aPS. Thus Perez-Vazquez et al. showed that the prevalence of APS increased from 10 to 23% after 15–18 years in a large cohort of SLE patients (Perez-Vazquez et al., 1993). A further study of 1000 APS patients has detailed the clinical features of the disorder (Cervera et al., 2002).

---

*Corresponding author.
Tel.: +44-207-188-3571; Fax: +44-207-620-2658
*E-mail address:* david.d'cruz@kcl.ac.uk

**Table 1**
Classification criteria for the antiphospholipid syndrome Miyakis et al. (2006)

Antiphospholipid antibody syndrome (APS) is present if at least one of the clinical criteria and one of the laboratory criteria that follow are met

Clinical criteria
  Vascular thrombosis
    One or more clinical episodes of arterial, venous, or small vessel thrombosis, in any tissue or organ. Thrombosis must be confirmed by objective validated criteria (i.e., unequivocal findings of appropriate imaging studies or histopathology). For histopathologic confirmation, thrombosis should be present without significant evidence of inflammation in the vessel wall
  Pregnancy morbidity
    (a) One or more unexplained deaths of a morphologically normal fetus at or beyond the 10th week of gestation, with normal fetal morphology documented by ultrasound or by direct examination of the fetus, or
    (b) One or more premature births of a morphologically normal neonate before the 34th week of gestation because of: (i) eclampsia or severe preeclampsia defined according to standard definitions, or (ii) recognized features of placental insufficiency, or
    (c) Three or more unexplained consecutive spontaneous abortions before the 10th week of gestation, with maternal anatomic or hormonal abnormalities and paternal and maternal chromosomal causes excluded
  In studies of populations of patients who have more than one type of pregnancy morbidity, investigators are strongly encouraged to stratify groups of subjects according to a, b, or c above

Laboratory criteria
  Lupus anticoagulant (LA) present in plasma, on two or more occasions at least 12 weeks apart, detected according to the guidelines of the International Society on Thrombosis and Haemostasis (Scientific Subcommittee on LAs/phospholipid-dependent antibodies)
  Anticardiolipin (aCL) antibody of IgG and/or IgM isotype in serum or plasma, present in medium or high titer (i.e., >40 GPL or MPL, or > the 99th percentile), on two or more occasions, at least 12 weeks apart, measured by a standardized ELISA
  Anti-$\beta$2 glycoprotein-I antibody of IgG and/or IgM isotype in serum or plasma (in titer > the 99th percentile), present on two or more occasions, at least 12 weeks apart, measured by a standardized ELISA, according to recommended procedures

An international consensus statement on classification criteria for definite APS has been validated (Table 1) (Wilson et al., 1999; Lockshin et al., 2000). The criteria were updated recently, but have yet to be validated (Miyakis et al., 2006). These classification criteria were developed for use in research studies rather than as diagnostic criteria, which as yet do not exist. Other well-recognized features of APS such as thrombocytopenia, hemolytic anemia, transient ischaemic attacks, transverse myelitis, livedo reticularis, valvular heart disease, demyelinating syndromes, chorea, and migraine were not thought to have as strong an association as the final criteria, and were excluded as classification criteria possibly resulting in lower sensitivity but higher specificity (Miyakis et al., 2006). In clinical practice, however, the physician should still consider the diagnosis in the right clinical context in the presence of persistently positive aPL, and commence treatment according to clinical judgment after exclusion of other causes of these clinical features.

There are however, numerous traps for the unwary and many other conditions can be associated with aPL but are not necessarily associated with thrombosis. Thus aPL may occur in infections such as HIV and syphilis and in association with malignancy or following exposure to certain drugs (Table 2). aPL in these circumstances are not necessarily pathogenic and these conditions should therefore be considered in any differential diagnosis of APS.

**Table 2**
Anti-phospholipid antibodies in other conditions

| Autoimmune connective tissue disorders | Drugs |
|---|---|
| Systemic vasculitides | Chlorpromazine |
| Malignancy | Quinine/quinidine |
| Crohn's disease | Hydralazine |
| Infection | Procainamide |
| Syphilis/Lyme | Phenytoin |
| Human immunodeficiency virus | Interferon-$\alpha$ |
| Hepatitis C | Anti-TNF$\alpha$ therapies |
| Cytomegalovirus | |
| Mycoplasma | |

APS has a significant impact on survival. For example in a retrospective study of 52 patients with aCL followed over 10 years, 29% of APS patients (31 patients) had recurrent events and in the asymptomatic group (21 patients) half developed APS: mortality was 10% (Shah et al., 1998). In another study, Jouhikainen et al. compared 37 LA positive SLE patients with 37 age- and sex-matched SLE patients without LA. During a median follow-up of 22 years, 30% in the LA group died in contrast to 14% in the control group (Jouhikainen et al., 1993). Among patients with venous thromboembolism, the mortality in Swedish patients was 15% at 4 years in those with aCL and 6% in those without antibodies (Schulman et al., 1998). The largest prospective study of 1000 SLE patients showed that after 10 years of follow-up there were 68 deaths of whom 18 (26.5%) died from thrombosis associated with aPL (Cervera et al., 1993). The most common thrombotic events were cerebrovascular accidents (11.8%), coronary occlusions (7.4%), and pulmonary emboli (5.9%).

There is increasing evidence that thrombosis contributes to the damage accrued in patients with SLE, which in turn may contribute to morbidity as well as mortality. Two recent studies have clearly demonstrated that APS with thrombotic manifestations independently contributes to irreversible organ damage as well as mortality in lupus patients (Soares et al., 2003; Ruiz-Irastorza et al., 2004). Thus, Ruiz-Irastorza's study of over 200 SLE patients extending over 25 years demonstrated both higher damage scores and increased mortality in APS patients, most of whom had suffered arterial thromboses (Ruiz-Irastorza et al., 2004).

## 3. Risk factors for thrombosis in APS: two hit hypothesis

It is clear that not all aPL positive patients will inevitably develop clinical features of APS. The precise reasons for this remain unclear and it seems likely that additional factors are required for a first thrombotic event or pregnancy-related feature. However, previous thromboses, in the context of persistent moderate to high aCL levels and/or LA, are the most powerful predictors of future events. In a cohort of 360 patients in the Italian aPL Registry, followed prospectively for 3.9 years with either a positive LA or aCL, 34 patients developed a thrombotic event: an incidence of 2.5%/patient-year, with a rate of 5.4%/patient-year in those with a previous thrombosis and 0.95%/patient-year in asymptomatic subjects (Finazzi et al., 1996). Clearly the mere presence of aPL is not sufficient for an event. Patients with aCL>40 units and previous thrombosis were important risk factors for future events. Similarly, the greater the different numbers of aPL detected in a given patient the greater the risk of thrombosis (Finazzi et al., 1996). The importance of previous thrombosis as a risk factor was highlighted by the recurrence rate in a retrospective study by Khamashta et al., where those with APS and previous thrombosis had a recurrence rate of 20%/patient-year of follow-up (Khamashta et al., 1995). In pregnancy, patients with a prior history of miscarriages or vascular occlusions have a significantly higher rate of adverse pregnancy outcomes (Finazzi et al., 1996).

Numerous other risk factors may contribute to the development of a first thrombotic event in the presence of aPL. A study of 404 patients with aPL showed that, at the time of the initial thrombosis, 50% of patients had coincident risk factors for thrombosis: previous surgery and prolonged immobilization were significantly associated with venous thrombosis, and hypercholesterolemia and arterial hypertension with arterial thrombosis (Giron-Gonzalez et al., 2004).

Virchow's observations on the three factors relevant to clot formation still hold good today: factors related to the blood (hypercoagulability), those related to the rate of flow, and factors related to the vessel wall itself. The complex mechanisms by which aPL may affect platelets and endothelial cells to produce a procoagulant state have been discussed in detail (Giannakopoulos et al., 2007). However, evidence is emerging of abnormalities of the vessel wall that may be relevant to APS. Accelerated atherosclerosis is undoubtedly a feature of SLE that contributes to mortality (Roman et al., 2003). However, studies in patients without lupus who are aPL positive have shown increased carotid intima-media thickness associated with an increased risk of arterial thrombosis (Medina et al., 2003). Another study found a higher prevalence of an abnormal ankle–brachial index in patients with primary APS compared to healthy controls, suggesting widespread vascular abnormalities (Baron et al., 2005). Similarly, the prevalence of an abnormal ankle–brachial index in young women with APS and pregnancy morbidity but without previous thrombosis was also higher than in healthy young female controls (Christodoulou et al., 2006). Further evidence of vessel wall abnormalities comes from data showing a higher prevalence of renal artery stenosis in association with aPL in patients with SLE (Sangle et al., 2003). This suggests that vessels that have high velocity turbulent flow may be at increased risk of vascular abnormality in the presence of aPL. Recent data suggests a similar phenomenon with coeliac artery stenosis in aPL positive patients (Sangle et al., 2006). Even at the capillary level there may be abnormalities. Nailfold video capillaroscopy in patients with primary APS showed abnormal morphology with smaller capillary diameters than controls, although these changes could not be correlated with impairment of functional parameters (Vaz et al., 2004). The authors suggested that the smaller capillary diameters resulted in lower local tissue perfusion and hypoxia, although these parameters were not directly measured. If correct though, these conditions would clearly favor a procoagulant state.

Several studies have shown that risk factors can be additive. In young adults with venous thrombosis, Rosendaal et al. found that the risk of thrombosis rose sharply with the number of risk factors and that fewer factors were required for thrombosis in older subjects (Rosendaal, 1997). Several groups have reported the additional presence of coagulation abnormalities, such as factor V Leiden, in patients with APS. Factor V Leiden and aCL can both cause the activated protein C resistance phenotype and, not surprisingly, the combination has been associated with severe thrombosis (Brenner et al., 1996; Ames et al., 1998). Methylenetetrahydrofolate reductase C 677→T substitution (leading to increased homocysteine) may also have an effect on age at first occlusive event (Ames et al., 1998). Furthermore, Peddi reported the development of catastrophic APS in a patient with SLE, aCL, and antithrombin III deficiency (Peddi and Kant, 1995).

## 4. Conditions associated with APS

A wide spectrum of disorders has been associated with APS. This is a common disorder and may even exceed the prevalence of APS associated with rheumatic disorders, especially if women who only have aPL related pregnancy morbidity are included. It has been estimated that up to half of patients with APS do not have an associated systemic disease (Asherson et al., 1989). The nomenclature of "primary" and "secondary" APS has been discarded on the grounds that the clinical features of APS are the same whether or not there is an associated autoimmune disorder (Miyakis et al., 2006). APS has been described in all the autoimmune rheumatic disorders including systemic vasculitides. However, thrombotic manifestations of APS are not usually seen with infection-or drug-associated aCL, although occasional reports of thrombosis in infections such as acquired immune deficiency syndrome (HIV/AIDS) and cytomegalovirus (CMV) suggests that in patients with APS, especially where there are atypical features, an underlying infection should be considered (Soweid et al., 1995; Labarca et al., 1997). Procainamide has been shown to produce β2-glycoprotein 1-dependent antibodies that are potentially pathogenic (Merrill et al., 1997).

## 5. Organ manifestations of APS

Any organ in the body may be affected by arterial, venous, or small vessel thrombosis. The most common manifestations include deep vein thromboses, pulmonary emboli, cerebral and myocardial infarctions. Table 3 summarizes the wide spectrum of these clinical features. The skin is often affected and a characteristic feature is livedo reticularis—an extremely useful clinical marker of the disease and a pointer towards a poorer prognosis (Fig. 1).

**Table 3**
Clinical associations

| | |
|---|---|
| CNS | Dego's disease |
|   Chorea | Splinter hemorrhages |
|   Migraine | Superficial thrombophlebitis |
|   Psychosis | Distal cutaneous ischemia |
|   Epilepsy | Bone |
|   CVA/TIA |   Avascular necrosis |
|   Hypoperfusion on SPECT scanning |   Bone marrow necrosis |
|   Sensorineural hearing loss |   Fractures |
|   Transverse myelopathy | Obstetric |
|   Cognitive impairment |   Recurrent miscarriage |
|   Pseudotumor cerebri |   Pre-eclampsia |
|   Cerebral vein/artery thrombosis |   Growth retardation |
|   Retinal venous thrombosis |   HELLP syndrome |
|   Multiple sclerosis like syndrome | Renal |
| Gastrointestinal |   Glomerular thrombosis |
|   Hepatic necrosis |   Renal artery stenosis |
|   Acalculous cholecystitis |   Renal insufficiency |
|   Budd–Chiari |   Renal artery thrombosis |
|   Intestinal ischemia |   Renal vein thrombosis |
|   Coeliac artery stenosis | Pulmonary |
| Vascular disease |   Pulmonary embolism |
|   Atherosclerosis |   Pulmonary hypertension |
|   Cardiac valvular disease |   ARDS |
|   Acute myocardial infarction | Endocrine |
|   Failed angioplasty |   Adrenal failure |
|   Diastolic dysfunction |   Hypopituitarism |
|   Intracardiac thrombosis | Haematological |
|   Cardiomyopathy |   Thrombocytopenia |
|   Buerger 's disease |   Autoimmune hemolytic anemia |
| Skin |   Thrombotic microangiopathy |
|   Livedo reticularis | |
|   Cutaneous ulcers | |
|   Skin necrosis | |

*Abbreviations used*: CVA, cerebrovascular accident; TIA, transient ischemic attack; SPECT, single position emission computerized tomography; HELLP, hemolytic anaemia, elevated liver function tests, and low platelets; ARDS, adult respiratory distress syndrome.

The focus of this chapter is however renal disease and the reader is referred to recent reviews for more details on the protean manifestations of this disorder.

## 6. Renal manifestations

The kidney may be affected in APS and renal thrombotic manifestations have been reported since the earliest descriptions of the syndrome. However, it is only in the last decade that the prognostic implications of aPL for renal function have been appreciated, particularly in aPL positive patients with lupus nephritis and in those undergoing renal transplantation.

## 7. Hypertension

Hypertension was one of the first major features described in association with livedo reticularis and aPL. In his Prosser-White oration, Graham Hughes noted: "These patients' blood pressure often fluctuates, apparently correlating with the severity of the livedo, suggesting a possible renovascular

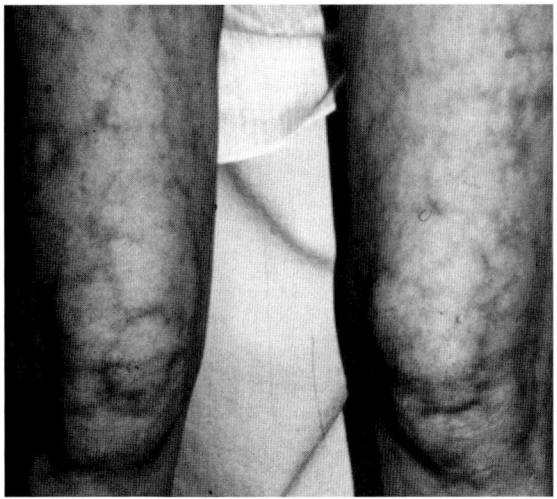

**Figure 1.** Livedo reticularis. This is the typical "broken" pattern of pathological livedo reticularis associated with APS as well as other conditions such as polyarteritis nodosa.

etiology. However, this group of patients rarely has primary renal disease" (Hughes, 1984). As time has gone on, the prevalence and spectrum of primary renal disease has increased considerably. Hypertension is common in aPL positive patients. For example, data in abstract form from our Lupus Clinic shows an overall prevalence of hypertension of 29% in 600 patients. Livedo reticularis was exceedingly common (86% of hypertensive patients) and appears to be a sensitive clinical marker in these patients (Sangle et al., 2004).

The major implication is that patients with aPL complicated by hypertension should be vigorously investigated for an underlying renal lesion, especially in the presence of livedo reticularis. In this context, particularly when the hypertension is difficult to control, the simple outpatient approach of urine dip testing and analysis of serum urea and creatinine may not be sensitive enough to detect early APS nephropathy. More detailed assessments such as glomerular filtration rate, renal ultrasound, nuclear medicine DMSA scans, and imaging of the renal arteries and veins should be considered, as well as the more standard tests such as quantification of urine protein excretion and searching for an active urine sediment. It has been well established that SLE patients who are aPL positive accumulate more damage than comparable aPL negative patients, increasing the risk of significant morbidity and death (Ruiz-Irastorza et al., 2004). Key markers of damage include arterial events such as strokes and myocardial infarction: the early diagnosis and treatment of hypertension is therefore critical in these patients.

## 8. Renal artery lesions

The etiology of renovascular hypertension has been difficult to define until recently. Early case reports usually described frank renal artery thrombosis and infarction where the clinical consequences were severe (Ostuni et al., 1990; Hernandez et al., 1996; Asherson et al., 1991; Ames et al., 1992; Rossi et al., 1992; Mandreoli and Zucchelli (1993); Godfrey et al., 2000; Cacoub et al., 1993). Renal artery stenosis was also described, though in these reports the patients also had symptomatic renal ischaemia (Mandreoli, 1992). The possibility that asymptomatic renal artery stenosis may be associated with "difficult" hypertension was explored in a case-controlled cohort study. Using magnetic resonance angiography, 26% of aPL positive patients with poorly controlled hypertension were found to have renal artery stenosis, a significantly higher prevalence compared to 8% of young patients attending a hypertension clinic and 3% of live-related renal donors (Sangle et al., 2003). The stenotic lesions were generally smooth non-critical stenoses in the mid-portion of the renal artery, quite distinct from either fibromuscular dysplasia or atherosclerosis (Fig. 2). A striking observation has been that in patients who were on warfarin, inadequate anticoagulation often led to poor outcomes with worsening of hypertensive control, stent re-occlusions, and renal impairment (Sangle et al., 2005). The nature of these stenotic lesions remains unclear. A post-mortem study of SLE patients who were all aPL positive found a high prevalence of intimal hyperplasia which may contribute to vascular stenosis (Sipek-Dolnicar et al., 2002). Our experience of the response to anticoagulation does suggest a thrombotic basis. Hypotheses include a process of on-going low-grade mural thrombus

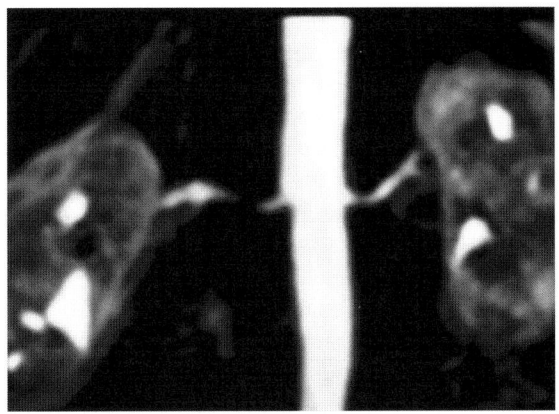

Figure 2. Right renal artery stenosis associated with hypertension in antiphospholipid syndrome (APS). The aorta is smooth suggesting that the stenosis is not related to atherosclerosis.

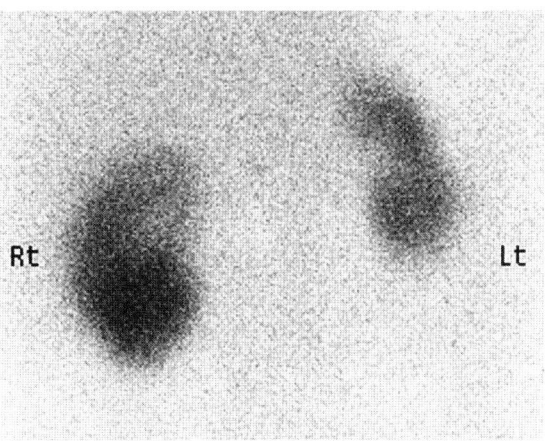

Figure 3. Nuclear medicine DMSA scan showing renal infarction in the right upper pole and small scarred left kidney in a patient with hypertension, renal impairment and APS.

within the renal arteries, or accelerated atherosclerosis, though the latter seems less likely given the appearances of the lesions. These studies have led to the concept that anticoagulation should be considered in hypertensive patients with aPL-related renal artery stenosis even in the absence of previous thrombotic events (Sangle et al., 2005).

Other vessels may also develop stenotic lesions in association with aPL. A study of vascular access in hemodialysis patients found a correlation between IgM aCL and Doppler evidence of stenosis in the vascular access sites (Adler et al., 2001). More recently, Sangle et al. have described a series of patients with coeliac artery stenosis, although a possible explanation in some patients may be compression from the median arcuate ligament of the diaphragm (Sangle et al., 2006). The concept that the vessel wall may be altered in APS is therefore gaining credence and indeed goes back to Virchow's triad of factors that may lead to thrombosis.

## 9. Cortical ischaemia/infarction

Thrombosis may occur in smaller diameter renal parenchymatous vessels resulting in areas of focal cortical ischaemia and/or necrosis (Amigo et al., 1992; Nochy et al., 1999). Clinically these may manifest as hypertension and renal impairment with imaging confirmation of small kidneys or cortical infarction on ultrasound or DMSA scanning (Fig. 3) (Calhoun et al., 2003). Histologically, glomerular ischaemia, interstitial fibrosis, tubular atrophy, and arterial and venous thrombus and sclerosis may be seen (Amigo et al., 1992; Nochy et al., 1999). Renal cortical ischaemia may present insidiously and progress slowly towards renal failure without overt glomerulonephritis, though there is often hypertension and mild proteinuria (Leaker et al., 1991).

## 10. Thrombotic microangiopathy

Thrombotic microangiopathy is perhaps the best known and most characteristic lesion of APS nephropathy, with distinctive microscopic and ultrastructural changes (Fig. 4) (Amigo et al., 1992; Nochy et al., 1999; Griffiths et al., 2000). The most common presenting clinical features include hypertension, proteinuria, and renal impairment. Proteinuria is often mild but can be nephrotic range (Amigo et al., 1992; Nochy et al., 1999; Griffiths et al., 2000). Histologically, there may be focal or diffuse microangiopathic changes affecting the whole intra-renal vascular tree and the glomerular tufts, with fresh as well as old and

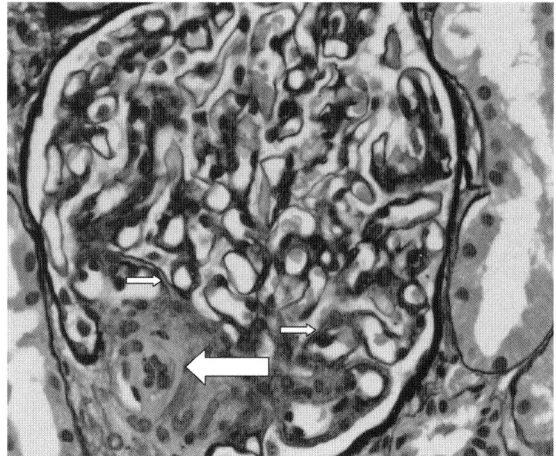

Figure 4. Thrombotic microangiopathy in APS. There is a hilar vessel thrombosis (large arrow) and basement membrane reduplications (small arrows) (Image courtesy of Dr. F. Tungekar).

recanalizing thrombi. Cortical atrophy is well described and is associated with focal atrophy and fibrosis (Amigo et al., 1992; Nochy et al., 1999; Griffiths et al., 2000). Ultrastructurally, a combination of glomerular basement membrane wrinkling and reduplication may be seen and electron microscopy can show redundant, wrinkled segments of basement membrane with straighter thin basement membrane sections adjacent to the endothelium (Griffiths et al., 2000). Although these ultrastructural changes have been described in lupus nephritis, there may well be pathognomonic of APS nephropathy. Small arterioles can also be affected by a non-inflammatory and frequently thrombotic vasculopathy, though these appearances may also be seen in a wide variety of conditions including thrombotic thrombocytopenic purpura, hemolytic uraemic syndrome, scleroderma renal crisis, malignant hypertension, pre-eclampsia, and post-partum renal failure, as well as complications arising from oral contraceptives, cyclosporin toxicity, chemotherapy, and renal transplant rejection (Amigo and Garcia-Torres, 2000).

Although glomerular capillary thrombosis has previously been described in detail in the early 1980s in association with the LA, these reports mainly concentrated on proliferative lupus nephritis and it is only recently that these appearances have been recorded in the primary APS (Kant et al., 1981; Glueck et al., 1985). It is now clear that the development of aPL-related thrombotic microangiopathy in the context of lupus nephritis increases the risk of a poor renal outcome due to hypertension, interstitial fibrosis, and renal impairment (Moss and Isenberg, 2001; Daugas et al., 2002). Clinicians should therefore consider the possibility of APS nephropathy when faced with a patient apparently having a flare of lupus nephritis, since anticoagulation as well as immunosuppression may be required.

## 11. Renal vein and inferior vena cava thrombosis

Thrombosis of the renal veins and inferior vena cava classically present with nephrotic range proteinuria and have been described in aPL positive patients with lupus nephritis, as well as in patients with the primary APS (Lai and Lan, 1997). Thus, in any patient with persistently positive aPL who develops sudden heavy proteinuria, careful Doppler studies of the renal vasculature should be considered. Of course, cause and effect cannot definitively be proven since nephrotic syndrome itself is a prothrombotic state and it is possible that, in aPL positive patients with nephrotic syndrome, the renal vein thrombosis may be a secondary event. Nevertheless, management will still include consideration of anticoagulation.

## 12. End-stage renal failure and renal transplantation

A small number of studies have rather curiously reported an unexpectedly high prevalence of aPL in patients undergoing hemodialysis for renal failure of unknown causes. The aPL were independent of age, length of time on dialysis, sex, type of dialysis membrane, drugs, and hepatitis B and C virus status. Of interest, vascular access thrombosis was significantly more frequent in patients with LA rather than aCL (Nied Prieto and Suki, 1994; Brunet et al., 1995).

There is increasing and convincing evidence that aPL positive patients undergoing renal transplantation are at significantly increased risk of renal vascular thrombosis and graft failure as well as systemic thrombosis. Quite apart from the usual thrombotic risks associated with any major abdominal surgery, and the renovascular thrombosis associated with renal transplant surgery, aPL seem to magnify this risk considerably (Stone et al., 1999; Vaidya et al., 1998). This has led some to suggest that all patients being considered for renal transplantation for renal failure of any cause should be screened for prothrombotic risks such as aPL, prothrombin gene G20210A polymorphisms, or a combined inherited thrombophilia (Andrassy et al., 2004). Given these risks, there are some who question whether aPL positive patients should undergo transplantation at all, since even when full anticoagulation is administered following renal allografting, the risks of graft loss and systemic thrombosis are not completely eliminated (Vaidya et al., 1998; Andrassy et al., 2004).

## 13. Treatment

### 13.1. General measures

Given the increased thrombotic risk of these patients and the possible association with atherosclerosis, vascular risk factors should be addressed. Lifestyle measures and reduction of risk factors such as obesity, smoking, hypertension, diabetes, and hyperlipidemia, are important. The combined oral contraceptive pill and hormone replacement therapy should be avoided.

### 13.2. Asymptomatic patients

Increasing numbers of asymptomatic or recurrent miscarriage patients are being detected due to improved awareness of the condition. A major dilemma is how these patients who have not had a thrombotic event but remain persistently aPL positive should be managed. There is no doubt that some of these patients will have a future event, but predicting those at high risk has proven difficult.

Many physicians recommend low-dose aspirin for management of those patients without previous thrombosis, particularly if titers of aPL are high; however, there is little objective evidence to support this. Indeed an on-going placebo-controlled study reported in abstract form has not shown any protective benefit against thrombosis so far (Erkan et al., 2004). Recent treatment recommendations suggest that in asymptomatic aPL positive individuals, not offering aspirin prophylaxis is a possible option while awaiting trial data (Lim et al., 2006). In SLE patients, there is some evidence supporting the use of hydroxychloroquine; in the LUMINA study, hydroxychloroquine use emerged as a protective factor against thrombosis in unvariate analysis, but this was not sustained in multivariate analysis (Ho et al., 2005).

Traveller's thrombosis has become topical and there is no doubt that prolonged journeys where passengers are seated for considerable periods increase the risk of venous thrombosis (Hughes et al., 2003). No studies have addressed the possible relevance of aPL in traveller's thrombosis, and in the absence of evidence, it seems reasonable to recommend simple measures such as support stockings, hydration, exercises, and ensuring therapeutic INRs for APS patients already on anticoagulation, for those undertaking long journeys by any transport mode. In very high-risk aPL positive patients with no previous thrombosis, some clinicians recommend a single injection of low molecular weight heparin prior to commencing the journey. Other high-risk periods include the post-operative period, especially after abdominal, gynecological, and orthopedic surgery, and particularly in the post-natal period where heparin prophylaxis is mandatory.

### 13.3. Thrombotic events

Arterial and venous events are treated conventionally with unfractionated or low molecular weight heparins, followed by oral anticoagulation with agents such as warfarin. If there is concern that the

APTT will not accurately reflect the degree of anticoagulation, in light of a raised pre-treatment APTT in APS, other indices can be used, such as the factor Xa inhibition test. Alternatively, low molecular weight heparins such as tinzaparin or enoxaparin can be used.

The current recommendation is that anticoagulation should be lifelong, given the risk of recurrent events, and several studies have supported this consensus view (Lim et al., 2006). However, lifelong anticoagulation is not without hazard, with major bleeding occurring in up to 40% in some long-term studies of non-APS patients (Fihn et al., 1993). Data from APS patients, from both retrospective cohort reviews and randomized controlled trials, suggests that the risk of recurrent thrombotic events exceeds the risk of bleeding, which is relatively low (Finazzi et al., 2005; Crowther et al., 2003).

The intensity of anticoagulation has been debated. Randomized controlled trials have suggested that INR levels of 2.0–3.0 may be sufficient in uncomplicated APS patients with only venous thrombotic events (Lim et al., 2006; Finazzi et al., 2005; Crowther et al., 2003). In patients with arterial events or with recurrent thrombotic events, however, higher INR ranges of 3.0–4.0 may be required (Lim et al., 2006; Finazzi et al., 2005; Crowther et al., 2003). In most instances, once patients are established on warfarin, aspirin does not confer any added advantage and can be discontinued.

The term catastrophic APS refers to a rare but very serious disorder characterized by accelerated thrombosis, multiple organ involvement including renal thrombotic microangiopathy, and death in the majority of patients (Fig. 5) (Bucciarelli et al., 2006). Treatment of catastrophic APS has involved glucocorticoids, cyclophosphamide, plasmapheresis, gammaglobulin, anticoagulation, and in the occasional patient, thrombolytic therapy. More than one modality has been tried in most patients. Although no clear approach has emerged the most recent study of mortality suggests that anticoagulation, corticosteroids, and plasma exchange may be useful treatments (Bucciarelli et al., 2006).

Thrombocytopenia is common in APS. Patients remain at risk of thrombosis despite this and

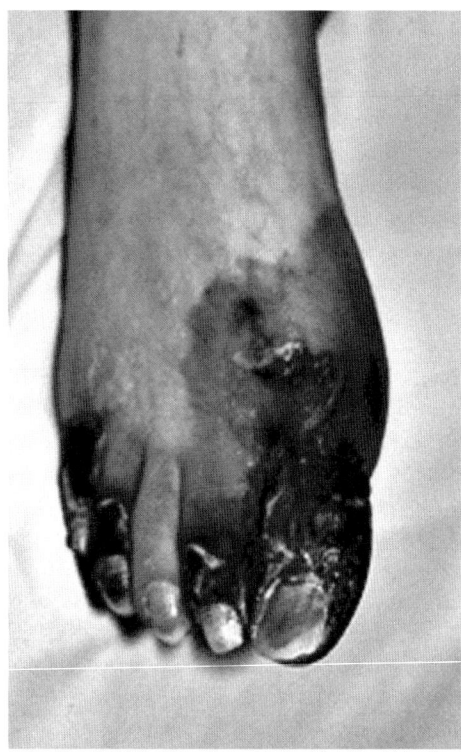

**Figure 5.** Severe gangrene in a patient with catastrophic APS complicated by thrombotic microangiopathy in the kidneys, cerebral infarction, and adult respiratory distress syndrome.

warfarin should be continued unless the platelet count falls below $50 \times 10^9$/L. Anticoagulation may be continued even when the platelet count is below $50 \times 10^9$/L, but the intensity of anticoagulation may need to be reduced. In patients with severe thrombocytopenia, glucocorticoids and intravenous immunoglobulins are usually effective. Other agents such as danazol, dapsone, and even aspirin have been tried. There is some debate as to the effectiveness of splenectomy in APS patients, although some studies suggest that splenectomy is successful in the long term (Hakim et al., 1998; Galindo et al., 1999).

A frequent problem in the management of female patients is menorrhagia, particularly when INRs are maintained at high levels. In this situation, the "Mirena" coil, an intrauterine coil with a silastic capsule containing levonorgestrel, has been found to be helpful (Pisoni et al., 2006).

## 13.4. Pregnancy

Women with previous renal disease from APS and renal impairment are at high risk of complications during pregnancy and so the management of pregnancy in women with APS is worth considering. These women will need very careful pre-conceptual counseling about the risk of pregnancy and the treatment changes needed to reduce the risk of pregnancy complications and fetal malformations.

The management of APS in pregnancy remains controversial, especially in light of recent animal studies suggesting that complement activation rather than thrombosis may be a major contributor to pregnancy morbidity (Girardi et al., 2006). In this model, blocking complement activation improved pregnancy outcome. In particular, these studies demonstrated that heparin at non-anticoagulant doses blocks complement activation, protecting against APS-related pregnancy loss. These studies remain to be confirmed in humans in an on-going study.

The current choice is aspirin or heparin, or both, and this has been reviewed in detail by Petri et al. (Petri and Qazi, 2006). This area remains controversial, especially since Farquharson et al. showed in a randomized controlled trial that high pregnancy success rates were achieved with low-dose aspirin and no advantage was gained by the addition of low molecular weight heparin (Farquharson et al., 2002). These data contrasted with previous controlled trials showing a significant benefit of heparin with aspirin over aspirin alone (Rai et al., 1997; Kutteh, 1996). Women with APS and previous thromboembolism are at extremely high risk in pregnancy and the puerperium, and should be given antenatal thromboprophylaxis with subcutaneous heparin with resumption of oral anticoagulation post-natally.

Warfarin exposure between 6 and 12 weeks of gestation can be associated with embryopathy, which is characterized by stippled epiphyses and nasal hypoplasia. Therefore, the change from warfarin to heparin should be achieved prior to 6 weeks gestation. Heparin does not cross the placenta and is not known to cause any adverse fetal effects. Baglin et al. have published guidelines for the use of heparin, including the use of low molecular weight heparin in pregnancy (Baglin et al., 2006). The risk of osteoporosis in the mother from long-term heparin use has probably been overestimated: a controlled study by Carlin et al. showed that bone loss is a feature of normal pregnancy and that low molecular weight heparin does not exacerbate this loss (Carlin et al., 2004).

There is a consensus that improved outcomes in APS pregnancies are associated with closer obstetric surveillance and multi-disciplinary clinics including nephrologists where appropriate. Viable APS pregnancies have a high incidence of obstetric and fetal complications, including intrauterine growth restriction, prematurity, and pre-eclampsia, hence close monitoring including uterine artery Doppler scans and timely delivery may improve fetal outcome in these women.

## 14. Summary

The identification of Hughes syndrome/APS has been a significant advance in the last 25 years, influencing nearly all branches of medicine. The implications of renal involvement have only recently been explored in detail. There is good evidence that APS nephropathy is a distinct entity with characteristic clinical and histological features. Whilst all renal vessels may be affected, thrombotic microangiopathy with glomerular lesions comprising basement membrane wrinkling and reduplications appear to be pathognomonic. As acute lesions heal, focal areas of fibrosis and atrophy may develop and depending on the extent and severity of these processes, may result in renal impairment. Recent studies have also confirmed the importance of livedo reticularis as a clinical marker of this syndrome in association with hypertension. Furthermore, asymptomatic renal artery stenosis may well be commoner than suggested by early case reports. Clinicians should thus review aPL positive patients very carefully for the development of renal disease. Crucially, patients with lupus nephritis who develop an additional antiphospholipid nephropathy should certainly be considered for long-term anticoagulation as well as immunosuppression to preserve renal function. Although anticoagulation is the mainstay of treatment, this remains imperfect and close attention to other risk factors especially hypertension may reduce the risk of end-stage renal failure in these patients.

---

**Key points**

- APS is a common condition that may occur on its own or in the context of other autoimmune connective tissue disorders such as systemic lupus erythematosus.
- Characteristic clinical features include arterial and venous thrombosis and pregnancy morbidity in association with autoantibodies against phospholipid-binding proteins. Livedo reticularis is a marker of poor prognosis.
- Renal manifestations often present non-specifically and may lead to hypertension, proteinuria, and renal impairment. Early recognition is critical as APS increases the risk of morbidity and mortality in patients with SLE.
- Treatment of thrombotic events is with long-term anticoagulation

---

# References

Adler, S., Szczech, L., Qureshi, A., Bollu, R., Thomas-John, R. 2001. IgM anticardiolipin antibodies are associated with stenosis of vascular access in hemodialysis patients but do not predict thrombosis. Clin. Nephrol. 56, 428–434.

Ames, P., Tommasino, C., D 'Andrea, G., Iannaccone, L., Brancaccio, V., Margaglione, M. 1998. Thrombophilic genotypes in subjects with idiopathic antiphospholipid antibodies—prevalence and significance. Thromb. Haemost. 79, 46–49.

Ames, P.R., Cianciaruso, B., Bellizzi, V., Balletta, M., Lubrano, E., Scarpa, R., Brancaccio, V. 1992. Bilateral renal artery occlusion in a patient with primary antiphospholipid antibody syndrome: thrombosis, vasculitis or both? J. Rheumatol. 19, 1802–1806.

Amigo, M.C., Garcia-Torres, R. 2000. Kidney disease in antiphospholipid syndrome. In: M.A. Khamashta (Ed.), Hughes Syndrome. Antiphospholipid Syndrome. Springer, pp. 70–81.

Amigo, M.C., García-Torres, R., Robles, M., Bochiccio, T., Reyes, P.A. 1992. Renal involvement in primary antiphospholipid syndrome. J. Rheumatol. 19, 1181.

Andrassy, J., Zeier, M., Andrassy, K. 2004. Do we need screening for thrombophilia prior to kidney transplantation? Nephrol. Dial. Transplant. 19 (Suppl. 4: iv), 64–68.

Asherson, R.A., Khamashta, M.A., Ordi-Ros, J., et al. 1989. The primary antiphospholipid syndrome: major clinical and serological features. Medicine 68, 366–374.

Asherson, R.A., Noble, G.E., Hughes, G.R. 1991. Hypertension, renal artery stenosis and the "primary" antiphospholipid syndrome. J. Rheumatol. 18, 1413–1415.

Baglin, T., Barrowcliffe, T.W., Cohen, A., Greaves, M. 2006. British Committee for Standards in Haematology. Guidelines on the use and monitoring of heparin. Br. J. Haematol. 133, 19–34.

Baron, M.A., Khamashta, M.A., Hughes, G.R., D'Cruz, D.P. 2005. Prevalence of an abnormal ankle-brachial index in patients with primary antiphospholipid syndrome: preliminary data. Ann. Rheum. Dis. 64 (1), 144–146.

Brandt, J.T., Triplett, D.A., Alving, B., Scharrer, I. 1995. Criteria for the diagnosis of lupus anticoagulants: an update. On behalf of the Subcommittee on Lupus Anticoagulant/Antiphospholipid Antibody of the Scientific and Standardisation Committee of the ISTH. Thromb. Haemost. 74, 1185–1190.

Brenner, B., Vulfsons, S.L., Lanir, N., Nahir, M. 1996. Coexistence of familial antiphospholipid syndrome and factor V Leiden: impact on thrombotic diathesis. Br. J. Haematol. 94, 166–167.

Brunet, P., Aillaud, M.F., San Marco, M., Philip-Joet, C., Dussol, B., Bernard, D., Juhan-Vague, I., Berland, Y. 1995. Antiphospholipids in hemodialysis patients: relationship between lupus anticoagulant and thrombosis. Kidney Int. 48, 794–800.

Bucciarelli, S., Espinosa, G., Cervera, R., Erkan, D., Gomez-Puerta, J.A., Ramos-Casals, M., Font, J., Asherson, R.A. 2006. European Forum on Antiphospholipid Antibodies. Mortality in the catastrophic antiphospholipid syndrome: causes of death and prognostic factors in a series of 250 patients. Arthritis Rheum. 54, 2568–2576.

Cacoub, P., Wechsler, B., Piette, J.C., et al. 1993. Malignant hypertension in antiphospholipid syndrome without overt lupus nephritis. Clin. Exp. Rheumatol. 11, 479–485.

Calhoun, W.B., Hartshorne, M.F., Servilla, K.S., Tzamaloukas, A.H. 2003. Renal cortical perfusion defects caused by antiphospholipid syndrome seen on fusion imaging. Clin. Nucl. Med. 28, 853–854.

Carlin, A.J., Farquharson, R.G., Quenby, S.M., Topping, J., Fraser, W.D. 2004. Prospective observational study of bone mineral density during pregnancy: low molecular weight heparin versus control. Hum. Reprod. 19, 1211–1214.

Cervera, R., Khamashta, M.A., Font, J., Sebastiani, G.D., Gil, A., Lavilla, P., Domenech, I., Aydintug, A.O., Jedryka-Goral, A., de Ramon, E., et al. 1993. Systemic lupus erythematosus: clinical and immunologic patterns of disease expression in a cohort of 1,000 patients. The European Working Party on Systemic Lupus Erythematosus. Medicine (Baltimore) 72, 113–124.

Cervera, R., Piette, J.C., Font, J., Khamashta, M.A., Shoenfeld, Y., Camps, M.T., Jacobsen, S., Lakos, G., Tincani, A., Kontopoulou-Griva, I., Galeazzi, M., Meroni, P.L., Derksen, R.H., de Groot, P.G., Gromnica-Ihle, E., Baleva, M., Mosca, M., Bombardieri, S., Houssiau, F., Gris, J.C., Quere, I., Hachulla, E., Vasconcelos, C., Roch, B., Fernandez-Nebro, A., Boffa, M.C., Hughes, G.R., Ingelmo, M. 2002. Euro-Phospholipid Project Group. Antiphospholipid syndrome: clinical and immunologic manifestations and patterns of disease expression in a cohort of 1,000 patients. Arthritis Rheum. 46, 1019–1027.

Christodoulou, C., Zain, M., Bertolaccini, M.L., Sangle, S., Khamashta, M.A., Hughes, G.R., D'Cruz, D.P. 2006. Prevalence of an abnormal ankle-brachial index in patients with antiphospholipid syndrome with pregnancy loss but without thrombosis: a controlled study. Ann. Rheum. Dis. 65, 683–684.

Crowther, M.A., Ginsberg, J.S., Julian, J., Denburg, J., Hirsh, J., Douketis, J., Laskin, C., Fortin, P., Anderson, D., Kearon, C., Clarke, A., Geerts, W., Forgie, M., Green, D., Costantini, L., Yacura, W., Wilson, S., Gent, M., Kovacs, M.J. 2003. A comparison of two intensities of warfarin for the prevention of recurrent thrombosis in patients with the antiphospholipid antibody syndrome. N. Engl. J. Med. 349, 1133–1138.

Daugas, E., Nochy, D., Huong du, L.T., Duhaut, P., Beaufils, H., Caudwell, V., Bariety, J., Piette, J.C., Hill, G. 2002. Antiphospholipid syndrome nephropathy in systemic lupus erythematosus. J. Am. Soc. Nephrol. 13, 42–52.

Erkan, D., Sammaritano, L., Levy, R., et al. 2004. APLASA Study 2004 update: primary thrombosis prevention in asymptomatic antiphospholipid antibody (APL) positive patients with low dose aspirin (ASA). Arthritis Rheum. 50 (Suppl. 9), S640.

Farquharson, R.G., Quenby, S., Greaves, M. 2002. Antiphospholipid syndrome in pregnancy: a randomized, controlled trial of treatment. Obstet. Gynecol. 100, 408–413.

Fihn, S.D., McDonell, M., Martin, D., Henikoff, J., Vermes, D., Kent, D., White, R.H. 1993. Risk factors for complications of chronic anticoagulation. A multicenter study. Warfarin Optimized Outpatient Follow-Up Study Group. Ann. Intern. Med. 118, 511–520.

Finazzi, G., Brancaccio, V., Moia, M., et al. 1996. Natural history and risk factors for thrombosis in 360 patients with antiphospholipid antibodies. A four year prospective study from the Italian Registry. Am. J. Med. 100, 530–536.

Finazzi, G., Marchioli, R., Brancaccio, V., Schinco, P., Wisloff, F., Musial, J., Baudo, F., Berrettini, M., Testa, S., D'Angelo, A., Tognoni, G., Barbui, T. 2005. A randomized clinical trial of high-intensity warfarin vs. conventional antithrombotic therapy for the prevention of recurrent thrombosis in patients with the antiphospholipid syndrome (WAPS). J. Thromb. Haemost. 3, 848–853.

Galindo, M., Khamashta, M.A., Hughes, G.R. 1999. Splenectomy for refractory thrombocytopenia in the antiphospholipid syndrome. Rheumatology (Oxford) 38, 848–853.

Giannakopoulos, B., Passam, F., Rahgozar, S., Krilis, S.A. 2007. Current concepts on the pathogenesis of the antiphospholipid syndrome. Blood 109, 422–430.

Girardi, G., Yarilin, D., Thurman, J.M., Holers, V.M., Salmon, J.E. 2006. Complement activation induces dysregulation of angiogenic factors and causes fetal rejection and growth restriction. J. Exp. Med. 203, 2165–2175.

Giron-Gonzalez, J.A., Garcia del Rio, E., Rodriguez, C., Rodriguez-Martorell, J., Serrano, A. 2004. Antiphospholipid syndrome and asymptomatic carriers of antiphospholipid antibody: prospective analysis of 404 individuals. J. Rheumatol. 31, 1560–1567.

Glueck, H.I., Kant, K.S., Weiss, M.A., Pollak, V.E., Miller, M.A., Coots, M. 1985. Thrombosis in systemic lupus erythematosus. Relation to the presence of circulating anticoagulants. Arch. Intern. Med. 145, 1389–1395.

Godfrey, T., Khamashta, M.A., Hughes, G.R. 2000. Antiphospholipid syndrome and renal artery stenosis. Q. J. Med. 93, 127–129.

Griffiths, M.H., Papadaki, L., Neild, G.H. 2000. The renal pathology of primary antiphospholipid syndrome: a distinctive form of endothelial injury. Q. J. Med. 93, 457–467.

Hakim, A.J., Machin, S.J., Isenberg, D.A. 1998. Autoimmune thrombocytopenia in primary antiphospholipid syndrome and systemic lupus erythematosus: the response to splenectomy. Semin. Arthritis Rheum. 28, 20–25.

Harris, E.N., Gharavi, A.E., Boey, M.L., Patel, B.M., Mackworth-Young, C.G., Loizou, S., Hughes, G.R. 1983. Anticardiolipin antibodies: detection by radioimmunoassay and association with thrombosis in systemic lupus erythematosus. Lancet 2, 1211–1214.

Hernandez, D., Dominguez, M.L., Diaz, F., Fernandez, M.L., Lorenzo, V., Rodriguez, A., Torres, A. 1996. Renal infarction in a severely hypertensive patient with lupus erythematosus and antiphospholipid antibodies. Nephron. 72 (2), 298–301.

Ho, K.T., Ahn, C.W., Alarcon, G.S., Baethge, B.A., Tan, F.K., Roseman, J., Bastian, H.M., Fessler, B.J., McGwin, G., Jr., Vila, L.M., Calvo-Alen, J., Reveille, J.D. 2005. Systemic lupus erythematosus in a multiethnic cohort (LUMINA): XXVIII. Factors predictive of thrombotic events. Rheumatology (Oxford) 44, 1303–1307.

Hughes, G.R.V. 1983. Thrombosis, abortion, cerebral disease, and the lupus anticoagulant. Br. Med. J. (Clin. Res. Ed.) 287, 1088–1089.

Hughes, G.R. 1984. The Prosser-White oration 1983. Connective tissue disease and the skin. Clin. Exp. Dermatol. 9, 535–544.

Hughes, R.J., Hopkins, R.J., Hill, S., Weatherall, M., Van de Water, N., Nowitz, M., Milne, D., Ayling, J., Wilsher, M., Beasley, R. 2003. Frequency of venous thromboembolism in low to moderate risk long distance air travellers: the New Zealand Air Traveller's Thrombosis (NZATT) study. Lancet 362, 2039–2044.

Jouhikainen, T., Stephansson, E., Leirisalo-Repo, M. 1993. Lupus anticoagulant as a prognostic marker in systemic lupus erythematosus. Br. J. Rheumatol. 32, 568–573.

Kant, K.S., Pollak, V.E., Weiss, M.A., Glueck, H.I., Miller, M.A., Hess, E.V. 1981. Glomerular thrombosis in systemic lupus erythematosus: Prevalence and significance. Medicine 60, 71–86.

Khamashta, M., Cuadrado, M., Mujic, F., Taub, N., Hunt, B., Hughes, G.R.V. 1995. The management of thrombosis in the antiphospholipid-antibody syndrome. N. Engl. J. Med. 332, 993–997.

Kutteh, W.H. 1996. Antiphospholipid antibody-associated recurrent pregnancy loss: treatment with heparin and low-dose aspirin is superior to low-dose aspirin alone. Am. J. Obstet. Gynecol. 174, 1584–1589.

Labarca, J., Rabaggliati, R., Radrigan, F., et al. 1997. Antiphospholipid syndrome associated with cytomegalovirus infection: case report and review. Clin. Infect. Dis. 24, 197–200.

Lai, N.S., Lan, J.L. 1997. Renal vein thrombosis in Chinese patients with systemic lupus erythematosus. Ann. Rheum. Dis. 56, 562–564.

Leaker, B., McGregor, A.O., Griffiths, M., Snaiyh, A., Neild, G.H., Isenberg, D. 1991. Insidious loss of renal function in patients with anticardiolipin antibodies and absence of overt nephritis. Br. J. Haematol. 30, 422–425.

Lim, W., Crowther, M.A., Eikelboom, J.W. 2006. Management of antiphospholipid antibody syndrome: a systematic review. J. Am. Med. Assoc. 295, 1050–1057.

Lockshin, M.D., Sammaritano, L.R., Schwartzman, S. 2000. Validation of the Sapporo criteria for antiphospholipid syndrome. Arthritis Rheum. 43, 440–443.

Mandreoli, M., Zuccala, A., Zucchelli, P. 1992. Fibromuscular dysplasia of the renal arteries associated with antiphospholipid autoantibodies: two case reports. Am. J. Kidney Dis. 20, 500–503.

Mandreoli, M., Zucchelli, P. 1993. Renal vascular disease in patients with primary antiphospholipid antibodies. Nephrol. Dial. Transplant. 8, 1277–1280.

Medina, G., Casaos, D., Jara, L.J., Vera-Lastra, O., Fuentes, M., Barile, L., Salas, M. 2003. Increased carotid artery intima-media thickness may be associated with stroke in primary antiphospholipid syndrome. Ann. Rheum. Dis. 62, 607–610.

Merrill, J.T., Shen, C., Gugnani, M., Lahita, R.G., Mongey, A.B. 1997. High prevalence of antiphospholipid antibodies in patients taking procainamide. J. Rheumatol. 24, 1083–1088.

Miyakis, S., Lockshin, M.D., Atsumi, T., Branch, D.W., Brey, R.L., Cervera, R., Derksen, R.H., de Groot, P.G., Koike, T., Meroni, P.L., Reber, G., Shoenfeld, Y., Tincani, A., Vlachoyiannopoulos, P.G., Krilis, S.A. 2006. International consensus statement on an update of the classification criteria for definite antiphospholipid syndrome (APS). J. Thromb. Haemost. 4, 295–306.

Moss, K.E., Isenberg, D.A. 2001. Comparison of renal disease severity and outcome in patients with primary antiphospholipid syndrome, antiphospholipid syndrome secondary to systemic lupus erythematosus (SLE) and SLE alone. Rheumatology (Oxford) 40, 863–867.

Nied Prieto, L., Suki, N.W. 1994. Frequent hemodyalisis graft thrombosis: association with antiphospholipid antibodies. Am. J. Kidney Dis. 23, 587–590.

Nochy, D., Daugas, E., Droz, D., et al. 1999. The intrarenal vascular lesions associated with primary antiphospholipid syndrome. J. Am. Soc. Nephrol. 10, 507–518.

Ostuni, P.A., Lazzarin, P., Pengo, V., Ruffatti, A., Schiavon, F., Gambari, P. 1990. Renal artery thrombosis and hypertension in a 13 year old girl with antiphospholipid syndrome. Ann. Rheum. Dis. 49, 184–187.

Peddi, V.R., Kant, K.S. 1995. Catastrophic secondary antiphospholipid syndrome with concomitant antithrombin III deficiency. J. Am. Soc. Nephrol. 5, 1882–1887.

Perez-Vazquez, M.E., Villa, A.R., Drenkard, C., Cabiedes, J., Alarcon-Segovia, D. 1993. Influence of disease duration, continued followup and further antiphospholipid testing on the frequency and classification category of antiphospholipid syndrome in a cohort of patients with systemic lupus erythematosus. J. Rheumatol. 20, 437–442.

Petri, M., Qazi, U. 2006. Management of antiphospholipid syndrome in pregnancy. Rheum. Dis. Clin. North Am. 32, 591–607.

Pisoni, C.N., Cuadrado, M.J., Khamashta, M.A., Hunt, B.J. 2006. Treatment of menorrhagia associated with oral anticoagulation: efficacy and safety of the levonorgestrel releasing intrauterine device (Mirena coil). Lupus 15, 877–880.

Rai, R., Cohen, H., Dave, M., Regan, L. 1997. Randomised controlled trial of aspirin and aspirin plus heparin in pregnant women with recurrent miscarriage associated with phospholipid antibodies (or antiphospholipid antibodies). Br. Med. J. 314, 253–257.

Roman, M.J., Shanker, B.A., Davis, A., Lockshin, M.D., Sammaritano, L., Simantov, R., Crow, M.K., Schwartz, J.E., Paget, S.A., Devereux, R.B., Salmon, J.E. 2003. Prevalence and correlates of accelerated atherosclerosis in systemic lupus erythematosus. N. Engl. J. Med. 349, 2399–2406.

Rosendaal, F. 1997. Thrombosis in the young: epidemiology and risk factors. A focus on venous thrombosis. Thromb. Haemost. 78, 1–6.

Rossi, E., Sani, C., Zini, M., Casoli, M.C., Restori, G. 1992. Anticardiolipin antibodies and renovascular hypertension. Ann. Rheum. Dis. 51, 1180–1181.

Ruiz-Irastorza, G., Egurbide, M.V., Ugalde, J., Aguirre, C. 2004. High impact of antiphospholipid syndrome on irreversible organ damage and survival of patients with systemic lupus erythematosus. Arch. Intern. Med. 164, 77–82.

Sangle, S., D'Cruz, D., Khamashta, M., Hughes, G.R.V. 2004. Prevalence of hypertension in 600 patients with antiphospholipid syndrome. Rheumatology (Oxford) 43 (Suppl. 2), 105.

Sangle, S.R., D'Cruz, D.P., Abbs, I.C., Khamashta, M.A., Hughes, G.R. 2005. Renal artery stenosis in hypertensive patients with antiphospholipid (Hughes) syndrome: outcome following anticoagulation. Rheumatology (Oxford) 44, 372–377.

Sangle, S.R., D'Cruz, D.P., Jan, W., Karim, M.Y., Khamashta, M.A., Abbs, I.C., Hughes, G.R. 2003. Renal artery stenosis in the antiphospholipid (Hughes) syndrome and hypertension. Ann. Rheum. Dis. 62, 999–1002.

Sangle, S.R., Jan, W., Lau, I.S., Bennett, A.N., Hughes, G.R., D'Cruz, D.P. 2006. Coeliac artery stenosis and antiphospholipid (Hughes) syndrome/antiphospholipid anti-bodies. Clin. Exp. Rheumatol. 24, 349.

Schulman, S., Svenungsson, E., Granqvist, S., Duration of Anticoagulation Study Group. 1998. Anticardiolipin antibodies predict early recurrence of thromboembolism and death among patients with venous thromboembolism following anticoagulant therapy. Am. J. Med. 104, 332–338.

Shah, N.M., Khamashta, M.A., Atsumi, T., Hughes, G.R.V. 1998. Outcome of patients with anticardiolipin anti-bodies: a 10 year follow up of 52 patients. Lupus 7, 3–6.

Sipek-Dolnicar, A., Hojnik, M., Bozic, B., Vizjak, A., Rozman, B., Ferluga, D. 2002. Clinical presentations and vascular histopathology in autopsied patients with systemic lupus erythematosus and anticardiolipin antibodies. Clin. Exp. Rheumatol. 20, 335–342.

Soares, M., Reis, L., Papi, J.A., Cardoso, C.R. 2003. Rate, pattern and factors related to damage in Brazilian systemic lupus erythematosus patients. Lupus 12, 788–794.

Soweid, A.M., Hajjar, R.R., Hewan-Lowe, K.O., Gonzalez, E.B. 1995. Skin necrosis indicating antiphospholipid syndrome in patient with AIDS. S. Med. J. 88, 778–786.

Stone, J.H., Amend, W.J., Criswell, L.A. 1999. Antiphospholipid antibody syndrome in renal transplantation: occurrence of clinical events in 96 consecutive patients with systemic lupus erythematosus. Am. J. Kidney Dis. 34, 1040–1047.

Vaidya, S., Wang, C.C., Gugliuzza, C., Fish, J.C. 1998. Relative risk of post-transplant renal thrombosis in patients with antiphospholipid antibodies. Clin. Transplant. 12, 439–444.

Vaz, J.L., Dancour, M.A., Bottino, D.A., Bouskela, E. 2004. Nailfold videocapillaroscopy in primary antiphospholipid syndrome (PAPS). Rheumatology (Oxford) 43, 1025–1027.

Wilson, W., Gharavi, A., Koike, T., et al. 1999. International consensus statement on preliminary classification for definite antiphospholipid syndrome. Report of an International Workshop. Arthritis Rheum. 42, 1309–1311.

CHAPTER 19

# Renal Involvement in Sjögren Syndrome

Michael Samarkos*, Haralampos M. Moutsopoulos

*Department of Pathophysiology, School of Medicine, National University of Athens, 115 27 Athens, Greece*

## 1. Introduction

Sjögren's syndrome (SS) is a common chronic autoimmune disorder described as "autoimmune epithelitis" or exocrinopathy (Moutsopoulos, 1994). It can be a primary disorder (pSS) or it can be secondary to other autoimmune diseases such as systemic lupus erythematosus (SLE). It usually involves the salivary and lacrimal glands, resulting in decreased production of saliva and tears (Kassan and Moutsopoulos, 2004). One distinguishing feature of SS is that patients have a significantly increased risk of B-cell lymphoproliferative disorders; thus, it can be thought of as "the crossroad of autoimmunity and lymphoid malignancy". The histopathological hallmark of SS is focal lymphoid cell infiltration of exocrine glands, while serologically it is characterized by the presence of various autoantibodies, such as anti-Ro, and anti-La. However, SS is not always an organ-specific disease and may involve extra-glandular tissue, leading to a systemic disease with synovitis, neuropathy, vasculitis, lung, kidney, and liver involvement (Kassan and Moutsopoulos, 2004).

Renal involvement in SS was initially thought to be rare. Occasional patients had been described with renal abnormalities including glomerular hyalinization and sclerosis, chronic pyelonephritis, and renal concentrating defects [quoted in Shearn and Tu (1965)]. However, during the 1960s more systematic study of SS revealed that interstitial disease, including renal tubular acidosis (RTA) and renal concentrating defects, was not rare in patients with SS. Over the years, larger studies elucidated the spectrum of renal involvement in primary Sjögren syndrome (pSS), which includes interstitial nephritis, distal renal tubular acidosis (dRTA), and other functional tubular defects, nephrocalcinosis, urinary calculi, and glomerulonephritis. The commonest renal manifestation of pSS is interstitial disease, while glomerulonephritis is infrequent. However, in a large percentage of patients, kidney involvement is not clinically significant and it can be detected only after specialized laboratory tests.

Renal involvement in secondary SS will not be discussed in this chapter, since it is difficult to decide whether renal involvement is the result of the SS process or the underlying disease, for example SLE.

The overall prevalence of renal involvement in pSS varies widely, ranging from 2 to 67% (Aasarod et al., 2000; Bloch et al., 1965; Bossini et al., 2001; Eriksson et al., 1995; Goules et al., 2000; Pertovaara et al., 1999; Pokorny et al., 1989; Siamopoulos et al., 1986; Vitali et al., 1991). This variation is probably due to several reasons: small numbers of patients studied, differences in patient selection, and different definitions of renal involvement. Most reports on renal involvement in SS have involved relatively small groups of patients, with the exception of Goules et al. (2000) and Vitali et al. (1991) who studied 471 and 104 patients with pSS, respectively. It is interesting that

---

*Corresponding author.
Tel.: +30-210-7462663; Fax: +30-210-7462664
E-mail address: msamarkos@otenet.gr

© 2008 Elsevier B.V. All rights reserved.
DOI: 10.1016/S1571-5078(07)07019-5

these two studies are among those with the lowest prevalence of renal involvement.

Patient selection might be another factor contributing to variations in the prevalence of renal involvement. Most studies lack clearly defined patient entry criteria, making selection bias possible. Indeed the highest prevalence of renal involvement has been reported by Eriksson et al. (1995), who included in their study patients already diagnosed with dRTA. Older studies have included patients with primary as well as secondary SS, so it is difficult to compare their results with more recent studies on patients with pSS only (Bloch et al., 1965; Shiozawa et al., 1987; Talal et al., 1968; Whaley et al., 1973).

Another problem is that there are several classification criteria for SS. The currently accepted classification criteria for SS are the so-called "European" criteria, which have been well defined and validated (Vitali et al., 1993). Many older studies have used alternative classification criteria. For example, Eriksson et al. (Enestrom et al., 1995; Eriksson et al., 1995) have used the Daniels–Talal criteria (Daniels and Talal, 1987). More recent and larger studies, such as that by Goules et al., have used the European criteria (Goules et al., 2000). As a result, some patients included in earlier studies as SS, do not fulfill current criteria. For example, in the study by Bloch et al. (1965). only 23 of the 62 patients fulfilled the current criteria for classification as pSS.

However, the major reason for the reported variation in the prevalence of renal disease in pSS is the different markers of renal involvement, which have been used. Each report defines renal involvement in a different way. Thus, some studies have defined it on the basis of rather subtle functional abnormalities, such as acidification defects detected by abnormal ammonium chloride loading test (Eriksson et al., 1995), while others define it based on markers suggesting clinically significant renal disease, such as elevated serum creatinine or proteinuria (Goules et al., 2000). Indeed, the highest prevalence of renal involvement in pSS has been reported by Eriksson et al. (1995), who studied several biochemical markers in patients with pSS and found overt or latent Type 1 or dRTA in 67% of 27 patients (Eriksson et al., 1995). On the other hand, the lowest prevalence of renal involvement has been reported in studies by Goules et al. (4.2%) and by Vitali et al. (2%), which used serum creatinine, creatinine clearance, proteinuria, and urinalysis to define renal involvement (Goules et al., 2000; Vitali et al., 1991). Consequently, discussing overall percentages of kidney involvement in pSS is not helpful. Instead one should focus on each individual abnormality (e.g., complete dRTA, and increased serum creatinine) and compare the results of different reports. Clinical and laboratory features in patients with pSS and renal involvement from major cohort studies are summarized in Table 1.

Table 1
Clinical and laboratory features in patients with pSS and renal involvement

|  | Pertovaara et al. (1999) | Goules et al. (2000) | Aasarod et al. (2000) | Bossini et al. (2001) |
| --- | --- | --- | --- | --- |
| Number of patients | 78 | 471 | 62 | 60 |
| dRTA | 18 (33%) | 12 (2.5%) | 7 (11%) | 3 (5%) |
| NDI | NR | 12 (2.5%) | 13 (21%) | 13/48 (27%) |
| Urolithiasis | 2 (2.5%) | 4 (0.8%) | 5 (8%) | 2 (3.3%) |
| Proteinuria | 34 (43%) | 10 (2.1%) | 1 (1.6%) | 12 (20%) |
| Hematuria | 13 (17%) | 7 (1.5%) | NR | 5 (8.3%) |
| Renal insufficiency | 9 (11.5%) | 5 (1%) | 13 (21%) | 8 (13.3%) |
| Renal biopsy | 3 | 18 | 1 | 9 |
| IN | 1 | 9 | 1 | 6 |
| GN | 2 | 8 | 0 | 1 |
| IN + GN | 0 | 1 | 0 | 2 |

*Abbreviations*: NDI, nephrogenic diabetes insipidus; NR, not reported; IN, interstitial nephritis; GN, glomerulonephritis.

## 2. Interstitial nephritis

The commonest form of renal involvement in pSS is interstitial nephritis presenting as overt or latent distal RTA, defects in urine concentrating ability (nephrogenic diabetes insipidus, NDI), nephrocalcinosis, and urolithiasis. Reports on renal tubular defects in patients with SS date back to the 1960s, when Kahn et al. (1962) reported renal concentrating defects in four patients with SS. Shearn and Tu (1965) described a patient with NDI which preceded SS, and Tu et al. (1968) reported interstitial nephritis in SS. There was also a report of RTA in patients with hyperglobulinemia but not clinically apparent SS (McCurdy et al., 1967). RTA, either latent or overt, was reported in small studies by Shearn and Tu (Shearn and Tu, 1968), Talal (Talal et al., 1968), and Shioji (Ren et al., 2001). However, the earliest report of renal involvement in SS in a significant number of patients was that of Bloch, who retrospectively studied 62 patients (Bloch et al., 1965). In this study transient or persistent hyposthenuria was detected in 16% of patients. However, as mentioned, only 23 of these patients would have been classified as pSS with the current classification (Vitali et al., 1993).

Other manifestations of interstitial disease, such as Type 2 or proximal RTA or Fanconi syndrome, have only occasionally been reported in patients with pSS (Bridoux et al., 2004), while there are reports of hypokalemia without dRTA in patients with pSS (Poux et al., 1992; Wrong et al., 1993).

### 2.1. Pathology and pathogenesis

Primary SS shows the histopathological characteristics of chronic tubulo-interstitial nephritis (Fig. 1). The interstitium is infiltrated focally or diffusely by small lymphocytes, plasma cells, and monocytes. A variable degree of tubular atrophy as well as interstitial fibrosis can be observed (Bossini et al., 2001).

The histopathological features of interstitial nephritis in pSS are not specific. Enestrom et al. (1995) have used a semiquantitative approach to analyze the kidney biopsies of 10 patients with pSS. In that report, interstitial inflammation was focal in 80% of patients. Unlike infection or drug-induced tubulo-interstitial nephritis, no eosinophils, neutrophils or lymphocytes were found in the interstitium. Interstitial fibrosis was found in 60% of patients, in the majority mild, and correlated with the degree of interstitial inflammation. Tubular atrophy was found in 80% of cases and it was slight or moderate.

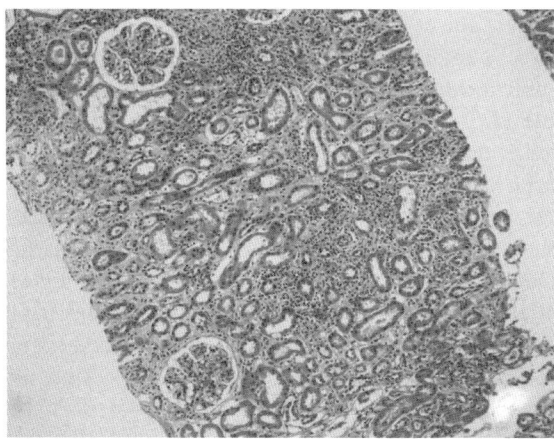

Figure 1. Tubulointerstitial nephritis. The interstitium is expanded by edema, focal fibrosis, and dense inflammatory infiltrates of mononuclear leukocytes and plasma cells (H&E stain, 200×).

The pathogenesis of interstitial nephritis in pSS is not clear. Several studies have looked at different pathogenetic aspects, including the nature of the infiltrating lymphocytes, hyperglobulinemia, autoantibodies against carbonic anhydrase II, and defects in the H-ATPase pump in the renal tubules. There are relatively few studies on the nature of the cells infiltrating the renal interstitium of patients with pSS. The earliest report was by Rosenberg et al. (1988) who found, using indirect immunofluorescence, that the infiltrating cells were predominantly helper/inducer T-cells, although nodules of B-cells were also identified. At the same time, Matsumura et al. (1988) reported that 66% of the infiltrating cells were CD5 positive T lymphocytes, while B-cells (CD19 positive) and monocytes (CD15 positive) constituted the rest of the cells. However, he identified T-cells as cytotoxic (CD8 positive) T-cells, rather than helper/inducer (CD4 positive) T-cells.

Murata et al. compared the TCR repertoire of T-cells infiltrating the kidney, with that of T-cells infiltrating the salivary glands and peripheral blood T lymphocytes. They found the TCR V$\beta$ gene repertoire to be more restricted in T-cells infiltrating kidneys of pSS patients, suggesting that these cells might recognize a different autoantigen than T-cells infiltrating labial salivary glands (Murata et al., 1995; Skopouli et al., 1991). Matsumura et al. also investigated the expression of adhesion and co-stimulatory molecules, as well as that of Fas–Fas ligand, in the kidneys of patients with pSS and interstitial nephritis. ICAM-1 was observed in and around interstitial inflammatory foci, while E-selectin and VCAM-1 were found in vessels with large cellular infiltrates (Matsumura et al., 1998b). Comparison of the expression of these molecules in salivary glands and kidneys suggests that the same inflammatory process operates in both tissues (Matsumura et al., 1988, 1998b). The co-stimulatory molecules CD80 (B7.1) and CD86 (B7.2) are aberrantly expressed on ductal epithelial cells of the salivary glands of patients with pSS (Manoussakis et al., 1999; Matsumura et al., 2001), while only CD86 is expressed in tubular epithelial cells (Matsumura et al., 2001). Whether this molecule is able to provide co-stimulation to T lymphocytes infiltrating the kidney, as occurs in the minor salivary glands (Manoussakis et al., 1999), remains to be investigated. Finally, a role for Fas–Fas ligand interactions in the pathogenesis of interstitial nephritis in pSS has been suggested, based on the expression of Fas by tubular epithelial cells and of Fas ligand by some of the infiltrating cells (Matsumura et al., 1998a).

Hyperglobulinemia has been historically associated with interstitial nephritis in patients with pSS. Talal et al. (1968) reported that patients with SS and RTA had higher levels of $\gamma$-globulins than patients with SS but without RTA; even a causative role of hyperglobulinemia has been proposed (Morris and Fudenberg, 1967). Subsequent studies failed to establish a pathogenetic role for hyperglobulinemia per se, as they gave conflicting results (Bossini et al., 2001; Pertovaara et al., 2001; Shioji et al., 1970; Skopouli, 2001). Pasternack et al. (1970) have showed that dRTA is absent in patients with rheumatoid arthritis and hyperglobulinemia.

Recently Takemoto et al. studied the association of antibodies against carbonic anhydrase II and renal disease in patients with pSS. Patients with pSS and dRTA had significantly elevated serum levels in comparison to patients with pSS without dRTA. It was noted that patients with pSS as a whole had significantly higher levels of antibodies against carbonic anhydrase II in comparison with normal controls (Takemoto et al., 2005). The authors suggested that these autoantibodies might be pathogenic. In fact an in vitro study has shown that antibodies against carbonic anhydrase I and II inhibit the catalytic activity of the enzyme, possibly in an isotype-specific manner (Botre et al., 2003). Supporting the pathogenetic role of antibodies against carbonic anhydrase is a study in which immunization of PL/J mice with carbonic anhydrase II induced autoimmune sialadenitis in association with the presence of serum antibodies against carbonic anhydrase II (Nishimori et al., 1995). Sialadenitis was induced in mice with specific H-2 halpotypes (H-$2^s$ and H-$2^u$). Based on these results the authors have speculated that carbonic anhydrase II might be one of the autoantigens in human SS (Nishimori et al., 1995).

Finally, another possible pathogenetic mechanism might be absence of the H-ATPase from tubular intercalated cells in patients with pSS, leading to defective tubular proton secretion and finally dRTA. At present, however, there are case reports of those patients in which immunohistochemistry showed absence of H-ATPase from the renal tubules (Bastani et al., 1995; Cohen et al., 1992).

## 2.2. Clinical presentation

There are few studies on the natural history of renal involvement in pSS. However, it seems that interstitial nephritis presents early in the disease process and only occasionally is a cause of renal insufficiency (Moutsopoulos et al., 1991; Rayadurg and Koch, 1990; Skopouli, 2001). Skopouli et al., in a study on the clinical evolution of 291 pSS patients, reported interstitial nephritis in 7% at diagnosis and in 9% after a mean followup of 3.6 years. Patients without systemic manifestations such as Raynaud's phenomenon, arthritis, liver involvement, and interstitial nephritis, at diagnosis were unlikely to develop these manifestations during followup (Skopouli et al., 2000). Kelly et al., in a cohort of 100 patients, found dRTA in three patients after a follow-up period of 34 months. However, all three patients had decreased serum bicarbonate at baseline (Kelly et al., 1991). In another study, Kruize et al. (1996) did not find any new clinically evident cases of renal involvement in a cohort of 21 patients with pSS after a median followup of 11 years.

### 2.2.1. Renal tubular acidosis

The prevalence of overt or latent dRTA ranges from 12% (Viergever and Swaak, 1991) to 67% (Eriksson et al., 1995), although most studies report dRTA in 26–35% of patients (Pavlidis et al., 1982; Shiozawa et al., 1987). It is noted, however, that the most recent and large studies have reported overt dRTA in only 2–6% of patients (Aasarod et al., 2000; Bossini et al., 2001; Goules et al., 2000; Pertovaara et al., 1999). On the other hand, SS is among the common causes of dRTA in adults (Caruana and Buckalew, 1988; Rodriguez, 2002). dRTA can be the presenting manifestation of SS; therefore, one should exclude pSS before labeling a case of dRTA as idiopathic (Rose, 2005a).

In almost all studies overt or complete dRTA is defined as the presence of an otherwise unexplained normal anion gap metabolic acidosis in association with inability to maximally lower urine pH ($<5.5$) in the face of acidemia (Rodriguez, 2002). The term latent or incomplete dRTA is applied to patients with impaired ability to excrete acid load but still able to maintain normal blood bicarbonate levels. Incomplete dRTA is usually detected by the oral acid load test with ammonium chloride (Buckalew et al., 1968; Rose, 2005a).

Although most studies do not report a plasma bicarbonate level in patients with dRTA, metabolic acidosis in dRTA is usually mild, with bicarbonate levels usually over 10 meq/l (Rose, 2005c). Aasarod et al. (2000) reported seven patients with dRTA who had base deficits ranging from 4.9 to 8.0 meq/l. More recently Takemoto et al. (2005) reported that patients with either complete or incomplete dRTA had mean serum bicarbonate levels of $21.5 \pm 0.8$ meq/l. Eriksson et al. (1996b) found that in patients with pSS, dRTA is associated with reduced glomerular filtration rate measured by $^{51}$Cr-EDTA. These patients also had histological evidence of interstitial nephritis.

### 2.2.2. Nephrocalcinosis and urolithiasis

Nephrocalcinosis is a recognized complication of dRTA (Buckalew, 1989) and occurs in almost 30% of patients according to an early study (Brenner et al., 1982). Moutsopoulos et al. described five patients with pSS and dRTA who subsequently developed nephrocalcinosis, urinary calculi, and renal insufficiency. On the other hand, Eriksson et al. (1996a) have described patients with pSS who presented with urolithiasis and dRTA. However, there are no data from cohort studies on the frequency of nephrocalcinosis in patients with pSS.

Urinary calculi can be the presenting manifestation of renal involvement in pSS and, in some cases, their presence antedates the development of Sicca symptoms (Eriksson et al., 1996a). The frequency of urinary calculi in pSS ranges from $<1$ to 8% (Aasarod et al., 2000; Goules et al., 2000; Pertovaara et al., 1999). Eriksson et al. (1995) reported that 11/27 patients with pSS had urolithiasis, but as has already been mentioned, selection bias is a major limitation to this study.

The formation of urinary calculi is attributed to dRTA, through multiple mechanisms (Buckalew, 1989). The primary event is acidemia, which increases calcium phosphate release from bone and decreases tubular resorption, leading to hypercalciuria. Another factor is high urinary pH, which favors calcium phosphate precipitation. Finally, hypocitraturia contributes to urolithiasis because urinary citrate inhibits calculi formation by solubilizing calcium phosphate and by inhibiting agglomeration of calcium crystals (Rose, 2005b). Eriksson et al. (1995) and Aasarod et al. (2000) documented hypocitraturia in 18/27 (74%) and 16/62 (25.8%) of their pSS patients, respectively.

## 2.2.3. Osteomalacia

Osteomalacia is a complication of proximal RTA (Brenner et al., 1982), while pSS is usually accompanied by dRTA. However, there are case reports of patients with pSS and osteomalacia. Some of these patients had dRTA (Diaz et al., 2004; Hajjaj-Hassouni et al., 1995; Okada et al., 2001), while others had evidence of proximal tubule dysfunction (Monte Neto et al., 1991). Patients with pSS without dRTA lack biochemical evidence of osteomalacia (Fulop and Mackay, 2004).

## 2.2.4. Nephrogenic diabetes insipidus

NDI presents with polyuria and polydipsia. It can be the presenting manifestation of pSS (Shearn and Tu, 1965), although pSS is an uncommon cause of NDI (Sasaki, 2004). Nonetheless, pSS should be excluded in patients with NDI who do not have the commonest causes of this syndrome, that is chronic lithium therapy and hypercalcemia.

NDI in pSS is usually mild and not clinically apparent. It is found in 21–48% of patients (Aasarod et al., 2000; Bossini et al., 2001; Eriksson et al., 1995). These studies have documented NDI using the water deprivation test or intranasal challenge with 1-desamino-8-d-arginine vasopressin; however, not all patients with low morning urine osmolality underwent the above tests (Bossini et al., 2001). Interestingly, maximal urine osmolality correlated with glomerular filtration rate and was lowest in patients with complete dRTA (Eriksson et al., 1995).

## 2.2.5. Hypokalemia

Although there are meticulous studies reporting several biochemical markers in patients with pSS and renal involvement, very few provide data on the potassium status of these patients. Among the major studies, only Bossini et al. (2001) reported that 7% of their patients had hypokalemia, while only 5% had complete dRTA. Takemoto et al. (2005), in a recent, study reported that potassium levels in patients with pSS and dRTA were $3.65 \pm 0.19$ meq/l. An unusual manifestation of pSS is hypokalemic periodic paralysis which can be the presenting symptom (al-Jubouri et al., 1999; Poux et al., 1992; Siamopoulos et al., 1994).

## 3. Glomerulonephritis

Glomerulonephritis in association with pSS was initially reported by Talal et al. (1968), while a more systematic approach was adopted by Moutsopoulos et al. who reported immune-complex glomerulonephritis in three patients with pSS. Glomerular involvement is rare in pSS; however, the exact prevalence is difficult to estimate. One reason is that the literature mainly consists of case reports, and most cohort studies of renal involvement in pSS include <10 patients with glomerulonephritis. An additional problem in studying glomerulonephritis is that in most patients with pSS and suspected renal involvement, the clinical manifestations are so mild that a kidney biopsy is not indicated. Indeed in the study by Goules et al. (2000) only 20 of 471 patients with pSS had clinically significant renal involvement; renal biopsy was performed in 18 and glomerulonephritis was found in 8, while 1 patient had both interstitial nephritis and glomerulonephritis.

In other cohort studies the number of renal biopsies in pSS is even smaller: Bossini et al. (2001) performed renal biopsy in 9/60 patients, Pertovaara et al. (1999) in 3/78, Aasarod et al. (2000) in 1/62, Eriksson et al. (1995) in 13/27, and Pavlidis et al. (1982) in 10/47. Histological findings of glomerulonephritis were found, respectively, in one, two, none, one, and three of the patients. It is noted that Bossini et al. (2001) found two patients and Pavlidis et al. found one patient with both interstitial nephritis and glomerulonephritis. In a follow-up study of patients with pSS, glomerulonephritis was found in only 1 patient of 265 at the time of diagnosis, but it had developed in 6 patients after a median followup of 3.6 years (Skopouli et al., 2000).

It is obvious from the above discussion that although glomerulonephritis is rare in pSS, the percentage of patients with glomerulonephritis among those who underwent renal biopsy, that is patients with clinically significant disease, ranges from approximately 10–45% (Bossini et al., 2001; Goules et al., 2000; Pavlidis et al., 1982).

## 3.1. Pathology and pathogenesis

The common histopathological forms are membranoproliferative (Cortez et al., 1995; Khan et al., 1988; Schlesinger et al., 1989) and membranous glomerulonephritis (Dabadghao et al., 1995; Yoshida et al., 1996), while there are reports of crescentic glomerulonephritis as well (Dabadghao et al., 1995; Dussol et al., 1994; Ghannouchi et al., 2006; Tatsumi et al., 1998, 2000). Goules et al. (2000) reported five patients with membranoproliferative glomerulonephritis, three of whom had IgM and C3 deposition, and four patients with mesangial proliferative glomerulonephritis (Fig. 2). Deposits of IgM and C3 were a common finding in six patients with glomerulonephritis reported by Skopouli et al. (2000). Dussol et al. (1994) reviewed 20 reported cases of GN; there were 10 patients with membranoproliferative and 6 with membranous glomerulonephritis while in 4 patients the type of glomerulonephritis was not specified. Tatsumi et al. (1998) quotes data published by Fujimoto and Dohi in a book chapter in Japanese (Fujimoto and Dohi, 1996). The authors studied glomerular histology in 109 patients with pSS. Glomeruli were normal in 43%; non-specific mesangial increase was found in 51%, thickening of the glomerular tuft in 2%, membranous glomerulonephritis in 3%, and IgA glomerulonephritis in 2% (Fujimoto and Dohi, 1996). Enestrom et al. (1995) noted glomerular sclerotic lesions in 5 of 10 renal biopsies from patients with pSS. They also noted small amounts of immune deposits, mainly IgM and C3, which were restricted to mesangium. No proliferative lesions were found in any of the patients.

The pathogenesis of glomerulonephritis in pSS most probably involves deposition of immune complexes. Moutsopoulos et al. (1978), in an early study, found circulating immune complexes in three patients with glomerulonephritis. The presence of immune deposits of IgM and C3 in the glomeruli has already been mentioned. On the other hand, the presence of glomerulonephritis has been associated with cryoglobulinemia. Dussol et al. (1994), reviewing the literature, found that cryoglobulins had been detected in 6/13 patients with glomerulonephritis and pSS. Similarly, Goules et al. (2000) established that the presence of mixed monoclonal cryoglobulinemia increased the odds of the biopsy diagnosis being glomerulonephritis, rather than interstitial nephritis, by 16-fold. It was suggested that glomerulonephritis was caused by the deposition of immune complexes consisting of IgMκ rheumatoid factor along with polyclonal IgG and IgA, similar to the glomerulonephritis of hepatitis C-associated mixed monoclonal cryoglobulinemia (Daghestani and Pomeroy, 1999; Goules et al., 2000).

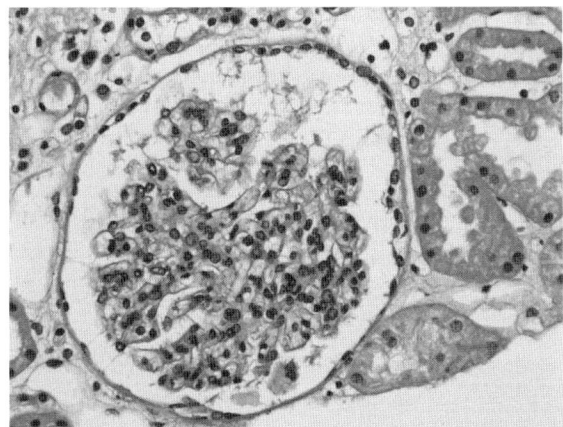

**Figure 2.** Mesangioproliferative glomerulonephritis. Mild segmental mesangial hypercellularity. The glomerular basement membranes appear normal (H&E stain, 400 ×).

## 3.2. Clinical presentation

In contrast to interstitial nephritis, glomerulonephritis is a relatively late manifestation of pSS. Skopouli et al. (2000), using Kaplan–Meier curves, showed that the estimated 5-year rate for glomerulonephritis was 2.3%. Clinical manifestations are not specific to pSS and include hypertension, proteinuria, and hematuria or impaired renal function. Goules et al. (2000) reported that 3/8 patients with glomerulonephritis had significantly increased serum creatinine (4.6–6.2 mg/dl) and two of them developed end-stage chronic renal failure necessitating hemodialysis. His review of the literature found only 3/9 patients with a creatinine clearance <50 ml/min and in two of these clearance increased to 50 ml/min after treatment. Thus, the prognosis of glomerulonephritis in pSS is not as benign as that of interstitial nephritis, as at least some patients may develop end-stage renal failure. In addition, the prognosis of patients with glomerulonephritis is aggravated due to the development of lymphoproliferative disorders (Goules et al., 2000).

When a patient with apparent pSS develops glomerulonephritis, it is important to rule out SLE, the presence of an overlap syndrome, and drug-induced glomerulonephritis (most frequently by non-steroidal anti-inflammatory drugs). This is especially true for membranous glomerulonephritis. Patients should be thoroughly re-evaluated, including full serological testing, and the pathologist should focus on immunofluorescence studies; glomerulonephritis associated with pSS reveals IgM and C3 deposits, while lupus nephritis is characterized by predominant IgG along with IgA, IgM, C3, C4, and C1q deposits. This so-called "full-house" immunofluorescence is found in a quarter of patients with lupus nephritis, but almost never in other forms of glomerulonephritis (Cameron, 1999).

## 4. Predictors of renal involvement and associations with other characteristics of pSS

As renal involvement in pSS is generally asymptomatic, investigators have looked for factors associated with or predictive for renal involvement (Table 2). Unfortunately, most studies are small and retrospective and were not specifically designed to investigate renal disease. Even studies with large number of patients have only a few with renal involvement (Goules et al., 2000). Hence, different studies report discrepant and sometimes contradictory results.

Bossini et al. (2001) compared several characteristics in a cohort of 60 patients with and without renal involvement. They found that the only significant differences were that patients with renal involvement were younger and had shorter disease duration. Factors such as clinical characteristics (arthralgia, Raynaud's phenomenon, vasculitis, neuropathy, and interstitial lung disease) or laboratory findings (cryoglobulinemia, hyperglobulinemia, rheumatoid factor, and anti-Ro and anti-La antibodies) did not differ significantly in the two groups (Bossini et al., 2001).

Pertovaara et al. (1999) compared patients with and without dRTA in their cohort of pSS patients. They found that patients with dRTA had longer disease duration, longer duration of xerostomia, and higher serum creatinine levels. In addition, they were more likely to be hypertensive and to have proteinuria. However, when these variables were entered in a logistic regression model, dRTA was associated with the presence of hypertension, proteinuria, and duration of xerostomia. Notably serum creatinine, age of the patient, or duration of disease did not seem to be associated with dRTA (Pertovaara et al., 1999). In the same study patients were divided into those with and without proteinuria. Univariate analysis revealed significant

Table 2
Association of renal involvement with other characteristics of pSS in various studies

| Study | Pertovaara et al. (2001) | Aasarod et al. (2000) | Skopouli et al. (2000) | Bossini et al. (2001) |
|---|---|---|---|---|
| Age | Yes | No | No | Yes |
| Disease duration | Yes | No | No | Yes |
| Salivary gland histology | No | Yes | NR | NR |
| Hypertension | Yes | NR | No | No |
| Anti-Ro/La | NR | Yes | No | No |
| Low C4 | NR | NR | Yes | No |
| Cryoglobulinemia | NR | NR | Yes | No |
| Hyperglobulinemia | Yes | No | No | No |
| Serum $\beta$2-microglobulin | Yes | NR | NR | NR |

*Abbreviation*: NR, not reported.

associations between proteinuria and systolic and diastolic blood pressures, duration of xerostomia, and increased serum $\beta2$ microglobulin ($\beta2m$). Logistic regression however showed that only duration of xerostomia and diastolic blood pressure were independently associated with proteinuria. Finally, it is important to note that there was also a significant association between the presence of proteinuria and dRTA (Pertovaara et al., 1999).

In a subsequent study on apparently the same cohort of patients, Pertovaara et al. (2001) focused exclusively on the factors predicting renal involvement in pSS. They studied different parameters of renal involvement at a time point at which the mean disease duration of their patient cohort was $9\pm4$ years, and they subsequently compared the baseline characteristics of their patients obtained from medical records. They reported that patients who subsequently developed dRTA had higher baseline levels of serum total $\gamma$-globulins and $\beta2m$. The association of increased serum levels of $\beta2$-m with dRTA has also been reported by Michalski et al. (1975). Serum $\beta2m$ levels were also associated with the development of proteinuria but the statistical significance of the association was marginal (Pertovaara et al., 2001). A possible explanation for the role of $\beta2m$ is that it is a marker of "active lymphoproliferation", which Pertovaara et al. (2001) consider as a hallmark of extraglandular manifestations in pSS.

In contrast, Aasarod et al. (2000) failed to confirm any of the above associations. Instead they found that patients with dRTA were significantly more likely to test positive for anti-Ro or anti-La, and that they had a higher number of inflammatory foci in labial salivary gland biopsies, a finding which was not present in a previous study (Pertovaara et al., 2001).

Skopouli et al. (2000) analyzed clinical evolution of pSS and they found that there was a strong association between glomerulonephritis and lymphoma development in the same patient, with a relative risk of 12.1 ($p=0.015$ by Fisher's exact test). Moreover, glomerulonephritis was strongly associated with peripheral neuropathy. Using Cox regression analysis of outcomes the authors established that purpura (in particular palpable purpura), low levels of C4, and mixed monoclonal cryoglobulinemia were significant predictors for the development of glomerulonephritis. It is noted that these variables were also predictors of lymphoma development (Skopouli et al., 2000).

In a large study, Goules took a different approach, comparing patients with interstitial nephritis to those with glomerulonephritis (Table 3). Patients with interstitial nephritis were younger and had shorter disease duration, as compared to patients with pSS and glomerulonephritis (Goules et al., 2000). Extraglandular manifestations as well as laboratory tests such as ANA, rheumatoid factor, complement, and anti-Ro and anti-La antibodies did not differ significantly between the groups. The association of glomerulonephritis with cryoglobulinemia and age remained significant in a multivariate regression model (Goules et al., 2000).

**Table 3**
Comparison of interstitial nephritis and glomerulonephritis in patients with pSS

| | Interstitial nephritis | Glomerulonephritis |
|---|---|---|
| Frequency | Common | Rare |
| Age of patients (years) | $36.8\pm11.9$ | $46\pm7.1^*$ |
| Years after onset | $2.2\pm3.3$ | $8.0\pm5.5^*$ |
| Prognosis | Benign | Unfavorable |
| Renal failure | Uncommon | Common |
| Raynaud phenomenon | 60% | 50% |
| Arthralgia/arthritis | 70% | 70% |
| Purpura | 30% | 30% |
| Lymphoma | 0% | 40% |
| Peripheral neuropathy | 0% | 20% |
| ANA | 100% | 100% |
| Anti-Ro | 80% | 70% |
| Anti-La | 50% | 50% |
| Low C3 | 0% | 20% |
| Low C4 | 30% | 50% |
| Cryoglobulins | 20% | 80%* |

Source: Modified from Goules et al. (2000).
$^*p<0.05$.

## 5. Treatment

No controlled studies exist on the treatment of the different forms of renal involvement in pSS. In patients with dRTA, the recommended treatment is oral alkali supplementation in the form of bicarbonate or citrate. Either sodium or potassium salts can be used. The target of therapy is normalization of plasma bicarbonate concentration. The usual alkali requirement in adults is 1–2 meq/kg daily. An additional aim of therapy should be correction of hypercalciuria and hypocitraturia, therefore it is prudent to monitor the urinary calcium to creatinine ratio or citrate to creatinine ratio, in order to adjust alkali supplementation. Appropriate alkali supplementation will prevent nephrocalcinosis, urolithiasis, and chronic renal insufficiency (Rodriguez, 2002). Patients with NDI due to pSS do not usually need treatment as the urine concentrating defect is mild. In patients with interstitial nephritis a course of corticosteroids might be of benefit, especially if plasma creatinine is elevated (Tu et al., 1968). Other forms of treatment have been used only when there was a concomitant problem, for example plasmapheresis and intravenous pulses of cyclophosphamide for cryoglobulinemia (Goules et al., 2000).

In patients with pSS and glomerulonephritis, various forms of treatment have been used, including the combination of corticosteroids with intravenous pulse cyclophosphamide (Goules et al., 2000; Khan et al., 1988), corticosteroids alone (Dussol et al., 1994; Ghannouchi et al., 2006; Moutsopoulos et al., 1978), methylprednisolone with azathioprine, (Goules et al., 2000), and plasmapheresis (Tatsumi et al., 1998). However the number of patients treated is small and no conclusions can be drawn about the effectiveness of each form of treatment.

## 6. Conclusions

Two major forms of renal involvement have been described in patients with pSS: interstitial nephritis and glomerulonephritis.

Interstitial nephritis presents as dRTA, nephrocalcinosis and urolithiasis, NDI and, in rare cases, as proximal RTA (Fanconi syndrome) or hypokalemia. Interstitial nephritis generally occurs early in young patients and in many cases is asymptomatic and has a benign prognosis. Histopathologically the renal interstitium is infiltrated by lymphocytes, which bear many similarities with those infiltrating the salivary glands.

Glomerulonephritis, on the other hand, is relatively rare and occurs late in the disease; its prognosis is not as benign as that of interstitial nephritis, as it can lead to significant loss of renal function. The histopathological forms include membranoproliferative, mesangial proliferative, and membranous glomerulonephritis. Glomerulonephritis is probably immune complex-mediated and the presence of cryoglobulins seems to play a central role. Of importance is the association of glomerulonephritis with the presence of lymphoma, a fact that worsens prognosis in these patients.

**Key points**

- Renal involvement in pSS is relatively frequent ranging from 2 to 67% in different studies.
- The most common form of renal involvement is interstitial nephritis manifesting as dRTA and NDI, and less frequently as nephrocalcinosis, urolithiasis, and hypokalemia.
- Interstitial nephritis occurs in younger patients, relatively early in the disease course, and has generally benign prognosis. It rarely leads to renal failure.
- Intestitial nephritis is characterized by a lymphocytic infiltrate very similar to that of salivary glands.
- Treatment of interstitial nephritis in usually symptomatic.
- Glomerulonephritis is rare in pSS.
- Glomerulonephritis occurs late in the disease course and may lead to renal failure. It is associated with lymphoproliferative disorders.
- Membranoproliferative and membranous glomerulonephritis are the commonest histological types of glomerulonephritis in pSS.
- Glomerulonephritis in pSS is treated by cyclophosphamide and/or corticosteroids.

## Acknowledgments

We thank Professor Lydia Nakopoulou (University of Athens Medical School, Department of Pathology) for providing the kidney histopathology figures.

## References

Aasarod, K., Haga, H.J., Berg, K.J., et al. 2000. Renal involvement in primary Sjogren's syndrome. QJM 93, 297.

al-Jubouri, M.A., Jones, S., Macmillan, R., et al. 1999. Hypokalaemic paralysis revealing Sjogren syndrome in an elderly man. J. Clin. Pathol. 52, 157.

Bastani, B., Haragsim, L., Gluck, S., et al. 1995. Lack of H-ATPase in distal nephron causing hypokalaemic distal RTA in a patient with Sjogren's syndrome. Nephrol. Dial. Transplant. 10, 908.

Bloch, K.J., Buchanan, W.W., Wohl, M.J., et al. 1965. Sjogren's syndrome. A clinical, pathological, and serological study of sixty-two cases. Medicine (Baltimore) 44, 187.

Bossini, N., Savoldi, S., Franceschini, F., et al. 2001. Clinical and morphological features of kidney involvement in primary Sjogren's syndrome. Nephrol. Dial. Transplant. 16, 2328.

Botre, F., Botre, C., Podesta, E., et al. 2003. Effect of anticarbonic anhydrase antibodies on carbonic anhydrases I and II. Clin. Chem. 49, 1221.

Brenner, R.J., Spring, D.B., Sebastian, A., et al. 1982. Incidence of radiographically evident bone disease, nephrocalcinosis, and nephrolithiasis in various types of renal tubular acidosis. N. Engl. J. Med. 307, 217.

Bridoux, F., Kyndt, X., bou-Ayache, R., et al. 2004. Proximal tubular dysfunction in primary Sjogren's syndrome: a clinicopathological study of 2 cases. Clin. Nephrol. 61, 434.

Buckalew, V.M. Jr. 1989. Nephrolithiasis in renal tubular acidosis. J. Urol. 141, 731.

Buckalew, V.M., Jr., McCurdy, D.K., Ludwig, G.D., et al. 1968. Incomplete renal tubular acidosis. Physiologic studies in three patients with a defect in lowering urine pH. Am. J. Med. 45, 32.

Cameron, S.J. 1999. Lupus nephritis. J. Am. Soc. Nephrol. 10, 413.

Caruana, R.J., Buckalew, V.M. Jr. 1988. The syndrome of distal (type 1) renal tubular acidosis. Clinical and laboratory findings in 58 cases. Medicine (Baltimore) 67, 84.

Cohen, E.P., Bastani, B., Cohen, M.R., et al. 1992. Absence of H(+)-ATPase in cortical collecting tubules of a patient with Sjogren's syndrome and distal renal tubular acidosis. J. Am. Soc. Nephrol. 3, 264.

Cortez, M.S., Sturgill, B.C., Bolton, W.K. 1995. Membranoproliferative glomerulonephritis with primary Sjogren's syndrome. Am. J. Kidney Dis. 25, 632.

Dabadghao, S., Aggarwal, A., Arora, P., et al. 1995. Glomerulonephritis leading to end stage renal disease in a patient with primary Sjogren syndrome. Clin. Exp. Rheumatol. 13, 509.

Daghestani, L., Pomeroy, C. 1999. Renal manifestations of hepatitis C infection. Am. J. Med. 106, 347.

Daniels, T.E., Talal, N. 1987. Diagnosis and differential diagnosis in Sjogren's syndrome. In: N. Talal, H.M. Moutsopoulos, S.S. Kassan (Eds.), Sjogren's Syndrome: Clinical and Immunological Aspects. Springer Verlag, Berlin, p. 193.

Diaz, R.C., Gonzalez, R.C., Trinidad San Jose, J.C., et al. 2004. Osteal complications as first manifestation in a patient with primary Sjogren's Syndrome and with associated distal tubular acidosis (type 1) and chronic renal insufficiency. Ther. Apher. Dial. 8, 160.

Dussol, B., Tsimaratos, M., Bolla, G., et al. 1994. Crescentic glomerulonephritis and primary Gougerot–Sjogren syndrome. [Article in French.]. Nephrologie 15, 295.

Enestrom, S., Denneberg, T., Eriksson, P. 1995. Histopathology of renal biopsies with correlation to clinical findings in primary Sjogren's syndrome. Clin. Exp. Rheumatol. 13, 697.

Eriksson, P., Denneberg, T., Enestrom, S., et al. 1996a. Urolithiasis and distal renal tubular acidosis preceding primary Sjogren's syndrome: a retrospective study 5–53 years after the presentation of urolithiasis. J. Intern. Med. 239, 483.

Eriksson, P., Denneberg, T., Granerus, G., et al. 1996b. Glomerular filtration rate in primary Sjogren's syndrome with renal disease. Scand. J. Urol. Nephrol. 30, 121.

Eriksson, P., Denneberg, T., Larsson, L., et al. 1995. Biochemical markers of renal disease in primary Sjogren's syndrome. Scand. J. Urol. Nephrol. 29, 383.

Fujimoto, T., Dohi, K. 1996. Renal involvement. In: K. Dohi (Ed.), Clinical Aspects of Sjogren's Syndrome. [Book in Japanese.]. Nankodo, Tokyo, p. 112.

Fulop, M., Mackay, M. 2004. Renal tubular acidosis, Sjogren syndrome, and bone disease. Arch. Intern. Med. 164, 905.

Ghannouchi, M., Bouajina, E., Zeglaoui, H., et al. 2006. Segmental and focal glomerulonephritis in the course of primitive Gougerot–Sjogren syndrome. [Article in French.]. Rev. Med. Intern. 27, 156.

Goules, A., Masouridi, S., Tzioufas, A.G., et al. 2000. Clinically significant and biopsy-documented renal involvement in primary Sjogren syndrome. Medicine (Baltimore) 79, 241.

Hajjaj-Hassouni, N., Guedira, N., Lazrak, N., et al. 1995. Osteomalacia as a presenting manifestation of Sjogren's syndrome. Rev. Rhum. Engl. Ed. 62, 529.

Kahn, M., Merritt, A.D., Wohl, M.J., et al. 1962. Renal concentrating defect in Sjogren's syndrome. Ann. Intern. Med. 56, 883.

Kassan, S.S., Moutsopoulos, H.M. 2004. Clinical manifestations and early diagnosis of Sjogren syndrome. Arch. Intern. Med. 164, 1275.

Kelly, C.A., Foster, H., Pal, B., et al. 1991. Primary Sjogren's syndrome in north east England—a longitudinal study. Br. J. Rheumatol. 30, 437.

Khan, M.A., Akhtar, M., Taher, S.M. 1988. Membranoproliferative glomerulonephritis in a patient with primary Sjogren's syndrome. Report of a case with review of the literature. Am. J. Nephrol. 8, 235.

Kruize, A.A., Hene, R.J., van der, H.A., et al. 1996. Long-term followup of patients with Sjogren's syndrome. Arthritis Rheum. 39, 297.

Manoussakis, M.N., Dimitriou, I.D., Kapsogeorgou, E.K., et al. 1999. Expression of B7 costimulatory molecules by salivary gland epithelial cells in patients with Sjogren's syndrome. Arthritis Rheum. 42, 229.

Matsumura, R., Kondo, Y., Sugiyama, T., et al. 1988. Immunohistochemical identification of infiltrating mononuclear cells in tubulointerstitial nephritis associated with Sjogren's syndrome. Clin. Nephrol. 30, 335.

Matsumura, R., Umemiya, K., Goto, T., et al. 2001. Glandular and extraglandular expression of costimulatory molecules in patients with Sjogren's syndrome. Ann. Rheum. Dis. 60, 473.

Matsumura, R., Umemiya, K., Kagami, M., et al. 1998a. Glandular and extraglandular expression of the Fas–Fas ligand and apoptosis in patients with Sjogren's syndrome. Clin. Exp. Rheumatol. 16, 561.

Matsumura, R., Umemiya, K., Nakazawa, T., et al. 1998b. Expression of cell adhesion molecules in tubulointerstitial nephritis associated with Sjogren's syndrome. Clin. Nephrol. 49, 74.

McCurdy, D.K., Cornwell, G.G. III., DePratti, V.J. 1967. Hyperglobulinemic renal tubular acidosis. Report of two cases. Ann. Intern. Med. 67, 110.

Michalski, J., Daniels, T.E., Talal, N., et al. 1975. Beta-2 microglobulin and lymphocytic infiltration in Sjogren's syndrome. N. Engl. J. Med. 293, 1228.

Monte Neto, J.T., Sesso, R., Kirsztajn, G.M., et al. 1991. Osteomalacia secondary to renal tubular acidosis in a patient with primary Sjogren's syndrome. Clin. Exp. Rheumatol. 9, 625.

Morris, R., Fudenberg, H. 1967. Impaired renal acidification in patients with hypergammaglobulinemia. Medicine (Baltimore) 46, 57.

Moutsopoulos, H.M. 1994. Sjogren's syndrome: autoimmune epithelitis. Clin. Immunol. Immunopathol. 72, 162.

Moutsopoulos, H.M., Balow, J.E., Lawley, T.J., et al. 1978. Immune complex glomerulonephritis in Sicca syndrome. Am. J. Med. 64, 955.

Moutsopoulos, H.M., Cledes, J., Skopouli, F.N., et al. 1991. Nephrocalcinosis in Sjogren's syndrome: a late sequela of renal tubular acidosis. J. Intern. Med. 230, 187.

Murata, H., Kita, Y., Sakamoto, A., et al. 1995. Limited TCR repertoire of infiltrating T cells in the kidneys of Sjogren's syndrome patients with interstitial nephritis. J. Immunol. 155, 4084.

Nishimori, I., Bratanova, T., Toshkov, I., et al. 1995. Induction of experimental autoimmune sialoadenitis by immunization of PL/J mice with carbonic anhydrase II. J. Immunol. 154, 4865.

Okada, M., Suzuki, K., Hidaka, T., et al. 2001. Rapid improvement of osteomalacia by treatment in a case with Sjogren's syndrome, rheumatoid arthritis and renal tubular acidosis type 1. Intern. Med. 40, 829.

Pasternack, A., Martio, J., Nissila, M., et al. 1970. Renal acidification and hypergammaglobulinemia. A study of rheumatoid arthritis. Acta Med. Scand. 187, 123.

Pavlidis, N.A., Karsh, J., Moutsopoulos, H.M. 1982. The clinical picture of primary Sjogren's syndrome: a retrospective study. J. Rheumatol. 9, 685.

Pertovaara, M., Korpela, M., Kouri, T., et al. 1999. The occurrence of renal involvement in primary Sjogren's syndrome: a study of 78 patients. Rheumatology (Oxford) 38, 1113.

Pertovaara, M., Korpela, M., Pasternack, A. 2001. Factors predictive of renal involvement in patients with primary Sjogren's syndrome. Clin. Nephrol. 56, 10.

Pokorny, G., Sonkodi, S., Ivanyi, B., et al. 1989. Renal involvement in patients with primary Sjogren's syndrome. Scand. J. Rheumatol. 18, 231.

Poux, J.M., Peyronnet, P., Le, M.Y., et al. 1992. Hypokalemic quadriplegia and respiratory arrest revealing primary Sjogren's syndrome. Clin. Nephrol. 37, 189.

Rayadurg, J., Koch, A.E. 1990. Renal insufficiency from interstitial nephritis in primary Sjogren's syndrome. J. Rheumatol. 17, 1714.

Ren, H., Chen, N., Chen, X., et al. 2001. Clinical and pathologic analysis of Sjogren's syndrome with renal impairment: a report of 84 cases. [Article in Chinese.]. Zhonghua Nei Ke Za Zhi 40, 367.

Rodriguez, S.J. 2002. Renal tubular acidosis: the clinical entity. J. Am. Soc. Nephrol. 13, 2160.

Rose, B.D. 2005a. Etiology and diagnosis of type 1 and type 2 renal tubular acidosis. In: B.D. Rose (Ed.), UpToDate. Waltham, MA.

Rose, B.D. 2005b. Nephrolithiasis in renal tubular acidosis. In: B.D. Rose (Ed.), UpToDate. Waltham, MA.

Rose, B.D. 2005c. Renal disease in Sjogren's syndrome. In: B.D. Rose (Ed.), UpToDate. Waltham, MA.

Rosenberg, M.E., Schendel, P.B., McCurdy, F.A., et al. 1988. Characterization of immune cells in kidneys from patients with Sjogren's syndrome. Am. J. Kidney Dis. 11, 20.

Sasaki, S. 2004. Nephrogenic diabetes insipidus: update of genetic and clinical aspects. Nephrol. Dial. Transplant. 19, 1351.

Schlesinger, I., Carlson, T.S., Nelson, D. 1989. Type III membranoproliferative glomerulonephritis in primary Sjogren's syndrome. Conn. Med. 53, 629.

Shearn, M.A., Tu, W.H. 1965. Nephrogenic diabetes insipidus and other defects of renal tubular function in Sjogren's syndrome. Am. J. Med. 39, 312–318.

Shearn, M.A., Tu, W.H. 1968. Latent renal tubular acidosis in Sjogren's syndrome. Ann. Rheum. Dis. 27, 27.

Shioji, R., Furuyama, T., Onodera, S., et al. 1970. Sjogren's syndrome and renal tubular acidosis. Am. J. Med. 48, 456.

Shiozawa, S., Shiozawa, K., Shimizu, S., et al. 1987. Clinical studies of renal disease in Sjogren's syndrome. Ann. Rheum. Dis. 46, 768.

Siamopoulos, K.C., Elisaf, M., Moutsopoulos, H.M. 1994. Hypokalaemic paralysis as the presenting manifestation of primary Sjogren's syndrome. Nephrol. Dial. Transplant. 9, 1176.

Siamopoulos, K.C., Mavridis, A.K., Elisaf, M., et al. 1986. Kidney involvement in primary Sjogren's syndrome. Scand. J. Rheumatol. (Suppl. 61), 156.

Skopouli, F.N. 2001. Kidney injury in Sjogren's syndrome. Nephrol. Dial. Transplant. 16 (Suppl. 6), 63.

Skopouli, F.N., Dafni, U., Ioannidis, J.P., et al. 2000. Clinical evolution, and morbidity and mortality of primary Sjogren's syndrome. Semin. Arthritis. Rheum. 29, 296.

Skopouli, F.N., Fox, P.C., Galanopoulou, V., et al. 1991. T cell subpopulations in the labial minor salivary gland histopathologic lesion of Sjogren's syndrome. J. Rheumatol. 18, 210.

Takemoto, F., Hoshino, J., Sawa, N., et al. 2005. Autoantibodies against carbonic anhydrase II are increased in renal tubular acidosis associated with Sjogren syndrome. Am. J. Med. 118, 181.

Talal, N., Zisman, E., Schur, P.H. 1968. Renal tubular acidosis, glomerulonephritis and immunologic factors in Sjogren's syndrome. Arthritis Rheum. 11, 774.

Tatsumi, H., Tateno, S., Hiki, Y., et al. 1998. Crescentic glomerulonephritis associated with membranous nephropathy in a case with primary Sjogren's syndrome. Nephrol. Dial. Transplant. 13, 2624.

Tatsumi, H., Tateno, S., Hiki, Y., et al. 2000. Crescentic glomerulonephritis and primary Sjogren's syndrome. Nephron. 86, 505.

Tu, W.H., Shearn, M.A., Lee, J.C., et al. 1968. Interstitial nephritis in Sjogren's syndrome. Ann. Intern. Med. 69, 1163.

Viergever, P.P., Swaak, T.J. 1991. Renal tubular dysfunction in primary Sjogren's syndrome: clinical studies in 27 patients. Clin. Rheumatol. 10, 23.

Vitali, C., Bombardieri, S., Moutsopoulos, H.M., et al. 1993. Preliminary criteria for the classification of Sjogren's syndrome. Results of a prospective concerted action supported by the European Community. Arthritis Rheum. 36, 340.

Vitali, C., Tavoni, A., Sciuto, M., et al. 1991. Renal involvement in primary Sjogren's syndrome: a retrospective-prospective study. Scand. J. Rheumatol. 20, 132.

Whaley, K., Webb, J., McAvoy, B.A., et al. 1973. Sjogren's syndrome. 2. Clinical associations and immunological phenomena. Q. J. Med. 42, 513.

Wrong, O.M., Feest, T.G., MacIver, A.G. 1993. Immune-related potassium-losing interstitial nephritis: a comparison with distal renal tubular acidosis. Q. J. Med. 86, 513.

Yoshida, K., Suzuki, J., Kume, K., et al. 1996. Membranous glomerulonephritis with primary Sjogren's syndrome detected by urine screening of school children. Clin. Nephrol. 45, 422.

# CHAPTER 20

# The Kidney in Systemic Sclerosis

Virginia D. Steen*

*Division of Rheumatology, Immunology and Allergy, Department of Medicine, Georgetown University, 3800 Reservoir Road, NW-LL, Gorman, Washington, DC 20007, USA*

Kidney involvement in systemic sclerosis (SSc) is primarily manifested by scleroderma renal crisis (SRC). Until recently, it was the most severe complication in scleroderma and was the most frequent cause of death in these patients. Fortunately, over the last l0–15 years, angiotensin converting enzyme (ACE) inhibitors have dramatically improved the outcome of SRC. Consequently, prompt diagnosis of renal crisis is critical so that immediate therapeutic intervention can achieve the best possible outcome. Renal abnormalities independent of renal crisis have been noted, but can usually be attributed to other problems. Further understanding of the pathogenesis of renal disease in scleroderma may lead to additional improvement in the therapy of renal crisis and perhaps the disease in general. This chapter reviews the pathogenesis, clinical setting, and therapy of this serious complication of SSc.

## 1. Pathogenesis of renal involvement

The pathogenesis of renal events in SSc remains incompletely understood, but the damage seems to evolve from a series of insults to the kidney (Fig. 1). The primary process, similar to that seen in vessels in other organs, is injury to the endothelial cells, which results in intimal thickening and proliferation of intralobular and arcuate arteries. Inflammatory cells, including lymphocytes and other mononuclear cells, are conspicuously absent in the pathologic examination of these arteries. The thickened abnormal vessel wall allows platelet aggregation and adhesion to occur. Release of platelet factors increases vascular permeability and may participate in the production of increased collagen and fibrin deposition contributing to the lumenal narrowing (Kahaleh and Leroy, 1999).

The narrowed arterial vessels are the primary cause of decreased renal perfusion, particularly cortical blood flow. Episodic vasospasm, or what has been called "renal Raynaud's" phenomenon, has been carefully demonstrated in early classic studies by Cannon although its significance is unclear (Cannon, 1974). Cannon showed that three of four patients had a significant reduction in cortical blood flow following cold water hand immersion. Additionally, Cannon found that patients with progressive renal failure had severely reduced cortical blood flow, whereas other patients had normal or only slightly diminished blood flow. A variety of techniques, including xenon-133 washout, $I^{131}$ hippurate, and static 99 mTc DTPA scans have been used to assess blood flow and renal dysfunction (Cannon, 1974; Desai et al., 1990; Sokoloff, 1952; Urai, 1958). Abnormalities have been documented in asymptomatic patients but none of these techniques have been successful in the early identification or prediction of renal crisis. Newer techniques using color flow Doppler sonography have looked at renal vessels in scleroderma patients. The resistance index (RI), a measure of renal blood flow, was abnormal

---

*Corresponding author.
Tel.: +202-687-8233; Fax: +202-687-8579
E-mail address: steev@georgetown.edu

© 2008 Published by Elsevier B.V.
DOI: 10.1016/S1571-5078(07)07020-1

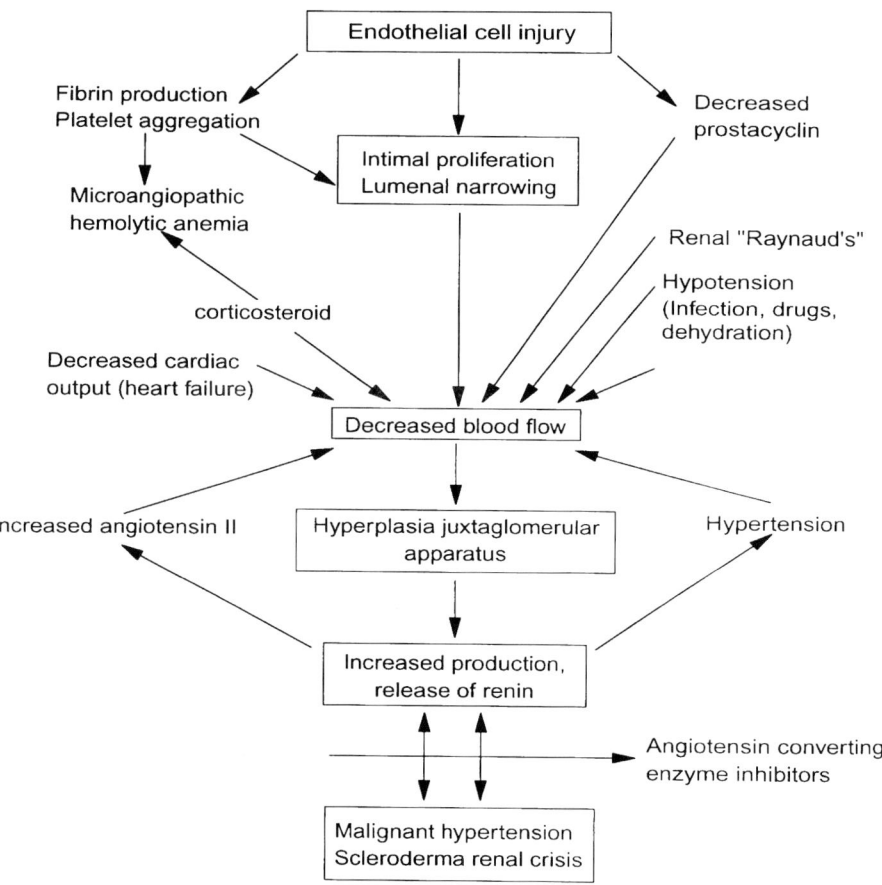

**Figure 1.** A potential pathogenetic mechanism for scleroderma renal crisis (SRC), with multiple factors contributing to a vicious cycle that results in malignant hypertension and renal failure.

in scleroderma patients and correlated with "renal" involvement (Nishijima et al., 2001) and disease duration (Rivolta et al., 1996). It improved with iloprost (Bugrova et al., 2001) and angiotensin converting enzyme inhibitors but not calcium channel blockers (Scorza et al., 1997). This technique, like other very sensitive measures of vascular involvement, may show vascular abnormalities but it is unlikely that it will predict renal crisis. Renal crisis occurs early in the disease and these studies showing that the RI abnormalities correlate with long disease duration (Rivolta et al., 1996).

Decreased blood flow leads to decreased perfusion of the juxtaglomerular apparatus, which causes hyperplasia of the juxtaglomerular apparatus as well as release of renin (Stone et al., 1974). Patients with renal crisis have markedly elevated peripheral levels of renin, which strongly supports the primary role of the renin–angiotensin system mediating the hypertension. Also, the dramatic improvement in hypertension following nephrectomy (Moorthy et al., 1978) demonstrates the importance of renin derived from the kidney in the pathogenesis of renal crisis (Cannon, 1974). Kovalchik found hyperreninemia and an exaggerated renin response to a cold pressor test in patients without clinical evidence of SRC although they had marked vascular changes on renal biopsy (Kovalchik et al., 1978). However, prior to the actual onset of renal crisis, hyperreninemia is not consistently present (Fleischmajer and Gould, 1975; Steen et al., 1984a) and when detected is not predictive of SRC

(Fleischmajer and Gould, 1975; Nussbaum, 1992; Steen et al., 1984a). Although hyperreninemia plays a major role in the pathogenesis of SRC, something else triggers the acute onset and rapid progression of renal failure, which is then fueled by the hyperreninemia.

Vascular changes are present in patients without renal crisis and, like plasma renin activity, do not predict the development of SRC (Kovalchik et al., 1978; Trostle et al., 1988). Kidney biopsies from diffuse scleroderma patients without renal abnormalities show vessels with the typical intimal proliferation and thickening that are seen in patients with renal crisis (Kovalchik et al., 1978). A case control autopsy series documented that even limited cutaneous scleroderma patients, who very rarely get renal crisis, had thickened vessels compared to the non-scleroderma controls (Trostle et al., 1988). Thickening of the vessels and the degree of lumenal occlusion were not correlated with age, disease duration, or last serum creatinine. Vascular changes are frequently present in scleroderma patients, but additional factors beyond the vascular changes and hyperreninemia must be present to trigger the acute crisis event.

The precipitation of SRC could result from situations in which renal blood flow is further compromised. Some authors have reported an increased frequency of SRC onset during cold months, suggesting the possibility of "renal Raynaud's" phenomenon (Cannon, 1974; Traub et al., 1983), although our clinical experience does not confirm this association (Steen et al., 1990). Cardiac dysfunction that decreases renal perfusion, i.e., large pericardial effusions, arrhythmias, or congestive heart failure, have preceded SRC in some patients (McWhorter and Leroy, 1974; Steen et al., 1984a), but they also can be the result of a hyperreninemic state (Follansbee, 1986). Pregnancy, with its alterations in blood volume and flow, has been reported to precipitate renal crisis (Karlen and Cook, 1974), but our extensive experience with scleroderma in pregnancy suggests that the association of renal crisis is primarily with early diffuse scleroderma and not with pregnancy (Steen et al., 1989).

Sepsis and dehydration causing hypotension could contribute to the problem. Drugs capable of causing decreased renal perfusion such as calcium channel blockers used in the management of Raynaud's phenomenon and ACE inhibitors may produce hypotension, but they have not been associated with increased frequency of renal crisis. Non-steroidal anti-inflammatory agents may deplete vasodilating prostaglandins, thus compromising renal blood flow. There is no convincing evidence that any of these drugs precipitate SRC, but cautious use of them is prudent in SSc patients at high risk for SRC.

Corticosteroids have long been implicated in the development of SRC (Lunseth, 1951; Sharnoff, 1951). However, since patients who are most likely to receive steroids are those with early inflammatory disease, they are the same patients who are at greatest risk for SRC. A significant association of antecedent *high* dose ($>40$ mg) prednisone or high-dose pulse methylprednisolone therapy (Helfrich et al., 1989; Kohno et al., 2000; Yamanishi et al., 1996) was noted in patients who had normotensive SRC. A case-control study of patients with renal crisis also found a significant association of high-dose prednisone ($>15$ mg prednisone) and renal crisis in the 6 months prior to renal crisis (Steen and Medsger, 1998). Because these compounds are capable of inhibiting prostacyclin production, increasing ACE activity, and altering endothelial function, they have the potential to play a role in the pathogenesis of SRC.

Narrowed arteries/arterioles and decreased blood flow caused by a variety of sources are likely to cause ischemia of the juxtaglomerular apparatus. Some additional factor triggers the acute release of large amounts of renin. This then causes increased angiotensin II, further vasoconstriction, elevated blood pressure, and renal ischemia. The end result is a vicious cycle as demonstrated in Fig. 1.

More recently, endothelial cell activation has been suggested to play a potential role in the development or progression of renal crisis. Increased levels of endothelin-1 (Vancheeswaran et al., 1994), soluble vascular adhesion molecules (s-VCAM-1), and soluble E-selectin (Stratton et al., 1998) have been shown to be associated with renal crisis. In one small series of scleroderma patients the highest level of E-selectin occurred in a renal crisis patient (Denton et al., 1995). Although there is no evidence that auto antibodies play a role in the pathogenesis of SRC, the striking dichotomy between the frequency of SRC in patients with anti-centromere antibody (<1%) and those with anti-RNA polymerase III (33%) is very intriguing (Steen et al., 2005). These antibody markers for disease subsets should lead us to ways to determine why some people get SRC and others do not.

## 2. Renal pathology

Pathologic changes of "scleroderma kidney" are very similar to those observed in other forms of malignant hypertension. Grossly, the capsule may show areas of infarction, hemorrhage, or even cortical necrosis. Microscopic changes are characteristically seen in the small interlobular and arcuate arteries (Fisher, 1958). The earliest change is intimal edema, followed by an intense proliferation of intimal cells and production of mucinous ground substance composed of glycoprotein and mucopolysaccharides. Lymphocytes and other mononuclear cells are absent. Fibrinoid necrosis may be present either in arterial walls or in a subintimal location in small arteries and arterioles. The resulting intimal thickening in interlobular arteries leads to narrowing and often total obliteration of the lumen (Fig. 2). In some

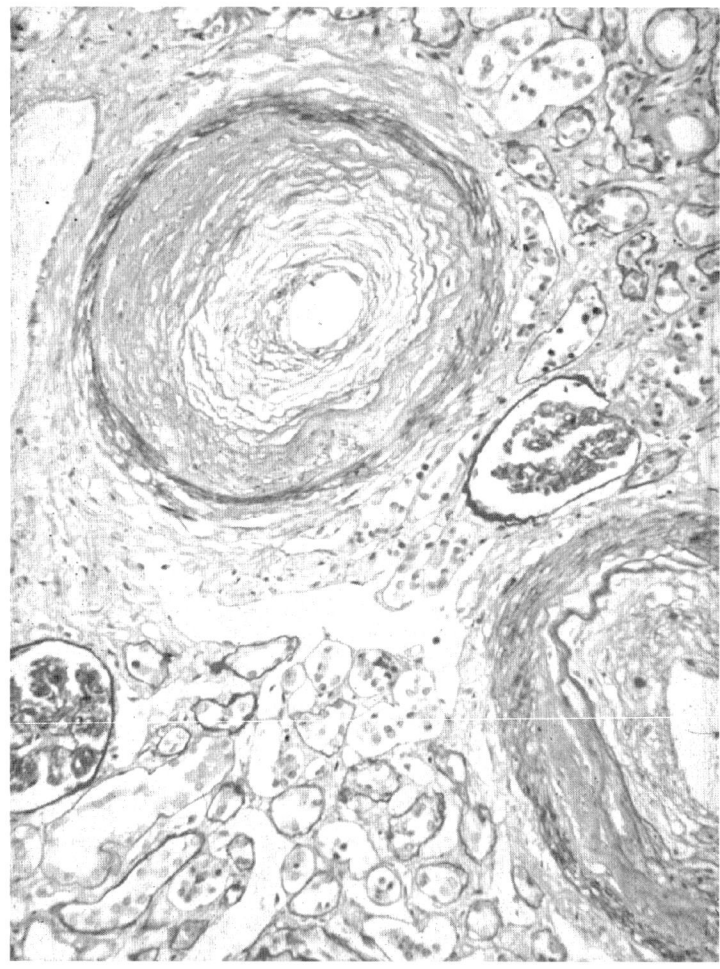

**Figure 2.** Medium-sized renal cortical artery of a patient with diffuse systemic sclerosis and renal crisis. There is severe concentric, edematous myxoid intimal proliferation with almost total obliteration of the lumen (Magnification ×275).

cases the media is thickened, but more often it appears stretched and thinned. Intramural fibrin deposition or fibrin thrombi have been noted, as in other forms of malignant hypertension, but can also be seen in scleroderma patients who are not hypertensive. Adventitial and peri-adventitial fibrosis are seen in SRC, but they are rarely noted in non-sclerodermatous malignant hypertension, making them helpful distinguishing features between the two entities (Shapiro, 1992). Large arteries may be normal or may show more typical atherosclerotic changes consistent with the patient's age.

Glomerular changes are variable and include thickening and collapse of capillary loops and other ischemic changes. Irregular thickening of glomerular basement membrane may result in more loop-like lesions. Juxtaglomerular cell hyperplasia is not specific to SSc but is consistent with the marked hyperreninemia characteristic of SRC (Fleischmajer and Gould, 1975; Stone et al., 1974). It is most prominent when arterial narrowing is severe. Tubules appear to be secondarily affected by vascular insufficiency from arterial lumenal occlusion. Flattening and degeneration of tubular cells are the most prominent changes.

Immunoglobulins (chiefly IgM) and complement components (C3) are non-specifically deposited in small renal arteries, but discrete electron-dense deposits consistent with immune complexes are absent (Kovalchik et al., 1978; Lapenas et al., 1978). Immune reactants are rarely found in the glomeruli although fibrinogen has been detected. The non-specificity of these findings is attributed to gross disruption of vascular integrity and increased permeability rather than immune injury.

Patients with diffuse scleroderma without renal crisis will have similar intimal proliferation in the arteries but to a lesser degree. Thus, a biopsy in a scleroderma patient without classic manifestations of renal crisis could very easily show the typical vascular changes. Even limited scleroderma patients, who rarely if ever get renal crisis, have more intimal proliferation than the non-scleroderma controls. Biopsy studies have shown that patients with these asymptomatic pathologic changes do not subsequently develop renal crisis (Clements et al., 1994; Kovalchik et al., 1978). Some non-renal crisis patients had extensive reduplication and proliferation of elastic fibers.

## 3. Renal crisis demographics

### 3.1. Definition

SRC is defined as the new onset of accelerated arterial hypertension and/or rapidly progressive oliguric renal failure during the course of SSc. One should not assume that non-malignant hypertension alone without azotemia or other renal abnormalities is renal crisis. Likewise, urine abnormalities and/or mild azotemia in a scleroderma patient are likely to have other explanations and should not be considered SRC.

### 3.2. Epidemiology

Renal crisis occurs in approximately 10% of the entire scleroderma population and 20–25% in patients with diffuse scleroderma. Interestingly, the incidence of renal crisis appears to have decreased since ACE-inhibitors have been available. Although calcium channel blockers and D-penicillamine have been associated with a decreased occurrence of renal crisis (Steen et al., 1982; Steen and Medsger, 1998), it is more likely that aggressive treatment with ACE-inhibitors has affected our ability to accurately diagnose this once fatal complication of scleroderma. There is no evidence that ACE-inhibitors prevent renal crisis. Several series have had patients who developed renal crisis while taking ACE-inhibitors (Denton and Black, 2000; Steen and Medsger, 1998). In one series of SRC patients 19 of 33 received "prophylactic" ACE inhibitors (Black C, unpublished data). Perhaps the low dose used in normotensive patients is inadequate to handle the surge of renin when SRC is triggered or gives a false sense of security so that the patient and physician are not as attentive as they would be otherwise.

Renal crisis is most often encountered early in the course of the disease, with 80% of SRC cases occurring less than 4 years after the first symptom attributable to scleroderma (Steen et al., 1994). However, late occurrences, even 20 years after

**Table 1**

Comparison of clinical characteristics in patients with renal crisis at time of renal crisis and those with diffuse cutaneous scleroderma without renal crisis at first visit

|  | Renal crisis ($n=227$) | No renal crisis ($n=777$) |
|---|---|---|
| Demographics | | |
| Age | 51 | 50 (at equivalent time) |
| Symptoms <4 years | 80% | 76% |
| Race, African American | 7.5% | 7.6% |
| Sex, male | 21% | 25% |
| Diffuse scleroderma | 83% | 95% |
| Anti-topoisomerase (Scl-70) | 19% | 34% |
| Anti-centromere antibody | 2% | 2% |
| Findings at time of renal crisis (or at time of first visit) | | |
| BP, mean | 184/108 | 120/74 |
| Papilledema | 29% (52% before ACE-I) | 0 |
| Seizures | 8% (11% before ACE-I) | 0 |
| 24 h urine, $>0.25$ g/24 h | 63% | 9% |
| Hematuria ($>5$ hpf) | 38% | 2% |
| Granular casts | 29% | 1% |
| Microangiopathic hemolytic anemia | 30% | 4% |
| Platelets <150,000 | 40% | <1% |
| ESR > 50 mm/h | 36% | 24% |
| Pericardial effusions | 27% | 10% |
| CHF/arrhythmias | 29% | 4% |

*Note*: All findings at the time of renal crisis occurred dramatically more frequently than in the no renal crisis patients ($p<0.0001$).

disease onset, have been seen. Some studies indicate that African-American patients are three times as likely as Caucasians to develop SRC, and (proportionately) males are more frequently affected than females. Our own statistics when only looking at diffuse scleroderma patients do not show these findings although only 6% of all our patients are African American (Table 1).

## 3.3. Factors predicting SRC

Patients with a greatly increased risk to develop this complication must be followed extremely closely for any hints of renal crisis (Tables 1 and 2). Patients with diffuse cutaneous scleroderma with skin thickening on the proximal extremities and/or the trunk are at greatest risk for SRC, with 20–25% of this patient subgroup getting SRC (Steen and Medsger, 1990). The rapid progression of skin thickening has been shown to be a good predictor of SRC (Steen et al., 1984a). These patients with early diffuse scleroderma should monitor their own

**Table 2**

Factors that occur prior to SRC that may be predictive for future SRC

| Predictive of SRC | Not predictive of SRC |
|---|---|
| Disease symptoms <4 years | Previous blood pressure elevations |
| Diffuse skin involvement | Abnormal urinalysis |
| Rapid progression of skin thickening | Stable mildly elevated serum creatinine |
| Anti-RNA polymerase III antibody | Anti-topoisomerase or anti-centromere antibodies |
| New anemia | Pathologic abnormalities in renal blood vessels |
| New cardiac events   Pericardial effusion   Congestive heart failure | |
| Antecedent high-dose corticosteroid | |

blood pressure regularly, and should know to notify their physicians immediately when their blood pressure is increased above their own normal levels. Only 1% of patients with limited cutaneous scleroderma (previously termed the CREST syndrome) who have long-standing Raynaud's and skin changes restricted to distal extremities ever develop renal crisis. Only a handful of renal crisis patients have limited scleroderma (Donohoe, 1992; Steen et al., 1984b). The vast majority of SRC cases (75–80%) occur in patients with obvious diffuse cutaneous changes at the time of renal crisis.

Another 15–20% of SRC cases occur in patients who are destined to develop typical diffuse scleroderma, although they only have minimal or even no skin changes at the time of the diagnosis of renal crisis. It is not infrequent for this type of patient with such minimal cutaneous and systemic findings to have the diagnosis of renal crisis made only at the time of kidney biopsy (Korzets et al., 1998; Molina et al., 1995; Phan et al., 1999). There are several distinguishing features that help to identify those patients who are likely to evolve to diffuse cutaneous disease (Table 3). These patients almost always have a short duration of symptoms, often less than 1 year. Polyarthritis/arthralgias, puffy or swollen hands and legs, carpal tunnel syndrome, new fatigue, or weight loss are a common complex of symptoms in patients with early diffuse scleroderma (Leroy et al., 1988). New onset of Raynaud's may be the only symptom present, although its absence in early diffuse scleroderma at the time of renal crisis is not uncommon. The presence of palpable tendon friction rubs, which occur in 65% of diffuse scleroderma patients, is an extremely helpful and predictive sign of diffuse scleroderma even prior to the development of diffuse cutaneous skin involvement (Steen and Medsger, 1997). Less than 5% of limited scleroderma patients ever have tendon rubs. Additionally, limited scleroderma patients typically have 5–10 years of Raynaud's phenomenon with minimal articular or systemic symptoms at initial diagnosis (Steen and Medsger, 1990). Patients not known to have scleroderma, who present with new isolated malignant hypertension and have some systemic symptoms should be carefully questioned for the presence of the aforementioned clinical features.

Autoantibodies may be helpful in predicting SRC. Anti-nuclear antibodies are seen in 95% of scleroderma so their presence may be helpful in determining whether a malignant hypertension patient could possible have scleroderma. The presence of the scleroderma specific antibody, anti-topoisomerase antibody or anti-Scl-70, suggests the diagnosis of diffuse scleroderma, but it is not a specific marker for renal crisis. There are similar percentages of patients with and without this antibody who have renal crisis (Steen and Medsger, 1990). The anti-centromere antibody, the classic limited scleroderma (or CREST syndrome) antibody is not a risk factor for renal crisis (Steen et al., 1984b). Anti-RNA polymerase III is another antibody that is seen almost exclusively in diffuse scleroderma, and 24–33% of patients with this antibody develop SRC (Bunn et al., 1998; Okano et al., 1993; Rivolta et al., 1996). In several patients with malignant hypertension and renal failure but without cutaneous manifestations of scleroderma, anti-RNA polymerase III was found prior to the documentation of renal crisis on biopsy (Molina et al., 1995; Phan et al., 1999). In contrast, renal crisis occurs in only 10% of patients with anti-topoisomerase antibody.

Antecedent hypertension is not usually present prior to SRC. Most often there is a very acute onset of markedly elevated blood pressure. Normal blood pressures have been documented within 24 h prior to the onset of SRC hypertension (Traub et al., 1983). Non-malignant hypertension without any urine, blood, or kidney abnormalities is seen in scleroderma patients and these patients have a good outcome. Our study identified this type of hypertension in 12% of patients, a mean of 5 years

**Table 3**
Rheumatic disease symptoms which would suggest scleroderma as the etiology of malignant hypertension in patients without the firm diagnosis of scleroderma

---

Recent onset of Raynaud's (although this may be absent at time of renal crisis)
Swollen stiff hands/fingers suggestive of arthritis
Carpal tunnel syndrome
Swollen lower legs without any obvious etiology
Tendon friction rubs and pain over distal extremity tendons
New onset of fatigue, weight loss, joint pains, weakness
Positive anti-nuclear antibody
Some skin thickening even if it confined to the distal extremities
Diagnosis of "CREST" syndrome in a patient with <18 months of symptoms

after onset of scleroderma. It was unassociated with proteinuria or renal insufficiency (Mallee et al., 1985). The frequency of non-malignant hypertension has not been shown to be higher than in the general population (Steen et al., 1984a), and it is hard to know whether it is part of the spectrum of scleroderma renal involvement. Patients developing non-malignant hypertension do not appear to be at increased risk for developing SRC, but the early use of ACE inhibitors has hampered our ability to determine the significance of this "mild" type of hypertension. New hypertension may occur after the initiation of corticosteroids, which may themselves precipitate renal crisis. However, to be on the safe side, ACE-inhibitors should be the first agent used in any diffuse scleroderma patient with hypertension.

Marked elevation of plasma renin is the hallmark of acute SRC. Often it is 10 times normal and occasionally reaches 100 times normal. Kovalchik and Gavras found abnormal plasma renin activity in scleroderma patients (Kovalchik et al., 1978; Gavras et al., 1977). However, in a 10-year prospective study, Clements did not find peripheral renal activity predictive of renal crisis (Clements et al., 1994). Because the use of ACE inhibitors interferes with the renin assay and results are often not available for weeks, this important finding is rarely used in the diagnosis or management of SRC. In isolation, abnormal urinalysis, increased serum creatinine, or a decreased creatinine clearance have not been helpful in predicting SRC. Such findings can usually be attributed to other causes or are only transient (Clements et al., 1994; Kovalchik et al., 1978; Steen et al., 1984a, 2005).

Several non-renal abnormalities may precede SRC. Asymptomatic pericardial effusion, congestive heart failure, and/or arrhythmias may antedate renal crisis (McWhorter and Leroy, 1974; Steen et al., 1984a). Some patients present with these symptoms and initial treatment is focused on the heart rather than the blood pressure. Hyperreninemia even without hypertension may be the cause of pulmonary edema and thus may be contributing to these cardiac problems (Wasner et al., 1978). New anemia, an uncommon manifestation of scleroderma, can be an early clue to renal crisis (Steen et al., 1984a), particularly when microangiopathic hemolysis and thrombocytopenia are present. Careful evaluation of any anemia or thrombocytopenia is necessary to avoid falsely attributing these findings to immune-mediated hemolytic anemia, drug toxicity, or other causes.

Prior use of high-dose corticosteroids (prednisone >40 mg/day) and pulse methylprednisolone have been reported to precede the development of SRC in some patients with normal blood pressure during renal crisis (Helfrich et al., 1989; Kohno et al., 2000; Yamanishi et al., 1996). A case control study matched 106 patients with renal crisis to other scleroderma patients based on features that would be associated with increased risk for renal crisis or the use of steroids (Steen and Medsger, 1998). Sex, disease subtypes, disease duration, extent of skin thickening, the presence of tendon friction rubs, and inflammatory myopathy were similar in both groups. Patients who received high-dose prednisone (>15 mg/day) were three times more likely to develop renal crisis in the next 6 months. High-dose steroids should be used with great caution and very close monitoring in patients with early diffuse scleroderma.

Cyclosporin A is another drug that has been implicated in precipitating renal crisis and can cause severe nephrotoxicity similar to that seen during the management of transplants (Denton et al., 1994; Ruiz et al., 1991). There must be particular caution and close monitoring of blood pressure and laboratory tests if this drug is chosen to be used in high-risk diffuse scleroderma patients.

## 3.4. Clinical findings

Patients may complain of severe headache, blurred vision, or other encephalopathic symptoms with the onset of accelerated hypertension. Seizures may be an early finding but, fortunately, early and effective therapy has decreased the frequency of these events. Non-specific complaints of increased fatigue or just not feeling well must be taken seriously and high-risk patients should check their own blood pressure if these symptoms occur.

Most patients have striking elevations of blood pressure at the onset of SRC. Ninety percent have blood pressure levels greater than 150/90 mm Hg, and 30% have diastolic recordings greater than 120 mm Hg. Up to 10% of cases have a normal blood pressure. An increase of 20 mm Hg in a blood pressure reading may be significantly elevated for that particular patient and yet may still remain in the normal range (95/60 to 140/85). This can represent renal crisis. Further testing and close monitoring are necessary for any changes in blood pressure. This event, called normotensive renal crisis, requires the presence of other features, primarily rapidly progressive unexplained azotemia and/or microangiopathic hemolytic anemia with thrombocytopenia. Pulmonary hemorrhage is a rare life-threatening problem, which has occurred in several of these patients (Bar et al., 2001; Helfrich et al., 1989). It complicates the diagnosis and is a poor prognostic sign.

In some situations, SRC symptoms are confused with other illnesses. Several cases of thrombotic thrombocytopenic purpura (TTP) have been reported in scleroderma patients, but it is unclear whether it was an isolated coexistent disease or just a different interpretation of SRC (Kapur et al., 1997; Kfoury Baz et al., 2001). A review of the eight cases of TTP and scleroderma in the literature found that there were few differences between the patient subsets. Although a few "responded" to plasmapheresis, most were also treated with ACE-inhibitors (Manadan et al., 2005). Fever and hemorrhagic manifestations were the only findings that were different. New research in the pathophysiology of TTP has led to the observation that vWF-cleaving protease activity is decreased or deficient in TTP (Lian, 2005). While it is not yet known whether this occurs in SRC, it may be helpful in separating these very similar entities. If a diagnosis of TTP is made in a scleroderma patient, an ACE-inhibitor should be used in conjunction with TTP treatment (Kfoury Baz et al., 2001).

## 4. Laboratory findings

### 4.1. Renal abnormalities

Patients rarely present with end stage renal disease. The serum creatinine is usually elevated and rises rapidly during the initial event. Although a slow increase of serum creatinine can occur over days to weeks, it is much more likely to increase by 0.5–1.0 mg/dl creatinine per day. It is important to recognize that serum creatinine often continues to rise even after the blood pressure is controlled. Control of the pressure means return of it to at least 120/80 mmHg, but preferably to their pre-renal crisis values. Since this is such an acute episode, rarely are there neurologic problems associated with a rapid decrease in blood pressure. The issue of whether the ACE-inhibitor itself contributes to increases in creatinine is often raised, but in the setting of confirmed renal crisis, I have not seen any patient who has had significant improvement in serum creatinine after stopping the ACE-inhibitor. Unfortunately, there are still situations where the serum creatinine continues to rise and the patient develops renal failure in spite of adequate control of the blood pressure with ACE-inhibitors. In these circumstances the addition of corticosteroids, immunosuppressive therapy, or plasmapheresis are never helpful. Routine urinalysis shows proteinuria (not usually exceeding 2 g/24 h), microscopic hematuria (5–100 rbc/hpf), and often granular casts.

### 4.2. Hematology

Microangiopathic hemolytic anemia, which is characterized by normochromic, fragmented red blood cells, schistocytes, reticulocytosis, and thrombocytopenia, occurs in almost half of patients with SRC. The platelet count is rarely lower than 20,000/mm$^3$ and its improvement is often the first sign of adequate response to therapy, even though the serum creatinine is continuing to increase. Patients are not usually symptomatic from this process except that the anemia may precipitate congestive heart failure.

### 4.3. Cardiac decompensation

SRC may present with congestive heart failure (dyspnea, paroxysmal nocturnal dyspnea, or even pulmonary edema), serious ventricular arrhythmias (even cardiac arrest); or large pericardial effusions (Follansbee, 1986; McWhorter and Leroy, 1974; Steen et al., 1984a). This is primarily from the stress of the hypertension on the heart, effects of hyperreninemia, and from fluid overload secondary to oliguric renal failure, although some patients with very severe disease also have primary scleroderma myocardial involvement contributing to these problems. Frequently, cardiac decompensation is thought to be the cause of the hypertension rather than the other way around. It is not unusual for physicians to focus on treating the heart failure or the pericardial effusion rather than the hypertension. It is important to recognize that until the blood pressure is better controlled, these cardiac problems will be difficult to treat. Severe pulmonary hypertension secondary to the malignant systemic hypertension is also seen, but has a different course than the more frequent chronic pulmonary hypertension seen in limited scleroderma patients. Prompt control of the blood pressure usually improves these cardiac problems and, if controlled, the patient is unlikely to have persistent pulmonary hypertension.

## 5. Management

### 5.1. ACE-inhibitors

The vicious cycle of decreased blood flow, ischemia, hyperreninemia, hypertension, and further vasoconstriction almost invariably resulted in a fatal outcome prior to the availability of ACE-inhibitors. In those days, only a small minority of SRC patients (<10%) survived more than 3 months. In the late 1970s, there were several reports of survival with very aggressive approach in controlling the blood pressure and dialysis (Leroy and Fleischmann, 1978; Wasner et al., 1978). However, persistent, uncontrollable hypertension, hyperreninemia, and resultant congestive heart failure made management even with dialysis very difficult. For a time, bilateral nephrectomy was performed to eliminate the hyperreninemia. This allowed the blood pressure, heart failure, and dialysis to be managed more successfully (Mitnick and Feig, 1978; Traub et al., 1983).

Also in the late 1970s, the first ACE-inhibitors were experimentally used in scleroderma. These drugs work by acting as competitive inhibitors of the conversion of angiotensin I to angiotensin II. Inhibition of angiotensin II production promptly lowers blood pressure in scleroderma patients. Although angiotensin I and renin continue to accumulate, they are not biologically active and do not increase blood pressure. These drugs also proteolyze bradykinins, which, as potent vasodilators, potentially could have a role in the hypotensive effect of these agents. In 1979, Lopez-Overjero described two scleroderma patients with dramatic reversal of malignant hypertension and normalization of renal dysfunction as the result of treatment with an oral ACE inhibitor (Lopez-Ovejero et al., 1979). Additional series confirmed this almost miraculous response (Thurm and Alexander, 1984; Zawada, et al., 1981). Survival was dramatically improved compared to the pre-captopril time.

### 5.2. Outcome with ACE-inhibitors

The use of ACE-inhibitors has dramatically changed the survival of patients with SRC. Prior to the availability of these drugs patients almost always died. Only 10% survived the first year. Most recently, the long-term outcome of 145 cases of SRC seen at the University of Pittsburgh who were treated with ACE-inhibitors showed that 61% had a good outcome as defined by not requiring or only requiring temporary dialysis (Steen and Medsger, 2000) (Figs. 3 and 4). Fifty-four of the 145 patients never required dialysis. Their serum creatinine peaked at 3.8 mg/dl and slowly decreased. Seven years after renal crisis, these patient's mean serum creatinine was 1.8 mg/dl. None of them went on to develop chronic renal failure and none required dialysis. There were 62 patients who required dialysis during the acute renal crisis episode, but more than half ($n = 34$) were successfully able to discontinue dialysis 3–18 months (mean 8 months) later. Their mean serum creatinine 6 years later was 2.2 mg/dl. Only two of

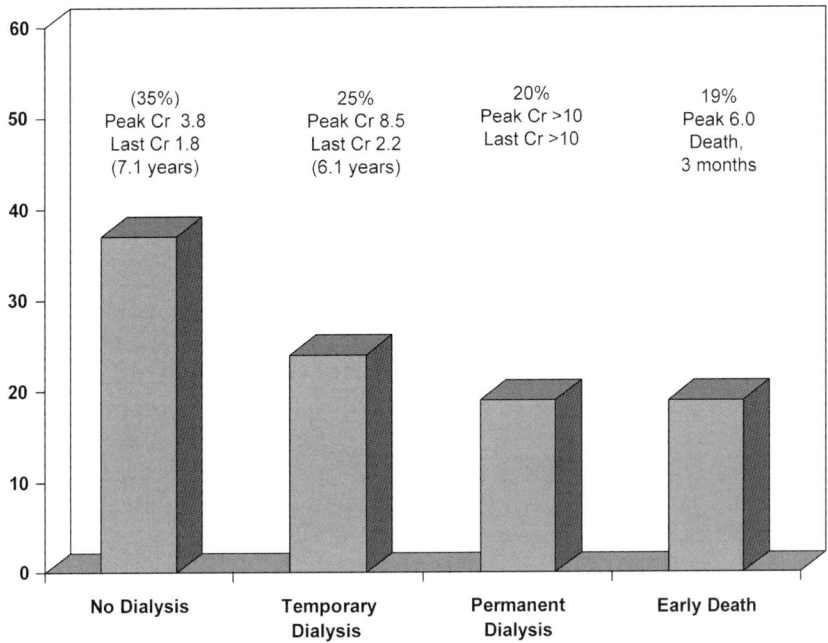

**Figure 3.** The frequency of different outcomes of renal crisis and serum creatinines (Cr) (mg/dl) at different time points after renal crisis in 145 patients with SRC. The duration since renal crisis is given for the last serum creatinine.

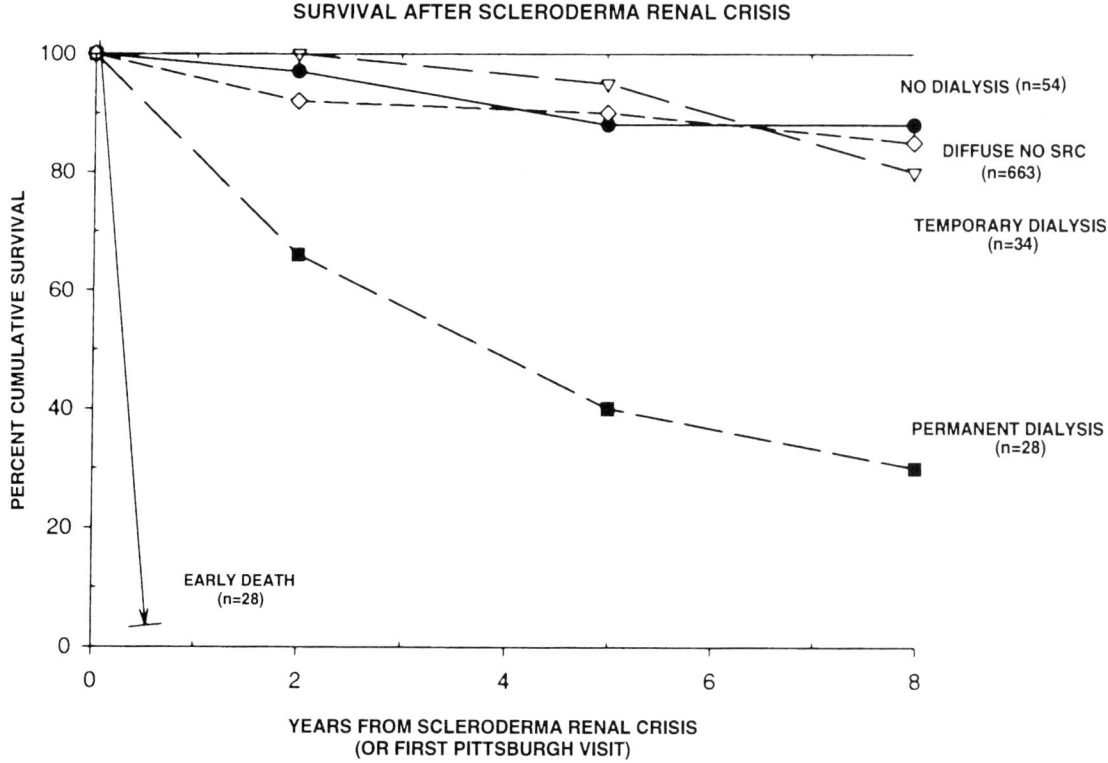

**Figure 4.** The percent cumulative survival rate for patients with different outcomes of SRC and patients with diffuse scleroderma without renal crisis.

them developed slowly progressive renal failure and went back on dialysis (4%). There were still 28 (19%) patients who had an early death, a mean of 3 months after SRC. This group was older, male, with cardiac involvement and had a higher serum creatinine at the start of treatment. Delay in diagnosis is the primary cause of a poor outcome in renal crisis today.

Renal crisis has gone from the most common cause of scleroderma related deaths, 40% in the 1970s, to only 8% in the in the last 10 years. The treatment of SRC is now so successful that SRC patients with a good outcome (no or temporary dialysis) had as good a survival as diffuse scleroderma patients who never had renal crisis (Fig. 4). The 5-year cumulative survival in these groups after renal crisis (or from the first visit) was around 90%, and was 80–85% at 8 years. SRC patients on permanent dialysis did not fair nearly as well but their 40% 5-year survival was still significantly better than survival of renal crisis prior to ACE-inhibitors.

## 5.3. Refractory renal crisis

Not all patients' blood pressures respond promptly to the ACE inhibitor. The goal should be to normalize the blood pressure (back to the normal value, 120/70–80 mmHg) in the first 3 days. Captopril has a shorter half-life and thus allows more flexibility with dosage changes early in the course but any agent can be used. There is no difference in the outcome of patients treated with the second-generation ACE-inhibitors compared to captopril. If the blood pressure is not adequately controlled with maximum amounts of an ACE inhibitor alone, other types of anti-hypertensive agents, including calcium channel blockers or clonidine can be added. Beta-blockers should be avoided since they aggravate Raynaud's symptoms. It is not unusual for the serum creatinine to continue to rise even though the blood pressure is controlled. Do NOT assume that the ACE-inhibitor is "not working" or is contributing to the deterioration. Although this may occur in other settings, stopping the ACE inhibitor during renal crisis never improves renal function. In the early stages, controlling the blood pressure is the major goal and once that is achieved, the renal outcome will depend on how much damage has occurred prior to the control of the blood pressure. Treatment with steroids, immunosuppressive agents, or plasmapheresis is NOT helpful at any time in the management of renal crisis. In some cases renal failure cannot be prevented (Whitman et al., 1982). The initial level of creatinine at the start of therapy plays a pivotal role in the final outcome. Starting an ACE-inhibitor when the serum creatinine is greater than 3 mg/dl, or not controlling the blood pressure within 3 days are associated with a bad outcomes (Steen et al., 1990). Males, older age, and presence of congestive heart failure are additional risk factors associated with a bad outcome.

## 5.4. Angiotensin receptor blockers

Although there is experimental evidence that the angiotensin receptor blockers (ARB) might have an additive effect to ACE-inhibitors, clinical experience with these agents has been variable (Caskey et al., 1997; Hasegawa et al., 2000). Some patients have had inadequate control of blood pressure, and others have had recurrence of hypertension when they have been switched from an ACE-inhibitor, or deterioration when an angiotensin-blocker was added to the ACE-inhibitor. The lack of a bradykinin effect which occurs with the ARB could explain why ARB may be less effective than ACE inhibitors. Experimentally, a rat model of hypertension (not scleroderma) treated with a combination of an ACE-inhibitor and an ARB showed they potentiated each other (Siragy, 2001). While this does not explain why the renal crisis patients receiving both drugs did not do well, bradykinin may have a more important role in renal crisis than realized. The use of ARB should not be the first line agent in the treatment of SRC but they may be used effectively. Patients should be monitored even more carefully if these agents are used. Although further study is necessary to confirm these observations, ARB in renal crisis should be used with extreme caution.

## 5.5. Normotensive renal crisis

Management of normotensive renal crisis is also with ACE inhibitors. Although those patients do not have significant increases in the blood pressure, the drugs can be life saving during acute SRC even in the absence of hypertension. Even in small doses they can reverse the process if given early enough in the course. Thus, it is very important to strongly consider SRC in the setting of patients with early diffuse scleroderma who have renal insufficiency or other suggestions of renal crisis even in the absence of malignant hypertension.

## 5.6. Renal crisis and pregnancy

The management of scleroderma during pregnancy is challenging, but it is particularly challenging for women who have survived renal crisis and wish to become pregnant. Although ACE-inhibitors have been reported to cause fatal, fetal renal atresia in many patients, the frequency of this occurrence is not known (Pryde and Barr, 2001). After an episode of renal crisis, ACE inhibitors are required to maintain blood pressure control and renal function indefinitely. Patients have had successful pregnancy outcomes while on ACE-inhibitors (Steen, 1999); however, their use during pregnancy, particularly during the third trimester, is associated with a high risk of serious kidney problems in the baby.

Ten women from our scleroderma cohort have had 12 pregnancies after an episode of renal crisis (Steen, 2002). Five healthy babies were born to four women who remained on ACE-inhibitors throughout the pregnancy. Two women discontinued ACE-inhibitors prior to or early in pregnancy and their blood pressure was successfully managed with other medications including calcium channel blockers. Their three pregnancies were successfully completed without maternal problems and resulted in premature but healthy babies. Three women who discontinued the ACE-inhibitors prior to pregnancy had major problems with uncontrolled hypertension in spite of aggressive non-ACE-inhibitor treatment. Off ACE-inhibitors, their blood pressure was not easily controlled and two had major increases in their serum creatinine. One of these women had a 29-week stillbirth. Another one was started on captopril during the 20th week of pregnancy in as low a dose as necessary along with other medications to control her blood pressure. At 31 weeks, she developed oligohydramnios, there was concern for the fetus and labor was induced. The 2.8-pound infant had some hypotension but did well. The third patient had very poor control of her blood pressure. Even though a very small dose of captopril was added in the 24th week, her blood pressure was still inadequately controlled. When her creatinine reached 2.9 mg/dl labor was induced. The 1.3 pound infant died after a 2-month struggle for life, but he did not have any renal problems. None of these infants had any significant evidence of ACE-inhibitor toxicity.

Pregnancy in patients after renal crisis may be successful but there are potential disastrous outcomes as well. There are several possible approaches that a patient can take if she desires a pregnancy after renal crisis but they each contain significant risk. If the patient discontinues the ACE-inhibitor and the blood pressure is not controlled with other medications, then the patient must be put back on an ACE-inhibitor. Otherwise, they are likely to experience severe deterioration in renal function and potential problems with the fetus as well. In the above small series, the worst outcomes occurred in patients who had very poor blood pressure control. Patients should consider a trial of ACE-inhibitors prior to pregnancy to see if they have any chance of successful blood pressure control without ACE-inhibitors. Another possible way of managing the pregnancy would be to use a small dose of ACE-inhibitor along with non-ACE-inhibitor medication to control blood pressure, combined with close monitoring for oligohydramnios or other signs of fetal abnormalities. In any situation, the patient and her spouse have to seriously consider their willingness to abort a pregnancy associated with a severely injured infant. The patient must discuss a variety of options and potential outcomes before deciding whether to become or continue a pregnancy. There are no easy answers.

## 5.7. Dialysis

Dialysis studies using the ESRD database have not shown the aforementioned 50% discontinuation rate in scleroderma patients on dialysis (Tsakiris et al., 1996). However, many patients discontinued dialysis before they entered the ESRD database and none of the database studies have included only patients treated aggressively with ACE-inhibitors. Patients requiring permanent dialysis had similar types and frequency of vascular access and peritoneal clearance problems compared to other dialysis patients. In our series of patients, the rate of hemodialysis complications, including thrombosis, ischemia, and revision was comparable to other non-scleroderma series (Donohoe, 1992; Rocco et al., 1996; Tsakiris et al., 1996). Only one of the 34 hemodialysis patients had new acute digital ulcers following graft placement and she had a history of prior severe digital ulcers (Steen and Medsger, 2000). Four of 18 patients did not have adequate clearance to do peritoneal dialysis, but those who were able to use peritoneal dialysis, did very well.

An ACE-inhibitor should be continued even while the patient is on dialysis, since so many patients have the potential of improvement in their renal function after renal crisis. Hyperreninemia may be an ongoing process causing further damage to kidneys and heart, preventing kidney recovery and possibly causing congestive heart failure, so it is important to continue to use an ACE-inhibitor even if it is only a small dose on non-dialysis days. Prior to ACE-inhibitors, even after kidney failure occurred, management of blood pressure, heart failure, and dialysis was so difficult that nephrectomies were necessary.

## 5.8. Transplant

Since there is a real possibility and hope for the return of adequate renal function and subsequent discontinuation of dialysis, plans for renal transplant should be kept on hold until at least 12 months have passed without return of kidney function. Recurrences of SRC have been reported in a few patients following renal transplant (Caplin et al., 1999; Pham et al., 2005; Woodhall et al., 1976). All have occurred in patients transplanted within the first year following the initial SRC episode (Pham et al., 2005). It is unclear what role ACE-inhibitors did or did not have in these recurrences. It is likely that the cause of these recurrences was persistent hyperreninemia from the native kidney. Thus, an ACE-inhibitor should probably be used after transplant if the native kidneys remain. Overall, renal transplant improved survival in scleroderma compared to those who remained on dialysis (Tsakiris et al., 1996). A review of outcomes of 50 kidney transplants in rare diseases from the United Network for Organ Sharing registry from 1987 to 1996 showed some decrease in graft and overall survival in scleroderma patients compared to those with analgesic nephropathy and diabetes. However, the survival was still better than the survival on dialysis alone.

## 6. Non-renal crisis kidney problems

### 6.1. Abnormal kidney function tests

Early literature suggests that 45–60% of all scleroderma patients have hypertension, proteinuria, or azotemia (Cannon, 1974; Leroy and Fleischmann, 1978; Steen et al., 2005). This was confirmed in a recent study, but no attempt was made to see if the abnormalities were scleroderma related or not (Donohoe, 1992). A similar frequency of renal abnormalities, including azotemia, proteinuria, hematuria, or hypertension, has been seen in our population of diffuse cutaneous scleroderma patients (Fig. 5). Fifty-two percent of 667 patients with diffuse scleroderma, followed for a mean of 9.5 years of disease, had evidence of renal abnormalities. Nineteen percent had classic SRC. Mild isolated hypertension requiring medication but without evidence of renal crisis occurred in 79 (12%). Half of them had new isolated hypertension as opposed to a prior history of hypertension and 173 (26%) had some non-SRC renal abnormality.

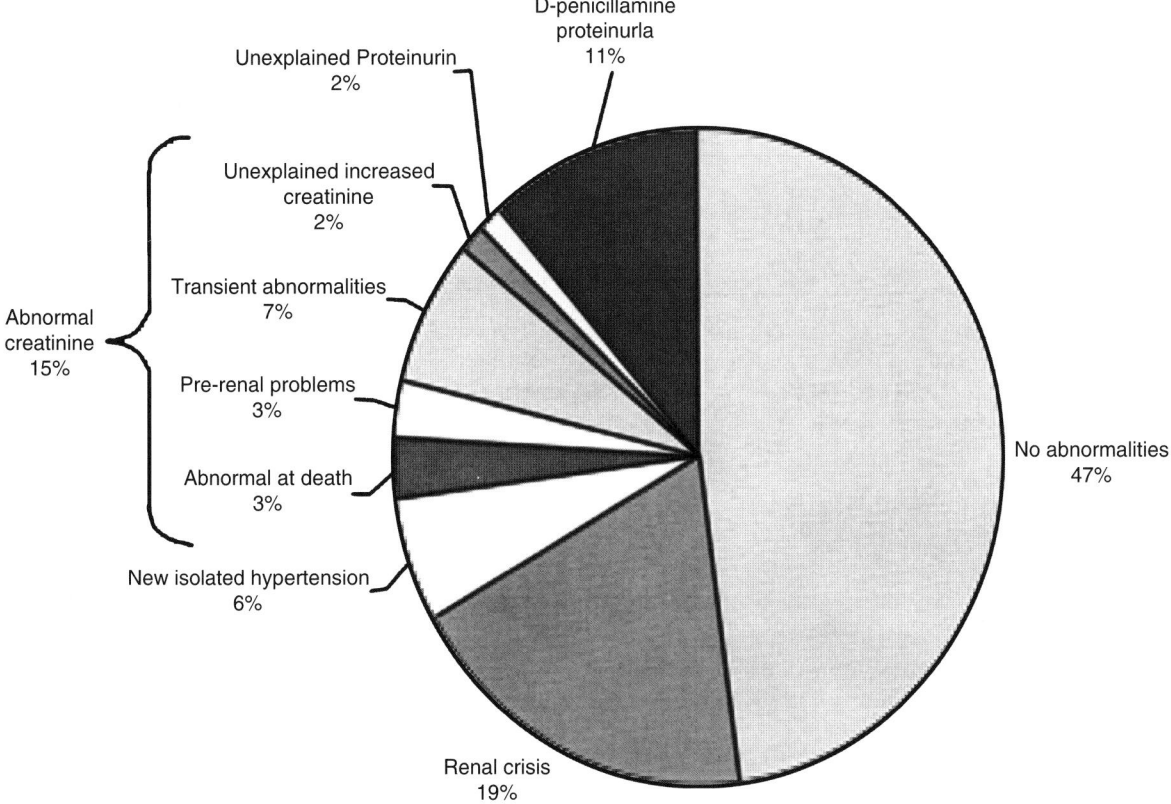

**Figure 5.** The cumulative frequency and etiology of kidney abnormalities in 667 diffuse scleroderma patients followed prospectively for 9 years.

One hundred and five patients (15% of diffuse scleroderma patients) without renal crisis had a creatinine greater than 1.3 mg/dl, at some point in their illness (Steen et al., 2005). However, the cause of most of these abnormalities could be explained by factors other than intrinsic scleroderma renal abnormalities. Twenty-two (21% of the 105 with serum creatinine increases) had their first abnormal creatinine during the hospitalization prior to their death, which was not due to renal crisis. Most of the causes were other scleroderma organ involvement including gastrointestinal, heart, or lung failure. Increased creatinine was explained in another 22 (21%) patients by events associated with pre-renal effects from severe congestive heart failure, scleroderma gastrointestinal involvement with diarrhea, and/or dehydration, volume depletion from acute illness or infection, diuretics, steroids, or drug reactions (cyclosporin, D-penicillamine, or non-steroidal anti-inflammatory medications). Transient increases in the serum creatinine occurred in 49 (47%) patients, but in all patients the last recorded creatinine, 5.9 years later, was normal. Only 12 (1.8%) of these 667 diffuse scleroderma patients had an elevation in serum creatinine, which was not easily explained by other causes. The mean highest creatinine in these patients was 2.4 mg/dl and the mean last creatinine was 1.6 mg/dl. Several patients had hypertension, but the increase in creatinine did not occur at the onset of the hypertension. Thus, chronic progressive azotemia independent of SRC is distinctly unusual in diffuse scleroderma patients.

Eighty-six diffuse scleroderma patients (12%) excreted more than 250 mg of protein in 24 h (or had +3 protein on dipstick). In 78% of these patients the urinary problems were thought to be secondary to a membranous nephropathy from D-penicillamine toxicity (Steen et al., 2005). Some of these patient's renal biopsies, performed after more than 6 months of persistent proteinuria, showed a membranous glomerulonephritis consistent with D-penicillamine toxicity. Only 12 (1.8%) of these 667 diffuse cutaneous scleroderma patients had unexplained proteinuria (mean 400 mg/24 h). None of them developed renal crisis. Others have also not found significant proteinuria or azotemia independent of renal crisis (Mallee et al., 1985).

## 6.2. Crescentic, ANCA positive glomerulonephitis

There have been several case reports of a necrotizing, crescentic glomerulonephritis associated with an anti-myeloperoxidase (MPO) anti-neutrophil cytoplasmic antibody (ANCA) occurring in scleroderma patients (Hillis et al., 1997). This was first reported as a drug toxicity in patients taking D-penicillamine, but more recently several cases have been reported in patients with limited scleroderma who have not been exposed to any potential drugs that could cause this problem (Anders et al., 1999; Karpinski et al., 1997; Maes et al., 2000). These patients are usually normotensive, have nephrotic range proteinuria, renal insufficiency, and do not have microangiopathic hemolytic anemia or thrombocytopenia. Thus, they are quite different from the usual renal crisis patient. However, kidney biopsy is necessary to make the diagnosis. Treatment with steroids and immunosuppressive agents, as in microscopic polyarteritis, may prevent progressive renal insufficiency (Martinez et al., 2000). The frequency of this is unknown. One series of 81 scleroderma patients found only 2 who had a perinuclear ANCAs with high titers of anti-MPO antibodies (Locke et al., 1997). Although there is nothing that suggests that this form of renal abnormality is related to scleroderma, the occurrence of two rare diseases makes us curious. Further study is necessary.

### Key points

- Scleroderma renal crisis with malignant hypertension and rapidly progressive renal failure is a life-threatening emergency and needs to be diagnosed and treated aggressively.
- Patients with early diffuse scleroderma, rapidly progressive skin thickening (or very early disease even before skin thickening is present), new onset congestive heart failure, or recent treatment with high-dose steroids, are at greatest risk for developing renal crisis.
- Urgent treatment with ACE-inhibitors can be life saving. Other anti-hypertensive therapy, steroids, plasmapharesis are not effective.
- More than half of the patients going on dialysis are able to discontinue it permanently. ACE-inhibitors should be continued even in very low doses while on dialysis.
- Kidney disease in diffuse scleroderma independent of renal crisis is rare and not progressive. Patients with renal abnormalities unassociated with renal crisis should be carefully evaluated for other non-scleroderma kidney problems.

## References

Anders, H.J., Wiebecke, B., Haedecke, C., Sanden, S., Combe, C., Schlondorff, D. 1999. MPO-ANCA-positive crescentic glomerulonephritis: a distinct entity of scleroderma renal disease? Am. J. Kidney Dis. 33, e3.

Bar, J., Ehrenfeld, M., Rozenman, J., Perelman, M., Sidi, Y., Gur, H. 2001. Pulmonary–renal syndrome in systemic sclerosis. Semin. Arthritis Rheum. 30, 403–410.

Bugrova, O.V., Kutyrina, I.M., Bagirova, V.V., Morozova, E.V., Gromova, M.M. 2001. Effects of acute pharmacological blockade of the renin–angiotensin system on intrarenal hemodynamics in patients with systemic lupus erythematosus and systemic sclerosis. Ter. Arkh. 73, 20–25.

Bunn, C.C., Denton, C.P., Shi-wen, X., Knight, C., Black, C.M. 1998. Anti-RNA polymerases and other autoantibody specificities in systemic sclerosis. Br. J. Rheumatol. 37, 15–20.

Cannon, P.J., Hassar, M., Case, D.B., Casarella, W.J., Sommers, S.C., LeRoy, E.C. 1974. The relationship of hypertension and renal failure in scleroderma (progressive systemic sclerosis) to structural and functional abnormalities of the renal cortical circulation. Medicine 53, 1–46.

Caplin, N.J., Dikman, S., Winston, J., Spiera, H., Uribarri, J. 1999. Recurrence of scleroderma in a renal allograft from an identical twin sister. Am. J. Kidney Dis. 33, e7.

Caskey, F.J., Thacker, E.J., Johnston, P.A., Barnes, J.N. 1997. Failure of losartan to control blood pressure in scleroderma renal crisis. Lancet 349, 620.

Clements, P.J., Lachenbruch, P.A., Furst, D.E., Maxwell, M., Danovitch, G., Paulus, H.E. 1994. Abnormalities of renal physiology in systemic sclerosis. A prospective study with 10-year followup. Arthritis Rheum. 37, 67–74.

Denton, C.P., Bickerstaff, M.C., Shiwen, X., Carulli, M.T., Haskard, D.O., Dubois, R.M., Black, C.M. 1995. Serial circulating adhesion molecule levels reflect disease severity in systemic sclerosis. Br. J. Rheumatol. 34, 1048–1054.

Denton, C.P., Black, C.M. 2000. Scleroderma and related disorders: therapeutic aspects. Baillieres Best. Pract. Res. Clin. Rheumatol. 14, 17–35.

Denton, C.P., Sweny, P., Abdulla, A., Black, C.M. 1994. Acute renal failure occurring in scleroderma treated with cyclosporin A: a report of three cases. Br. J. Rheumatol. 33, 90–92.

Desai, Y., Ghanekar, M.A., Siquera, R.D., Joshi, V.R. 1990. Renal involvement in scleroderma. J. Assoc. Physicians India 38, 768–770.

Donohoe, J.F. 1992. Scleroderma and the kidney. Kidney Int. 41, 462–477.

Fisher, E.R., Rodnan, G.P. 1958. Pathologic observations concerning renal involvement in progressive systemic sclerosis. Arch. Pathol. 65, 29–39.

Fleischmajer, R., Gould, A.B. 1975. Serum renin and renin substrate levels in scleroderma. Proc. Soc. Exp. Biol. Med. 150, 374–379.

Follansbee, W. 1986. The cardiovascular manifestations of systemic sclerosis (scleroderma). In: R.A. O'Rourke (Ed.), Current Problems in Cardiology. Yearbook Medical Publishers, Inc., Chicago, pp. 245–298. Ref Type: Serial (Book, Monograph).

Gavras, H., Gavras, I., Cannon, P.J., Brunner, H.R., Laragh, J.H. 1977. Is elevated plasma renin activity of prognostic importance in progressive systemic sclerosis? Arch. Intern. Med. 137, 1554–1558.

Hasegawa, S., Iesato, K., Tsukahara, T., Yamamoto, S., Kondou, Y., Ogawa, M., Ueda, S. 2000. Successful use of angiotensin II receptor antagonist (losartan) in a patient with scleroderma renal crisis. Nippon. Jinzo Gakkai Shi 42, 60–65.

Helfrich, D.J., Banner, B., Steen, V.D., Medsger, T.A., Jr. 1989. Normotensive renal failure in systemic sclerosis. Arthritis Rheum. 32, 1128–1134.

Hillis, G.S., Khan, I.H., Simpson, J.G., Rees, A.J. 1997. Scleroderma, D-penicillamine treatment, and progressive renal failure associated with positive antimyeloperoxidase antineutrophil cytoplasmic antibodies. Am. J. Kidney Dis. 30, 279–281.

Kahaleh, M.B., Leroy, E.C. 1999. Autoimmunity and vascular involvement in systemic sclerosis (SSc). Autoimmunity 31, 195–214.

Kapur, A., Ballou, S.P., Renston, J.P., Luna, E., Chung-Park, M. 1997. Recurrent acute scleroderma renal crisis complicated by thrombotic thrombocytopenic purpura. J. Rheumatol. 24, 2469–2472.

Karlen, J.R., Cook, W.A. 1974. Renal scleroderma and pregnancy. Obstet. Gynecol. 44, 349–354.

Karpinski, J., Jothy, S., Radoux, V., Levy, M., Baran, D. 1997. D-penicillamine-induced crescentic glomerulonephritis and antimyeloperoxidase antibodies in a patient with scleroderma. Case report and review of the literature. Am. J. Nephrol. 17, 528–532.

Kfoury Baz, E.M., Mahfouz, R.A., Masri, A.F., Jamaleddine, G.W. 2001. Thrombotic thrombocytopenic purpura in a case of scleroderma renal crisis treated with twice-daily therapeutic plasma exchange. Ren. Fail. 23, 737–742.

Kohno, K., Katayama, T., Majima, K., Fujisawa, M., Iida, S., Fukami, K., Ueda, S., Nishida, H., Sata, M., Kato, S., Morimatsu, M., Okuda, S. 2000. A case of normotensive scleroderma renal crisis after high-dose methylprednisolone treatment [in process citation]. Clin. Nephrol. 53, 479–482.

Korzets, Z., Schneider, M., Savin, H., Ben Chetrit, S., Bernheim, J., Shitrit, P., Bernheim, J. 1998. Intriguing presentation of scleroderma renal crisis (scleroderma renal crisis sine scleroderma sine hypertension). Nephrol. Dial. Transplant. 13, 2953–2956.

Kovalchik, M.T., Guggenheim, S.J., Silverman, M.H., Robertson, J.S., Steigerwald, J.C. 1978. The kidney in progressive systemic sclerosis: a prospective study. Ann. Intern. Med. 89, 881–887.

Lapenas, D., Rodnan, G.P., Cavallo, T. 1978. Immunopathology of the renal vascular lesion of progressive systemic sclerosis (scleroderma). Am. J. Pathol. 91, 243–258.

LeRoy, E.C., Black, C., Fleischmajer, R., Jablonska, S., Krieg, T., Medsger, T.A., Jr., Rowell, N., Wollheim, F. 1988. Scleroderma (systemic sclerosis): classification, subsets and pathogenesis. J. Rheumatol. 15, 202–205.

LeRoy, E.C., Fleischmann, R.M. 1978. The management of renal scleroderma: experience with dialysis, nephrectomy and transplantation. Am. J. Med. 64, 974–978.

Lian, E.C. 2005. Pathogenesis of thrombotic thrombocytopenic purpura: ADAMTS13 deficiency and beyond. Semin. Thromb. Hemost. 31, 625–632.

Locke, I.C., Worrall, J.G., Leaker, B., Black, C.M., Cambridge, G. 1997. Autoantibodies to myeloperoxidase in systemic sclerosis. J. Rheumatol. 24, 86–89.

Lopez-Ovejero, J.A., Saal, S.D., D'Angelo, W.A., Cheigh, J.S., Stenzel, K.H., Laragh, J.H. 1979. Reversal of vascular and renal crises of scleroderma by oral angiotensin-converting-enzyme blockade. N. Engl. J. Med. 300, 1417–1419.

Lunseth, J.H., Baker, L.A., Shifrin, A. 1951. Chronic scleroderma with acute exacerbation during corticotropin therapy. Arch. Intern. Med. 88, 783–792.

Maes, B., Van Mieghem, A., Messiaen, T., Kuypers, D., Van Damme, B., Vanrenterghem, Y. 2000. Limited cutaneous systemic sclerosis associated with MPO-ANCA positive renal small vessel vasculitis of the microscopic polyangiitis type. Am. J. Kidney Dis. 36, E16.

Mallee, C., Meijers, K.A., Cats, A. 1985. Renal scleroderma, value of clinical markers. Clin. Exp. Rheumatol. 3, 287–290.

Manadan, A.M., Harris, C., Block, J.A. 2005. Thrombotic thrombocytopenic purpura in the setting of systemic sclerosis. Semin. Arthritis Rheum. 34, 683–688.

Martinez, A.J., Picazo, M.L., Torre, A., Pascual, D., Diaz, R.C., Rinon, C. 2000. Progressive systemic sclerosis associated with anti-myeloperoxidase ANCA vasculitis with renal and cutaneous involvement. Nefrologia 20, 383–386.

McWhorter, J.E., Leroy, E.C. 1974. Pericardial disease in scleroderma (systemic sclerosis). Am. J. Med. 57, 566–575.

Mitnick, P.D., Feig, P.U. 1978. Control of hypertension and reversal of renal failure in scleroderma. N. Engl. J. Med. 299, 871–872.

Molina, J.F., Anaya, J.M., Cabrera, G.E., Hoffman, E., Espinoza, L.R. 1995. Systemic sclerosis sine scleroderma: an unusual presentation in scleroderma renal crisis. J. Rheumatol. 22, 557–560.

Moorthy, A.V., Wu, M.J., Beirne, G.J., Sundstrom, W.S. 1978. Control of hypertension with acute renal failure in scleroderma without nephrectomy. Lancet 1, 563–564.

Nishijima, C., Sato, S., Hasegawa, M., Nagaoka, T., Hirata, A., Komatsu, K., Takehara, K. 2001. Renal vascular damage in Japanese patients with systemic sclerosis. Rheumatology (Oxford) 40, 406–409.

Nussbaum, A.I., LeRoy, E.C. 1992. Renal involvement in scleroderma. In: The kidney and rheumatic disease. Butterworth, London. pp. 282–296.

Okano, Y., Steen, V.D., Medsger, T.A., Jr. 1993. Autoantibody reactive with RNA polymerase III in systemic sclerosis. Ann. Intern. Med. 119, 1005–1013.

Pham, P.T., Pham, P.C., Danovitch, G.M., Gritsch, H.A., Singer, J., Wallace, W.D., Hayashi, R., Wilkinson, A.H. 2005. Predictors and risk factors for recurrent scleroderma renal crisis in the kidney allograft: case report and review of the literature. Am. J. Transplant. 5, 2565–2569.

Phan, T.G., Cass, A., Gillin, A., Trew, P., Fertig, N., Sturgess, A. 1999. Anti-RNA polymerase III antibodies in the diagnosis of scleroderma renal crisis sine scleroderma. J. Rheumatol. 26, 2489–2492.

Pryde, P.G., Barr, M., Jr. 2001. Low-dose, short-acting, angiotensin-converting enzyme inhibitors as rescue therapy in pregnancy. Obstet. Gynecol. 97, 799–800.

Rivolta, R., Mascagni, B., Berruti, V., Quarto, D.P., Elli, A., Scorza, R., Castagnone, D. 1996. Renal vascular damage in systemic sclerosis patients without clinical evidence of nephropathy. Arthritis Rheum. 39, 1030–1034.

Rocco, M.V., Bleyer, A.J., Burkart, J.M. 1996. Utilization of inpatient and outpatient resources for the management of hemodialysis access complications. Am. J. Kidney Dis. 28, 250–256.

Ruiz, J.C., Val, F., de Francisco, A.L., de Bonis, E., Zubimendi, J.A., Prieto, M., Canga, E., Sanz, d.C., Arias, M. 1991. Progressive systemic sclerosis and renal transplantation: a contraindication to the use of cyclosporine A? Transplant. Proc. 23, 2211–2212.

Scorza, R., Rivolta, R., Mascagni, B., Berruti, V., Bazzi, S., Castagnone, D., Quarto, d.P. 1997. Effect of iloprost infusion on the resistance index of renal vessels of patients with systemic sclerosis. J. Rheumatol. 24, 1944–1948.

Shapiro, A.P., S.M.T.J. 1992. Renal involvement in systemic sclerosis. In: Diseases of the Kidney. Little, Brown and Co, Boston. pp. 2039–2048.

Sharnoff, J.G., C.H.S.I. 1951. Cortison-treated scleroderma. J. Am. Med. Assoc. 145, 1230–1232.

Siragy, H.M., de Gasparo, M., El Kersh, M., Carey, R.M. 2001. Angiotensin-converting enzyme inhibition potentiates angiotensin II type 1 receptor effects on renal bradykinin and cGMP. Hypertension 38, 183–186.

Sokoloff, L. 1952. Some aspects of the pathology of collagen disease. Bull. N. Y. Acad. Med. 32, 760–767.

Steen, V.D. 1999. Pregnancy in women with systemic sclerosis. Obstet. Gynecol. 94, 15–20.

Steen, V.D. 2002. Management of pregnancy in scleroderma renal crisis. Arthritis Rheum. 52, s45. Ref Type: Abstract.

Steen, V.D., Conte, C., Day, N., Ramsey-Goldman, R., Medsger, T.A., Jr. 1989. Pregnancy in women with systemic sclerosis. Arthritis Rheum. 32, 151–157.

Steen, V.D., Costantino, J.P., Shapiro, A.P., Medsger, T.A., Jr. 1990. Outcome of renal crisis in systemic sclerosis: relation to availability of angiotensin converting enzyme (ACE) inhibitors [see comments]. Ann. Intern. Med. 113, 352–357.

Steen, V.D., Lanz, J.K., Jr., Conte, C., Owens, G.R., Medsger, T.A., Jr. 1994. Therapy for severe interstitial lung disease in systemic sclerosis. A retrospective study [see comments]. Arthritis Rheum. 37, 1290–1296.

Steen, V.D., Medsger, T.A., Jr. 1990. Epidemiology and natural history of systemic sclerosis. Rheum. Dis. Clin. N. Am. 16, 1–10.

Steen, V.D., Medsger, T.A., Jr. 1997. The palpable tendon friction rub: an important physical examination finding in patients with systemic sclerosis [see comments]. Arthritis Rheum. 40, 1146–1151.

Steen, V.D., Medsger, T.A., Jr. 1998. Case-control study of corticosteroids and other drugs that either precipitate or protect from the development of scleroderma renal crisis. Arthritis Rheum. 41, 1613–1619.

Steen, V.D., Medsger, T.A., Jr. 2000. Long-term outcomes of scleroderma renal crisis. Ann. Intern. Med. 133, 600–603.

Steen, V.D., Medsger, T.A., Jr., Osial, T.A., Jr., Ziegler, G.L., Shapiro, A.P., Rodnan, G.P. 1984a. Factors predicting development of renal involvement in progressive systemic sclerosis. Am. J. Med. 76, 779–786.

Steen, V.D., Medsger, T.A., Jr., Rodnan, G.P. 1982. D-Penicillamine therapy in progressive systemic sclerosis (scleroderma): a retrospective analysis. Ann. Intern. Med. 97, 652–659.

Steen, V.D., Syzd, A., Johnson, J.P., Greenberg, A., Medsger, T.A., Jr. 2005. Kidney disease other than renal crisis in patients with diffuse scleroderma. J. Rheumatol. 32, 649–655.

Steen, V.D., Ziegler, G.L., Rodnan, G.P., Medsger, T.A., Jr. 1984b. Clinical and laboratory associations of anticentromere antibody in patients with progressive systemic sclerosis. Arthritis Rheum. 27, 125–131.

Stone, R.A., Tisher, C.C., Hawkins, H.K., Robinson, R.R. 1974. Juxtaglomerular hyperplasia and hyperreninemia in progressive systemic sclerosis complicated acute renal failure. Am. J. Med. 56, 119–123.

Stratton, R.J., Coghlan, J.G., Pearson, J.D., Burns, A., Sweny, P., Abraham, D.J., Black, C.M. 1998. Different patterns of endothelial cell activation in renal and pulmonary vascular disease in scleroderma. Q. J. Med. 91, 561–566.

Thurm, R.H., Alexander, J.C. 1984. Captopril in the treatment of scleroderma renal crisis. Arch. Intern. Med. 144, 733–735.

Traub, Y.M., Shapiro, A.P., Rodnan, G.P., Medsger, T.A., McDonald, R.H., Jr., Steen, V.D., Osial, T.A., Jr., Tolchin, S.F. 1983. Hypertension and renal failure (scleroderma renal crisis) in progressive systemic sclerosis. Review of a 25-year experience with 68 cases. Medicine (Baltimore) 62, 335–352.

Trostle, D.C., Bedetti, C.D., Steen, V.D., al Sabbagh, M.R., Zee, B., Medsger, T.A., Jr. 1988. Renal vascular histology and morphometry in systemic sclerosis. A case-control autopsy study. Arthritis Rheum. 31, 393–400.

Tsakiris, D., Simpson, H.K., Jones, E.H., Briggs, J.D., Elinder, C.G., Mendel, S., Piccoli, G., dos Santos, J.P., Tognoni, G., Vanrenterghem, Y., Valderrabano, F. 1996. Report on management of renal failure in Europe, XXVI, 1995. Rare diseases in renal replacement therapy in the ERA-EDTA Registry. Nephrol. Dial. Transplant. 11 (Suppl. 7), 4–20.

Urai, l.S., G.N.Z.W.W. 1958. Renal function in scleroderma. Br. Med. J. 2, 1264–1266.

Vancheeswaran, R., Magoulas, T., Efrat, G., Wheeler-Jones, C., Olsen, I., Penny, R., Black, C.M. 1994. Circulating endothelin-1 levels in systemic sclerosis subsets—a marker of fibrosis or vascular dysfunction? [see comments]. J. Rheumatol. 21, 1838–1844.

Wasner, C., Cooke, C.R., Fries, J.F. 1978. Successful medical treatment of scleroderma renal crisis. N. Engl. J. Med. 299, 873–875.

Whitman, H.H., III, Case, D.B., Laragh, J.H., Christian, C.L., Botstein, G., Maricq, H., Leroy, E.C. 1982. Variable response to oral angiotensin-converting-enzyme blockade in hypertensive scleroderma patients. Arthritis Rheum. 25, 241–248.

Woodhall, P.B., McCoy, R.C., Gunnells, J.C., Seigler, H.F. 1976. Apparent recurrence of progressive systemic sclerosis in a renal allograft. J. Am. Med. Assoc. 236, 1032–1034.

Yamanishi, Y., Yamana, S., Ishioka, S., Yamakido, M. 1996. Development of ischemic colitis and scleroderma renal crisis following methylprednisolone pulse therapy for progressive systemic sclerosis. Intern. Med. 35, 583–586.

Zawada, E.T., Jr., Clements, P.J., Furst, D.A., Bloomer, H.A., Paulus, H.E., Maxwell, M.H. 1981. Clinical course of patients with scleroderma renal crisis treated with captopril. Nephron. 27, 74–78.

# CHAPTER 21

# Amyloidosis

Julian D. Gillmore*, Philip N. Hawkins

*National Amyloidosis Centre, Centre for Amyloidosis and Acute Phase Proteins, Department of Medicine, University College London, Hampstead Campus, Rowland Hill Street, London NW3 2PF, UK*

## 1. Introduction

Amyloidosis is a clinical disorder caused by extracellular deposition of insoluble abnormal fibrils, derived from aggregation of misfolded normally soluble protein. Over 20 different unrelated proteins are known to form amyloid fibrils in vivo, which share a pathognomonic ultrastructure and tinctorial properties. Systemic amyloidosis, in which amyloid deposits are present in the viscera, blood vessel walls, and connective tissues, is progressive and frequently fatal and is the cause of about one per thousand deaths in developed countries. There are also various localized forms of amyloidosis in which the deposits are confined to specific foci or to a particular organ or tissue. These may be clinically silent or trivial and discovered incidentally, or they may be associated with serious disease, such as hemorrhage in local respiratory or urogenital tract AL amyloidosis. In addition there are important diseases associated with local amyloid deposition in which the pathogenetic role of the amyloid remains unclear, notably including Alzheimer's disease, the prion disorders, and type II diabetes mellitus.

In addition to the fibrils, amyloid deposits always contain the normal plasma protein serum amyloid P component (SAP), because it binds specifically to an as yet uncharacterized ligand expressed by all amyloid fibrils. Radiolabelled SAP is a specific, quantitative tracer for imaging amyloid deposits scintigraphically (Hawkins, 2002). Treatment of amyloidosis comprises measures to support impaired organ function, including renal replacement therapy and organ transplantation, along with vigorous efforts to control underlying conditions responsible for production of fibril precursors. Serial SAP scintigraphy has demonstrated that reduction of the supply of amyloid fibril precursor proteins leads to regression of amyloid deposits and clinical benefit in many cases.

## 2. Pathogenesis of amyloidosis

Amyloidogenesis involves substantial refolding of the native structures of the various amyloid precursor proteins, which enables them to auto-aggregate in a highly ordered manner to form fibrils with a characteristic $\beta$-sheet structure (Sunde et al., 1997). Amyloid fibrils may contain the intact amyloidogenic protein or be composed of cleavage fragments. Structurally normal transthyretin (TTR) is inherently amyloidogenic and even at normal concentrations it forms amyloid fibrils in almost all individuals over 80 years of age, sometimes causing senile systemic amyloidosis. The other protein precursors with wild-type sequence which can form amyloid fibrils in vivo, serum amyloid A protein (SAA) and $\beta_2$-microglobulin ($\beta_2$m), do so only when they have been

---

*Corresponding author.
Tel.: +44-20-7433-2726; Fax: +44-20-7433-2817
*E-mail address:* j.gillmore@medsch.ucl.ac.uk

© 2008 Elsevier B.V. All rights reserved.
DOI: 10.1016/S1571-5078(07)07021-3

present at grossly supraphysiological concentrations for prolonged periods. Variant proteins with enhanced amyloidogenicity can be acquired, as with the monoclonal immunoglobulin light chains responsible for AL amyloidosis, or inherited as in familial amyloidosis. There is always a lag period, often of many years, between first appearance of a potentially amyloidogenic protein and the deposition of clinically significant amyloid, but accumulation of amyloid can nevertheless occur very rapidly once the process has begun, probably reflecting a seeding phenomenon. Amyloidosis is exceptionally rare in children and even young adults, and increasing age may thus favor amyloid deposition, although the underlying mechanisms are not known.

All amyloid deposits contain abundant heparan sulfate and dermatan sulfate proteoglycans and glycosaminoglycan chains, some of which are tightly bound to the fibrils and may contribute to amyloid fibrillogenesis as well as stabilization of the fibril structure (Kisilevsky and Fraser, 1996). All amyloid deposits also contain amyloid P component, which is identical to and derived from the normal circulating plasma protein SAP. SAP undergoes avid (Kd~1 µmol/l), specific, calcium dependent, reversible binding to amyloid fibrils of all types leading to its remarkable specific concentration in amyloid deposits. SAP binds both to glycosaminoglycans and to protein ligands specifically present on all types of amyloid fibril, and may also promote formation and/or stabilize the fibrils (Tennent et al., 1995; Pepys et al., 2002). Other plasma proteins, such as apolipoprotein E, are sometimes detectable in amyloid deposits, but none with the universality and abundance of SAP.

The mechanisms by which amyloid deposits damage tissues and compromise organ function are incompletely understood. Massive deposits, which may amount to kilograms, are structurally disruptive and incompatible with normal function, as are strategically located small deposits, for example, in the glomeruli or nerves. However, the relationship between quantity of amyloid and organ dysfunction differs greatly between individuals, and there is a suggestion that the rate of new amyloid deposition may be more important a determinant of progressive organ failure than the amyloid load itself. In vitro studies have suggested that certain isolated amyloid fibrils have cytotoxic properties (Bucciantini et al., 2002).

Major unanswered questions concern the tissue distribution and time of appearance of amyloid deposits as well as their variable clinical consequences. Although many features of the various forms of amyloidosis overlap, the clinical phenotype associated with a particular fibril type can be enormously variable, even between family members with identical amyloidogenic mutations. There are clearly major genetic or environmental factors that influence amyloidogenesis in vivo, other than simply the presence of an adequate supply of amyloidogenic protein precursor.

## 3. Clinical amyloidosis

### 3.1. Localized amyloidosis

The commonest form of local amyloidosis is caused by foci of otherwise benign monoclonal B-cells or plasma cells producing monoclonal immunoglobulin light chains (L) that are deposited as AL amyloid, most frequently in the respiratory tract, urogenital tract, or skin. (Amyloidosis nomenclature comprises the letter A to designate amyloid, followed by an abbreviation of the name of the fibril protein.) Local amyloid composed of $\beta$-protein within the walls of cerebral blood vessels can be responsible for Congophilic amyloid angiopathy causing cerebral hemorrhage and stroke. Peptide hormones forming amyloid deposits in benign or malignant tumors of endocrine tissue, and microscopic senile amyloid deposits, composed of various different proteins in the arterial wall, the heart, the seminal vesicles, and the prostate, are incidental histological findings with little evidence that the amyloid causes disease.

### 3.2. Acquired systemic amyloidosis

Acquired systemic amyloidosis is the cause of death in about 1 in 1000 of the British population, and is probably much under-diagnosed in the elderly population in which it probably occurs most frequently. Systemic AL amyloidosis is the most serious and commonly diagnosed form, outnumbering referrals of AA amyloidosis to the UK National Amyloidosis Centre by fourfold. Although less serious, dialysis-related $\beta_2$-microglobulin amyloidosis causes much suffering in about one million patients receiving long-term renal replacement therapy worldwide. Senile systemic amyloidosis, which predominantly involves the heart and is often referred to as senile cardiac amyloidosis, occurs in about one-quarter of individuals over the age of 80 years, a sector of the population that is ever rising.

*Systemic AA amyloidosis* formerly known as secondary amyloidosis, is a complication of chronic infections and inflammatory conditions characterized by a sustained acute phase response in which there is persistently increased production of SAA. SAA is an apolipoprotein of high-density lipoprotein particles, produced predominantly in the liver, and is, together with C-reactive protein, the most dynamic acute phase protein. SAA concentration rises from less than 5 mg/l in healthy subjects to as much as 2000 mg/l at the peak of a severe acute phase response. In rheumatoid arthritis, juvenile rheumatoid arthritis, other inflammatory arthritides, Crohn's disease, familial Mediterranean fever, and the various hereditary periodic fever syndromes, the SAA concentration typically remains markedly elevated for months and years unless the inflammatory activity spontaneously remits or is suppressed by therapy. Up to around 5% of individuals with sustained high SAA values may eventually develop AA amyloidosis. In hereditary periodic fever syndromes, the genetic bases of which are increasingly being elucidated, the incidence of AA amyloidosis can be much higher. A small number of patients with AA amyloidosis have no clinically overt inflammatory disease, although some are carriers of inherited fever syndrome genes.

AA amyloid involves the viscera but may be widely distributed without causing clinical symptoms. More than 95% of patients present with non-selective proteinuria, or renal impairment (Lachmann et al., 2005). Hematuria, isolated tubular defects, nephrogenic diabetes insipidus, and diffuse renal calcification occur rarely. Kidney size is typically normal, but may be enlarged, or, in advanced cases, reduced. End-stage chronic kidney disease and its complications are the cause of death in 40–60% of patients with AA amyloidosis. Amyloidotic kidneys are overly sensitive to insults and acute renal failure may be easily precipitated by hypotension and/or salt and water depletion following surgery, excessive use of diuretics, or intercurrent infection. The second most common presentation is with organ enlargement, such as hepatosplenomegaly or occasionally thyroid goiter, with or without overt renal abnormality, but in such cases amyloid deposits are almost always widespread at the time of presentation (Lovat et al., 1998). Clinically significant involvement of the heart is rare in AA amyloidosis, as is liver failure, but gastrointestinal amyloid deposits resulting in dysfunction, including bleeding, are common in advanced disease (Lovat et al., 1997).

The median duration of inflammatory disorders associated with AA amyloidosis is 17 years, but latency can be as short as just 1 year. The prognosis is closely related to the degree of renal dysfunction (Lachmann et al., 2005) and the effectiveness of anti-inflammatory treatment (Gillmore et al., 2001), although availability of hemodialysis and renal transplantation prevents early death from uraemia per se.

*Systemic AL amyloidosis* previously known as primary amyloidosis, is the most common form of clinical amyloid disease in developed countries. AL fibrils are derived from monoclonal immunoglobulin light chains and consist of the whole or part of the variable (VL) domain. Almost any B-cell dyscrasia, including myeloma, lymphomas, and macroglobulinaemia, may be complicated by AL amyloidosis, but over 80% of cases are associated with subtle and otherwise "benign" monoclonal gammopathies. Histologically, amyloid deposition occurs in up to 15% of patients with myeloma, but usually in clinically insignificant amounts, and about 2% of patients with "benign" monoclonal gammopathy develop clinical amyloidosis. A monoclonal paraprotein or free light chain can be detected in serum or urine by conventional electrophoresis and immunofixation in only about 80–90% patients with AL amyloidosis (Kyle and Greipp, 1983), but high sensitivity serum free light chain assays can confirm a monoclonal gammopathy in most remaining cases. Until recently it was common practice to diagnose apparent "primary" cases of amyloidosis, with no previous predisposing inflammatory condition or family history of amyloidosis, as AL type by exclusion. However, it has lately been recognized that hereditary amyloidosis is often poorly penetrant and can have a late onset, so that there may be no family history (Lachmann et al., 2002). The coincident occurrence of a monoclonal gammopathy may then be gravely misleading and it is essential to exclude all known amyloidogenic mutations (see below) when immunohistochemical or biochemical identification of the amyloid fibril protein has not given positive results.

AL amyloid occurs equally in men and women, usually over the age of 50 but as early as the third decade. The clinical manifestations are protean, as virtually any tissue other than the brain may be directly involved (Kyle and Gertz, 1995). Uraemia, heart failure, or other effects of the amyloid usually cause death within 1–2 years of diagnosis, unless the underlying B-cell clone is suppressed. The heart is affected pathologically in up to 90% of AL patients, in 30% of whom restrictive cardiomyopathy is the presenting feature. Renal AL amyloid has the same manifestations as renal AA amyloid, but the prognosis is worse. Gut involvement may cause motility disturbances (often secondary to autonomic neuropathy), malabsorption, perforation, hemorrhage, or obstruction. Macroglossia occurs rarely but is almost pathognomonic. Hyposplenism sometimes occurs in both AA and AL amyloidosis. Painful sensory polyneuropathy with early loss of pain and temperature sensation followed later by motor deficits is seen in 10–20% of cases and carpal tunnel syndrome in 20%. Autonomic neuropathy leading to orthostatic hypotension, impotence, and gastrointestinal disturbances may occur alone or together with peripheral neuropathy, and has a very poor prognosis. Skin involvement takes the form of papules, nodules, and plaques usually on the face and upper trunk, and involvement of dermal blood vessels results in purpura occurring either spontaneously or after minimal trauma and is quite common. Articular amyloid is rare but the symptoms may mimic an inflammatory polyarthritis. Infiltration of the glenohumeral joint and surrounding soft tissues occasionally produces the characteristic "shoulder pad" sign. A rare but serious manifestation of AL amyloid is an acquired bleeding diathesis that may be associated with deficiency of factor X and sometimes also factor IX; this does not occur in AA amyloidosis, but vascular deposits in all types of systemic amyloidosis may cause serious bleeding in the absence of a clotting factor deficiency.

*Dialysis associated amyloidosis* ($A\beta_2m$) is a complication of long-term dialysis for end-stage renal failure. $\beta_2$-microglobulin ($\beta_2m$), the invariant chain of the MHC class I molecule, is cleared and catabolized only by the kidney and is very poorly cleared by peritoneal or hemodialysis. In end stage renal failure its circulating concentration rises from 1–2 to around 50–70 mg/l. Histological studies have shown the presence of early subclinical $\beta_2m$ amyloid deposits among 20–30% of patients within 3 years of commencing dialysis. Some individuals develop symptoms within 3–5 years and by 20 years the prevalence is almost 100% (Drüeke, 1998). $\beta_2m$ amyloid is preferentially deposited in articular and peri-articular structures and its manifestations are largely confined to the locomotor system. Carpal tunnel syndrome is usually the presenting feature and is frequently followed by amyloid arthropathy. The arthralgia of $A\beta_2m$ affects the shoulders, knees, wrists, and small joints of the hand and is associated with joint swelling, chronic tenosynovitis, and occasionally hemarthroses. Although $A\beta_2m$ is a systemic form of amyloid, and there have been occasional reports of congestive cardiac failure, gastrointestinal symptoms and macroglossia, manifestations outside the musculoskeletal system are rare. $A\beta_2m$ is an intractable complication of long-term dialysis, for which the only effective treatment is renal transplantation. However the incidence is apparently now falling, possibly due to use of new dialysis membranes, cleaner dialysis fluids, and higher flux dialysis.

*Senile transthyretin amyloidosis (ATTR).* Over the age of 80 years wild-type TTR amyloid deposits in the heart, kidneys, and respiratory tract are an almost universal incidental finding at autopsy, but some elderly patients with more extensive TTR amyloid deposits in the heart develop a clinically significant restrictive cardiomyopathy. This syndrome, often known as senile cardiac amyloidosis is untreatable, other than by heart transplantation in rare younger patients. Occasionally, amyloid deposits derived from genetically variant TTR are deposited predominantly in the heart and present in a similar manner, notably including TTR Ile122 in black Africans (see Hereditary amyloidosis below).

## 3.3. Hereditary systemic amyloidosis

This disorder is rare but can sometimes be treated very effectively, and its study has provided invaluable information on amyloid fibrillogenesis and pathogenetic mechanisms, leading to development of new potential therapies for amyloidosis. The most common cause of hereditary amyloidosis is a mutation in the gene for TTR, which affects around perhaps 10,000 individuals worldwide. The other amyloid fibril proteins that cause hereditary amyloidosis are apolipoproteins AI and AII, fibrinogen A α-chain, gelsolin, and lysozyme in systemic amyloidosis, cystatin C in the Icelandic form of hereditary cerebral hemorrhage with amyloidosis and β-protein in the Dutch form of this disease. Over 80 mutations, most of which are amyloidogenic, are known in TTR and new amyloidogenic mutations in the other proteins listed continue to be discovered.

Severe and ultimately fatal peripheral and/or autonomic neuropathy are major features of hereditary TTR amyloidosis (familial amyloid polyneuropathy) but fatal cardiac and subtle but significant renal involvement are also common. ApoAI amyloidosis sometimes causes neuropathy but this is not a feature of the other hereditary amyloid types which typically involve the viscera. Age of onset, distribution of amyloid deposits, and clinical presentation can vary widely both within and between families, even with the same mutation. All the amyloidogenic mutations are dominant but they are variably penetrant and there may be no family history. AL amyloidosis is sometimes diagnosed by exclusion because rigorous positive immunohistochemical identification of AL type fibrils is not possible in some cases. Without use of the new sensitive and reliable test for free immunoglobulin light chains in serum, the amyloid deposits may be the only sign of monoclonal gammopathy. Thus, there is scope for misdiagnosis of hereditary amyloidosis as AL type, and the inappropriate use of dangerous cytotoxic regimens aimed at ablation of clonal B-cell disease. It is mandatory that the amyloid fibril type is positively identified in all systemic amyloidosis patients and/or that there is comprehensive testing for all known amyloidogenic mutations (Lachmann et al., 2002).

### 3.3.1. Familial amyloidotic polyneuropathy
Familial amyloidotic polyneuropathy (FAP) is caused by point mutations in the gene for the plasma protein TTR and is an autosomal dominant syndrome with variable penetrance. Symptoms typically present between the third and seventh decades. The disease is characterized by progressive and disabling peripheral and autonomic neuropathy, and varying degrees of visceral amyloid involvement. Severe cardiac amyloidosis is common. Deposits within the vitreous of the eye occur in a proportion of cases and are very characteristic, but renal, thyroid, splenic and adrenal deposits are usually asymptomatic. There are well-recognized foci in Portugal, Japan, and Sweden but FAP has been reported in most ethnic groups throughout the world. There is considerable phenotypic variation in the age of onset, rate of progression, involvement of different systems, and disease penetrance generally, although within families the pattern may be quite consistent. More than 80 variant forms of TTR are associated with FAP, the most frequent of which is Met30. TTR Ala60 is the most frequent cause of FAP in the British population, and usually presents after age 50 years, often with predominant cardiac amyloidosis.

### 3.3.2. Hereditary lysosyme amyloidosis

Hereditary non-neuropathic systemic amyloidosis has been described in association with five lysozyme variants, His67, Thr56, Ile57, Asn70, and Arg64. Most patients present in middle age with proteinuria, very slowly progressive renal impairment and sometimes hepatosplenomegaly with or without purpuric rashes. Virtually all patients have substantial gastrointestinal amyloid deposits, and although these are often asymptomatic, they are important since gastrointestinal hemorrhage or perforation is a frequent cause of death (Gillmore et al., 1999).

### 3.3.3. Hereditary apolipoprotein AI amyloidosis

About a dozen amyloidogenic variants are known, which variably present with massive abdominal visceral amyloid involvement, predominant cardiomyopathy, hoarseness, skin amyloid, or an FAP-like syndrome. The majority of patients eventually develop renal failure but despite extensive hepatic amyloid deposition, liver function usually remains well preserved (Joy et al., 2003). Normal wild-type apolipoprotein AI amyloid is itself weakly amyloidogenic, and is the precursor of small amyloid deposits that occur quite frequently in aortic atherosclerotic plaques (Westermark et al., 1995).

### 3.3.4. Hereditary fibrinogen A alpha chain amyloidosis

Fibrinogen A alpha chain was first isolated from amyloid fibrils in 1993. Four amyloidogenic mutations have been described in eight unrelated kindreds. These include Leu554 and two frame shifting deletion mutations. However, the commonest variant is Val526, which is now known to have low penetrance in most families. Indeed, 5% of patients referred to the UK National Amyloidosis Centre with a diagnosis of acquired AL amyloidosis have been shown on further investigation to have hereditary fibrinogen A alpha chain Val526 amyloidosis. Most patients present in middle age with proteinuria or hypertension and progress to end-stage renal failure over 4–10 years. Amyloid deposition is seen in the kidneys, spleen, and sometimes the liver but is usually asymptomatic in the latter two sites. Renal grafts frequently fail within 7 years due to recurrent amyloidosis.

### 3.4. The kidneys in systemic amyloidosis

Amyloid is frequently deposited in the kidneys in nearly all forms of systemic amyloidosis. Amyloid deposition is the major finding in 2.5% of all native renal biopsies. Over 90% of patients with AA amyloidosis present with renal manifestations, typically proteinuria and/or renal impairment. Approximately 50% of patients with systemic AL amyloidosis are diagnosed by histological examination of a renal biopsy specimen and a renal presentation is typical in patients with hereditary fibrinogen A alpha chain, apolipoprotein AI, apolipoprotein AII, and lysozyme amyloid types. Renal amyloid is a cause of very heavy proteinuria although occasionally renal function may remain normal despite substantial parenchymal deposits demonstrable by SAP scintigraphy, particularly in hereditary TTR and hereditary gelsolin amyloidosis. The susceptibility of amyloid-laden kidneys to acute insults is undoubtedly increased and their capacity to recover following an episode of acute renal failure is substantially reduced compared to acute renal failure in the absence of amyloid.

The natural history of renal disease due to amyloid is variable, usually reflects the natural history of the extra-renal disease and is dependent, in part, upon amyloid type. Renal progression in hereditary apolipoprotein AI amyloidosis is typically very slow. The median time from presentation to end-stage renal failure in one study was 8 years (Gillmore et al., 2006), contrasting with systemic AL amyloidosis, in which the median time to end-stage renal failure is usually around 1 year (Gertz et al., 1992).

Progression to end-stage renal failure in renal amyloidosis is common and occurs in approximately one third of patients with AA, one quarter of patients with AL and all patients with hereditary renal amyloidosis. The survival of patients requiring dialysis partly depends on amyloid type and is excellent among those with hereditary renal amyloidosis but poor among patients with AL type (median 8 months in some series (Gertz et al., 1992)). Dialysis modality is not particularly influenced by the presence of amyloid, although patients with severe cardiac and/or autonomic nerve involvement by amyloid may be exquisitely sensitive to intravascular volume change and therefore tolerate hemodialysis poorly.

Replacement of failing organs in systemic amyloidosis has been controversial due to concerns regarding accumulation of amyloid in the graft and progressive amyloid accumulation in other organs (Pasternack et al., 1986). Patient survival after cardiac transplantation for AL amyloid cardiomyopathy is reduced compared to survival following cardiac transplantation for other causes (Dubrey et al., 2004), and patient survival after renal transplantation is reportedly reduced in patients with amyloidosis compared to patients with other causes of end-stage renal failure (Celik et al., 2006). Recurrence of amyloid causing graft failure is unusual in AA amyloidosis and occurs only very slowly after renal transplantation in apolipoprotein AI and apolipoprotein AII amyloidosis (Magy et al., 2003; Gillmore et al., 2006).

Experience with renal transplantation at the UK National Amyloidosis Centre has generally been favorable. Among 30 patients with AA amyloidosis followed up at our unit who underwent renal transplantation, 1 year patient and graft survival was 93 and 83% respectively, with 5 year patient and graft survivals of 93 and 74% respectively. Median graft survival was over 12 years. Among 17 patients with AL amyloidosis who received renal transplants, 1 year patient and graft survivals were both 93%, with 5 year patient and graft survival of 71 and 68% respectively. Among patients with hereditary renal amyloidosis 1 and 5 year patient and graft survivals were all around 90% (data unpublished).

Therapy to suppress the production of the fibril precursor protein can favorably alter the natural history and outcome of renal amyloidosis, which may include complete resolution of nephrotic range proteinuria, improvement in renal excretory function and prevention of amyloid recurrence causing renal allograft failure (Gillmore et al., 2001, 2006). In addition, such therapy frequently halts the progression of extra-renal amyloid deposits, even among patients who may already be dialysis dependent, thereby prolonging overall patient survival. Further details regarding available therapies are outlined in the management section below.

## 4. Diagnosis of amyloidosis

Until recently amyloidosis was an exclusively histological diagnosis, and green birefringence of deposits stained with Congo red when viewed in cross-polarized light remains the gold standard. Immunohistochemical staining of amyloid-containing tissue is the simplest method for identifying the amyloid fibril type. However, biopsies provide small samples that cannot provide information on the extent, localization, progression, or regression of amyloid deposits, aspects in which histology is complemented by whole body radiolabeled SAP scintigraphy.

### 4.1. Histochemical diagnosis of amyloid

Amyloid may be an incidental finding on biopsy of the kidneys, liver, heart, bowel, peripheral nerve, lymph node, skin, thyroid, or bone marrow. When amyloidosis is suspected clinically, biopsy of rectum or subcutaneous fat is least invasive with a sensitivity of more than 90% in cases of systemic AA or AL. Alternatively, a clinically affected tissue may be biopsied directly. Many cotton dyes, fluorochromes, and metachromatic stains have been used, but Congo red staining is the pathognomonic histochemical test for amyloidosis. The stain is unstable and must be freshly prepared every 2 months or less. Section thickness of 5–10 μm and inclusion in every staining run of a positive control tissue containing modest amounts of amyloid are critical.

### 4.1.1. Immunohistochemistry

Although many amyloid fibril proteins can be identified immunohistochemically, demonstration of amyloidogenic proteins in tissue does not, on its own, establish the presence of amyloid. Congo red staining and green birefringence are always required. Commercially available antibodies to SAA and $\beta_2$M generally yield definitive results, but AL deposits are stainable with standard antisera to $\kappa$ or $\lambda$ light chains in only about half of fixed biopsies. Immunohistochemical staining of amyloid may require pre-treatment of sections with formic acid or alkaline guanidine or deglycosylation.

### 4.1.2. Electron microscopy

Transmission electron microscopy reveals the typical fibrillar ultrastructure of tissue amyloid deposits, but fibrils cannot always be convincingly identified, and electron microscopy alone is not sufficient to confirm the diagnosis of amyloidosis. Isolated purified amyloid fibrils can be imaged by negatively stained electron microscopy as straight, non-branching fibrils of indeterminate length, and about 10 nm in diameter.

## 4.2. Non-histological investigations

Two-dimensional echocardiography showing small, concentrically hypertrophied ventricles, generally impaired contraction, dilated atria, homogeneously echogenic valves, and increased echodensity of ventricular walls is virtually diagnostic of cardiac amyloidosis. However, clinically significant restrictive diastolic impairment may be difficult to detect even by comprehensive Doppler and other functional studies. Imaging after injection of isotope-labeled calcium-seeking tracers has poor sensitivity and specificity and is of no routine clinical value. Recent studies of cardiac magnetic resonance imaging seem promising.

In cases of known or suspected hereditary amyloidosis the gene defect must be characterized, but it remains essential to corroborate DNA findings by confirming one way or another that the respective protein is indeed the main constituent of the amyloid.

A high sensitivity latex enhanced serum immunoassay has lately been developed which can quantify circulating free immunoglobulin light chains with remarkable sensitivity of < 5 mg/l (Bradwell et al., 2001). This compares with typical detection limits of 150–500 mg/l by immunofixation, and 500–2000 mg/l by electrophoresis. In a series of 262 patients undergoing assessment at the UK National Amyloidosis Centre, a monoclonal immunoglobulin could not be detected at presentation by electrophoresis or immunofixation, in either serum or urine, in 21% of cases. In a further 26% monoclonal light chains could only be detected qualitatively by immunofixation. By contrast, monoclonal free immunoglobulin light chains were quantified using the serum free light chain immunoassay in 98% of patients. This assay has a major application in monitoring the response to chemotherapy of the clonal disease in patients with AL amyloidosis, enabling such treatment to be given on a much more rational basis than previously.

### 4.2.1. SAP scintigraphy

SAP is a highly conserved, invariant plasma glycoprotein of the pentraxin family that becomes specifically and highly concentrated in amyloid deposits of all types as a result of its calcium dependent binding to amyloid fibrils. Following intravenous injection, radiolabeled SAP distributes between the circulating and the amyloid-bound SAP pools in proportion to their size and can then be imaged and quantified (Hawkins et al., 1990). This safe non-invasive method uniquely provides invaluable information on the diagnosis, distribution and extent of amyloid deposits throughout the body, and serial scans monitor progress and response to therapy. Serial SAP scans have unequivocally demonstrated that amyloid deposits of all types can regress when the supply of the respective amyloid fibril precursor protein is sufficiently reduced (Fig. 1) (Gillmore et al., 1998, 2001; Rydh et al., 1998). This technique is not available commercially but is used routinely in the UK National Amyloidosis Centre.

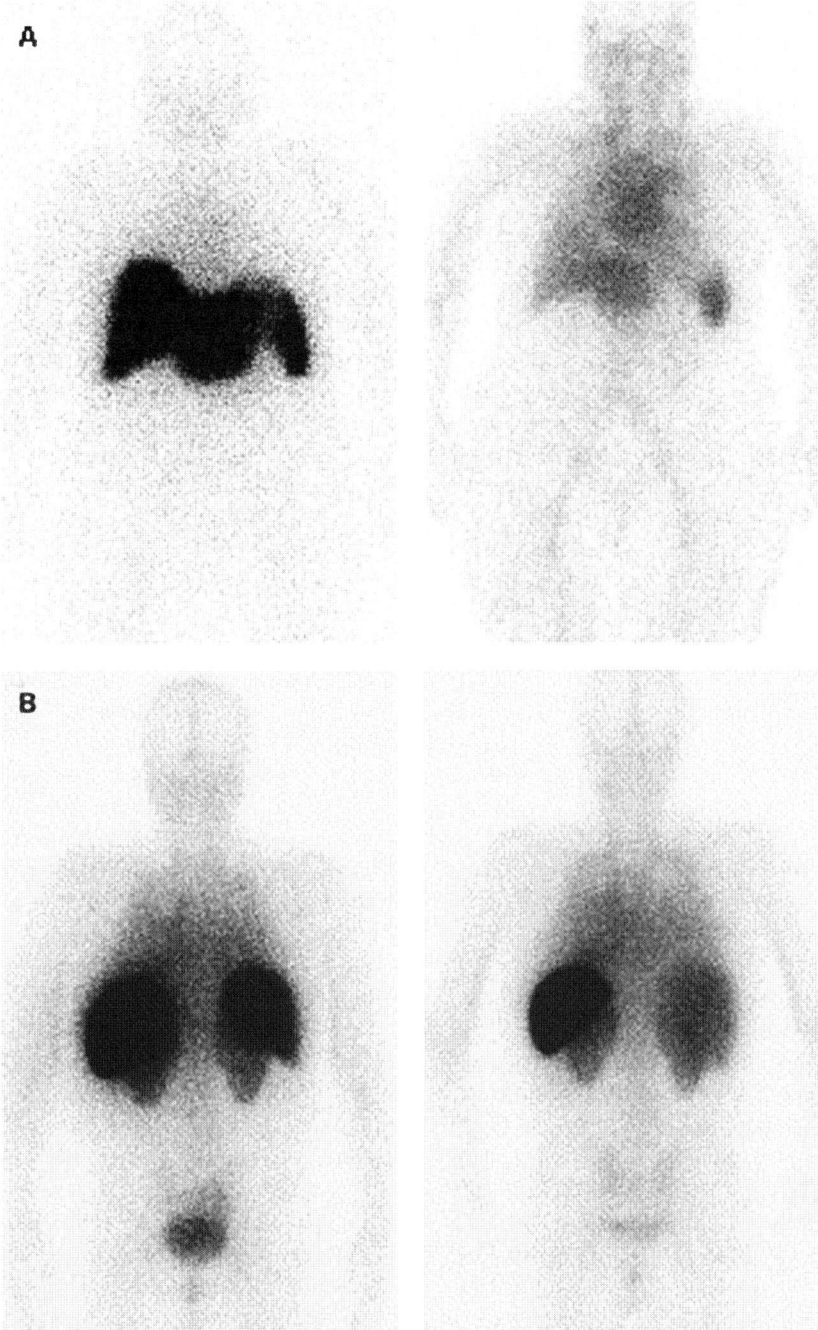

**Figure 1.** (A) Serial anterior whole-body scintigraphs in a patient with AL amyloidosis treated with oral melphalan and corticosteroids: baseline scan (left) showed extensive amyloid deposits in the liver and spleen obscuring the signal from the kidneys; follow-up scintigraphy 6 months later (right) showed complete regression of amyloid from the liver and marked regression from the spleen with a reciprocal increase in the blood-pool signal. (B) Serial posterior whole-body $^{123}$I-labelled SAP scintigraphy in a 19-year-old man with sustained remission from juvenile rheumatoid arthritis. Median SAA values were < 10 mg/l during this 2-year interval: baseline scan (left) showed extensive amyloid deposits in liver, spleen, and kidneys which had regressed very prominently in the liver at follow-up (right). The patient had not voided before the baseline scan, which shows radioactive degradation products in the urinary bladder.

## 5. Management of amyloidosis

Localized amyloid masses can only be treated surgically. In the absence of available generic anti-amyloid therapy, the twin aims of management in systemic amyloidosis are reduction of the supply of the respective amyloid fibril precursor protein so that amyloid deposition ceases and regression of existing deposits may occur, and scrupulous supportive care, including dialysis and organ transplantation. The prognosis of systemic amyloidosis remains poor for many patients, especially those with AL type in whom there is often a significant delay before diagnosis by which time there is substantial visceral and/or neural involvement, but recent advances have greatly extended median survival times. Awareness of the compromised functional reserve of amyloidotic organs and extreme care to protect renal function are critically important. Outcomes are much better in centers with specialist expertise.

Rational management has been greatly improved by recent availability of routine assays for circulating SAA in AA, and immunoglobulin free light chains in AL amyloidosis. Treatment of the underlying inflammatory disorder in AA amyloidosis, to reduce SAA values ideally to normal, dramatically improves survival, halts ongoing amyloid accumulation, and slows or even reverses the decline in renal function (Gillmore et al., 2001). The new biologic agents that neutralize tumor necrosis factor (TNF) and interleukin-1, potently suppress the acute phase response in many patients with rheumatoid arthritis, seronegative spondyloarthropathies, Crohn's disease, and some hereditary periodic fever syndromes. Treatment with colchicine prevents AA amyloidosis in familial Mediterranean fever (Zemer et al., 1986). Excision of solitary Castleman's disease masses that produce IL-6 can be every effective when this condition is complicated by AA amyloidosis (Vigushin et al., 1994).

Suppression of the B-cells producing amyloidogenic monoclonal immunoglobulin light chains through chemotherapy is associated with arrest of amyloid deposition, regression of deposits, preservation of organ function, and enhanced survival in many patients with systemic AL amyloidosis (Kyle et al., 1997). Availability of the robust, sensitive, Freelite™ immunoassay for immunoglobulin free light chains in serum has been one of the most important advances in management of AL amyloidosis (Bradwell et al., 2001; Lachmann et al., 2003). The AL fibril precursor protein can now be monitored prospectively and chemotherapy tailored accordingly. Sustained reduction of the serum concentration of free monoclonal light chains reduces amyloid deposition, and although suppression by 50% or more was associated with enhanced survival in a cohort of patients with AL amyloidosis, the degree of suppression required to prevent ongoing amyloid accumulation varies substantially between individuals (Lachmann et al., 2003). Unfortunately, many patients with AL amyloidosis tolerate chemotherapy poorly, and a proportion of plasma cell clones are refractory to high-dose therapy. Oral melphalan and prednisolone is better tolerated than more aggressive treatment regimens but responses are few and often very delayed (Gertz et al., 1991). Intermediate dose infusional chemotherapy regimens, such as vincristine, adriamycin, and dexamethasone, or melphalan and dexamethasone can induce swifter responses (Goodman et al., 2004, 2005). High-dose chemotherapy with peripheral stem cell rescue has lately been used quite widely, but treatment related mortality is extremely high at 15–25% in this setting, especially outside specialist amyloidosis centers (Comenzo and Gertz, 2002). Other current approaches include thalidomide alone or in combination with cyclophosphamide and dexamethasone (Wechalekar et al., 2006), Rituximab™ in patients with CD20 positive clones, and new agents including the proteasome inhibitor bortezomib. The satisfactory response to less intense chemotherapy indicates that high-dose regimens are excessive in some cases, but there is presently no way to identify which individuals will tolerate and respond best to which treatment. The key point is to sufficiently suppress production of the amyloidogenic free light chain without unacceptable toxicity, and this requires careful individual monitoring.

At present, apart from transplantation to replace failed organs and liver transplantation to remove the source of amyloidogenic proteins of hepatic origin, only symptomatic treatment is available for hereditary systemic amyloidosis. The liver is the source of plasma TTR and over 700 liver transplants have been performed for treatment of hereditary TTR amyloidosis since this "surgical gene therapy" approach was introduced in 1991 (Herlenius et al., 2004). In younger patients carrying the common Met30 amyloidogenic mutation the outcome is generally good, with arrest of neuropathy, but paradoxical acceleration of TTR amyloid deposition following liver transplantation may occur in the heart and certain other sites in some patients. This unexpected phenomenon has been best documented in older patients with non Met30 variants (Stangou et al., 1998). A few combined heart and liver transplants have been performed.

The livers of patients with hereditary TTR amyloidosis contain only microscopic amyloid deposits in the blood vessels and interstitial tissues, and retain normal liver function. A large number of domino liver transplants have therefore been conducted in recipients with various terminal liver diseases for whom normal livers were not available. This has certainly prolonged their lives but the first such recipient has now developed symptomatic systemic TTR amyloidosis 8 years after transplantation (Stangou et al., 2005).

Combined liver and kidney transplantation was dramatically effective in a patient with hereditary fibrinogen amyloidosis, who had received two consecutive renal transplants and then developed amyloidotic liver failure (Gillmore et al., 2000), and several more AFib patients have now received combined liver and kidney transplants. These operations have demonstrated that the liver is the sole site of synthesis of plasma fibrinogen, but the appropriate roles of liver versus renal, and/or combined liver plus kidney transplantation in management of this disease have yet to be determined. Patients with apoAI amyloidosis can develop kidney, liver and cardiac amyloidosis, and organ transplants have been performed in several such patients visiting the UK National Amyloidosis Centre with excellent results, including dual organ transplants in four cases (Gillmore et al., 2006). After a median follow up of 9 years from transplantation, 7 of 10 patients with apoAI amyloidosis had functioning grafts. A single renal transplant failed due to recurrent amyloid after 25 years in a patient in whom there had been no intervention to reduce production of the amyloidogenic protein and two patients died with functioning transplants, including one from progressive systemic amyloidosis 13 years after renal transplantation. Reducing the production of the amyloidogenic protein by liver transplantation in two patients with apoAI amyloidosis has resulted in overall amyloid regression and, to date, prevented development of graft amyloid (Fig. 2). This contrasts sharply with a patient with hereditary lysozyme amyloidosis and a marked familial phenotype of hepatic amyloidosis leading to liver rupture, in whom liver transplantation, which does not appreciably alter the concentration of amyloidogenic variant lysozyme, was followed by fatal re-accumulation of liver amyloid. Liver transplantation has also been performed in a very small number of patients with hepatic failure due to systemic AL amyloidosis, most of whom have fared badly.

Elucidation of aspects of the molecular pathogenesis of amyloid and amyloidosis has generated a variety of novel approaches to therapy. We have developed a drug that targets SAP with the goal of eliminating SAP from amyloid deposits, in the hope that this may reduce amyloid deposition and/or accelerate amyloid clearance (Pepys et al., 2002). Preliminary open label studies are in progress in patients with systemic amyloidosis to optimize dosing and SAP depletion. Neurochem Inc. have just completed a double blind controlled clinical trial in AA amyloidosis of eprodisate, a small molecule glycosaminoglycan analogue aimed at blocking the pro-amyloidogenic interaction between SAA and glycosaminoglycans (Kisilevsky et al., 1995). One hundred and eighty-three patients with AA amyloidosis and renal involvement were randomized to receive eprodisate or placebo for 24 months. Primary composite endpoints were an assessment of renal function and death. Adverse events were similar in the two groups. Fewer patients in the eprodisate group

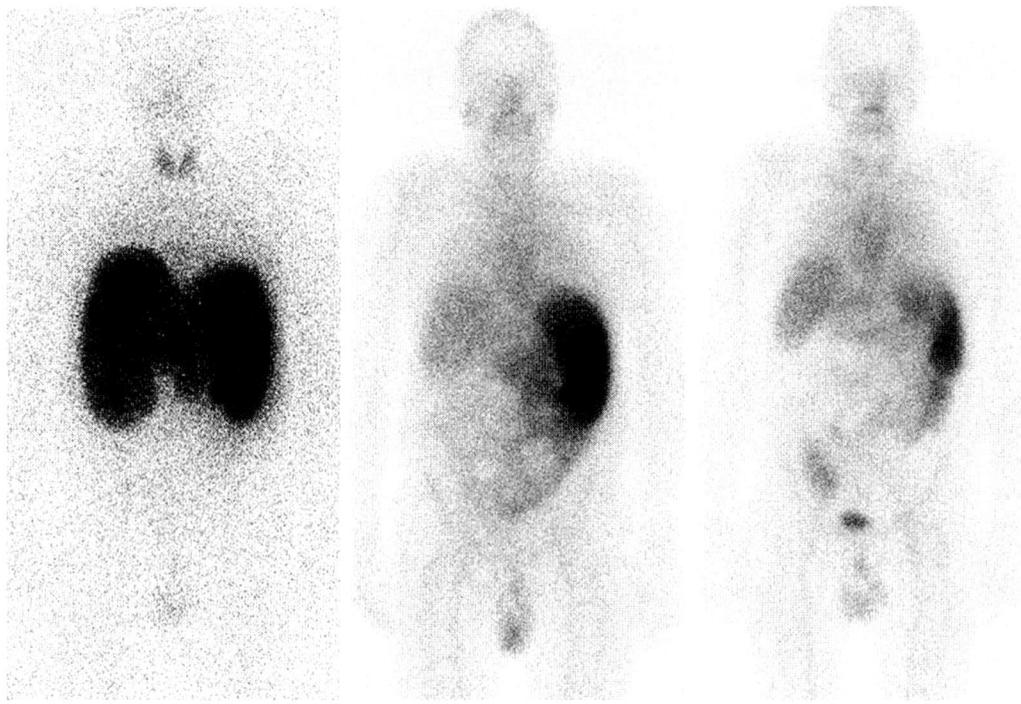

**Figure 2.** Serial anterior whole body $^{123}$I-SAP scintigraphy in a patient with hereditary apoAI amyloidosis. Prior to liver transplantation (left) there was extensive amyloid in the liver and spleen obscuring the kidneys and adrenal glands. One year after liver transplantation (middle), there was regression of amyloid from the spleen. Three and a half years after liver transplantation and 8 months after cadaveric renal transplantation (right) there had been further substantial regression of splenic amyloid without evidence of amyloid in either graft; the normal transplant kidney is apparent in the right iliac fossa.

compared to the placebo group had worsened disease at 24 months with a relative risk of 0.58 (CI: 0.37–0.93, $P = 0.025$) and the rate of renal decline was slower in the eprodisate group. Eprodisate is currently being evaluated for approval by the US Food and Drug Administration (FDA). Small molecule ligands that stabilize the native tetrameric structure of TTR and prevent its fibrillogenesis are being actively investigated for prophylaxis and therapy in TTR amyloidosis. Other strategies include stabilizing native structures of other amyloidogenic proteins and preventing and reversing fibrillogenesis, as well as disrupting established deposits, using antibodies, synthetic peptides and small molecule drugs. Some of these potential new therapies may enter clinical trials within the next few years and offer exciting prospects for improvements in treatment (Gillmore and Hawkins, 2006).

### Key points

- Amyloidogenesis involves refolding of the native structures of amyloid fibril precursor proteins.
- Green birefringence with Congo red staining remains the pathognomonic histochemical test for amyloidosis.
- The amyloid fibril type should be determined by immunohistochemistry and, where necessary, genetic analysis should be undertaken in all cases of amyloidosis.
- Management of systemic amyloidosis consists of reduction of the supply of the respective amyloid fibril precursor protein and supportive care.
- Novel approaches to therapy include stabilizing amyloidogenic proteins and disrupting established deposits using antibodies, synthetic peptides, and small molecule drugs.

## Acknowledgments

The work of the Centre for Amyloidosis and Acute Phase Proteins is supported by Medical Research Council Programme Grant G79/00051 and NHS R&D funds. The National Health Service National Amyloidosis Centre is funded entirely by the UK Department of Health.

## References

Bradwell, A.R., Carr-Smith, H.D., Mead, G.P., et al. 2001. Highly sensitive, automated immunoassay for immunoglobulin free light chains in serum and urine. Clin. Chem. 47, 673.

Bucciantini, M., Giannoni, E., Chiti, F., et al. 2002. Inherent toxicity of aggregates implies a common mechanism for protein misfolding diseases. Nature 416, 507.

Celik, A., Saglam, F., Dolek, D., et al. 2006. Outcome of kidney transplantation for renal amyloidosis: a single-center experience. Transplant. Proc. 38, 435.

Comenzo, R.L., Gertz, M.A. 2002. Autologous stem cell transplantation for primary systemic amyloidosis. Blood 99, 4276.

Drüeke, T.B. 1998. Dialysis-related amyloidosis. Nephrol. Dial. Transplant. 13 (Suppl. 1), 58.

Dubrey, S.W., Burke, M.M., Hawkins, P.N., et al. 2004. Cardiac transplantation for amyloid heart disease: the United Kingdom experience. J. Heart Lung Transplant. 23, 1142.

Gertz, M.A., Kyle, R.A., Greipp, P.R. 1991. Response rates and survival in primary systemic amyloidosis. Blood 77, 257.

Gertz, M.A., Kyle, R.A., O'Fallon, W.M. 1992. Dialysis support of patients with primary systemic amyloidosis. A study of 211 patients. Arch. Intern. Med. 152, 2245.

Gillmore, J.D., Booth, D.R., Madhoo, S., et al. 1999. Hereditary renal amyloidosis associated with variant lysozyme in a large English family. Nephrol. Dial. Transplant. 14, 2639.

Gillmore, J.D., Booth, D.R., Rela, M., et al. 2000. Curative hepatorenal transplantation in systemic amyloidosis caused by the Glu526Val fibrinogen a-chain variant in an English family. Q. J. Med. 93, 269.

Gillmore, J.D., Davies, J., Iqbal, A., et al. 1998. Allogeneic bone marrow transplantation for systemic AL amyloidosis. Br. J. Haematol. 100, 226.

Gillmore, J.D., Hawkins, P.N. 2006. Emerging drug therapies for amyloidosis. Nature Clin. Practice Nephrol. 2, 263.

Gillmore, J.D., Lovat, L.B., Persey, M.R., et al. 2001. Amyloid load and clinical outcome in AA amyloidosis in relation to circulating concentration of serum amyloid A protein. Lancet 358, 24.

Gillmore, J.D., Stangou, A.J., Lachmann, H.J., et al. 2006. Organ transplantation in hereditary apolipoprotein AI amyloidosis. Am. J. Transplant. 6, 2342.

Goodman, H.J.B., Lachmann, H.J., Hawkins, P.N. 2004. Intermediate dose intravenous melphalan and dexamethasone treatment in 144 patients with systemic AL amyloidosisBlood 104, 755A. [abstract].

Goodman, H.J.B., Wechalekar, A.D., Lachmann, H.J., et al. 2005. Survival and responses in 229 patients with AL amyloidosis treated with VAD or VAD-like chemotherapyHematologica 90 (Suppl. 1), 201. [abstract].

Hawkins, P.N. 2002. Serum amyloid P component scintigraphy for diagnosis and monitoring amyloidosis. Curr. Opin. Nephrol. Hypertens. 11, 649.

Hawkins, P.N., Lavender, J.P., Pepys, M.B. 1990. Evaluation of systemic amyloidosis by scintigraphy with 123I-labeled serum amyloid P component. N. Engl. J. Med. 323, 508.

Herlenius, G., Wilczek, H.E., Larsson, M., et al. 2004. Ten years of international experience with liver transplantation for familial amyloidotic polyneuropathy: results from the Familial Amyloidotic Polyneuropathy World Transplant Registry. Transplantation 77, 64.

Joy, T., Wang, J., Hahn, A., et al. 2003. APOA1 related amyloidosis: a case report and literature review. Clin. Biochem. 36, 641.

Kisilevsky, R., Fraser, P. 1996. Proteoglycans and amyloid fibrillogenesis. Ciba Found. Symp. 199, 58.

Kisilevsky, R., Lemieux, L.J., Fraser, P.E., et al. 1995. Arresting amyloidosis in vivo using small molecule anionic sulphonates or sulphates: implications for Alzheimer's disease. Nature Med. 1, 143.

Kyle, R.A., Gertz, M.A. 1995. Primary systemic amyloidosis: clinical and laboratory features in 474 cases. Semin. Hematol. 32, 45.

Kyle, R.A., Gertz, M.A., Greipp, P.R., et al. 1997. A trial of three regimens for primary amyloidosis: colchicine alone, melphalan and prednisone, and melphalan, prednisone, and colchicine. N. Engl. J. Med. 336, 1202.

Kyle, R.A., Greipp, P.R. 1983. Amyloidosis (AL): clinical and laboratory features in 229 cases. Mayo Clin. Proc. 58, 665.

Lachmann, H.J., Booth, D.R., Booth, S.E., et al. 2002. Misdiagnosis of hereditary amyloidosis as AL (primary) amyloidosis. N. Engl. J. Med. 346, 1786.

Lachmann, H.J., Gallimore, R., Gillmore, J.D., et al. 2003. Outcome in systemic AL amyloidosis in relation to changes in concentration of circulating free immunoglobulin light chains following chemotherapy. Br. J. Haematol. 122, 78.

Lachmann, H.J., Goodman, H.J.B., Gallimore, J. et al. 2005. Characteristic and clinical outcome of 340 patients with systemic AA amyloidosis. In: G. Grateau, R.A. Kyle, M. Skinner (Eds.), Amyloid and Amyloidosis. CRC Press, Boca Raton, FL, p. 173.

Lovat, L.B., Pepys, M.B., Hawkins, P.N. 1997. Amyloid and the gut. Dig. Dis. 15, 155.

Lovat, L.B., Persey, M.R., Madhoo, S., et al. 1998. The liver in systemic amyloidosis: insights from $^{123}$I serum amyloid P component scintigraphy in 484 patients. Gut 42, 727.

Magy, N., Liepnieks, J.J., Yazaki, M., et al. 2003. Renal transplantation for apolipoprotein AII amyloidosis. Amyloid 10, 224.

Pasternack, A., Ahonen, J., Kuhlback, B. 1986. Renal transplantation in 45 patients with amyloidosis. Transplantation 42, 598.

Pepys, M.B., Herbert, J., Hutchinson, W.L., et al. 2002. Targeted pharmacological depletion of serum amyloid P component for treatment of human amyloidosis. Nature 417, 254.

Rydh, A., Suhr, O., Hietala, S.-O., et al. 1998. Serum amyloid P component scintigraphy in familial amyloid polyneuropathy: regression of visceral amyloid following liver transplantation. Eur. J. Nucl. Med. 25, 709.

Stangou, A.J., Hawkins, P.N., Heaton, N.D., et al. 1998. Progressive cardiac amyloidosis following liver transplantation for familial amyloid polyneuropathy: implications for amyloid fibrillogenesis. Transplantation 66, 229.

Stangou, A.J., Heaton, N.D., Hawkins, P.N. 2005. Transmission of systemic transthyretin amyloidosis by domino liver transplantation. N. Engl. J. Med. 352, 2356.

Sunde, M., Serpell, L.C., Bartlam, M., et al. 1997. Common core structure of amyloid fibrils by synchrotron X-ray diffraction. J. Mol. Biol. 273, 729.

Tennent, G.A., Lovat, L.B., Pepys, M.B. 1995. Serum amyloid P component prevents proteolysis of the amyloid fibrils of Alzheimer's disease and systemic amyloidosis. Proc. Natl. Acad. Sci. USA. 92, 4299.

Vigushin, D.M., Pepys, M.B., Hawkins, P.N. 1994. Rapid regression of AA amyloidosis following surgery for Castleman's disease. In: R. Kisilevsky, M.D. Benson, B. Frangione et al. (Eds.), Amyloid and Amyloidosis 1993. Parthenon Publishing, Pearl River, New York, p. 48.

Wechalekar, A.D., Goodman, H.J.B., Lachmann, H.J., et al. 2006. Safety and efficacy of risk adapted cyclophosphamide, thalidomide and dexamethasone in systemic AL amyloidosis. Blood 109, 457.

Westermark, P., Mucchiano, G., Marthin, T., et al. 1995. Apolipoprotein A1-derived amyloid in human aortic atherosclerotic plaques. Am. J. Pathol. 147, 1186.

Zemer, D., Pras, M., Sohar, E., et al. 1986. Colchicine in the prevention and treatment of amyloidosis of familial Mediterranean fever. N. Engl. J. Med. 314, 1001.

# CHAPTER 22

# Inflammatory Arthritis, Behçet's Syndrome, and Sarcoidosis

Olivier Harari*

*UCB Celltech, Bath Road, Slough SL1 3WE, UK*

## 1. Introduction

The inflammatory arthritides are a group of autoimmune diseases, sub-classified into two principal groups, based on the presence or absence of the autoantibody, rheumatoid factor (RF) (Table 1). Together, they comprise the most prevalent of all the systemic autoimmune conditions. Their foremost clinical feature is chronic synovial inflammation, but in addition a variety of extra-articular lesions can occur. Target organs usually include the eye, the lung interstitium, the skin, and the bowel, but the kidney is infrequently directly involved. Glomerulonephritis (GN) can occur, and when it does, the type of lesion is highly variable. However, renal AA amyloidosis as a sequel of chronic inflammation is seen more frequently, in all the inflammatory arthritides. Nevertheless, the most common cause of renal dysfunction in this group of diseases is pharmacotoxicity, and the leading class of agent responsible is that of the non-steroidal anti-inflammatory drugs (NSAID). Sarcoidosis is a systemic disease characterized by non-caseating granulomatous inflammation, principally involving the lung and the peripheral lymph nodes. A granulomatous interstitial nephritis (GIN) can occur, as can nephrocalcinosis, as a result of increased vitamin D metabolism and resultant hypercalciuria. Behçet's disease is a chronic relapsing inflammatory illness primarily affecting mucosa, skin, eye, and brain. Renal manifestations are unusual, but reported. This chapter seeks to review in detail the significant part played by renal involvement in this miscellaneous group of conditions (Table 2).

## 2. Inflammatory arthritis

### 2.1. Rheumatoid arthritis

Rheumatoid arthritis (RA) is the most prevalent inflammatory arthritis worldwide. It is characterized by a chronic synovitis occurring at many joint areas in a symmetric distribution, usually involving metacarpophalangeal joints and/or wrists. Extra-articular features occur principally amongst the 75% of patients who are RF seropositive.

Table 1
Classification of the inflammatory arthritides

Rheumatoid arthritis
   Seropositive for rheumatoid factor
      Without systemic vasculitis
      With systemic vasculitis
   Seronegative for rheumatoid factor
Seronegative spondyloarthropathies
   Ankylosing spondylitis
   Psoriatic arthritis
   Reactive arthritis
   Enteropathic arthritis
   Undifferentiated spondyloarthropathy
Juvenile idiopathic arthritis
   Oligoarticular
   Polyarticular
   Spondyloarthritis
   Systemic (Still's disease)

*Corresponding author.
Tel.: +44-208-383-1173; Fax: +44-208-383-1930
E-mail address: o.harari@imperial.ac.uk

**Table 2**
Renal lesions in rheumatic diseases

|  | RA | AS | BD | Sarcoid | NSAID |
|---|---|---|---|---|---|
| Glomerulosclerosis |  |  |  | + |  |
| IgA nephropathy | + | + | + | + |  |
| Membranous | + |  |  |  |  |
| Mesangiocapillary | + | + |  | + |  |
| Crescentic | + |  | + |  |  |
| Interstitial |  |  | + | + + | + + + |
| Amyloidosis | + + | + + | + | + |  |
| Nephrocalcinosis |  |  |  | + + |  |

*Symbols*: +, several case reports/small series; + +, significant percentage of cases in several series; + + +, common manifestation.

*Abbreviations*: RA, rheumatoid arthritis; AS, ankylosing spondylitis; BD, Behçet's disease; NSAID, non-steroidal anti-inflammatory drugs.

RF is an autoantibody targeted at the Fc portion of the IgG molecule. RF isotype can be, in order of frequency, IgM, IgA, or IgG. Extra-articular clinical features can be relatively benign, such as subcutaneous nodulosis, nail-fold vasculitis, secondary Sjogren's syndrome, and Raynaud's phenomenon. However, significant damage, progressing to organ failure, can be seen in cases of ocular scleritis, interstitial pneumonitis, and cardiac valve involvement. The most feared complication of RA is the development of systemic rheumatoid vasculitis, which can cause a catastrophic multi-organ involvement including digital gangrene and mononeuritis multiplex. Strikingly, renal involvement in any of these scenarios is rare. This is surprising when one considers the very high rate of RF seropositivity, and the accompanying depletion of complement C3, seen in patients with rheumatoid vasculitis (Voskuyl et al., 2003). These factors would suggest that rheumatoid vasculitis is mediated by immune complex deposition, an observation which would lead to the expectation of frequent renal involvement. Nevertheless, the number of cases of RA with GN, reported in the literature since 1990, and excluding patients with a history of significant nephrotoxic drug ingestion, is small.

The renal pathology in these patients is evenly split between mesangial, crescentic, and membranous GN. Although the number of cases is low, almost all are associated with RF seropositivity.

The cases of mesangial GN are usually associated with immune deposits in the glomeruli. The most common pattern is of isolated IgM deposition, followed by IgA, with associated C3 deposition in under half the cases (Korpela et al., 1997). In the cases of mesangial IgA deposition, there is a significant correlation between the degree of IgA deposition and the total serum IgA level. This has prompted some observers to note that these patients may have two unassociated but relatively common conditions, RA and IgA nephropathy (IgAN) (Nakano et al., 1996). Similarly, the majority of patients with crescentic GN in RA have detectable circulating pANCA reactivity, and show clinical manifestations of extra-renal systemic vasculitis (Harper et al., 1997). In these cases, immune complex deposition is present in half, while the remainder evince a pauci-immue nephritis. These may be cases of microscopic polyangiitis developing in cases of pre-existing RA, as has been observed with cases of Wegener's granulomatosis (Douglas et al., 2003).

The striking paucity of renal vasculitis in association with RA, in the literature that reflects recent clinical practice, is in contrast to historical autopsy and renal biopsy series. Here, the picture is less consistent. Some studies report a high incidence of GN of up to 50% (Adu et al., 1993; Boers et al., 1987; Helin et al., 1995; Ramirez et al., 1981). Others find little or no evidence of direct renal involvement (Pollak et al., 1962; Brun et al., 1965). It has been suggested that some of the former studies included patients with infections or drug nephrotoxicity, or were subject to selection bias due to referral patterns (Adu et al., 2001). Most authorities allow that renal vasculitis can occur, albeit rarely, in the context of rheumatoid vasculitis. It is perhaps not surprising that historical studies show a higher prevalence, as the overall incidence of rheumatoid vasculitis appears to have diminished over the last few decades (Ward, 2004; Watts et al., 2004). It has been suggested that this is occurring because of more effective treatments. Alternatively, there may be a secular trend towards a reduction in severity of RA, due to other environmental factors, such as changing infective disease patterns. In support of this, RF seropositivity rate, in a homogenous population of Pima

Indians, has been diminishing over time (Enzer et al., 2002). In summary, RA can progress to a multi-organ vasculitic disease characterized by immune complex deposition and complement fixation, although this is becoming increasingly unusual. However, even in such cases, it would appear that the kidney is relatively spared from involvement. The mechanisms by which this might occur are currently unknown.

### 2.1.1. Anti-rheumatic drugs

In the 30-year period approximately spanning 1970–1990, membranous nephritis was frequently encountered in RA patients, as a result of the use of oral and intramuscular gold compounds, and the metal chelators, D-penicillamine and bucillamine, as anti-rheumatic drugs. The emergence of the dihydrofolate reductase inhibitor, methotrexate, as the first-line anti-rheumatic drug, and the use of combination drug strategies including sulphasalazine, hydroxychloroquine, and biologic agents, has all but ended the use of gold and D-penicillamine in the treatment of RA. Concomitantly, the prevalence of membranous GN in RA has fallen sharply. Even the most recent case series show that the majority of cases are associated with gold or D-penicillamine treatment, with only small numbers or isolated reports in which there was no history of chelator or chrysotherapy (Yoshida et al., 1994; Zarza et al., 1996). Gold and D-penicillamine are also a cause of mesangial GN in RA; in a large recent series, 85% of cases were associated with a history of treatment with one or both classes of drugs. NSAID are now the most common cause for renal dysfunction in the RA population (for details, see chapter 6). Ciclosporin, the calcineurin inhibitor, is occasionally used in RA treatment regimes. These patients can experience significant elevation in plasma creatinine, as a result of vascular and tubulointerstitial changes (chapter 6) (Schiff and Whelton, 2000).

The last decade has witnessed the arrival of biologic (parenterally delivered recombinant protein) therapy for RA. The most successful and only widely used strategy so far has been the inhibition of the inflammatory cytokine, TNFα. Infliximab and adalumimab are neutralizing IgG antibodies (chimeric and humanized, respectively), and etanercept is a p75 TNFα receptor-Ig fusion protein that acts as a soluble decoy. Use of these agents is associated with the development of anti-nuclear antibodies (ANA) in some patients. Rarely, drug-induced lupus can occur (Charles et al., 2000; Shakoor et al., 2002). Furthermore, a small number of cases are reported in which GN developed as a result of TNF inhibitor treatment (Roux et al., 2004; Kemp et al., 2001). Four cases of crescentic, two of mesangial, and one of membranous nephritis are described (Stokes et al., 2005; Doulton et al., 2004). Five were associated with ANA positivity, and one with pANCA positivity. Nevertheless, this consequence of TNFα inhibition appears to be rare, and in spite of the continuing growth in use of these therapies, it is unlikely that a significant nephrotoxicity problem will emerge in clinical practice as a result.

### 2.1.2. AA amyloidosis

Renal amyloidosis has been an important contributor to the excess mortality seen in RA patients (see chapter 21) (Table 3). It has been estimated that, of the excess deaths due to RA, 20% are

**Table 3**

Rheumatic diseases significantly associated with the development of AA amyloidosis

---

Inflammatory arthritis
  Rheumatoid arthritis
  Seronegative spondyloarthitis
    Ankylosing spondylitis
    Psoriatic arthritis
    Reactive arthritis
  Adult-onset Still's disease
  Juvenile idiopathic arthritis
Auto-inflammatory syndromes
  Familial Mediterranean fever
  TRAPS
  Familial cold urticaria syndrome
  Muckle Wells syndrome
Connective tissue disease
  Systemic lupus erythematosus
  Mixed connective tissue disease
  Systemic sclerosis
Miscellaneous
  Behçet's disease
  Sarcoidosis
  Polymayalgia rheumatica/giant cell arteritis

---

*Abbreviation*: TRAPS, TNF receptor-associated periodic syndrome.

attributable to amyloidotic renal failure (Thomas et al., 2003). However, the picture has changed dramatically over the last two decades, with the near disappearance of amyloidosis as a clinical problem in RA. In the 1950s and 1960s, 13–26% of autopsies on RA patients showed evidence of amyloid disease (Missen and Taylor, 1956). The same authors, reporting at the close of the 1970s, put the prevalence at 4% (Wright and Calkins, 1981). Further detailed studies from Finland have described this trend (Myllykangas-Luosujarvi et al., 1999). One Finnish hospital reported 1779 biopsies performed on clinical suspicion of AA amyloidosis in 1987, with 181 positive. Ten years later, only 59 biopsies were deemed necessary, with 3 positive (Laiho et al., 1999). It is worth mentioning that most of these biopsies took the form of sub-cutaneous fat aspirations, which, if anything, over-estimate clinically significant amyloidosis (Gomez-Casanovas et al., 2001). It has been suggested that the decline in RA-associated amyloidosis is due to improvement in treatment for the underlying arthritis, or to a gradual reduction in the incidence of infective co-morbidities, such as tuberculosis (Hazenberg and van Rijswijk, 2000). Clearly, the fall in amyloidosis is in keeping with the improved outlook for RA patients in terms of progressive joint destruction and severe extra-articular manifestations.

## 2.2. Seronegative spondyloarthritis

The seronegative spondyloarthritides are a group of inflammatory arthritides characterized by several common features. RF is absent, the *HLA B27* gene is often present, the spine is frequently involved as are tendon entheses, and inflammation occurs in the anterior chamber of the eye, as well as the joints. The group comprises ankylosing spondylitis (AS), psoriatic arthritis, reactive arthritis, enteropathic arthritis, and undifferentiated spondyloarthropathy (Table 1). As with RA, the most common cause of renal dysfunction in this group is interstitial nephritis secondary to NSAID use, followed by glomerulosclerosis caused by amyloid deposition. GN is unusual, with a few cases in the literature of membranous and mesangial GN (Strobel and Fritschka, 1998). By far the commonest form described in association with AS is IgAN (Shu et al., 1986). This is intriguing, as both AS and IgAN have a male preponderance, a peak incidence in the second and third decades of life, and increased serum IgA level of the IgA1 sub-class (Montenegro and Monteiro, 1999; Barratt and Feehally, 2005). It has been suggested that these common features might indicate common pathogenic mechanisms. However, there are important differences. The IgA1 elevation in serum is monomeric in AS but polymeric in IgAN (Hocini et al., 1992). Secretory IgA level increases in AS but falls in IgAN (Collado et al., 1991). Ninety five percent of AS patients carry HLA B27, but there is no association between this allele and IgAN. The relationship between these two conditions remains unclear. IgAN is a common disease, and its occurrence in the context of inflammatory arthritis might be co-incidental (Matsuda et al., 2006; D'Amico, 2004). It is nevertheless striking that, unlike in RA, IgAN is by far the most common form of GN in the seronegative arthritis group (Nadir et al., 2003).

## 3. Sarcoidosis

Sarcoidosis is a non-caseating granulomatous inflammatory disease that comes in two distinct forms, acute and chronic. Peripheral lymph nodes are commonly involved, and the disease can also affect tissue interstitia, most commonly the lung, the skin, the eye, and the nervous system, and less frequently, the joints and the liver. Ten percent of sarcoidosis patients develop renal impairment. The most common cause is calcium precipitation in the kidney and renal tract, followed by granuloma formation in the renal interstitium. A number of unusual sequelae of sarcoidosis can also occur, such as GN and renal amyloidosis.

## 3.1. Disorders of calcium metabolism

Patients with active sarcoidosis often have abnormal calcium metabolism, with 40–62% of patients developing hypercalciuria (Conron et al., 2000). This abnormality fluctuates with disease, and 24-h urinary calcium can be used as a marker of disease activity. Hypercalciuria correlates with the serum ionized calcium level, but only 10% of patients develop hypercalcaemia, and this is rarely clinically significant (Hamada et al., 2002; Sharma, 1996). These abnormalities are caused by an elevated level of the active vitamin $D_3$ metabolite, calcitriol, a hormone that signals through nuclear hormone receptors (vitamin D receptor/retinoid X receptor heterodimer) to influence gene transcriptional activity. In the GI tract, the effect of this is to increase dietary calcium absorption, by increasing transport across the intestinal epithelia. Calcitriol also acts in bone, influencing the differentiation status of both osteoclast and osteoblast cells in a way that results in an overall increase in bone resorption, and release of calcium from the bone reservoir into the circulation (van Driel et al., 2004; Blair et al., 2005). Calcitriol (1,25 di-hydroxycholecalciferol; $1,25(OH)_2$ $D_3$) is synthesized from 25-hydroxycholecalciferol by the action of $25(OH)D_3$ 1α-hydroxylase. In health, this enzyme is restricted in expression to the proximal renal tubular cells. This pathway is exquisitely sensitive to negative feedback by calcitriol itself, and is furthermore dependent on an induction signal from parathyroid hormone, which in turn is suppressed by elevation in serum calcium concentration. In this way, calcitriol production is tightly regulated.

The abnormally raised calcitriol level in sarcoidosis is caused by the aberrant expression of $25(OH)D_3$ 1α-hydroxylase in macrophages, in the lung, and in other tissues affected by sarcoid inflammation (Adams et al., 1983; Inui et al., 2001; Mason et al., 1984). A key cellular constituent of a sarcoid granuloma is the activated macrophage (or "epithelioid histiocyte"). Macrophage activation is driven by the lymphocyte-derived cytokine, interferon-$\gamma$. It is therefore perhaps unsurprising to find that interferon-$\gamma$ has been shown to upregulate 1α-hydroxylase in monocyte/macrophages (Stoffels et al., 2006). The upregulation of calcitriol production appears to be one of the manifestations of activated macrophage phenotype in sarcoidosis. Dendritic cells are also found in sarcoid granulomata, and express 1α-hydroxylase upon stimulation (Ota et al., 2004; Fritsche et al., 2003). Other than interferon-$\gamma$, the other known stimulus for monocyte/macrophage 1α-hydroxylase induction is an activation signal delivered through Toll-like receptors (TLR). This receptor family detects the presence of invading micro-organisms by binding to pathogen-associated molecular patterns (Iwasaki and Medzhitov, 2004; Liu et al., 2006). The bacterial lipopolysaccharide receptor, TLR4, appears to be a major determinant of 1α-hydroxylase induction (Fritsche et al., 2003; Stoffels et al., 2006). This may not be relevant in sarcoidosis, as there are currently no mechanistic studies implicating TLR activation in the pathogenesis of sarcoidosis. However, there is evidence, albeit conflicting, to suggest that *tlr4* gene polymorphisms in the population modulate the incidence of sarcoidosis (Pabst et al., 2006; Veltkamp et al., 2006).

To summarize (see Fig. 1), calcitriol production is an important consequence of the macrophage and dendritic cell activation that occurs in sarcoidosis. Crucially, this calcitriol production differs from the physiological production from the proximal renal tubule, in that macrophage 1α-hydroxylase expression is insensitive to the negative feedback effect of calcitriol. It is also independent of parathyroid hormone. This dysregulation allows increases in circulating ionized calcium and increased calcium flow through the kidney as functional consequences of the increase in calcitriol. Why is calcitriol production induced by inflammatory stimuli in macrophages? It may have a beneficial, regulatory role: calcitriol signaling has been shown to have anti-inflammatory effects, specifically, the downregulation of the production of cytokines interferon-$\gamma$ and interleukin-2, and the downregulation of the expression of TLR2 (Sadeghi et al., 2006; Reichel et al., 1987; Manolagas et al., 1990). Calcitriol might thus be playing a modulatory role in macrophage-induced inflammation and elevated levels have been detected in tuberculosis, candidiasis, leprosy, silicone-induced granulomatous disease, Crohn's disease, Wegener granulomatosis, coccidiocidomycosis, histoplasmosis, berylliosis, and eosinophilic granuloma (Sharma, 2000). However, in sarcoidosis, the negative corollary of calcitriol production is hypercalciuria, and this leads to nephrocalcinosis in 5% of sarcoidosis

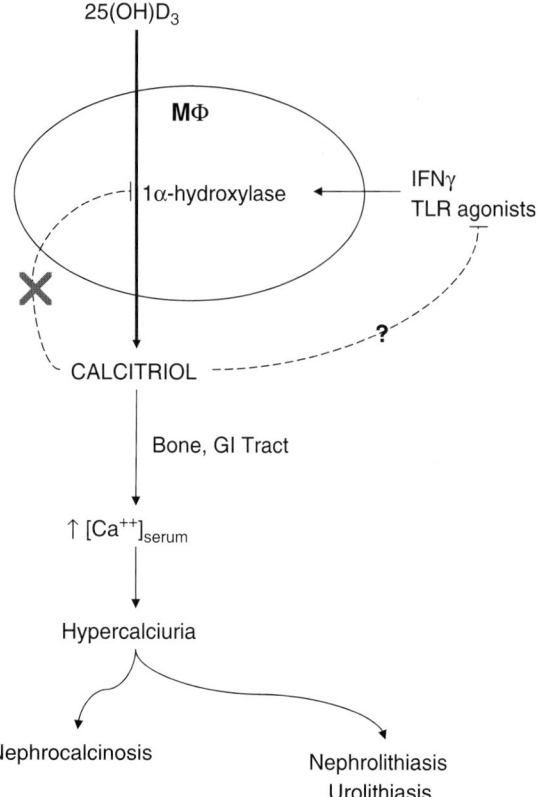

**Figure 1.** Calcium homeostatic pathway alteration in sarcoidosis. $25(OH)D_3$ 1-hydroxylase is induced in macrophages (M$\phi$) in sarcoidosis by the action of inflammatory mediators such as cytokines (interferon-$\gamma$, IFN$\gamma$) and possibly Toll-like receptor (TLR) agonists. Calcitriol is synthesized from 25-hydroxycholecalciferol ($25(OH)D_3$) by the action of 1$\alpha$-hydroxylase. Calcitriol then acts on bone and intestinal epithelia to release calcium into the circulation. This leads to hypercalciuria and calcium precipitation in the renal tract. Macrophage 1$\alpha$-hydroxylase is not sensitive to the negative feedback action of calcitriol. Calcitriol may have immunomodulating effects by inhibiting IFN$\gamma$ and TLR signaling pathways.

patients, and represents the most common cause of chronic renal failure in this condition. A further 10% of patients develop nephrolithiasis or urolithiasis, requiring intervention to prevent an obstructive nephropathy.

It is unclear how best to manage elevated calcitriol levels so as to prevent renal damage. In patients with high serum calcitriol but no significant hypercalciuria, it is probably sufficient to ensure sufficient oral intake of fluid, avoid prolonged exposure to sunlight (to limit cholecalciferol synthesis), and avoid ergocalciferol (vitamin $D_2$)-rich foods such as cod liver oil and oily fish. Patients with hypercalciuria and additional evidence of active sarcoid inflammation should be treated with corticosteroids, together with a steroid-sparing agent such as methotrexate. Steroids usually effectively suppress calcitriol levels, and the steroid-sparing agent is introduced to minimize dose-dependent iatrogenic hypercortisolism. If this strategy is ineffective, contraindicated or unacceptably toxic, there is some evidence for the use of ketoconazole, hydroxychloroquine, or bisphosphonates as second-line agents (Sinha et al., 1997; O'Leary et al., 1986; Glass et al., 1990). Patients with clinically significant hypercalcaemia should be adequately hydrated and treated with a loop diuretic in the acute phase, and a thiazide diuretic can be added to the maintenance drug regime if necessary. Hypercalciuria, without any other clinical evidence for active sarcoidosis can be a difficult problem. It is unknown whether exposure to the risk of steroid-induced side effects is justified, or whether a high fluid intake, and addition of thiazide diuretic without immunosuppression, can prevent renal damage.

## 3.2. Interstitial granulomatous nephritis

Sarcoidosis is the cause of 29% of cases of GIN (Table 4). The commonest cause of GIN is drug toxicity, and a further 11% of cases are idiopathic (Bijol et al., 2006). The incidence of GIN in sarcoidosis varies in published series between 5 and 40%, and is even higher in historical autopsy studies (Longcope and Freiman, 1952). Patients are usually over the age of 40 and there is a male preponderance. In the majority of cases, there is clinically evident sarcoidosis elsewhere, but GIN can occur as the only manifestation of sarcoidosis (Miyoshi et al., 2004; O'Riordan et al., 2001; Robson et al., 2003). GIN is frequently subclinical, or detected as a low-grade proteinuria, hematuria, or pyuria (Ikeda et al., 2001). Significant impairment of renal function can occur chronically or acutely. Intriguingly, this often occurs in the presence of a second, accompanying manifestation of renal sarcoidosis, usually nephrocalcinosis, but also GN (see the following section). In two reported cases, GIN presented as an inflammatory renal pseudotumor, and in one case GIN was linked to multiple tubular defects including nephrogenic diabetes insipidus (Muther et al., 1980; Rohatgi et al., 1990). Histologically, granulomata are found in the tubulo-interstitium and juxtaglomerular apparatus (Rheault et al., 2006). An accompanying interstitial lymphocytosis can be present (see Fig. 2). Sarcoid GIN is responsive to corticosteroid treatment in most cases, although once renal impairment has developed, function usually does not return to normal (Rajakariar et al., 2006). Refractory cases have been treated with steroid plus mycophenolate mofetil or infliximab with some success (Moudgil et al., 2006; Thumfart et al., 2005; Ahmed et al., 2006).

## 3.3. Other lesions

GN is rare in sarcoidosis, and reports exist of membranous GN, focal and segmental glomerulosclerosis, mesangial proliferative GN, IgAN and crescentic GN (Morita and Yoshimura, 2006). Renal AA amyloidosis complicating sarcoidosis is extraordinarily rare, with only five cases in the literature (Komatsuda et al., 2003). Another unusual manifestation of sarcoidosis is ureteric obstruction and hydronephrosis caused by extrinsic compression by retroperitoneal lymphadenopathy (Miyazaki et al., 1996). Finally, neurological sarcoidosis has been reported to present with polyuria and polydipsia, caused by cranial diabetes insipidus due to sarcoid infiltration of the pituitary gland (Bullmann et al., 2000).

## 4. Behçet's disease

Behçet's disease (BD) is a rare, chronic relapsing inflammatory illness characterized primarily by severe oro-genital ulceration, and ocular

**Table 4**
Causes of granulomatous interstitial nephritis (Bijol et al., 2006)

Infective
  Tuberculosis
  Histoplasmosis
  Leprosy
  Hydatid disease
Vasculitis
  Wegener's granulomatosis
  Microscopic polyangiitis
  Churg–Strauss vasculitis
Sarcoidosis
Oxaluria
Drugs
  Antibiotics
  NSAIDs
Xanthogranulomatous pyelonephritis
Idiopathic

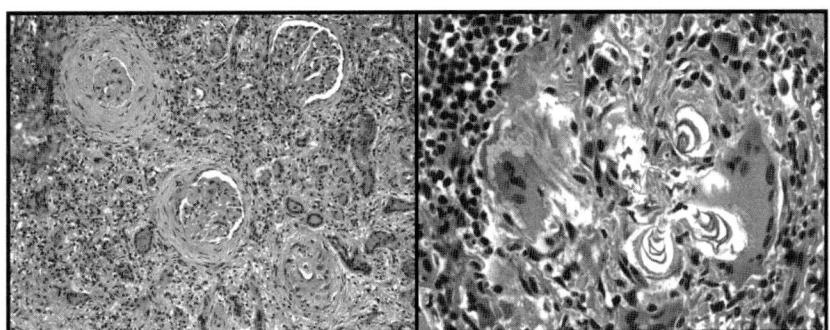

**Figure 2.** Histology of granulomatous interstitial nephritis due to sarcoidosis. Right panel: Non-caseating granulomata and an interstitial nephritis characterized by lymphocyte and scattered multi-nucleated giant cell infiltration. Tubular atrophy is also present (hematoxylin and eosin, original magnification × 200). Left panel: A non-caseating granuloma consisting of epithelioid histiocytes, multi-nucleated giant cells and calcified laminated concretions (Schaumann bodies) (hematoxylin and eosin, original magnification × 600). Reproduced with kind permission of Dr. Alan Sinaiko and Springer Science and Business Media (Rheault et al., 2006).

inflammation in the anterior and/or posterior uveal tract (Yurdakul et al., 2004). Various additional features can occur: inflammatory skin lesions, vasculitis with arterial or venous thrombosis, non-erosive arthritis, fatigue, and depression (Table 5) (Pickering and Haskard, 2000). Renal involvement is present in a minority of patients, although the precise prevalence has been difficult to assess due to the rarity of the condition, and possible ethno-geographic variation. Estimates have ranged in different series from 0 to 55% (Table 6) (Akpolat et al., 2002). The most common renal lesion is amyloidosis. AA amyloidosis occurs in up to 5% of BD patents, and accounts for just over half of all cases with renal involvement. This is apparently less common in the Japanese population. As with other causes of AA amyloidosis, patients progress through proteinuria and nephrotic syndrome to renal failure (Akpolat et al., 2000). GN can also occur in BD. The most common form is proliferative nephritis with crescent formation. IgG, IgA, IgM, and C3 deposition is found in the glomerulus. IgAN is also reported, but less commonly than in other rheumatic disorders (Hemmen et al., 1997). GN in the context of BD presents with hematuria and low-grade proteinuria. Pyuria is frequent, and the prognosis in terms of renal function is poor. BD frequently manifests as a vasculitis that affects medium-sized arteries, sometimes with aneurysm formation. Superficial and deep venous thrombosis often occurs, possibly secondary to inflammatory venulitis. Twenty percent of renal BD patients have renovascular disease, with aneurysms or stenoses of the medium-sized renal arteries. Systemic hypertension is the presenting feature, and aneurysmal rupture with significant hemorrhage can occur, as can acute renal infarction. A microangiopathy is described, but is more unusual. Patients present with hematuria and mild proteinuria (Angotti et al., 2003). Renal vein thrombosis is rare. This is perhaps surprising, given the frequency of deep vein thrombosis affecting the limbs, intracranial cortical veins, and inferior vena cava. When renal vein thrombosis does occur it is always in the context of other significant renal involvement, by amyloidosis, GN, or arteritis. Finally, there is one reported case of an inflammatory pseudotumor in BD (Aessopos et al., 2000).

**Table 5**
Diagnostic classification of Behçet's disease

Recurrent major or minor aphthous or herpetiform ulceration of the mouth
*Plus*
    Recurrent genital ulceration
    Erythema nodosum
    Pseudofolliculitis
    Papulopustular eruption
    Acneiform nodules
    Positive pathergy test
    Anterior or posterior uveitis
    Retinal vasculitis

*Note*: In the absence of other clinical explanations, patients must have recurrent oral ulceration observed by the physician and occurring at least three times in one 12-month period, plus two of the minor criteria (International Study Group for Behçet's Disease, 1990).

**Table 6**
Renal manifestations of Behçet's disease

Renal amyloidosis
Crescentic glomerulonephritis
IgA nephropathy
Medium-sized renal artery aneurysm/stenosis
Ischaemic renal microangiopathy
Interstitial nephritis
Renal inflammatory pseudotumor

---

**Key points**

- Inflammatory arthritis as a direct cause of renal disease is becoming increasingly infrequent.
- Arthritis-associated amyloidosis and vasculitis are declining in prevalence.
- NSAID nephrotoxicity continues to be the most significant problem for these patients.
- GN has declined with the fall-off in use of gold and D-penicillamine.
- Sarcoidosis causes hypervitaminosis D3, hypercalciuria, and nephrocalcinosis.
- Sarcoidosis can also manifest as granulomatous interstitial nephritis.
- Behcet's disease can cause a vasculitis of medium-sized arteries affecting the kidney.

# References

Adams, J.S., Sharma, O.P., Gacad, M.A., Singer, F.R. 1983. J. Clin. Invest. 72, 1856–1860.
Adu, D., Berisa, F., Howie, A.J., Emery, P., Bacon, P.A., McConkey, B., McGonigle, R.J., Michaels, J., Popert, A.J. 1993. Br. J. Rheumatol. 32, 1008–1011.
Adu, D., Emery, P., Madaio, M.P. 2001. Rheumatology and the kidney. Oxford University Press, Oxford.
Aessopos, A., Alatzoglou, K., Korovesis, K., Tassiopoulos, S., Lefakis, G., Ismailou-Parassi, A. 2000. Am. J. Nephrol. 20, 217–221.
Ahmed, M.M., Mubashir, E., Dossabhoy, N.R. 2006. *Clin. Rheumatol.* 26(8), 1346–1349.
Akpolat, T., Akkoyunlu, M., Akpolat, I., Dilek, M., Odabas, A.R., Ozen, S. 2002. Semin. Arthritis Rheum. 31, 317–337.
Akpolat, T., Akpolat, I., Kandemir, B. 2000. Am. J. Nephrol. 20, 68–70.
Angotti, C., D'Cruz, D.P., Abbs, I.C., Hughes, G.R. 2003. Rheumatology (Oxford) 42, 1416–1417.
Barratt, J., Feehally, J. 2005. J. Am. Soc. Nephrol. 16, 2088–2097.
Bijol, V., Mendez, G.P., Nose, V., Rennke, H.G. 2006. Int. J. Surg. Pathol. 14, 57–63.
Blair, H.C., Robinson, L.J., Zaidi, M. 2005. Biochem. Biophys. Res. Commun. 328, 728–738.
Boers, M., Croonen, A.M., Dijkmans, B.A., Breedveld, F.C., Eulderink, F., Cats, A., Weening, J.J. 1987. Ann. Rheum. Dis. 46, 658–663.
Brun, C., Olsen, T.S., Raaschou, F., Sorensen, A.W. 1965. Nephron. 2, 65–81.
Bullmann, C., Faust, M., Hoffmann, A., Heppner, C., Jockenhovel, F., Muller-Wieland, D., Krone, W. 2000. Eur. J. Endocrinol. 142, 365–372.
Charles, P.J., Smeenk, R.J., De Jong, J., Feldmann, M., Maini, R.N. 2000. Arthritis Rheum. 43, 2383–2390.
Collado, A., Sanmarti, R., Serra, C., Gallart, T., Canete, J.D., Gratacos, J., Vives, J., Munoz-Gomez, J. 1991. Scand. J. Rheumatol. 20, 153–158.
Conron, M., Young, C., Beynon, H.L. 2000. Rheumatology (Oxford) 39, 707–713.
D'Amico, G. 2004. Semin. Nephrol. 24, 179–196.
Douglas, G., Bird, K., Flume, P., Silver, R., Bolster, M. 2003. J. Rheumatol. 30, 2064–2069.
Doulton, T.W., Tucker, B., Reardon, J., Velasco, N. 2004. Clin. Nephrol. 62, 234–238.
Enzer, I., Dunn, G., Jacobsson, L., Bennett, P.H., Knowler, W.C., Silman, A. 2002. Arthritis Rheum. 46, 1729–1734.
Fritsche, J., Mondal, K., Ehrnsperger, A., Andreesen, R., Kreutz, M. 2003. Blood 102, 3314–3316.
Glass, A.R., Cerletty, J.M., Elliott, W., Lemann, J., Jr. Gray, R.W., Eil, C. 1990. J. Endocrinol. Invest. 13, 407–413.
Gomez-Casanovas, E., Sanmarti, R., Sole, M., Canete, J.D., Munoz-Gomez, J. 2001. Arthritis Rheum. 44, 66–72.
Hamada, K., Nagai, S., Shigematsu, M., Nagao, T., Hayaschi, M., Tsutsumi, T., Izumi, T. 2002. Sarcoidosis Vasc. Diffuse Lung Dis. 19, 71–77.
Harper, L., Cockwell, P., Howie, A.J., Michael, J., Richards, N.T., Savage, C.O., Wheeler, D.C., Bacon, P.A., Adu, D. 1997. Q. J. Med. 90, 125–132.
Hazenberg, B.P., van Rijswijk, M.H. 2000. Ann. Rheum. Dis. 59, 577–579.
Helin, H.J., Korpela, M.M., Mustonen, J.T., Pasternack, A.I. 1995. Arthritis Rheum. 38, 242–247.
Hemmen, T., Perez-Canto, A., Distler, A., Offermann, G., Braun, J. 1997. Br. J. Rheumatol. 36, 696–699.
Hocini, H., Iscaki, S., Benlahrache, C., Vitalis, L., Chevalier, X., Larget-Piet, B., Bouvet, J.P. 1992. Ann. Rheum. Dis. 51, 790–792.
Ikeda, A., Nagai, S., Kitaichi, M., Hayashi, M., Hamada, K., Shigematsu, M., Nagao, T., Izumi, T. 2001. Intern. Med. 40, 241–245.
International Study Group for Behcet's Disease. 1990. Lancet 335, 1078–1080.
Inui, N., Murayama, A., Sasaki, S., Suda, T., Chida, K., Kato, S., Nakamura, H. 2001. Am. J. Med. 110, 687–693.
Iwasaki, A., Medzhitov, R. 2004. Nat. Immunol. 5, 987–995.
Kemp, E., Nielsen, H., Petersen, L.J., Gam, A.N., Dahlager, J., Horn, T., Larsen, S., Olsen, S. 2001. Clin. Nephrol. 55, 87–88.
Komatsuda, A., Wakui, H., Ohtani, H., Maki, N., Nimura, T., Takatsu, H., Yamaguchi, A., Imai, H., Sawada, K. 2003. Clin. Nephrol. 60, 284–288.
Korpela, M., Mustonen, J., Teppo, A.M., Helin, H., Pasternack, A. 1997. Br. J. Rheumatol. 36, 1189–1195.
Laiho, K., Tiitinen, S., Kaarela, K., Helin, H., Isomaki, H. 1999. Clin. Rheumatol. 18, 122–123.
Liu, P.T., Stenger, S., Li, H., Wenzel, L., Tan, B.H., Krutzik, S.R., Ochoa, M.T., Schauber, J., Wu, K., Meinken, C., Kamen, D.L., Wagner, M., Bals, R., Steinmeyer, A., Zugel, U., Gallo, R.L., Eisenberg, D., Hewison, M., Hollis, B.W., Adams, J.S., Bloom, B.R., Modlin, R.L. 2006. Science 311, 1770–1773.
Longcope, W.T., Freiman, D.G. 1952. Medicine (Baltimore) 31, 1–132.
Manolagas, S.C., Hustmyer, F.G., Yu, X.P. 1990. Kidney Int. (Suppl. 29), S9–S16.
Mason, R.S., Frankel, T., Chan, Y.L., Lissner, D., Posen, S. 1984. Ann. Intern. Med. 100, 59–61.
Matsuda, M., Suzuki, A., Miyagawa, H., Shimizu, S., Ikeda, S. 2006. Clin. Rheumatol. 25, 415–418.
Missen, G.A., Taylor, J.D. 1956. J. Pathol. Bacteriol. 71, 179–192.
Miyazaki, E., Tsuda, T., Mochizuki, A., Sugisaki, K., Ando, M., Matsumoto, T., Sawabe, T., Kumamoto, T. 1996. Intern. Med. 35, 579–582.
Miyoshi, K., Okura, T., Manabe, S., Watanabe, S., Fukuoka, T., Higaki, J. 2004. Clin. Exp. Nephrol. 8, 279–282.
Montenegro, V., Monteiro, R.C. 1999. Curr. Opin. Rheumatol. 11, 265–272.
Morita, H., Yoshimura, A. 2006. Clin. Exp. Nephrol. 10, 85–86.
Moudgil, A., Przygodzki, R.M., Kher, K.K. 2006. Pediatr. Nephrol. 21, 281–285.

Muther, R.S., McCarron, D.A., Bennett, W.M. 1980. Clin. Nephrol. 14, 190–197.

Myllykangas-Luosujarvi, R., Aho, K., Kautiainen, H., Hakala, M. 1999. Rheumatology (Oxford) 38, 499–503.

Nadir, I., Topcu, S., Kaptanoglu, E., Icagasioglu, S. 2003. Clin. Exp. Rheumatol. 21, 410.

Nakano, M., Ueno, M., Nishi, S., Suzuki, S., Hasegawa, H., Watanabe, T., Kuroda, T., Ito, S., Arakawa, M. 1996. Ann. Rheum. Dis. 55, 520–524.

O'Leary, T.J., Jones, G., Yip, A., Lohnes, D., Cohanim, M., Yendt, E.R. 1986. N. Engl. J. Med. 315, 727–730.

O'Riordan, E., Willert, R.P., Reeve, R., Kalra, P.A., O'Donoghue, D.J., Foley, R.N., Waldek, S. 2001. Clin. Nephrol. 55, 297–302.

Ota, M., Amakawa, R., Uehira, K., Ito, T., Yagi, Y., Oshiro, A., Date, Y., Oyaizu, H., Shigeki, T., Ozaki, Y., Yamaguchi, K., Uemura, Y., Yonezu, S., Fukuhara, S. 2004. Thorax 59, 408–413.

Pabst, S., Baumgarten, G., Stremmel, A., Lennarz, M., Knufermann, P., Gillissen, A., Vetter, H., Grohe, C. 2006. Clin. Exp. Immunol. 143, 420–426.

Pickering, M.C., Haskard, D.O. 2000. J. R. Coll. Physicians Lond. 34, 169–177.

Pollak, V.E., Pirani, C.L., Steck, I.E., Kark, R.M. 1962. Arthritis Rheum. 5, 1–9.

Rajakariar, R., Sharples, E.J., Raftery, M.J., Sheaff, M., Yaqoob, M.M. 2006. Kidney Int. 70, 165–169.

Ramirez, G., Lambert, R., Bloomer, H.A. 1981. Nephron. 28, 124–126.

Reichel, H., Koeffler, H.P., Tobler, A., Norman, A.W. 1987. Proc. Natl. Acad. Sci. USA 84, 3385–3389.

Rheault, M.N., Manivel, J.C., Levine, S.C., Sinaiko, A.R. 2006. Pediatr. Nephrol. 21, 1323–1326.

Robson, M.G., Banerjee, D., Hopster, D., Cairns, H.S. 2003. Nephrol. Dial. Transplant. 18, 280–284.

Rohatgi, P.K., Liao, T.E., Borts, F.T. 1990. Urology 35, 271–275.

Roux, C.H., Brocq, O., Albert, C.B.V., Euller-Ziegler, L. 2004. Joint Bone Spine 71, 444–445.

Sadeghi, K., Wessner, B., Laggner, U., Ploder, M., Tamandl, D., Friedl, J., Zugel, U., Steinmeyer, A., Pollak, A., Roth, E., Boltz-Nitulescu, G., Spittler, A. 2006. Eur. J. Immunol. 36, 361–370.

Schiff, M.H., Whelton, A. 2000. Semin. Arthritis Rheum. 30, 196–208.

Shakoor, N., Michalska, M., Harris, C.A., Block, J.A. 2002. Lancet 359, 579–580.

Sharma, O.P. 1996. Chest 109, 535–539.

Sharma, O.P. 2000. Curr. Opin. Pulm. Med. 6, 442–447.

Shu, K.H., Lian, J.D., Yang, Y.F., Lu, Y.S., Wang, J.Y., Lan, J.L., Chou, G. 1986. Clin. Nephrol. 25, 169–174.

Sinha, R.N., Fraser, W.D., Casson, I.F. 1997. J. R. Soc. Med. 90, 156–157.

Stoffels, K., Overbergh, L., Giulietti, A., Verlinden, L., Bouillon, R., Mathieu, C. 2006. J. Bone Miner. Res. 21, 37–47.

Stokes, M.B., Foster, K., Markowitz, G.S., Ebrahimi, F., Hines, W., Kaufman, D., Moore, B., Wolde, D., D'Agati, V.D. 2005. Nephrol. Dial. Transplant. 20, 1400–1406.

Strobel, E.S., Fritschka, E. 1998. Clin. Rheumatol. 17, 524–530.

Thomas, E., Symmons, D.P., Brewster, D.H., Black, R.J., Macfarlane, G.J. 2003. J. Rheumatol. 30, 958–965.

Thumfart, J., Muller, D., Rudolph, B., Zimmering, M., Querfeld, U., Haffner, D. 2005. Am. J. Kidney Dis. 45, 411–414.

van Driel, M., Pols, H.A., van Leeuwen, J.P. 2004. Curr. Pharm. Des. 10, 2535–2555.

Veltkamp, M., Grutters, J.C., van Moorsel, C.H., Ruven, H.J., van den Bosch, J.M. 2006. Clin. Exp. Immunol. 145, 215–218.

Voskuyl, A.E., Hazes, J.M., Zwinderman, A.H., Paleolog, E.M., van der Meer, F.J., Daha, M.R., Breedveld, F.C. 2003. Ann. Rheum. Dis. 62, 407–413.

Ward, M.M. 2004. Arthritis Rheum. 50, 1122–1131.

Watts, R.A., Mooney, J., Lane, S.E., Scott, D.G. 2004. Rheumatology (Oxford) 43, 920–923.

Wright, J.R., Calkins, E. 1981. Medicine (Baltimore) 60, 429–448.

Yoshida, A., Morozumi, K., Takeda, A., Koyama, K., Oikawa, T. 1994. Clin. Ther. 16, 1000–1006.

Yurdakul, S., Hamuryudan, V., Yazici, H. 2004. Curr. Opin. Rheumatol. 16, 38–42.

Zarza, L.P., Sanchez, E.N., Acin, P.A., Ara, J.M., Banos, J.G. 1996. Clin. Rheumatol. 15, 385–388.

# Index

## A

$\beta_2$ glycoprotein I 298
$\beta_2$-microglobulin ($\beta_2$m) 357, 383, 386
A alpha chain amyloidosis 388
AA amyloid 183
AA amyloidosis 179, 388–389, 399, 403–404
AASV
   investigations 146
   renal involvement 143
   treatment 147
abatacept 331
abdominal pain 242
accelerated
   atherosclerosis 179, 186
   hypertension 370
ACE-inhibitors 262, 329, 367, 372, 374–376
acquired systemic amyloidosis 384
acute
   nephritic syndrome 220, 230
   renal failure 187, 230, 273
   tubulointerstitial nephritis 318
adalumimab 399
ADAMTS (a disintegrin and metalloprotease with thrombospondin type 1 domains) 271
ADAMTS 13 271
   deficiency 274
   deficiency in TTP 272
adaptive immunity 24
adriamycin 392
advanced sclerotic lupus nephritis 318
adverse effects 107
aetiology 200
aHUS – pathogenesis 266
AL amyloidosis 383, 389
alemtuzumab 151, 209
alfa-interferon (IFN-α) monotherapy 223
alpha 1 anti-trypsin 141
Alport's syndrome 209
alternative pathway 44
alternatively activated macrophages 82
alveolar capillaritis 144
Alzheimer's disease 383
ampicillin 241
amyloidogenesis 383

amyloidosis 181–183, 383
ANCA 123, 141, 146, 152
   and leukocyte transmigration 130
   and neutrophils 127
   and pathogenesis 141
   associated systemic vasculitides 123
   associated vasculitis 64
   associated vasculitis-clinical features 139, 142
   disease activity 126
   induced PMN activation 129
   testing 141
anemia 370
aneurysm formation 178
aneurysms 176, 180, 183, 186
angiography 177
angiotensin
   converting enzyme inhibitors 364
   receptor antagonists 329–330, 374
angiotensin receptor
   antagonists 333
   blockers 329
ankylosing spondylitis 400
anterior ischemic optic neuropathy 176
anti-nuclear antibodies (ANA) 399
anti-TNFα antibodies 132
antibiotics 261
antibody-associated glomerulonephritis (GN) 64
anti-C5 monoclonal antibodies 267
anticardiolipin antibodies 337
anti-CD20 monoclonal antibody 151, 223
anti-CD20 antibody 328
anti-CD40 ligand 329
anti-centromere antibody 369
anticoagulation 342
anti-DNA antibodies 286
anti-double stranded DNA 3
anti-GBM antibodies 144, 198, 204
anti-GBM disease 140
antigen presentation 294
antigen presenting cells 25
anti-glomerular basement membrane (anti-GBM) disease 8, 64, 195
anti-HCV therapy 223
anti-La 286
anti-lymphocyte globulin 209

anti-MPO antibodies 130
anti-MPO induced glomerulonephritis 132
anti-myeloperoxidase antibodies 3
anti-neutrophil cytoplasm antibodies 3, 140, 199, 245
anti-nuclear antibodies 369
anti-phospholipid antibodies 298, 333
antiphospholipid syndrome
   mortality 298, 333, 335
   nephropathy 338, 340
   related pregnancy loss 343
anti-PR3 antibodies 134
anti-rheumatic drugs 399
anti-RNA polymerase III 369
anti-Ro 286
anti-Scl-70 369
anti-Sm 286
anti-thymocyte globulin 151
anti-topoisomerase antibody 369
anti-tumor necrosis factor therapy 115, 179
antiviral therapy 223
aPL in SLE 333
apoAI amyloidosis 393
apolipoproteins AI and AII 387
apoptosis 287, 289, 292–293
APS nephropathy 338, 340
APS-related pregnancy loss 343
aspirin 181, 187, 343
atherosclerosis 176, 179, 335, 338
atypical HUS 262
autoantibodies 3, 43
autoimmune haemolytic anemia 298
autoimmune lymphoproliferative syndrome (ALPS) 292
autoimmune responses 23
autologous stem cell transplantation 328
autonomic neuropathy 387
autoreactive
   B-cells 4
   T lymphocytes 4
azathioprine 110, 147, 149, 179, 181–182, 206–207, 250, 326–327, 329, 358

# B

bacteremia 261
bacterial infection 142
B-cells 81, 200
   activity factor (BAFF) 295, 298, 329
   depletion 148
   epitopes 201
   hyperactivation 218, 296
   non-Hodgkin lymphoma 218
   receptor 25
   tolerance 25, 289
bcl-2 292
Behcet's disease (BD) 183, 403
Behcet's syndrome 175, 397
beta-blockers 374
bicarbonate 358
Birmingham Vasculitis Activity Score 143
bisphosphonates 402
BLyS 298
bortezomib 392
bronchoscopy 144
bucillamine 399
BXSB/yaa mouse 286, 297

# C

C1q 218, 312
   deficiency 286, 294
   deficient mice 293, 299
C2 deficiency 286
C3 312
   mutations 266
C3a 245
C4 312
   deficiency 286
C4a 245
C4A null allele 286
C5b-9 complex 242
calcineurin inhibitors 112
calcitriol 401
calcium channel blockers 364–365, 367, 374–375
c-ANCA 124
captopril 374
carbonic anhydrase II 352
cardiac
   amyloidosis 390
   arrhythmias 370
   complications 219
   dysfunction 365
cardiovascular risk 330
CARMA-1 293
carotid intima-media thickness 336
carotidynia 176
cataract 176
catastrophic APS 342
$CD4^+$ effector cells 134
CD19 297
CD22 297
CD80 (B7.1) 352
CD83 162
CD86 (B7.2) 352

CD95 (Fas) 292
cell-mediated immunity 134
  + T cells 134
central B-cell tolerance 293
central nervous system 245
cerebral and myocardial infarctions 336
cerebral vasculitis 251
chemokines 64, 260
chlorambucil 250
chronic renal failure 179, 219, 244, 274, 327, 355, 372
chronic tubulo-interstitial nephritis 351
Churg–Strauss
  angiitis 139
  Syndrome 123, 125
ciclosporin 150, 399
cigarette smoking 197
citrate 358
class II MHC 196
classical
  macrophage activation 82
  pathway 44
classification
  of cryoglobulins 216
  of lupus glomerulonephritis 312–313
  of vasculitis 139
clonodine 374
clopidogrel 268
CMV 336
  infection 262
Cogan's syndrome (CS) 175, 181
colchicine 392
collagen IV 200
complement 96, 204, 242, 286, 312, 367
  activation 44, 245, 301, 343
  deficiency 285
  proteins 33
  receptors 299
  regulation 45
  system 43, 311
complementary
  PR3 127
  protein 12
computed tomography angiography 177
conditions associated with APS 336
congestive heart failure 370–371
congophilic amyloid angiopathy 384
coronary artery aneurysms 187
corticosteroid 147–148, 181, 183, 187, 206,
    249, 324, 358, 365, 371, 402
  toxicity 181
  plasmapheresis 226
co-stimulatory molecules 26

coxsackie
  A 268
  B 268
C-reactive protein 151
crescentic glomerulonephritis 132, 140
crescentic nephritis 198
  cellular crescents 315
  complement 199
crescentic, ANCA positive glomerulonephritis 378
cryoglobulinemia 355
  laboratory findings complement 220
  glomerulonephritis 221
  vasculitis hypertension 227
  vasculitis 218
cryoglobulins 215
cryosupernatant plasma 275
crystalcryoglobulinemia 230
CTLA4-Ig (abatacept) 208, 329
cyclophosphamide 3, 142, 147–149, 152, 179, 182, 187,
    206–207, 226, 250, 326–327, 329, 342, 358, 392
cyclosporin A 182, 187, 207, 250–251, 370
cytokines 63
cytokine profile 82
cytoplasmic ANCA 141

D

danazol 250
deep vein thromboses 336
deep venous thrombosis 404
dendritic cells 25, 81, 159–160, 162, 294
deoxyspergualin 142, 150
dexamethasone 392
diabetes mellitus 100
Diagnosis 177, 198, 248
  of amyloidosis 389
diagnostic criteria 267
dialysis 372
  associated amyloidosis 386
  related $\beta_2$-microglobulin amyloidosis (A$\beta_2$m) 385
diffuse
  alveolar haemorrhage 150
  lupus nephritis 316
  proliferative 327
  proliferative glomerulonephritis 182
  type of inflammation 163
dilute Russell viper venom test 333
dipyridamole 250
directly pathogenic antibodies 298
disease monitoring 151
distal renal tubular acidosis 349
D-penicillamine 114, 367, 399

drug-induced
  anti-phospholipid antibodies 334
  atypical HUS 262
  TTP 267
  tubulointerstitial nephritis 318

# E

*E. coli* serotype O 157
echocardiography 390
eculizimab 267
elastin-associated calcification 163
electron microscopy 320, 390
end-stage renal failure 251
endobronchial inflammation 144
endocarditis 267
endothelial
  cell activation 363, 365
  damage and dysfunction 269
  injury 260
end-stage renal
  disease 220
  failure and renal transplantation 340
enoxaparin 342
enteropathic arthritis 400
environmental factors 287
epidemiology 241, 257, 262, 367
  and classification 267
  of vasculitis 140
episcleritis 146
epithelial crescent formation 247
eprodisate 393
Epstein Barr virus infection 218, 288
erythema nodosum 176, 182
erythematous papules 242
erythrocyte sedimentation 151
erythromycin 241
*Escherichia coli* (*E. coli*) 257
etanercept 151, 399
etiology 257
etoposide 150
European lupus nephritis trial 324
European vasculitis study group (EUVAS) 143, 147
experimental allergic glomerulonephritis 205
extra-renal disease 219

# F

factor B 265
factor H 263, 274
  autoantibodies 264
  deficiency 263

factor I 265
familial amyloidotic polyneuropathy 387
Fas 293
  ligand 293
Fc receptors 311
Fcγ receptor 95, 129, 286–287, 296, 299
Fcγ receptors IIb (FcγRIIb) 292, 294, 296–297
FcγRII 299
FcγRIIa 295, 299
FcγRIIa polymorphisms 299
FcγRIIb polymorphism 297
FcγRIII 141, 299
FcγRIIIb polymorphisms 300
fibrinoid necrosis 246, 314, 316, 366
fibromuscular dysplasia 338
fish oil 250
five factor score 143
focal lupus nephritis 315
focal segmental glomerulonephritis 181
foreign-body giant cells 160, 163, 169
Freelitet™ immunoassay 392
fresh-frozen plasma as 275
future treatments 208

# G

gammaglobulin 342
genetic
  factors associated with aHUS 285, 263
  influence 241, 205
  manipulation of macrophages 88
  predisposition 242
giant cell arteritis 140, 159, 175, 180
  pathogenesis 160
giant cells 169
glaucoma 176
glomerular
  capillary thrombosis 340
  haematuria 219
  necrosis 199
glomerulonephritis 183, 199, 233, 244, 251, 301, 349, 354
glucocorticoids 7, 186, 342
gold 399
Goodpasture's syndrome 196, 198, 204–205
  epidemiology 195
group A streptococcal antigen 241

# H

H7 257
HCV 217, 232

*Helicobacter pylori* 241
hematology 371
hemodialysis 227, 267, 340, 376
hemolytic uremic syndrome 187, 257–258, 320
Henoch–Schönlein purpura 140, 241
heparin 250, 343
hepatic involvement 219
hepatitis
   B virus 142, 186
   C virus 142, 186, 215
hereditary
   apolipoprotein AI amyloidosis 388
   fibrinogen 388
   lysosyme amyloidosis 388, 393
   periodic fever syndromes 385
   renal amyloidosis 388–389
   systemic amyloidosis 387, 393
   TTP 272
histology 246–247
histopathology 259
   glomerular lesions 259
HIV 334, 336
   infection 220, 262
HLA
   B27 400
   class II gene polymorphisms 286
   class II 205
   DR15 196, 203
   DRB1*01 242
   haplotypes 218
   linkage 203
HMG CoA reductase inhibitors 330
hormonal factors 288
Hughes syndrome 333
human immunodeficiency virus type 1 268
human leukocyte antigen 286
hyaline thrombus 314
hydralazine 126, 142, 287
hydroxychloroquine 341, 399, 402
hypercalcaemia 401
hypercalciuria 353, 400
hypercholesterolemia 103
hyperglobulinemia 352
hyperglycemia 103
hyperlipidemia 324, 330
hyperreninemia 364, 372, 376
hypertension 179, 185, 220, 230, 324, 337–339, 404
hypertensive retinopathy 176
hypocitraturia 353
hypogammaglobulinaemia 151
hypokalemia 354

## I

idiopathic crescentic glomerulonephritis 125
idiopathic necrotizing and crescentic glomerulonephritis 123
IFN-α 295
IgA 245
   ANCA 246
   glomerulonephritis 248
   immune complexes 242
   immune deposits 248
   dominant immune deposits 241, 245
   mediated inflammation 241
IgA nephropathy 400, 404
IgM rheumatoid factor 217
IL-8 260
IL-12 204
iloprost 364
immune cell activation 83
immune complexes 43, 94, 298, 300, 311, 355
   clearance 298
   deposition 300
immunoadsorption 208
immunofluorescence microscopy 248
immunoglobulins 367
immunohistochemistry 390
immunosuppressants 107
immunosuppressive
   drugs 226
   therapy 371
induction of ANCA 126
induction therapy
   with cyclophosphamide 324
   with mycophenolate mofetil 325
inflammatory Arthritis 397
infliximab 151, 181, 187, 399, 403
initiation of the autoimmune response 203
innate immunity 24
interferon gamma (IFN-γ) 159, 170, 204
internal elastic membrane 163
International Society of Nephrology (ISN)
   classification 323
   classification of lupus nephritis 323
interstitial granulomatous nephritis 402
interstitial nephritis 183, 187, 199, 349, 351
interstitial pulmonary disease 245
intimal hyperplasia 160
intravenous gamma globulin 328
intravenous immunoglobulin 111, 148, 150, 187, 250, 342
involvement 222
ischemic damage in GCA 170

ischemic renal disease 179
IVIG 251

## J

juxtaglomerular 365

## K

karyorrhexis 314
Kawasaki's disease (KD) 175, 186
ketoconazole 402
kidney 247
Klinefelter's syndrome 288

## L

Langhans
   giant cells 160, 169
   type of giant cell 163
lectin pathway 44
leflunomide 150
*Legionella pneumophila* 268
leukocyte transmigration 132
leukocytoclastic vasculitis 246, 248
LJP-934 (Riquent, abetimus) 328
limited cutaneous scleroderma 365, 368
linkage disequilibrium 286
livedo reticularis 336, 338
localized amyloidosis 384
low molecular weight heparin 341, 343
low-dose aspirin 341
LUNAR
   trial 328
luminal stenosis 178
lupus anti-coagulant 333
lupus nephritis 318
   adjunctive therapy 333
   maintenance therapy 327
   nove therapies 327
   vascular lesions 318
lymphocyte depletion 148, 151
lymphocytolytic therapies 209
lymphoma 267, 385
lymphopaenia 298
lymphoplasmacytic 218

## M

macroglobulinaemia 385
macrophage infiltration 84

macrophages 5, 25, 81
macroscopic
   haematuria 197
   hematuria 243
magnetic resonance
   angiography 177
   imaging (MRI) 178
major histocompatibility complex 25
malignant hypertension 367
MAINTAIN nephritis trial 327
management of
   aHUS 267
   amyloidosis 392
mast cells 81
matrix metalloproteinases 160
melphalan 392
membrane
   cofactor protein 264
   PR3 127
membrane-attack complex (MAC) 242
membranoproliferative glomerulonephritis 182, 263, 355
membranous
   glomerulonephritis 181, 312, 355
   lupus nephritis (MLN) 316, 329
   nephritis 399
menorrhagia 342
mesangial
   glomerulonephritis 311
   proliferation 247
   proliferative glomerulonephritis 355
   proliferative lupus nephritis 314
methotrexate 147–148, 179, 181–182, 339, 402
   pneumonitis 149
methyl prednisolone 207, 224, 226, 324, 365, 370
MHC class III genes 286
microangiopathic
   hemolysis 272, 370
   hemolytic anemia 371
microscopic
   haematuria 197, 243
   polyangiitis 123, 125, 139–140, 142, 144
migratory superficial thrombophlebitis 183
minimal mesangial lupus nephritis 314
minocycline 142
MMF 326, 327, 329
Mönckeberg-type of calcifications 163
monoclonal IgM rheumatoid factor 218
monocyte chemoattractant protein-1 (MCP-1) 260
mononeuritis multiplex 219
MRL/lpr 297–298, 301
   mouse 286
murine models of SLE 286

mycophenolate 179
  mofetil 4, 149–150, 207, 325, 403
*mycoplasma pneumoniae* 268
myeloma 385
myeloperoxidase (MPO) 124, 141
  ANCA 131
  deficient mice 131
myofibroblasts 160
myointimal proliferation 176

# N

nailfold video capillaroscopy 336
necrotizing glomerulonephritis 181
necrotizing vasculitis 131, 320
neovascularization 170, 178
nephrectomy 206, 267, 364
nephritis-associated plasmin receptor 241
nephrocalcinosis 182, 349, 351, 353, 401
nephrogenic diabetes insipidus 351, 354
nephrotic syndrome 179, 181, 187, 197, 220, 230, 243, 312, 317–318, 340
nephrotoxic nephritis 85
neutropaenia 298
neutrophils 246
nitric oxide 93
NKT cells 296
noninflammatory necrotizing vasculopathy 319
non-malignant hypertension 369
non-steroidal anti-inflammatory drugs (NSAID) 241, 399–400
normotensive renal crisis 375
NZB/W-F1 mouse 286, 294, 297–298, 301

# O

oestrogen 288
oral alkali 358
organ manifestations of APS 336
osteomalacia 354
oxidative stress 93

# P

p-ANCA 124
paracetamol 241
pathogenesis 159, 260, 269
  of amyloidosis 383
  of renal involvement 363
pathogenic autoantibodies 298
pathogenicity of ANCA
  in vivo models 130

pauciimmune
  crescentic glomerulonephritis 124, 131
  glomerulonephritis 182
  necrotizing glomerulonephritis 144
PE 269
pegylated IFN-α 2b 225
penicillamine 142
penicillin 241
pericardial effusion 370, 372
peri-nuclear ANCA 141
peripheral
  nervous system 245
  neuropathy 146
peritoneal dialysis 227, 267, 376
pexelizumab 267
plasma exchange 148, 150, 206–208, 235, 251, 267, 269, 275
plasmacytoid dendritic cells 295
plasmapheresis 4, 225, 250, 342, 358, 371
platelet-derived growth factor (PDGF) 160, 170
*pneumocystis jiruvecii* 152
polyarteritis nodosa 149, 184
polyclonal IgM rheumatoid factor 218
positron emission tomography 177
predictors of renal involvement 356
prednisolone 148, 207, 226, 250, 329, 365, 370
pregnancy 179, 262, 267, 343, 365
premature menopause 324
primary forms of TTP 268
primary systemic vasculitis 139
prion disorders 383
procainamide 287
pro-calcitonin 152
prodrome 143
programmed cell death gene-1 297
pro-inflammatory cytokines 94
prolactin 288
proliferative
  glomerulonephritis 247, 300, 312, 316
  lupus nephritis 3, 314
  nephritis 324
propyl thiouracil 142, 126
proteinase 3 124, 141
proteinuria 219, 244, 339
psoriatic arthritis 400
pulmonary
  biopsy 200
  cavitation 146
  disease 196
  emboli 336
  fibrosis 146
  hemorrhage 196, 199, 219

hypertension 372
involvement 177
pulsed intravenous corticosteroids 187, 235, 250
pulsed intravenous steroids 235
pulsed methylprednisolone 250
purpura 242

## R

RANTES 260
rapidly progressive
   crescentic glomerulonephritis 131
   glomerulonephritis 139–140, 250
Raynaud's phenomenon 365
reactive
   arthritis 400
   oxygen species 93
refractory renal crisis 374
regulators of complement activation 46
regulatory CD25+ T-cells 84
regulatory T-cells 9, 202, 208, 295–296
remission and relapse 148
renal
   abnormalities 371
   AL amyloid 386
   amyloidosis 399
   biopsy 143, 198–199
   impairment 339
   infarctions 185
   injury 301
   insufficiency 243
   involvement 179–180, 182–184, 186, 216, 243, 269, 387
   ischaemic renal infarction 339
   manifestations 219, 337
   microaneurysms 185
   pathologic changes 311
   pathology 221
   thrombotic microangiopathy 342
   transplantation 251, 262, 267, 341, 389
   tubular acidosis 351–353, 356
   vein and inferior vena cava thrombosis 340
   vein thrombosis 183, 404
renal artery
   aneurysm 183
   lesions 338
   stenosis 179, 182–183, 336, 338
   thrombosis 338
renal crisis
   demographics 367
   management 372
renal disease 197, 219
   in mixed (type II) cryoglobulinemia 217

renin 370
renovascular hypertension 184, 187
retinal
   infarction 170
   vein thrombosis 146
rheumatoid
   arthritis 267, 270, 397
   arthritis-renal involvement 398
   factor 398
ribavirin 224–225
risk factors for thrombosis in APS
rituximab 4, 151, 226, 228, 235, 275, 392
Rituximabt™ 392

## S

SAP scintigraphy 390
sarcoid vasculitis 182
sarcoidosis 175, 182, 397, 400, 402
scleroderma renal crisis 363, 370
   and pregnancy 375
scrotal swelling 245
secondary
   hypertension 179
   TTP 267
senile
   systemic amyloidosis 385
   transthyretin amyloidosis (ATTR) 386
seronegative spondyloarthritis-renal involvement 400
serum amyloid
   A protein (SAA) 383, 385
   P component (SAP) 383–384
shear stress 271
Shiga-like toxins 257
   Stx-1 and -2 260
*Shigella dysenteriae* 258, 260
silica exposure 126
sirolimus 150
Sjögren's syndrome 267, 270, 349
   clinical presentation 352
skin 246
splenectomy 342
*Staphylococcus aureus* 127
stem-cell transplantation 148
*Streptococcus pneumoniae* 262
stroke 180
sub-glottic stenosis 144
sulfamethoxazole 142
sulfasalazine 114, 399
syphilis 334
systemic
   AA amyloidosis 385
   AL amyloidosis 385, 388

amyloidosis 383
ANCA- vasculitis 3
lupus erythematosus (SLE) 64, 140, 267, 270, 285, 311, 323
sclerosis 363, 366

## T

tacrolimus 150, 327
Taipan snake venom tests 333
Takayasu's arteritis 140, 159, 175–176
   surgery 179
T-cells 81, 151, 200, 202, 204, 351
   hyperactivity 295
   receptors 25
   tolerance 27
temporal artery biopsy 180
TGF-$\beta$ 100, 208
thalidomide 392
the ALMS (Aspreva Lupus Management Study) 326
the CD40 330
Thomsen–Friedenreich antigen 262
thrombocytopaenia 298, 272, 342, 370
thrombolytic therapy 342
thrombomodulin 246
thrombotic
   events 341
   microangiopathy 259, 262, 274, 320, 339–340
   Thrombocytopenic Purpura (TTP) 267, 320, 371
ticlopidine 268
tinzaparin 342
tissue damage and fibrosis 301
tissue resident mDCs 295
TLR7 287, 294–295
TLR9 287, 294–295
TLRs 294
TNF-$\alpha$ 242
tolerance 23, 292
toll-like receptors (TLR) 30, 64, 82, 96, 287, 294, 401
transplantation 209
transthyretin 383
treatment
   of type II cryoglobulinemia 223
   recommendations 328
   TTP 274
trimethoprim 142

TTP-clinical features 268
TTR 387
tubulointerstitial nephritis 318
tumor necrosis
   alpha (TNF$\alpha$) blockade 148
   factor (TNF) blockade 151
twin studies 285
type I and type II cryoglobulins 217
type I
   cryoglobulinemia-renal disease 228
   cryoglobulinemic GN 228, 230–231, 235
   cryoglobulinemia 230–231, 233, 235
   cryoglobulins 215
   IFNs 288
type II
   activation 82
   (or mixed) cryoglobulins 215
   cryoglobulinemia 217
   diabetes mellitus 383
type III cryoglobulins 215, 217

## U

undifferentiated spondyloarthropathy 400
Upshaw–Schulman syndrome 272
urokinase 250, 353
UV light 287
uveitis 182

## V

vascular endothelial growth factor 160
vascular lesions in lupus nephritis 319
ventricular arrhythmias 371
vincristine 392
vitamin $D_3$ 401
von Willebrand factor 246, 270
VWF cleavage 271

## W

warfarin 250, 341, 343
Wegener's granulomatosis (WG) 123–125, 134, 139–140, 142, 144
WGET study 151